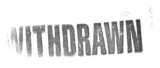

DIABETES AND THE BRAIN

CONTEMPORARY DIABETES

ARISTIDIS VEVES, MD, DSc

SERIES EDITOR

The Diabetic Foot: *Second Edition,* edited by *Aristidis Veves, MD, John M. Giurini, DPM, and Frank W. LoGerfo, MD, 2006*

The Diabetic Kidney, edited by *Pedro Cortes, MD and Carl Erik Mogensen, MD, 2006*

Obesity and Diabetes, edited by *Christos S. Mantzoros, MD, 2006*

Diabetic Retinopathy, edited by *Elia J. Duh, MD, 2008*

Diabetes and Exercise: edited by *Judith G. Regensteiner, PhD, Jane E.B. Reusch, MD, Kerry J. Stewart, EDD, Aristidis Veves, MD, DSc, 2009*

Diabetes and the Brain, edited by *Geert Jan Biessels, MD, PhD, Jose A. Luchsinger, MD, MPH*

DIABETES AND THE BRAIN

Edited by

Geert Jan Biessels, MD, PhD
University Medical Center, Utrecht, The Netherlands

Jose A. Luchsinger, MD, MPH
Columbia University College of Physicians and Surgeons,
New York, NY, USA

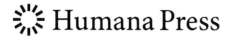 Humana Press

Editors
Geert Jan Biessels
Department of Neurology
Rudolf Magnus Institute of Neuroscience
University Medical Center Utrecht
PO Box 85500
Utrecht
3508 GA Utrecht
The Netherlands
g.j.biessels@umcutrecht.nl

Jose A. Luchsinger
Columbia University
Medical Center
Presbyterian Hospital
622 West 168th St.
New York, NY 10032
USA
jal94@columbia.edu

ISBN 978-1-60327-849-2   e-ISBN 978-1-60327-850-8
DOI 10.1007/978-1-60327-850-8

Library of Congress Control Number: 2009933948

springer.com

Preface

Diabetes, particularly type 2 or adult onset diabetes, is increasing in prevalence in the world. In the United States the prevalence of diabetes is over 12% in persons of age 60 years and older. The prevalence in Europe is 8–10% and catching up with the United States. The trend worldwide is for this prevalence to increase given the epidemic of overweight and obesity (2/3 of the adult United States population is overweight or obese). Thus, the fact that diabetes affects the brain is of enormous public health importance.

While acute cerebral complications of diabetes, such as hypoglycemia or stroke, are well recognized, more chronic cerebral conditions, such as cognitive and mood disorders, have failed to be recognized until recently. The last few decades have yielded new insights linking type 2 diabetes to dementia and other cognitive disorders and into the cognitive consequences of type 1 diabetes. Hence, the impact of diabetes on the brain has become a very multifaceted topic. Clinical care and research on cerebral complications of diabetes now involve internists, neurologists, psychiatrists, psychologists, and basic scientists. There has been a surge in pre-clinical and clinical research papers ranging from topics such as management of hyperglycemia in acute stroke to disturbances in insulin signaling in Alzheimer's disease. This has led to substantial progress in the field, but it also makes it more difficult for those involved to keep track of all relevant developments.

This book provides an update on the acute and chronic consequences of diabetes in the brain. We brought together experts from around the world in order to provide a helicopter view of this intriguing topic. The book offers not only in-depth reviews on cerebral complications of diabetes, but also introductory chapters on current insights into the pathophysiology and clinical management of diabetes and its complications and on stroke, neuropsychological assessment and dementia. With these "update on diabetes for neurologists" and "update on stroke and dementia for diabetologists" we hope to offer relevant and easily accessible background information that puts the cerebral complications of diabetes into context.

The target audience of this book is broad and includes medical specialists taking care of persons with diabetes and researchers in the diabetes field. It is important to point out that most clinicians and researchers think that the only complications of diabetes are microvascular (retinopathy, renal, neuropathy) and macrovascular (heart disease and stroke). Given increased longevity, the aging of our societies, and the increasing prevalence of diabetes, the chronic consequences of diabetes in the brain are at least as important but have failed to acquire the recognition that more traditional complications have. We believe that this book will bring the consequence of diabetes in the brain to the mainstream and thus has the potential to change the field.

We thank Aristidis Veves, from Harvard Medical School, Boston, for inviting us to put together this book for the Humana Press "Contemporary Diabetes" series, for which he is the series editor. We would also like to thank Paul Dolgert and Connie Walsh from Springer Science and Business Media for their help and support. Finally, we thank the authors, all internationally distinguished in their fields, for their invaluable contributions to this book.

Geert Jan Biessels
José A. Luchsinger

Contents

PART V EXPERIMENTAL MODELS AND PATHOPHYSIOLOGY

Contributors

GEERT JAN BIESSELS • *Department of Neurology, G03.228, Rudolf Magnus Institute of Neuroscience, University Medical Center, 3508 GA Utrecht, The Netherlands,* g.j.biessels@umcutrecht.nl

AUGUSTINA M.A. BRANDS, *PhD • Regional Psychiatric Centre/Zuwe Hofpoort Hospital, Woerden, The Netherlands; Helmholtz Institute, Utrecht University, Utrecht, The Netherlands,* i.brands@altrecht.nl

SUZANNE CRAFT, *PhD • Veterans Affairs Puget Sound, University of Washington, Geriatric Research, Education, and Clinical Center, Seattle, WA 98108, USA,* scraft@u.washington.edu

SUSANA EBNER, *MD • Medicine Department, Columbia University, New York, NY, USA,* sae2103@columbia.edu

HERMES JOSE FLOREZ, *MD, MPH, PhD • Associate Professor of Clinical Medicine and Epidemiology, Clinical Director Geriatric Research, Education and Clinical Center (GRECC), University of Miami Miller School of Medicine, Miami Veterans Affairs Healthcare System, Medicine Department, Divisions of Endocrinology and Geriatric Medicine, Miami, FL, USA,* hflorez@med.miami.edu

MATTHEW FREEBY, *MD • Department of Medicine, Columbia University, New York, NY, USA,* mf2314@columbia.edu

BRIAN M. FRIER, *BSc (Hons), MD, FRCP (Edin), FRCP (Glas) • Diabetes Department, Edinburgh, Scotland EH16 4SA, UK,* brian.frier@luht.scot.nhs.uk

RAJIV A. GANDHI, *MBChB, MRCP • Sheffield Teaching Hospitals, NHS Trust, Diabetes, Sheffield S10 2JF, UK,* rajiv.gandhi@sth.nhs.uk

L. JAAP KAPPELLE • *Department of Neurology, Rudolf Magnus Institute of Neuroscience, University Medical Center Utrecht, 3584 CX Utrecht, The Netherlands,* l.kappelle@umcutrecht.nl

ROY P.C. KESSELS • *Radboud University Nijmegen, Donders Centre for Cognition, 6500 HE Nijmegen, The Netherlands; Helmholtz Institute, Utrecht University, The Netherlands; Donders Institute for Brain,*

Cognition and Behaviour, Radboud University Nijmegen and Radboud University Nijmegen Medical Centre, Nijmesen, The Netherlands, r.kessels@ger.umcn.nl, r.kessels@donders.ru.nl

NYIKA D. KRUYT, *MD • Department of Neurology, University of Amsterdam, 1100 DE Amsterdam, The Netherlands,* n.d.kruijt@amc.uva.nl

MARIA D. LLORENTE, *MD • Chief, Psychiatry Service, Miami VA Healthcare System, Miller School of Medicine, University of Miami, Miami, FL, USA,* maria.llorente@med.va.gov

JOSÉ ALEJANDRO LUCHSINGER, *MD, MPH • Florence Irving Associate Professor of Medicine and Epidemiology, Gertrude H. Sergievsky Center, Columbia Univeristy Medical Center, New York, NY, USA,* jal94@columbia.edu

JULIE E. MALPHURS, *PhD • Health Science Specialist, Miami VA Healthcare System, Assistant Professor of Psychiatry, Miller School of Medicine, University of Miami, Miami, FL, USA, julie.malphurs@va.gov*

BORIS N. MANKOVSKY, *MD • Institute of Endocrinology, Kiev Ukraine,* mankovsky1964@yahoo.com

JENNIFER B. MARKS, *MD • University of Miami Miller School of Medicine, Miami Veterans' Affairs Medical Center, Miami, FL, USA,* jmarks@miami.edu

YAEL D. REIJMER • *Department of Neurology, G03.228, Rudolf Magnus Institute of Neuroscience, University Medical Center, 3508 GA Utrecht, The Netherlands, y.d.reijmer@umcutrecht.nl*

YVO W.B.M. ROOS, *MD, PhD • Department of Neurology, H2-218, Academic Medical Centre, University of Amsterdam, 1100 DE Amsterdam, The Netherlands,* Y.B.Roos@amc.uva.nl

CHRISTOPHER M. RYAN, *PhD • Department of Psychiatry, University of Pittsburgh School of Medicine, Pittsburgh, PA, USA,* ryancm@upmc.edu

ALEX AURELIO SANCHEZ, *MD • Advanced Geriatrics Fellow, University of Miami Miller School of Medicine, Medicine Geriatrics, Miami, FL, USA,* carot732003@yahoo.com

PHILIP SCHELTENS, *MD, PhD • VU University Medical Center, Alzheimer Center, Department of Neurology, Amsterdam 1007 MB, The Netherlands,* p.scheltens@vumc.nl

DINESH SELVARAJAH, *MBChB, MRCP* • *University of Sheffield, Diabetes Research, Royal Hallamshire Hospital, Sheffield S102JF, Yorkshire, UK,* dinesh.selvarajah@sth.nhs.uk

ANDERS A.F. SIMA • *Department of Pathology, Wayne State University School of Medicine, Detroit, MI 48201, USA,* asima@med.wayne.edu

ALINE M.E. STADES, *MD, PhD* • *Department of Internal Medicine, University Medical Center Utrecht, Utrecht, The Netherlands,* A.Stades@umcutrecht.nl

EDITH W.M.T. TER BRAAK, *MD, PhD* • *Department of Internal Medicine, University Medical Center Utrecht, Utrecht, The Netherlands,* e.terbraak@umcutrecht.nl

SOLOMON TESFAYE, *MD, FRCP* • *Diabetes Department, Sheffield Teaching Hospitals, Sheffield S10 2JF, Yorkshire, UK,* solomon.tesfaye@sth.nhs.uk

ESTHER VAN DEN BERG • *Department of Neurology, G03.228, Rudolf Magnus Institute of Neuroscience, University Medical Center Utrecht, 3508 GA Utrecht, The Netherlands,* e.vandenberg-6@umcutrecht.nl

WIESJE M. VAN DER FLIER, *PhD* • *VU University Medical Center, Alzheimer Center, Department of Neurology, Department of Epidemiology and Biostatistics, Amsterdam 1007 MB, The Netherlands,* wm.vdflier@vumc.nl

LAURA A. VAN DE POL, *MD* • *VU Medical Centre, Department of Neurology, 1007 MB Amsterdam, The Netherlands,* l.vandepol@vumc.nl

H. BART VAN DER WORP, *MD, PhD* • *Department of Neurology, Rudolf Magnus Institute of Neuroscience, University Medical Center Utrecht, 3584 CX Utrecht, The Netherlands,* h.b.vanderworp@umcutrecht.nl

G. STENNIS WATSON, *PhD* • *University of Washington, Psychiatry and Behavioral Sciences, Seattle, WA 98108, USA,* gswatson@u.washington.edu

IAIN D. WILKINSON, *MSc, PhD, FIPEM, ARCP* • *University of Sheffield, Academic Radiology, Royal Hallamshire Hospital, Sheffield S102JF, UK,* i.d.wilkinson@sheffield.ac.uk

I UPDATE ON DIABETES FOR NEUROLOGISTS

1

Type 1 Diabetes

*Edith W.M.T. ter Braak
and Aline M.E. Stades*

CONTENTS

ABSTRACT

Type 1 diabetes is a life long metabolic disorder that is characterized by absolute insulin deficiency resulting in hyperglycemia and lipolysis. Type 1 diabetes accounts for 5–10% of the total diabetes population, the majority of the other patients has type 2 diabetes. Insulin deficiency originates with autoimmune mediated β-cell destruction. Without insulin treatment, type 1 diabetes leads to dehydration and ketoacidosis and can ultimately be fatal. Prolonged exposure to hyperglycemia is responsible for microvascular damage in the eye, kidneys and nervous system and contributes to macrovascular disease of the coronary, cerebral and peripheral arteries. Limited joint mobility and the diabetic foot are other complications related to chronic hyperglycemia. Currently, the corner stone of the treatment of type 1 diabetes is exogenous insulin substitution aiming to restore near-normal glycemia in order to prevent or delay long-term complications. Recurrent hypoglycemia is a frequent complication and a serious burden for both patients and their significant others. Additional therapeutic interventions consist of lifestyle modifications, particularly aiming

From: *Contemporary Diabetes: Diabetes and the Brain*
Edited by: G. J. Biessels, J. A. Luchsinger (eds.), DOI 10.1007/978-1-60327-850-8_1
© Humana Press, a part of Springer Science+Business Media, LLC 2009

to reduce cardiovascular risk factors. In the future,the necessity for substitution with exogenous insulin may be replaced by β-cell transplantation or even preventive β-cell preservation. Patients must receive proper education and support, since they have to manage their chronic disease on a daily basis.

Key words: Type 1 Diabetes; Insulin; Ketoacidosis; Hyperglycemia; Hypoglycemia; Autoimmune; β-cells; Long-term complications; Education; Self-care.

INTRODUCTION

The current classification of diabetes in different subtypes is based on the defect(s) that causes hyperglycemia, namely, aberrant or deficient insulin secretion or insufficient insulin action *(1)*. Type 1 diabetes (T1D) originates from autoimmune-mediated destruction of the pancreatic β-cells that normally produce insulin, thus resulting in absolute insulin deficiency. Other types of pancreatic disease involving destruction of the β-cells, such as alcoholic pancreatitis, are classified otherwise. Previously, T1D was also known as juvenile-onset diabetes or insulin-dependent diabetes mellitus (IDDM). However, these expressions may result in misclassification and indistinct prognosis and therapeutic options. Criteria to diagnose T1D are shown in Table 1 *(1)*. Note that diagnostic criteria do not include HbA1c levels, which are exclusively used to follow glycemic control, but not diagnosis.

Table 1
Diagnostic criteria for diabetes mellitus (ADA)

Diabetes mellitus (overall)
Symptoms of polyuria, polydipsia, unexplained weight loss
or
Random plasma glucose ≥ 11.1 mmol/l (200 mg/dl) on 2 subsequent days
or
Fasting (>8 h) plasma glucose ≥ 7.0 mmol/l (126 mg/dl) on 2 subsequent days

Type 1 diabetes mellitus
Autoantibody GAD positive and/or autoantibody tyrosine phosphatase
    IA-2/IA-2β
or
Presenting with ketoacidosis

Additional criteria for diabetes mellitus type 1 (used for research purposes)
Fasting C-peptide <0.1 nmol/l
2 mg Glucagon IV-stimulated C-peptide < 0.3 nmol/l

Adapted from ADA Position Statement *(23)* and an interpretation of data from Service et al. *(63)*.

EPIDEMIOLOGY

Several studies report T1D incidence numbers of 0.1–36.8/100,000 subjects worldwide (2). Above the age of 15 years ketoacidosis at presentation occurs on average in 10% of the population; in children ketoacidosis at presentation is more frequent (3, 4). Overall, publications report a male predominance (1.8 male/female ratio) and a seasonal pattern with higher incidence in November through March in European countries. Worldwide, the incidence of T1D is higher in more developed countries (1, 2, 4–6). Throughout the last decades the overall incidence of T1D has not changed. Recent reports from several European countries, however, suggest that the median age at diagnosis decreased over the last decades. After asthma, T1D is a leading cause of chronic disease in children.

A diagnosis of T1D at the age of 30 or above was formerly referred to as latent-onset autoimmune diabetes in adults (LADA). This is not infrequent and it is estimated that about 10% of the population with a phenotype of type 2 diabetes actually had (autoimmune-mediated) T1D (7). This specific population has anti-GAD or IA-2 antibodies by definition, albeit that in the first 6 months to 6 years after diagnosis these patients do not depend on insulin and that part of them is overweight resulting in concomitant (relative) insulin resistance. In this particular subpopulation, β-cell destruction is only slowly progressive and may take up to 12 years to be complete. An association of the occurrence of T1D with viral infections in early childhood or with vaccination could not be confirmed in recent studies (8).

PATHOPHYSIOLOGY

Genetics and Autoimmunity

T1D is a cell-mediated autoimmune disease with destruction of β-cells that are located in the pancreatic islets of Langerhans. Several islet cell autoantibodies have been isolated: glutamic acid decarboxylase (GAD) and tyrosine phosphatases IA-2 and IA-2β. The majority of type 1 diabetic patients (75–95%) have positive autoantibodies at the time of manifestation. In addition, observations in families have shown an association with the HLA complex, especially the class 2 molecules, suggesting a predominant role in aberrances in T-cell-mediated responses via cytotoxic and helper T cells (6). T1D is strongly associated with HLA DQA and DQB genes, but this can differ among various populations throughout the world. In contrast, twin studies show a low concordant prevalence of T1D of only 30–55%.

Associated Autoimmune Diseases

Diabetes mellitus type 1 may be sporadic or associated with other autoimmune diseases within patients or within families. The latter has been classified as autoimmune polyglandular syndrome type II (APS-II). APS-II is a polygenic disorder with a female preponderance which typically occurs between the ages of 20 and 40 years *(9)*. In clinical practice, anti-thyroxine peroxidase (TPO) positive hypothyroidism is the most frequent concomitant autoimmune disease in type 1 diabetic patients, therefore all type 1 diabetic patients should annually be screened for the presence of anti-TPO antibodies. Other frequently associated disorders are atrophic gastritis leading to vitamin B12 deficiency (pernicious anemia) and vitiligo. Rare disorders in APS-II are presented in Table 2.

Table 2
Autoimmune polyglandular syndrome type II (APS-II)

Disease	Autoantibodies
Diabetes mellitus type 1	Anti-GAD
Autoimmune hypothyroidism	Anti-TPO
Addison's disease	Anti-adrenal cortex
Hypoparathyroidism	Unknown
Vitiligo	Anti-melanocyte
Alopecia	Unknown
Celiac disease	Anti-transglutaminase
	Anti-endomysium
Autoimmune hepatitis	Anti-nuclear antibody (ANA)
	Increased immunoglobulin G
Pernicious anemia/atrophic gastritis	Anti-parietal cell Anti-intrinsic factor
Idiopathic thrombocytic purpura	Unknown
Myasthenia gravis	Anti-acetylcholine receptor

Normal Glucose Homeostasis

Glucose and fatty acids are the main energy sources in most cells, each accounting for 40–45% of the total energy expenditure. In the fasting state, basal glucose turnover is 1.8–2.2 mg/kg/min of which the brain, being almost fully dependent on glucose, consumes 80% *(10)*. The gut absorbs glucose, lipids, and proteins and transports them to the liver. Glucose uptake in the liver takes place via glucose transporter 2 (GLUT2) and is insulin independent. Insulin promotes glycogen storage in the liver and insulin-dependent glucose uptake via glucose transporter 4 (GLUT4) in muscle and adipocytes for glycogen storage and triglyceride formation *(11)*. The remainder of glucose is used for basal energy in the whole body. During change from the postprandial anabolic state to the catabolic (fasting) state between meals and during exercise, insulin is down-regulated and glucagon is up-regulated in order to maintain a stable glucose plasma concentration. In the fasting state, the plasma glucose level is maintained via glycogenolysis in the liver. The liver glycogen storages are depleted after a 12–24 h fast, after which proteins are consumed for gluconeogenesis in the liver. However, even then plasma insulin concentrations are not completely suppressed, because glucose uptake for basal cell metabolism is insulin dependent and thus inhibits the liver from ketogenesis. The liver, brain, and pancreas are considered to have insulin-independent glucose uptake via glucose transporters (GLUT 1, GLUT2) *(12)*. The brain does not feature an alternate energy source such as lipid β-oxidation, but can adapt slowly in the long-fasting state to ketone bodies as fuel. In contrast, muscle tissue switches to β-oxidation of triglycerides (lipolysis), and proteins are degraded to amino acids, which can be used by the liver for gluconeogenesis for basal metabolism *(10)*. In nondiabetic subjects this process is well balanced by a decreased insulin/glucagon ratio, without an excess of ketogenesis and free fatty acids.

Insulin Deficiency

The normal human pancreas contains a superfluous amount of β-cells. In T1D, β-cell destruction therefore remains asymptomatic until a critical β-cell reserve is left. This destructive process takes months to years *(6, 7)*. After the asymptomatic period, gluconeogenesis cannot be suppressed due to partial insulin deficiency, resulting in hyperglycemia and limited ketogenesis. If plasma glucose concentration exceeds the threshold for renal glucose reabsorption (about 10 mmol/l), the urinary glucose concentration further increases and the first clinical signs become manifest. Due to glucosuria, clinical signs of polyuria, polydipsia, and weight loss subsequently evolve into hypovolemia, along with lipolysis and expenditure of amino acids, resulting in a catabolic state. The body is able to keep the production of ketone bodies limited until a critically low insulin level is reached. This process may be accelerated by intercurrent infections or by other co-morbidity that increases insulin resistance. Absolute insulin deficiency leads to a life-threatening vicious circle of hyperglycemia, dehydration, and ketoacidosis, which is described below in the paragraph on *Short-Term Complications* and in *Hyperglycemic Hyperosmolar State*, Chapter 7. Only in a minority of type 1 diabetic patients does the disease begin with diabetic ketoacidosis, the majority presents with a milder course that may be mistaken as type 2 diabetes *(7)*.

Interplay of Insulin with Other Hormones

Insulin is the main regulator of glucose metabolism by stimulating glucose uptake in tissues and glycogen storage in liver and muscle and by inhibiting gluconeogenesis in the liver *(11)*. Moreover, insulin is a growth factor for cells and cell differentiation, and acting as anabolic hormone insulin stimulates lipogenesis and protein synthesis. Glucagon is the counterpart of insulin and is secreted by the α-cells in the pancreatic islets in an inversely proportional quantity to the insulin concentration. Glucagon, being a catabolic hormone, stimulates glycolysis and gluconeogenesis in the liver as well as lipolysis and uptake of amino acids in the liver. Epinephrine and norepinephrine have comparable catabolic effects and act nearly simultaneously in the physiologic counter regulatory response during hypoglycemia (see *Hypoglycemia in People with Diabetes*, Chapter 6) *(13)*. Glucagon secretion is not completely understood, but is supposed to be a consequence of an intra-islet decrement of insulin *(14)*. This hypothesis is sustained by the observation that T1D patients lose the glucagon response to hypoglycemia after several years, when all β-cells are destroyed, while glucagon secretion, in response to other stimuli such as certain intravenously administered secretagogues, is preserved in T1D.

Insulin is secreted by the β-cell in response to an increased plasma glucose level via a sensing mechanism of the β-cell using the insulin-independent GLUT 2 transporter *(12, 13)*. Another mechanism of insulin secretion has been clarified based on the observation that insulin concentrations show a higher rise after oral glucose loading than after a comparable intravenous glucose load. The gut-derived hormones glucose-dependent insulin-releasing polypeptide (GIP) and glucagon like peptide-1 (GLP-1) are secreted within minutes after food ingestion and act on multiple tissues, since GLP-1 receptors are located on islet cells (α and β-cells), liver, adipocytes, brain, muscle, and stomach. GLP-1 promotes insulin release and inhibits glucagon release, but only in the postprandial state. GLP-1 analogs are, however, not of therapeutic interest in T1D, because GLP-1 relies on the availability of endogenous insulin secretion *(15)*.

SHORT-TERM COMPLICATIONS

Hyperglycemia, Ketoacidosis

Diabetic ketoacidosis (DKA) is a life-threatening complication of T1D caused by an absolute deficiency of insulin and often revealing the diagnosis *(16)*. DKA is also frequently observed in patients with preexisting T1D due to intercurrent infections, ischemia, or inappropriate adherence to treatment. All patients with nausea or vomiting should be warned to seek medical care, because they are at risk for DKA. This risk may be aggravated when patients are inclined to postpone insulin injections intending to avoid hypoglycemia when they are not eating. Importantly, nausea and vomiting may also be the first symptoms of DKA. In addition, patients with DKA typically present with hyperventilation due to respiratory compensation of metabolic acidosis, severe dehydration, and coma, but DKA may also mimic acute abdomen. Laboratory tests reveal a high plasma glucose level and metabolic acidosis, with either increased or decreased potassium values. The treatment of ketoacidosis consists of rehydration with saline and intravenous insulin substitution to suppress ketogenesis. Major electrolyte shifts occur because of rehydration and recovering from acidosis, therefore potassium and other electrolytes should be closely monitored and substituted if necessary (see also *Hyperglycemic Hyperosmolar State*, Chapter 7).

Hypoglycemia

Hypoglycemia is a common problem in T1D due to relatively overdosing of insulin in combination with underestimating the energy expenditure of physical exercise. It may also be related to concomitant medications such as the use of (nonselective) β-blocking agents. Besides the risk of hypoglycemic coma and (very seldom) death, fear of hypoglycemia restrains patients to strive for optimal glycemic control. The risk of hypoglycemia increases with improved glycemic control, autonomic neuropathy, longer duration of diabetes, and the presence of long-term complications *(17)*.

Hypoglycemia is defined as an event with a glucose concentration below 3.9 mmol/l, with symptoms that recover after glucose normalization. Severe hypoglycemia is defined as any hypoglycemic event requiring help from another person to recover and may be complicated by seizure or coma *(18)*. Classical autonomous warning symptoms include sweating, palpitations, anxiety, hunger, and tremor. When plasma glucose concentration decreases further symptoms can progress toward neuroglycopenic symptoms consisting of drowsiness, paralysis, and cognitive dysfunction precluding appropriate self-management by glucose ingestion. When hypoglycemia remains untreated and blood glucose concentrations further decrease, this ultimately results in coma and/or convulsion. During hypoglycemia the cardiac QT interval is lengthened by sympathoadrenal stimulation directly on the myocardium and decreased serum potassium; this supposedly contributes to (fatal) cardiac arrhythmia during hypoglycemia *(19, 20)* (see also *Hypoglycemia in People with Diabetes*, Chapter 6).

LONG-TERM COMPLICATIONS

T1D may ultimately lead to such dreadful conditions as blindness, limb amputations, and renal failure calling for dialysis or renal transplantation. Hence, for both patients and health care workers prevention and delay of long-term complications are important incentives in striving for good glycemic control. Long-term complications in type 1 diabetic patients (see Table 3) are traditionally divided into microvascular complications, comprising retinopathy, nephropathy, and neuropathy, and macrovascular damage, including peripheral vascular disease (PVD), coronary artery disease (CAD), and cerebral vascular disease (CVD). Moreover, musculoskeletal complications and the diabetic foot are clinical entities that are multicausal and/or for which causes are not yet fully understood. Long-term complications are prevalent in any population of type 1 diabetic patients with increasing prevalence and severity in relation to disease duration and glycemic control and other risk factors.

Table 3
Overview of long-term complications and associated conditions of type 1 diabetes

Microvascular	Retinopathy
	Neuropathy
	Nephropathy
Macrovascular (atherosclerosis)	Coronary heart disease (CHD)
	Peripheral vascular disease (PVD)
	Cerebral vascular disease (CVD)
	Diabetic foot (multi causal)
Co-existing risk factors for atherosclerosis	Hypertension
	Dyslipidemia
	Smoking
	Obesity
	Family history
Miscellaneous	Musculoskeletal
	Diabetic foot (multicausal)

Although clinicians and scientists believed for decades that the level of glycemic control is crucial for the risk of future complications, it was not until 1993 before the publication of the first randomized-controlled trial (widely known as the diabetes control and complications trial (DCCT)) which supplied evidence that better glycemic control is actually able to reduce the risk of microvascular complications, making intensive insulin treatment worthwhile *(21)*. A follow-up study (the Epidemiology of

Diabetes Interventions and Complications (EDIC) study) showed comparable results for macrovascular sequelae *(22)*.

The pathogenesis of diabetic complications is multifactorial, complicated, and not yet fully elucidated. In brief, focusing on the role of hyperglycemia, so-called advanced glycation end products (AGEs) and sorbitol are considered to contribute to tissue damage. In addition there may be more tissue-specific factors that contribute to tissue damage, like protein kinase C in the kidney. An overview of current insights into the pathogenesis of long-term diabetic complications is supplied by Michael Brownlee *(23)*.

Retinopathy

Diabetic retinopathy is the most widespread cause of visual loss in the Western world and probably the most feared complication of diabetes. It is caused by microangiopathic lesions of the retinal precapillary arterioles, capillaries, and venules. Damage is caused both by microvascular leakage from breakdown of the inner blood–retinal barrier and by microvascular occlusion.

Prevalence of retinopathy at 8–10 years after the onset of diabetes in more recent reports varies between 30 and 60%. This is lower than may be expected from older cohort studies. Data support the conclusion that this may be attributed to better levels of glycemic control that are achieved during the last decades *(24)*. It was already known from previous intervention studies that the development and progression of diabetic retinopathy in T1D can be prevented by better glycemic control *(25)*. An important observation from these trials is that retinopathy may actually worsen during the first year of tightened glycemic control. This observation is even more relevant with respect to women planning to become pregnant: this usually calls for intensified insulin treatment in order to achieve adequate glycemic control before conception. Although the risk of progression during pregnancy is increased in women with the highest initial HbA1c values and in those with the greatest reduction in HbA1c values, probably factors related to pregnancy per se also contribute. Apart from glycemic control other factors that increase the risk of, or are associated with, retinopathy include diabetes duration, albuminuria and nephropathy, and hypertension. Lowering blood pressure has been shown to decrease the progression of retinopathy in type 2 diabetes. Epidemiological data suggest that the same is probably true for T1D.

Several systems for the classification of the severity of diabetic retinopathy and diabetic macular edema exist. An international group of experts reached consensus about a five-stage disease severity classification that was developed for clinical purposes aiming to improve screening of people with

diabetes and in order to facilitate proper communication and discussion
among health care providers (Table 4) *(26)*.

Table 4
Diabetic retinopathy (DR) disease severity scale[1]

Severity level of DR	Ophthalmoscopic findings
No apparent retinopathy	No abnormalities
Mild nonproliferative	Microaneurysms only
Moderate nonproliferative	More than just microaneurysms but less than severe nonproliferative retinopathy
Severe nonproliferative	>20 intraretinal hemorrhages in 4 quadrants or definite venous beading in ≥2 quadrants or prominent intraretinal microvascular abnormalities in ≥1 quadrant NO signs of proliferative retinopathy
Proliferative	≥1 of: neovascularization, vitrous/preretinal hemorrhage

[1] Adapted from Wilkinson et al. and the Global Diabetic Retinopathy Project Group *(26)*.

Screening for diabetic retinopathy with dilated pupils by an ophthal-
mologist is recommended within 5 years after the onset of diabetes and
annually thereafter. Screening is necessary because retinopathy remains
asymptomatic until macular edema and/or proliferative diabetic retinopathy
are present and by then it may be too late for effective treatment aiming at
symptom relief and slowing progression. Macular edema results from capillary leakage and can develop at all stages of retinopathy. It typically presents
with the gradual onset of blurring of near and distant vision in patients
who have other evidence of microvascular eye disease, such as perimacu-
lar microaneurysms. Apart from glycemic control hypertension is also a risk
factor for retinopathy. The efficacy of laser photocoagulation in preventing
visual loss from proliferative diabetic retinopathy is well-established in randomized trials.

Importantly, the presence of retinopathy should not be considered a con-
traindication to the prescription of salicylates which may be indicated for
other reasons, because this treatment does not increase the risk of retinal
hemorrhage.

Apart from retinopathy, other eye diseases are related to diabetes.
Cataract is much more frequent in patients with diabetes and tends to
become clinically significant at a younger age. Glaucoma is markedly
increased in diabetes too.

Diabetic Neuropathy

The ultimate consequences of diabetic neuropathy include such grave conditions as impaired mobility, limb amputation, and progressive deformities particularly of the feet. Diabetic neuropathies are heterogeneous with diverse clinical manifestations including symmetric polyneuropathy, autonomic neuropathy, radiculopathies, mononeuropathies, and mononeuropathy multiplex. However, not all peripheral neuropathy in diabetes patients is caused by diabetes (27, 28). Attention should be paid to other potential causes of neuropathy, such as monoclonal gammopathy, folic acid or vitamin B_{12} deficiency, extensive use of alcohol, and co-existing chronic inflammatory demyelinating polyneuropathy (CIDP). The need for annual screening for diabetic neuropathy in all patients is discussed in the subsection of foot care. Diabetic polyneuropathy is primarily a symmetrical sensory neuropathy that gradually causes the typical "stocking-glove" sensory loss at progression. Various staging systems for use in research and for clinical purposes exist. Diabetes is the most common cause of neuropathic (Charcot) arthropathy in the Western world. A warm, swollen foot in a diabetic patient with long-standing neuropathy without local or systemic signs of infection is consistent with Charcot's disease and calls for abstinence from putting weight on the foot until symptoms subside.

Major clinical manifestations of diabetic autonomic neuropathy include resting tachycardia, orthostatic hypotension, disturbances of gastrointestinal motility, erectile dysfunction, sudomotor dysfunction, impaired neurovascular function, and hypoglycemic autonomic failure resulting in impaired glucose counterregulation in case of hypoglycemia. Bladder dysfunction may affect renal function and should be distinguished from worsening nephropathy. Referral to an urologist is warranted to assess the potential need for intermittent self-catheterization.

Nephropathy and Hypertension

In up to 40% of type 1 diabetic patients, diabetic nephropathy may ultimately result in end-stage renal disease (ESRD). ESRD necessitates renal function replacement by hemodialysis, peritoneal dialysis, or renal transplantation if possible. Fortunately, chances of renal function preservation have dramatically improved over the last few decades because of better glycemic control and appropriate blood pressure management.

Early stages of nephropathy tend to become clinically detectable about 10–12 years after diagnosis (Table 5). Annual screening for urinary albumin excretion and monitoring of serum creatinine level are recommended for all patients with a diabetes duration of 5 years or longer. Once nephropathy has progressed to persistent macroalbuminuria, prognosis worsens: about half

Table 5
Diabetic nephropathy

Stages of diabetic nephropathy	Albuminuria Albumin in first morning urine sample	Albumin/creatinine ratio Albumin and creatinine in first morning urine sample: ACR, mg/mmol	Glomerular filtration rate[1] Estimated from serum creatinine level: eGFR, ml/min/1.73 m^2
1 Glomerular hyperfiltration and renal enlargement	<30 mg/24 h		Increased
2 Silent preclinical. Early glomerular lesions	<30 mg/24 h		Normal or increased
3 Incipient	30–299 mg/24 h (microalbuminuria)[2]	> 2.5 (men) > 3.5 (women)	Normal (>90)
4 Overt	≥300 mg/24 h (macroalbuminuria)	> 30 (men or women)	Decreased Mild renal impairment 60–89 Moderate 30–59 Severe 15–29
5 End-stage renal disease	≥300 mg/24 h (macroalbuminuria)	> 30 (men or women)	<15

[1] Use Cockcroft- and Gault-formula or MDRD (modification of diet in renal disease).
[2] Confirm diagnosis within 2 months or with two out of three samples within 1 year.

of patients with macroalbuminuria develop ESRD within 10 years and 75% within 20 years *(29)*.

Occasionally other potential causes of renal disease apart from nephropathy must be considered in patients with albuminuria. More specifically this should be the case in the presence of an active urine sediment (if urinary tract infection has been excluded) or when clinical presentation is atypical with acute or rapidly declining renal function, early onset renal impairment within 5 years after the diagnosis of diabetes, or in the absence of diabetic retinopathy or neuropathy.

Risk factors for diabetic nephropathy for which specific interventions are available include glycemic control, blood pressure, early glomerular hyperfiltration, and smoking. In addition, several studies suggest that genetic susceptibility may play a role with a variety of underlying mechanisms, including ACE polymorphism. In the presence of chronic hyperglycemia the risk for diabetes-associated kidney disease seems to be magnified by risk alleles at several susceptibility loci, some of which differ between men and women *(30)*. Hypertension is more prevalent in certain populations, such as people from African descent and Native Americans.

At the time nephropathy is diagnosed, nearly all T1D patients have other signs of microvascular damage, such as retinopathy and neuropathy. Usually, retinopathy precedes the onset of overt nephropathy. Intensive insulin treatment aiming for near-normoglycemia has been demonstrated to delay the onset of microalbuminuria and the progression of microalbuminuria to macroalbuminuria *(31)*. Furthermore, progression of renal impairment may be delayed by several interventions of which anti-hypertensive treatment is the most important. Angiotensin-converting enzyme inhibitors (ACEi) are widely considered the type of drug of first choice. ACEi have been shown to be able to slow the decline in GFR in patients once macroalbuminuria has developed *(32, 33)*. Even in normotensive patients with microalbuminuria prescription of an ACEi may be considered. When these drugs are not tolerated, angiotensin II receptor blockers (ARBs) are recommended. When ACEi or ARBs are prescribed, monitoring of serum potassium levels in addition to serum creatinine levels is indicated, especially after introducing these anti-hypertensive medications for the first time. Depending on the clinical context, thiazide diuretics, β-blocking agents, and calcium channel blockers may also be used in addition or as a substitution, but they are generally second-choice agents. Multiple drugs are generally needed to achieve adequate blood pressure control in the majority of patients. Importantly, caution has to be taken in women who consider pregnancy: ACEi inhibitors and ARBs are contraindicated around conception and during pregnancy because they cause damage to the fetus.

The main treatment goal in order to preserve renal function as long as possible is striving for blood pressure control below 130/80 mmHg and preferably even lower in patients with albuminuria. A repeat systolic blood pressure ≥130 mmHg or diastolic blood pressure ≥80 mmHg confirms a diagnosis of hypertension. In patients without albuminuria pharmacological treatment is recommended in the case of systolic blood pressure ≥ 140 mmHg and/or diastolic blood pressure ≥ 90 mmHg in addition to lifestyle therapy. The latter may suffice when systolic blood pressure is between 130 and 139 mmHg and diastolic blood pressure between 80 and 89 mmHg. Caution not to lower diastolic blood pressure below 75 mmHg in patients with known cardiovascular disease is called for on the other hand.

In addition to normalization of blood pressure lifestyle adjustments are recommended, especially smoking cessation. Protein restriction is advocated by some authors and may especially be considered when nephropathy is worsening despite good glycemic control and blood pressure regulation in the presence of ACE inhibitor and/or ARBs.

Macrovascular Complications

T1D should be considered as an independent risk factor for atherosclerosis, potentially resulting in clinically apparent cardiovascular disease, peripheral vascular disease, and cerebrovascular disease. An older study shows that the cumulative mortality of coronary heart disease in T1D was 35% by the age 55 *(34)*. In comparison, the Framingham Heart Study showed a cardiovascular mortality of 8% of men and 4% of women without diabetes, respectively. Comparable data were observed with respect to nonfatal myocardial infarction and angina.

Although the DCCT initially failed to show a reduction in macrovascular complications by intensified insulin treatment and more tight glycemic control, the follow-up study (EDIC) to the DCCT demonstrated that intensive insulin therapy in patients with T1D is able to decrease fatal and nonfatal cardiovascular events. Interestingly, these results indicate that a sustained period of glycemic control has lasting benefit in reducing cardiovascular morbidity and mortality in T1D *(35, 36)*. These results are supported by similar findings from other studies.

Cardiovascular risk factors in diabetic patients without manifest cardiac disease should be assessed at least once a year. These risk factors include dyslipidemia, hypertension, smoking, a positive family history of premature coronary disease, and the presence of microalbuminuria or macroalbuminuria that, in this context, serves as an epidemiological marker for endothelial damage. Established risk factors should be treated accordingly using ACEi, statins, and salicylates. Screening for asymptomatic coronary artery disease remains somewhat controversial but is not recommended *(37)*. However, perception of ischemic pain may be blunted or atypical in some patients due to autonomous neuropathy.

PVD interacts with diabetic neuropathy in the pathogenesis of diabetic foot ulcers and gangrene. In symptomatic patients claudication can present in buttock and hip, thigh, calf, or foot depending on the localization(s) of the arteriosclerotic lesion(s).

Atherosclerosis is basically a systemic disease. Patients with one clinically apparent localization are at risk for other manifestations. Interventions therefore should always simultaneously include appropriate assessment and management of potential risk factors.

Musculoskeletal Complications

The so-called musculoskeletal complications of diabetes comprise a rather heterogeneous group of ailments that are often present concurrently (see Table 6). They are foremost observed in patients with long-standing diabetes in whom microvascular and macrovascular complications also result in complaints and symptoms. It is therefore often difficult to attribute signs and complaints to one diagnosis or another.

Although musculoskeletal complications are quite prevalent in long-standing diabetes, generally less attention is paid to these conditions both clinically and in research. For patients these ailments may cause a lot of discomfort in daily life and comprise considerable uncertainty with respect to cause, prognosis, and therapeutic options. This becomes even more marked since diabetologists and primary care physicians may consider a variety of specialists for referral, such as a rheumatologist, orthopedic surgeon, neurologist, plastic surgeon, rehabilitation specialist, or physiotherapist. In the literature these complications are infrequently approached as a group or as a systemic disorder, but rather from a "limb-oriented" perspective. To make matters even more complicated from the clinician's and patient's perspectives, some of these diseases such as cheiroarthropathy are almost exclusively seen in patients with diabetes, while others, such as carpal tunnel syndrome or Dupuytren's are also quite common in a variety of other conditions and are also seen without any known underlying disorder.

Musculoskeletal disease in diabetes is best viewed as a systemic disorder with involvement of connective tissue. Potential pathophysiological mechanisms that play a role are glycosylation of collagen, abnormal cross-linking of collagen, and increased collagen hydration *(38)*. In addition, other mechanisms like neuropathy and microangiopathy and hormonal abnormalities such as high insulin levels may play a role as well.

Table 6
Clinical syndromes of musculoskeletal disease associated with diabetes

	Clinical Syndrome		Diagnosis	Treatment options
Hand	Limited Joint Mobility (LJM)	Also called: diabetic cheiroarthropathy or stiff hand syndrome	Clinical (see text)	Probably irreversible, relation to glycemic control controversial but optimizing control is advocated
	Carpal Tunnel Syndrome (CTS)	Median nerve entrapment CTS is frequently present in LJM Differentiate from polyneuropathy	Clinical Nerve conduction studies confirming selective impairment of median nerve conduction Check for thenar muscle atrophy	Splinting, local corticosteroid[1] injection Ergonomic adjustments (e.g., computer workstations) Surgical decompression
	Dupuytren's contracture	Due to thickening of the palmar fascia Other organs may be involved (see text)	Clinical	Physiotherapy and local corticosteroid injection may be considered Flexion deformities >40 degrees at the metacarpophalangeal or >20 degrees at the proximal interphalangeal joint are suggested as indications for surgery; high recurrence rates

Table 6
(Continued)

Clinical Syndrome		Diagnosis	Treatment options
	Flexor tenosynovitis	"Trigger finger"	Clinical, "locking phenomenon"	Immobilization in acute stage Local corticosteroid injection Surgery (outcome may be less successful in diabetes)
	Diabetic sclerodactyly	Thickening and waxiness of the dorsal skin of the fingers Associated with LJM but also seen separately	Clinical	No treatment known
Shoulder	Adhesive capsulitis	"Frozen shoulder" Reversible contraction of the glenohumeral joint capsule	Clinical	Corticosteroid injections Physiotherapy Often self-limited condition in 6–18 months
	Calcific periarthritis Limited Joint Mobility (LJM)	Often asymptomatic	Calcium deposits on shoulder X-ray	

Table 6
(Continued)

Clinical Syndrome		Diagnosis	Treatment options
Reflex sympathetic dystrophy	"Shoulder hand syndrome" Association with diabetes uncertain	Clinical Autonomic testing, imagining studies May be associated with adhesive capsulitis	Regional sympathetic nerve block (may also be used diagnostically)
Skeleton Diffuse idiopathic skeletal hyperostosis (DISH)	Also called: ankylosing hyperostosis or Forestier's disease Metaplastic calcification and osteophyte formation of spinal ligaments and entheses (where tendons and ligaments attach to bone), mainly thoracic spine Association with diabetes uncertain	Distinctive radiographic findings: flowing linear calcification and ossification of paravertebral ligaments	Physical therapy Analgesics

[1]Note: Even locally injected corticosteroids may lead to considerable blood glucose disturbances

For practical purposes, a "limb-oriented" overview of these conditions is given in Table 6. It should be stressed, however, that this may be an oversimplification. A classical example is Dupuytren's disease, which may be observed in up to 42% of adults with diabetes mellitus, typically in patients with long-standing T1D. Dupuytren's is characterized by thickening of the palmar fascia due to fibrosis with nodule formation and contracture, leading to flexion contractures of the digits, most commonly affecting the fourth and fifth digits. These abnormalities are quite readily observed during routine office visits and patients tend to bring up their complaints in an early stage because of perceived limitations in daily life. However, in fact there may be other related fibrosing diseases present as well that are more easily overlooked while patients may not bring forward complaints spontaneously. Other fibrosing conditions that are often seen concurrently with the palmar fibrosis of Dupuytren's are nodular plantar fibrosis of the feet, nodular fasciitis of the popliteal fascia, and Peyronie's disease of the penis (39).

Limited joint mobility or diabetic cheiroarthropathy is attributed to abnormal collagen in connective tissue around joints and is readily recognized by the "prayer sign": when asked to place opposite palmar sides of the hands and fingers together there is an inability to completely close the gap due to contractures in the metacarpophalangeal, proximal interphalangeal, and distal interphalangeal joints (40, 41). At the "table top test" the patient is unable to flatten the palm of the hand when pressing it against the surface of a table.

It is obvious that one or more of the above-mentioned conditions of the hand, especially when concurring in the presence of distal symmetric sensorimotor polyneuropathy (or one of the other clinical syndromes of neuropathy with involvement of the hands), lead to incapacities with respect to many aspects of daily life, including self-monitoring of blood glucose levels and injecting insulin.

Foot Care

Foot problems in diabetes are common and comprise ulceration, infection, and gangrene, thus resulting in serious morbidity and disability that may ultimately lead to amputation and even death. The lifetime risk of a foot ulcer for diabetic patients is about 15% (42). Amputation is predictive of a severely diminished life expectation, which in part reflects serious co-morbidity and high age. In addition this may be indicative of the accessibility to appropriate care and the standard of delivered care (43).

Screening, education, and early recognition are the mainstay of the prevention of more serious problems. All patients with diabetes should have an annual foot exam to assess risk factors for ulceration and amputation. At the same time, appropriate education with regard to foot self-care and risk factors can be delivered (Table 7) (44).

Table 7
Annual preventive foot care visit in primary care

Assessment of neuropathy, including a quantitative somatosensory threshold test	Semmes–Weinstein 5.07 (10 g) monofilament at specific sites
Visual inspection of the foot and footwear	Skin lesions, especially between the toes and under the metatarsal heads
	Nail care
	Erythema, warmth, callus formation
	Bony deformities, joint mobility, gait and balance
	Shoes and socks
Screening for peripheral arterial disease	History for claudication
	Assessment of pedal pulses
	Ankle brachial index
Address educational issues	Selection of appropriate footware
	Avoiding walking on bare feet
	Daily self-inspection of feet in case of diminished protective sensibility
	Importance to seek medical help in case of skin lesions and/or infection
Assessment of self-care ability and involving a family member if indicated	Visual impairment
	Diminished movement ability
	Impaired cognitive function

Once ulcers or infections are present, health care providers for diabetic patients should have a broad view on therapeutic possibilities. Since foot ulcers are generally multicausal in origin they call for a multidisciplinary approach, preferably using a protocol. In addition, effective record keeping and communication between team members are essential *(45)*.

Several classification systems for diabetic foot ulcers exist, but there is no consensus yet with respect to classifying or even describing foot ulcers. For clinical purposes, description of an ulcer should be thorough and clear including a photograph, if possible. Descriptions of wounds should include depth, extent, area, location, appearance, temperature, and odor. Wound depth is an important determinant of outcome *(46, 47)*. Deep ulcers with cellulitis or abscess formation often involve osteomyelitis. From this stage on parenteral administration of antibiotics and hospitalization are indicated. Radiologic changes occur late in the course of osteomyelitis and negative radiographs certainly do not exclude it. In addition to osteomyelitis, assessment of arterial vascular disease is called for. Revascularization may be indicated in order to promote wound healing. Aggressive revascularization has been shown to decrease amputation at all levels *(48, 49)*.

TREATMENT

Insulin

Insulin therapy is mandatory for survival in T1D. The ideal insulin regimen mimics the physiological pattern of insulin secretion with low fasting insulin levels, a slow rise in insulin concentration in the early morning, and with postprandial peaks that closely follow the ingestion of carbohydrates and other food. The blood glucose profile over the day is preferably targeted to near normal glycemia with avoidance of hypoglycemia (see Table 8). The percentage of glucose binding to hemoglobin (HbA1c) reflects glucose concentrations in the preceding 4–8 weeks *(50)*. The therapeutic goal is an HbA1c concentration around 7.0% to prevent microvascular and possibly macrovascular complications, unless hypoglycemia interferes *(51, 52)*. The best approach to reach good glycemic control is either a multiple daily injection (MDI) regimen (also called basal bolus regimen) or continuous subcutaneous insulin infusion (CSII) using a pump. In MDI and CSII a prepandial bolus of rapid- or short-acting insulin is injected to prevent postprandial hyperglycemia. For basal insulin supply, intermediate- or long-acting insulin is administered or with CSII low doses of rapid-acting insulin are continuously infused *(53)*.

The dose of long- or intermediate-acting insulin is adjusted according to the fasting glucose concentration, but is limited by nocturnal hypoglycemia. In contrast, some patients show high fasting glucose concentration, which may be attributed to the so-called dawn phenomenon: the physiological early morning cortisol peak results in increased insulin resistance. Another pitfall

Table 8
Typical algorithm for insulin dosage adjustment aiming at near normal glycemia

Blood Glucose (BG, mmol/L) target level		Preprandial dose of rapid/short acting insulin	Bedtime dose of intermediate/long acting insulin
Fasting BG	4–6		Increase if BG > 6 (unless nocturnal hypoglycemia)
Preprandial BG	4–6	Increase dose before previous meal if BG > 6	
Postprandial BG (2 hours after)	5–7	Increase if BG > 7	
BG at bedtime	7–9	Small extra bolus if BG > 9, review evening snacks	

is a rebound high fasting glucose after undetected nocturnal hypoglycemia, especially in MDI. One of the advantages of CSII is the possibility of a programmed increase of early morning insulin infusion and variable basal insulin infusion in accordance with exercise.

Most currently available human insulin and insulin analogs are manufactured through recombinant DNA technology. Before DNA technology emerged, chemically modified pork insulin was used (derived from its pancreas) and is still available in some countries *(54)*. Insulin analogs have a change in amino acid sequence of the β chain that influences the absorption rate *(55)*. Insulin compounds are categorized by the rate of acting.

Rapid-acting insulin analogs (lispro [Humalog], aspart [NovoRapid], and glulisine [Apidra]) are available as three different formulations, all showing comparable absorption rates.

The peak insulin concentration is 40 min after injection and comes close to the postprandial insulin profile in healthy volunteers. The rapid-acting analogs show a rapid waning of action in 3–4 h. The advantage for patients is more flexibility since the time of injection is just before the meal and the frequency of hypoglycemia may be reduced with preservation of comparable HbA1c levels. The manufacturer of inhaled insulin Exubera, an effective alternative for rapid-acting subcutaneous insulin, recently stopped its production for financial economic reasons. Exubera was expensive and might have caused long-term adverse events with respect to alveolar function by inhaling insulin which is a potent growth factor.

Regular short-acting insulin is unchanged human insulin. Due to its tendency to form hexamers in the subcutis, preparations of normal human insulin have a slower absorption rate after injection than the rapid-acting insulin analogs. The maximum insulin peak concentration is lower, occurs after 90 min, and the waning of action is 4–6 h. Due to a lag time for the onset of action, patients have to inject regular insulin 30 min before the meal, and because of its longer duration of action, patients often have to take a snack between meals to avoid hypoglycemia before the next meal.

Intermediate-acting insulin is used as basal insulin since it results in a prolonged, relatively low insulin concentration. Neutral protamine Hagedorn (NPH) is human insulin in a buffered solution and has to be stirred before injection. Unfortunately, its absorption rate is quite variable. With an insulin peak level 6 h after an injection with NPH insulin, there is an increased risk of nocturnal hypoglycemia.

Insulin detemir is an analog with a fatty acid chain that binds to albumin. Its time of action is 17.5 h and patients often end up with a twice daily regimen. Patients who use insulin detemir have less nocturnal hypoglycemia, lower fasting glucose, and less weight gain in a once daily regimen, compared to NPH. Disappointingly, recent data with a twice daily regimen of insulin detemir in type 2 diabetes did not show a difference in weight gain compared to other basal insulin regimens *(56)*. Long-acting insulin glargine is an analog that is less soluble in the subcutaneously pH neutral environment because of a changed isoelectric point. The time of action is about 24 h and it results in lower fasting glucose concentration and less frequent nocturnal hypoglycemia. Results of a study reporting a head-to-head comparison of detemir and glargine in T1D are expected to be published soon.

Both long-acting insulin analogs detemir and glargine may cause dermal irritation locally around the injection site. Mixtures of rapid- or short-acting insulin in combination with NPH are available and these are given twice daily. Its use is no longer indicated in the majority of type 1 patients. However, a mixture can be a solution in T1D patients with a short life expectancy or difficulties with the management of an MDI regimen, e.g., in the presence of cognitive impairment.

Metformin is potentially of use in overweight T1D patients with decreased insulin sensitivity calling for high insulin dosages. Metformin inhibits gluconeogenesis and possibly improves insulin sensitivity. A mean decrease of HbA1c levels of about 1% or a decrement of insulin dosages and weight loss has been reported in studies with metformin added to insulin therapy in T1D *(57, 58)*. Most patients with CSII use a rapid-acting insulin analog, since postprandial glucose is better controlled. A recent meta-analysis reported that CSII improved metabolic control (HbA1c), in combination with a decreased frequency of severe hypoglycemia, especially in patients suffering from frequent severe hypoglycemia *(53)*. However, patients eligible for CSII should be motivated by proper education from their health care providers, to perform frequent self-monitoring of blood glucose (SMBG) in order to engage in taking responsibility for self-management. In patients on CSII there is an increased risk of ketoacidosis due to the absence of a subcutaneous insulin reservoir, especially in case of potential technical problems with the pump or its supplies. Currently pumps are becoming available that are able to continuously measure subcutaneous glucose levels and that notify patients by an alarm in case of high or low glucose values. However, closed-loop systems are not available yet.

Devices

Patients receive instructions for SMBG using a small portable meter. Insulin administration is then adjusted using algorithms based on fasting, preprandial, postprandial, and evening glucose concentrations to reach target blood glucose values (see Table 3). Blood glucose measurement devices are reasonably accurate and precise in the euglycemic range, but less exact in the hypoglycemic range. In patients with frequent hypoglycemia or extremely variable blood glucose values use of a continuous glucose monitoring system (CGMS) in combination with a diary may uncover underlying problems and give patients insight into their behavioral actions and reactions as well as the way their body responds.

Insulin injection systems are available in a variety of disposable or reusable devices. For patients with impaired vision, magnifying or sensible-audible options are available, which enable patients to keep track of their adjusted insulin doses and ultimately may help them to preserve their independence in daily life. Patient's preferences should be the predominant determinants for the injection system used and the type of insulin within its class that is prescribed.

In-Hospital Blood Glucose Monitoring

Intercurrent morbidity, such as infections or trauma, frequently worsens hyperglycemia by means of a temporarily diminished sensitivity for insulin, while on the other hand hypoglycemia is at stake in the presence of abdominal discomfort and diminished food intake. Consequently, in order to prevent ketoacidosis due to the absolute deficiency of insulin, patients should obtain either a low dose of basal insulin (50% of their usual dosage) or continuous intravenous insulin infusion. In critical care, currently, blood glucose target levels < 6.1 mmol/l are widely implemented because of accumulating evidence for improved survival. Some studies show conflicting data of the hazards of hypoglycemia and related mortality (see also *Hypoglycemia in People with Diabetes*, Chapter 6) *(51)*. Glycemic targets in medical–surgical wards are not definite, but data suggest improved outcome at lower levels (see also *Treatment of Hyperglycemia*, Chapter 9). In general, glucose levels below 10 mmol/l are advised in hospitalized patients with avoidance of hypoglycemia.

LIFESTYLE

Patients are encouraged to maintain an active lifestyle and to exercise. They should receive advice on how to modify insulin dosage according to the amount and duration of exercise to avoid related hypoglycemia and potential late hypoglycemia at night. Vigorous exercise can deteriorate severe hypertension, retinopathy, and autonomic neuropathy and should be avoided without previous medical consultation *(51)*.

Diet

Patients with normal body weight do not have dietary restrictions with respect to carbohydrate intake, but even so they should monitor their carbohydrate intake and adjust the dose of short-acting insulin based on experience or a personalized calculation of carbohydrate/insulin ratio. Both lean and obese patients should be advised to restrict saturated fats and *trans*-fats. The use of alcohol is not prohibited, but should be moderate. Binge drinking of alcoholic beverages can induce late hypoglycemia *(51)*. Smoking should be discouraged at all times, and patients should be offered both mental and pharmacological support to quit.

Management of Risk Factors for Cardiovascular Disease

According to current standards, blood pressure is monitored routinely at every visit *(51)*. Measurement of fasting lipids should be obtained annually. If the recommended LDL target value < 2.6 mmol/l is not met after 6 months with lifestyle modifications consisting of diet and exercise, pharmacological therapy with statins is indicated. If statins are not tolerated, a 40% reduction from baseline is alternatively considered a reasonable goal *(51)*. Combination therapy to reach treatment targets may be prescribed but their effect is not (yet) confirmed in trials with hard endpoints. Aspirin therapy is indicated in patients with cardiovascular disease and may also be considered in case of increased cardiovascular risk, such as in diabetic nephropathy *(51)*.

β-Cell Transplantation

For years, combined renal and pancreatic transplantation has been performed in type 1 diabetic patients with end-stage renal failure or dialysis. Those patients received a renal graft and a pancreas anastomosis on the bladder for secretion of exocrine pancreas hormones and digestive fluids *(59)*. After transplantation, patients initially become independent of insulin. Transplantation of pancreas tissue only, without renal transplantation, is not being performed because of an alleged disadvantageous balance between profits of insulin independence and disproportional low graft survival with recurrent insulin dependence and because of adverse effects of immunosuppression such as hypertension, dyslipidemia, neurotoxicity and nephrotoxicity, peripheral edema, and mouth ulcers. During the last decade, β-cell or islet transplantation is gaining terrain by improvement of the technical procedures involved in the isolation of islets without exocrine pancreatic tissue by the injection and infusion of islets in the portal vein area.

With islet transplantation, the graft survival for complete independence of insulin has improved from 20% graft survival after 1 year to 20% insulin independence after 3 years *(59, 60)*. However, if insulin substitution is needed again after β-cell transplantation, good metabolic control is much easier to reach with far less hypoglycemia and with restoration of hypoglycemia awareness. This strategy is severely limited by the requirement of about five donors in order to harvest enough islets for one recipient.

Recent research also shows possibilities to preserve β-cell function: Short-term treatment with CD3 antibody was shown to preserve residual β-cell function for at least 18 months in patients with recent-onset T1D *(61)*.

LIVING WITH DIABETES

Being diagnosed with T1D has lifetime consequences for daily life for the patient himself (who is at that time often still a child) and for his or her family, friends, and other acquaintances, e.g., at school, work, and during sports. Such widely accepted social activities as having a meal in a restaurant, having a drink or two in a café, and even hurrying to catch a train have a different impact on people with diabetes than on those who are not dependent on exogenous insulin. In addition, diabetes also influences the perspective on diverse matters as career choices, starting a family, and getting a mortgage. Having diabetes raises issues concerning one's driver's license, job applications, and absence from work or school due to visiting the doctor and other health care workers or related to intercurrent sequelae such as (nightly) hypoglycemic spells. Insurances (medical, disability, life insurance) generally have strict policies resulting in more difficult and sometimes denied admittance and charge higher rates even for applicants with well-controlled diabetes without complications.

The above may clearly result in stress, grief, frustration, and disappointment, as may be the case in many other chronic conditions. In T1D this is further complicated by the fact that managing the disease on a day-to-day basis is based on self-care consisting of regular insulin injections and an extensive set of do's and do not's regarding lifestyle. Psychological distress in its turn may have negative effects on one's ability to adhere to self-care and may thus further worsen quality of life, in terms of mental health with respect to short- and long-term complications. More specifically, anxiety related to hypoglycemia may result in a vicious circle ensuing in self-treatment strategies with avoidance of low blood glucose levels and poor glycemic control.

Appropriate education and support with respect for the autonomy of persons with diabetes is therefore extremely important. Paternalism and moralism should be avoided, and health care workers caring for patients with diabetes and their families need to be trained in counseling techniques.

Psychological interventions including psychoanalytically informed therapies, cognitive behavior therapy, and family systems therapy are widely used attempting to improve both psychological well-being and glycemic control. A meta-analysis of the results of psychological interventions showed a small but significant absolute reduction in glycated hemoglobin levels in children (including adolescents) of nearly 0.5% and an improvement with respect to psychological distress *(62)*. Unfortunately, neither of these was the case in adults.

Education of people with diabetes is a comprehensive task and involves teamwork by a team that comprises at least a nurse educator, a dietician, and a physician. It is, however, essential that individuals with diabetes assume an active role in their care themselves, since appropriate self-care behavior is the cornerstone of the treatment of diabetes.

REFERENCES

1. American Diabetes Association. Diagnosis and classification of diabetes mellitus. Diabetes Care 2008; 31(Suppl 1):S55–S60.
2. Karvonen M, Viik-Kajander M, Moltchanova E, Libman I, LaPorte R, Tuomilehto J. Incidence of childhood type 1 diabetes worldwide. Diabetes Mondiale (DiaMond) Project Group. Diabetes Care 2000; 23(10):1516–1526.
3. Neu A, Willasch A, Ehehalt S, Hub R, Ranke MB. Ketoacidosis at onset of type 1 diabetes mellitus in children–frequency and clinical presentation. Pediatr Diabetes 2003; 4(2): 77–81.
4. Ostman J, Lonnberg G, Arnqvist HJ, et al. Gender differences and temporal variation in the incidence of type 1 diabetes: results of 8012 cases in the nationwide Diabetes Incidence Study in Sweden 1983–2002. J Intern Med 2008; 263(4):386–394.
5. Bruno G, Merletti F, Biggeri, A, et al. Increasing trend of type 1 diabetes in children and young adults in the province of Turin (Italy). Analysis of age, period and birth cohort effects from 1984 to 1996. Diabetologia 2001; 44(1):22–25.
6. Eisenbarth GS. Update in type 1 diabetes. J Clin Endocrinol Metab 2007; 92(7):2403–2407.
7. Stenstrom G, Gottsater A, Bakhtadze E, Berger B, Sundkvist G. Latent autoimmune diabetes in adults: definition, prevalence, beta-cell function, and treatment. Diabetes 2005; 54(Suppl 2):S68–S72.
8. Cardwell CR, Carson DJ, Patterson CC. No association between routinely recorded infections in early life and subsequent risk of childhood-onset Type 1 diabetes: a matched case-control study using the UK General Practice Research Database. Diabet Med 2008; 25(3):261–267.
9. Dittmar M, Kahaly GJ. Polyglandular autoimmune syndromes: immunogenetics and long-term follow-up. J Clin Endocrinol Metab 2003; 88(7):2983–2992.
10. Kruszynska YT. Normal metabolism: the physiology of fuel homeostasis. In: Pickup JC, Williams G, eds. Textbook of Diabetes. Oxford: Blackwell Science Ltd, 2006.
11. Saltiel AR, Kahn CR. Insulin signalling and the regulation of glucose and lipid metabolism. Nature 2001; 414(6865):799–806.
12. Shepherd PR, Kahn BB. Glucose transporters and insulin action–implications for insulin resistance and diabetes mellitus. N Engl J Med 1999; 341(4):248–257.
13. Gibson TB, Lawrence MC, Gibson CJ, et al. Inhibition of glucose-stimulated activation of extracellular signal-regulated protein kinases 1 and 2 by epinephrine in pancreatic beta-cells. Diabetes 2006; 55(4):1066–1073.
14. Cryer PE. Mechanisms of hypoglycemia-associated autonomic failure and its component syndromes in diabetes. Diabetes 2005; 54(12):3592–3601.
15. Drucker DJ, Nauck MA. The incretin system: glucagon-like peptide-1 receptor agonists and dipeptidyl peptidase-4 inhibitors in type 2 diabetes. Lancet 2006; 368(9548):1696–1705.

16. Hyperglycemic crises in diabetes. Diabetes Care 2004; 27(Suppl 1):S94.
17. ter Braak EW, Appelman AM, van de LM, Stolk RP, van Haeften TW, Erkelens DW. Clinical characteristics of type 1 diabetic patients with and without severe hypoglycemia. Diabetes Care 2000; 23(10):1467–1471.
18. Defining and reporting hypoglycemia in diabetes: a report from the American Diabetes Association Workgroup on Hypoglycemia. Diabetes Care 2005; 28(5):1245–1249.
19. Robinson RT, Harris ND, Ireland RH, Lee S, Newman C, Heller SR. Mechanisms of abnormal cardiac repolarization during insulin-induced hypoglycemia. Diabetes 2003; 52(6): 1469–1474.
20. Murphy NP, Ford-Adams ME, Ong KK, et al. Prolonged cardiac repolarisation during spontaneous nocturnal hypoglycaemia in children and adolescents with type 1 diabetes. Diabetologia 2004; 47(11):1940–1947.
21. The Diabetes Control and Complications Trial Research Group. The Effect of Intensive Treatment of Diabetes on the Development and Progression of Long-Term Complications in Insulin-Dependent Diabetes Mellitus. N Engl J Med 1993; 329(14):977–986.
22. Intensive Diabetes Treatment and Cardiovascular Disease in Patients with Type 1 Diabetes. N Engl J Med 2005; 353(25):2643–2653.
23. Brownlee M. The pathobiology of diabetic complications: A unifying mechanism. Diabetes 2005; 54(6):1615–1625.
24. Lecaire T, Palta M, Zhang H, Allen C, Klein R, D'Alessio D. Lower-than-expected prevalence and severity of retinopathy in an incident cohort followed during the first 4–14 years of type 1 diabetes: the Wisconsin Diabetes Registry Study. Am J Epidemiol 2006; 164(2): 143–150.
25. The Diabetes Control and Complications Trial Research Group. The effect of intensive treatment of diabetes on the development and progression of long-term complications in insulin-dependent diabetes mellitus. N Engl J Med 1993; 329(14):977–986.
26. Wilkinson CP, Ferris FL, Klein RE, et al. Proposed international clinical diabetic retinopathy and diabetic macular edema disease severity scales. Ophthalmology 2003; 110(9):1677–1682.
27. American Diabetes Association. Standards of Medical Care in Diabetes –2008. Diabetes Care 2008; 31(Suppl 1):S12–S54.
28. Boulton AJM, Vinik AI, Arezzo JC, et al. Diabetic Neuropathies: A statement by the American Diabetes Association. Diabetes Care 2005; 28(4):956–962.
29. Molitch ME, DeFronzo RA, Franz MJ, et al. Nephropathy in diabetes. Diabetes Care 2004; 27(Suppl 1):S79–S83.
30. Freedman BI, Bostrom M, Daeihagh P, Bowden DW. Genetic Factors in Diabetic Nephropathy. Clin J Am Soc Nephrol 2007; 2(6):1306–1316.
31. The Diabetes Control and Complications Trial Research Group. The effect of intensive treatment of diabetes on the development and progression of long-term complications in insulin-dependent diabetes mellitus. N Engl J Med 1993; 329(14):977–986.
32. Freedman BI, Bostrom M, Daeihagh P, Bowden DW. Genetic Factors in Diabetic Nephropathy. Clin J Am Soc Nephrol 2007; 2(6):1306–1316.
33. American Diabetes Association. Standards of Medical Care in Diabetes – 2008. Diabetes Care 2008; 31(Suppl 1):S12–S54.
34. Krolewski AS, Kosinski EJ, Warram JH, et al. Magnitude and determinants of coronary artery disease in juvenile-onset, insulin-dependent diabetes mellitus. Am J Cardiol 1987; 59(8): 750–755.
35. Krolewski AS, Kosinski EJ, Warram JH, et al. Magnitude and determinants of coronary artery disease in juvenile-onset, insulin-dependent diabetes mellitus. Am J Cardiol 1987; 59(8): 750–755.
36. The Diabetes Control and Complications Trial Research Group. The effect of intensive treatment of diabetes on the development and progression of long-term complications in insulin-dependent diabetes mellitus. N Engl J Med 1993; 329(14):977–986.
37. American Diabetes Association. Standards of Medical Care in Diabetes – 2008. Diabetes Care 2008; 31(Suppl 1):S12–S54.

38. Hordon LD. Musculoskeletal complications in diabetes mellitus. UpToDate version 16.2. 15-9-2006. http://www.uptodate.com/online/content/topic.do?topicKey=muscle/10289& selectedTitle=2~150&source=search_result. Accessed April 6, 2009.

39. Wooldridge WE. Four related fibrosing diseases. When you find one, look for another. Postgrad Med 1988; 84(2):269–271, 274.

40. Kim RP, Edelman SV, Kim DD. Musculoskeletal complications of diabetes mellitus. Clinical Diabetes 2001; 19: 132–135.

41. Browne DL, McCrae FC, Shaw KM. Musculoskeletal disease in diabetes. Pract Diab Int 2001; 18:62–64.

42. Jeffcoate WJ, Harding KG. Diabetic foot ulcers. Lancet 2003; 361(9368):1545–1551.

43. American Diabetes Association. Standards of Medical Care in Diabetes – 2008. Diabetes Care 2008; 31(Suppl 1):S12–S54.

44. American Diabetes Association. Standards of Medical Care in Diabetes – 2008. Diabetes Care 2008; 31(Suppl 1):S12–S54.

45. van Houtum WH. Barriers to the delivery of diabetic foot care. The Lancet 2005; 366(9498):1678–1679.

46. American Diabetes Association. Standards of Medical Care in Diabetes – 2008. Diabetes Care 2008; 31(Suppl 1):S12–S54.

47. Consensus Development Conference on Diabetic Foot Wound Care: 7-8 April 1999, Boston, Massachusetts. American Diabetes Association. Diabetes Care 1999; 22(8): 1354–1360.

48. American Diabetes Association. Standards of Medical Care in Diabetes – 2008. Diabetes Care 2008; 31(Suppl 1):S12–S54.

49. Consensus Development Conference on Diabetic Foot Wound Care: 7-8 April 1999, Boston, Massachusetts. American Diabetes Association. Diabetes Care 1999; 22(8): 1354–1360.

50. Test of glycemia in diabetes. American Diabetes Association. Diabetes Care 2004; 27(Suppl 1):S91–S93.

51. American Diabetes Association. Standards of medical care in diabetes – 2008. Diabetes Care 2008; 31(Suppl):S12–S54.

52. Robinson RT, Harris ND, Ireland RH, Macdonald IA, Heller SR. Changes in cardiac repolarization during clinical episodes of nocturnal hypoglycaemia in adults with Type 1 diabetes. Diabetologia 2004; 47(2):312–315.

53. Pickup JC, Sutton AJ. Severe hypoglycaemia and glycaemic control in Type 1 diabetes: meta-analysis of multiple daily insulin injections compared with continuous subcutaneous insulin infusion. Diabet Med 2008; 25(7):765–774.

54. Insulin administration. American Diabetes Association. Diabetes Care 2004; 27(Suppl 1):S106–S109.

55. Hirsch IB. Insulin analogues. N Engl J Med 2005; 352(2):174–183.

56. Rosenstock J, Davies M, Home PD, Larsen J, Koenen C, Schernthaner G. A randomised, 52-week, treat-to-target trial comparing insulin detemir with insulin glargine when administered as add-on to glucose-lowering drugs in insulin-naive people with type 2 diabetes. Diabetologia 2008; 51(3):408–416.

57. Khan AS, McLoughney CR, Ahmed AB. The effect of metformin on blood glucose control in overweight patients with Type 1 diabetes. Diabet Med 2006; 23(10):1079–1084.

58. Lund SS, Tarnow L, Astrup Asb, et al. Effect of adjunct metformin treatment in patients with type-1 diabetes and persistent inadequate glycaemic control. A randomized study. PLoS ONE 2008; 3(10):e3363.

59. Bertuzzi F, Ricordi C. Beta-cell replacement in immunosuppressed recipients: old and new clinical indications. Acta Diabetol 2007; 44(4):171–176.

60. Merani S, Shapiro AM. Current status of pancreatic islet transplantation. Clin Sci (Lond) 2006; 110(6):611–625.

61. Keymeulen B, Vandemeulebroucke E, Ziegler AG, et al. Insulin needs after CD3-antibody therapy in new-onset type 1 diabetes. N Engl J Med 2005; 352(25):2598–2608.

62. Winkley K, Ismail K, Landau S, Eisler I. Psychological interventions to improve glycaemic control in patients with type 1 diabetes: systematic review and meta-analysis of randomised controlled trials. BMJ 2006; 333(7558):65.
63. Service FJ, Rizza RA, Zimmerman BR, Dyck PJ, O'Brien PC, Melton LJ 2rd. The classification of diabetes by clinical and C-peptide criteria. A prospective population-based study. Diabetes Care 1997; 20(2):198–201.

2

Type 2 Diabetes

Hermes J. Florez, Alex A. Sanchez, and Jennifer B. Marks

CONTENTS

ABSTRACT

Type 2 diabetes (T2D) is the most common form of diabetes, a metabolic disorder characterized by hyperglycemia resulting from defects in insulin action, insulin secretion, or both. Early diagnosis of T2D and the high-risk category of pre-diabetes may help reduce the associated public health and clinical burden. Available diagnostic strategies include fasting plasma glucose, oral glucose tolerance test, and casual plasma glucose in the presence of symptoms of hyperglycemia. Potential use of hemoglobin A1c as part of the strategy for screening and diagnosis has been recently proposed. Those with risk factors for T2D should be targeted including patients with overweight/obesity, those with family history of T2D, those aged 45 years and older, race/ethnic minorities (such as Native Americans, African Americans, Latinos, and Asian Americans), women with history of gestational diabetes, and those with metabolic syndrome abnormalities (high blood pressure, low HDL cholesterol, and high triglycerides). Lifestyle modification (i.e., weight loss through diet and increased physical activity) has proven effective in reducing incident T2D in high-risk groups. Prevention trials using pharmacological therapy (metformin, α-glucosidase

From: *Contemporary Diabetes: Diabetes and the Brain*
Edited by: G. J. Biessels, J. A. Luchsinger (eds.), DOI 10.1007/978-1-60327-850-8_2
© Humana Press, a part of Springer Science+Business Media, LLC 2009

inhibitors, or thiazolidinediones) have also reported a significant lowering of the incidence of T2D. As a chronic condition, T2D requires continuous care to prevent damage to various organs, including the eyes, kidney, nervous system, and cardiovascular system. Appropriate glycemic control, blood pressure and lipid management, nutrition and physical activity, taking into account functional status and comorbidities, are needed to prevent microvascular and macrovascular complications. A variety of oral antihyperglycemic agents, which target different mechanisms in the pathogenesis of T2D, are as follows: insulin sensitizers, insulin secretagogues, α-glucosidase inhibitors, and the new dipeptidyl peptidase (DPP)-IV inhibitors. Injectable agents for the treatment of insulin-deficient T2D include traditional insulin preparations, newer insulin analogs, amylin, and incretin mimetics. Additional aspects of T2D management in the older adult include the assessment of geriatric syndromes and psychosocial screening. Efforts to improve T2D care following recommended guidelines are still very much needed.

Key words: Type 2 Diabetes; Diagnosis; Epidemiology; Prevention; Management; Insulin resistance; Insulin secretion.

INTRODUCTION

Diabetes mellitus is a group of metabolic disorders characterized by hyperglycemia, which can result from defects in insulin secretion, insulin action, or both. Diabetes is a chronic illness that requires continuing medical care and patient self-management education to prevent acute complications and to reduce long-term complications.

DIAGNOSIS

The American Diabetes Association (ADA) diagnostic criteria for diabetes and the two high-risk categories of pre-diabetes, impaired fasting glucose (IFG) and impaired glucose tolerance (IGT), updated in 2003 are defined in Table 1 (1). There are three ways to diagnose diabetes. Because of simplicity of use, acceptability to patients, and low cost, the fasting plasma glucose (PG) is the preferred diagnostic test. In the presence of symptoms of diabetes (polyuria, polydipsia, weight loss, etc.), a casual plasma glucose of greater or equal than 200 mg/dl is diagnostic. The 75-g oral glucose tolerance test (OGTT) is more sensitive and modestly more specific than fasting PG, but it is less reproducible and less frequently performed in clinical settings. In the absence of unequivocal hyperglycemia, any test used to diagnose diabetes must be confirmed on a subsequent day by a PG measured either in the fasting state or 2 h after an oral glucose load.

Table 1
The diagnostic criteria for diabetes and the classification of impaired fasting
glucose (IFG) and impaired glucose tolerance (IGT)

	FPG (mg/dl)	*2-HPG (mg/dl)*	*Sx of diabetes + CPG*
Normal	<100	<140	–
IFG	≥100 and <126	–	–
IGT	–	≥140 and < 200	–
Diabetes	≥126	≥200	+ and CPG≥200 mg/dl

FPG, fasting plasma glucose (FPG); 2-HPG, plasma glucose 2 h after a challenge with 75 g glucose; CPG, casual plasma glucose; Sx (symptoms) of diabetes: polydipsia, polyuria, and unexplained weight loss.
Adapted from American Diabetes Association *(1)*.

The 2006 joint report from the World Health Organization (WHO) and International Diabetes Federation (IDF) also provides an update on guidelines for diagnosis of diabetes *(2)*. Their diagnostic criteria (i.e., fasting PG ≥ 7.0 mmol/l [126 mg/dl] or 2-h PG ≥ 11.1 mmol/l [200 mg/dl])remained unchanged since these criteria distinguish a group with significantly increased premature mortality and higher risk of microvascular and cardiovascular complications.

Recently, a committee of experts in the area of diagnosis, monitoring, and management of diabetes provided a review of the available evidence and made recommendations regarding the screening and diagnosis of diabetes using hemoglobin A1c (HbA1c) *(3)*. The main factors in support of using HbA1c as a screening and diagnostic test included (a) HbA1c does not require patients to be fasting; (b) HbA1c reflects longer-term glycemia than does PG; (c) HbA1c laboratory methods are now well standardized and reliable (more information in the National Glycohemoglobin Standardization Program web site at www.ngsp.org); (d) errors caused by non-glycemic factors affecting HbA1c, such as hemoglobinopathies, are infrequent and can be minimized by confirming the diagnosis of diabetes with a PG-specific test. Several recommendations were made: (1) screening standards should be established that prompt further testing and closer follow-up, including fasting PG ≥100 mg/dl, random PG ≥130 mg/dl, or HbA1c > 6.0% (2) HbA1c ≥ 6.5–6.9%, confirmed by a PG-specific test (fasting PG or OGTT), should establish the diagnosis of diabetes; (3) HbA1c ≥ 7%, confirmed by another HbA1c or a PG-specific test (FPG or OGTT) should establish the diagnosis of diabetes.

Hyperglycemia insufficient to meet the diagnostic criteria for diabetes is categorized as either IFG or IGT, depending on whether it is identified by a fasting PG or by an OGTT. According to the ADA, IFG is diagnosed when the fasting PG level is ≥ 100 mg/dl (≥ 110 mg/dl based on WHO/IDF criteria) but <126 mg/dl. IGT exists when the PG level 2 h after a 75-g oral glucose load is ≥ 140 mg/dl but <200 mg/dl. These are considered to be pre-diabetic states. Furthermore, an international committee (IDF/ADA/EASD) reported that a HbA1c $\geq 6\%$ but $< 6.5\%$ helps identifying people at very high-risk of developing diabetes (http://care.diabetesjournals.org/content/32/7/1327)

EPIDEMIOLOGY

Diabetes and its complications constitute a significant public health problem worldwide and are an important cause of morbidity and mortality. In fact, diabetes has reached epidemic proportions throughout the world, and the prevalence is expected to continue to rise. The International Diabetes Federation estimates that more than 245 million people around the world have diabetes (4). This total is expected to rise to 380 million within 20 years. Each year a further 7 million people develop diabetes. Diabetes, mostly type 2 diabetes (T2D), now affects 5.9% of the world's adult population with almost 80% of the total in developing countries. The regions with the highest rates are the Eastern Mediterranean and Middle East, where 9.2% of the adult population is affected, and North America (8.4%). The highest numbers, however, are found in the Western Pacific, where some 67 million people have diabetes, followed by Europe with 53 million.

According to new 2007 prevalence data estimates recently released by the Centers for Disease Control and Prevention (CDC), diabetes now affects nearly 24 million people in the United States (USA), an increase of more than 3 million in approximately 2 years (5). Among adults, diabetes increased in both men and women and in all age groups, but still disproportionately affects the elderly. Almost 25% of the population aged 60 years and older had diabetes in 2007. Another 57 million people are estimated to have pre-diabetes. It has been projected that one in three Americans born in 2000 will develop diabetes, with the highest estimated lifetime risk among Latinos (males, 45.4% and females, 52.5%) (6).

A rise in obesity rates is to blame for much of the increase in T2D (7). Nearly two-thirds of American adults are overweight or obese (8). The prevalence of abdominal obesity (i.e., large waist circumference) among US adults has increased continuously during the past 15 years. Over one-half of US adults have abdominal obesity (9). This is a major concern given the strong association between measures reflecting abdominal obesity and the development of T2D (10).

The risk of developing diabetes rises not only with overweight/obesity (body mass index, BMI≥ 25 kg/m^2) and lack of physical activity, but with increasing age (≥45 years) and family history *(1)*. Specific population sub-groups have a higher prevalence of diabetes than the population as a whole. Recent data showed that compared to white non-Hispanics (6.6%) diabetes remains higher in race/ethnic minority groups: Native Americans and Alaska Natives (16.5%), African Americans (11.8%), Latinos (10.4%), which includes rates for Puerto Ricans (12.6%), Mexican Americans (11.9%), and Cubans (8.2%), and Asian Americans (7.5%) *(11)*. Women with a history of prior gestational diabetes or polycystic ovarian syndrome are at increased risk. Also, the predictive value of traditional and non-traditional risk factors has been evaluated in cohort studies *(12, 13)*. In addition to age, family history of diabetes, obesity and pre-diabetes, and those with other metabolic syndrome components (high blood pressure, low HDL cholesterol, and high triglycerides) are at higher risk. The greater the number of these metabolic risk factors in a given person, the higher the chance of that individual developing diabetes.

PATHOGENESIS

There are two underlying mechanism that lead to the onset of clinical T2D: inadequate insulin action in target tissues (insulin resistance) and inadequate secretion from pancreatic β-cells (Fig. 1) *(14)*. Insulin resistance arises prior to the onset of clinical disease, but predicts the development of diabetes *(15–17)*. Environmental factors, particularly obesity and a sedentary lifestyle, are important contributors to the development of diabetes, largely because of their effects on insulin sensitivity *(18–20)*. When target tissues become insulin resistant, glucose uptake is decreased, hepatic glucose production increases, and lipolysis is enhanced. In muscle, the increased free fatty acid (FFA) availability accelerates fat oxidation, resulting in decreased insulin-mediated glucose uptake and disposal. In the liver, elevated FFAs promote gluconeogenesis and increase hepatic glucose output.

When inadequate insulin secretion from pancreatic β-cell dysfunction is also present, hyperglycemia develops, heralding the onset of T2D *(14–17)*. In the natural history of progression to diabetes, β-cells initially increase insulin secretion in response to insulin resistance and, for a period of time, are able to effectively maintain glucose levels below the diabetic range. However, when β-cell function begins to decline, insulin production is inadequate to overcome the insulin resistance, and blood glucose levels rise. Insulin resistance, once established, remains relatively stable over time. Therefore, progression of T2D is a result of worsening β-cell function with pre-existing insulin resistance.

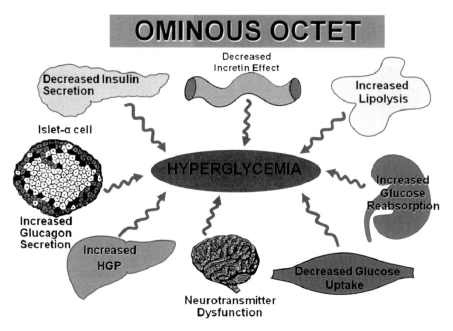

Fig. 1. Defects in the pancreas and in target tissues for insulin action in type 2 diabetes. In the non-diabetic individual, insulin suppresses hepatic glucose output, stimulates glucose uptake and utilization in muscle and adipose tissue, and suppresses lipolysis in adipose tissue. When these tissues become resistant to the actions of insulin, hepatic glucose production increases, glucose uptake is decreased, and lipolysis is enhanced. Increased free fatty acids (FFAs) from lipolysis stimulate cellular uptake of FFAs and lipid oxidation. In muscle, the increased FFA availability accelerates fat oxidation, resulting in decreased insulin-mediated glucose uptake and utilization. In the liver, elevated FFAs stimulate gluconeogenesis and increase hepatic glucose output. When β-cell dysfunction is present, insulin resistance in the target tissues leads to hyperglycemia and to the development of type 2 diabetes. (From DeFronzo, R. From the triumvirate to the ominous octet: a new paradigm for the treatment of type 2 diabetes mellitus. Copyright © 2009 American Diabetes Association from Diabetes, 2009; 58:773–795. Reprinted with permission from the American Diabetes Association.)

Despite major advances in understanding the pathophysiology of T2D, unraveling the complex link between genetic risk and environmental factors in this burgeoning epidemic has proven difficult *(21)*. Linkage approaches have clarified the etiology of monogenic diabetic syndromes and congenital lipodystrophies, and candidate gene association studies have identified a number of common variants implicated in T2D. Several genetic loci have now been reproducibly associated with T2D in genome-wide scans. For example, common variants in the gene that encodes the transcription factor 7-like 2 (TCF7L2), involved in the control of insulin secretion, have been strongly associated with T2D *(22)*. At the individual level, carrying the TCF7L2-risk allele increases T2D risk 50%. However, at the population level, the attributable risk is lower than 25% and varies with the allele frequency. The presence of the TCF7L2 rs7903146-risk allele increases TCF7L2 gene expression in β-cells, possibly impairing glucagon-like peptide-1-induced insulin secretion and/or the production of new mature β-cells. It is expected that the detection of other such genes in genome-wide association scans will help elucidate the genetic architecture and pathophysiology of T2D.

PREVENTION OR DELAY OF TYPE 2 DIABETES

Prevention efforts may start with promotion of healthy lifestyle and appropriate screening in those at higher risk: individuals $\geq$ 45 years of age and those with a BMI $\geq$ 25 kg/m^2 *(22)*. Screening should also be considered for people who are <45 years of age and are overweight if they have another risk factor for diabetes: physical inactivity, first-degree relative with diabetes, members of high-risk ethnic populations (e.g., African American, Latino, Native American, Asian American, Asian American, and Pacific Islander), women who delivered a baby weighing > 9 lb or were diagnosed with gestational diabetes, hypertension, low HDL cholesterol, high triglycerides, women with polycystic ovarian syndrome, IGT, or IFG on previous testing, other clinical conditions associated with insulin resistance (e.g., severe obesity and acanthosis nigricans), and history of cardiovascular disease (CVD). Repeat testing may be carried out at 3-year intervals.

Lifestyle modification (i.e., weight loss through diet and increased physical activity) has proven effective in reducing incident T2D in high-risk groups. The Da Qing Study (China) randomly allocated 33 clinics (557 persons with IGT) to 1 of 4 study conditions: control, diet, exercise, or diet plus exercise *(23)*. Compared with the control group, the incidence of diabetes was reduced in the three intervention groups by 31, 46, and 42%, respectively, and with a modest weight loss in study participants. The Finnish Diabetes Prevention Study evaluated 522 obese persons with IGT randomly allocated on an individual basis to a control group or a lifestyle intervention group that emphasized physical activity, weight loss, limited total dietary intake and intake of saturated fat, and increased intake of dietary fiber *(24)*. During the trial, the incidence of diabetes was reduced by 58% in the lifestyle group compared with the control group. The US Diabetes Prevention Program is the largest trial of primary prevention of diabetes to date and was conducted at 27 clinical centers with 3,234 overweight and obese participants with IGT randomly allocated to 1 of 3 study conditions: control, use of metformin, or intensive lifestyle intervention *(25)*. The goal of lifestyle intervention was to achieve and maintain 7% or greater weight loss through a low-calorie, low-fat diet and 150 or more minutes of moderate physical activity weekly. Nearly half the participants were African American, Hispanic American, Asian American, or Native American. Over 3 years, the incidence of diabetes was reduced by 31% in the metformin group and by 58% in the lifestyle group; the latter value is identical to that observed in the Finnish Study. To prevent 1 case of diabetes, only 7 patients needed to be treated with lifestyle change, compared with 14 patients treated with metformin. The magnitude of risk reduction in the lifestyle intervention group was similar across all ethnic groups, and participants in all age and BMI subgroups achieved a clinically significant reduction in risk. In contrast, metformin was relatively ineffective in older and less obese participants.

Type 2 diabetes prevention trials using other forms of pharmacological therapy have also reported a significant lowering of the incidence of diabetes. The α-glucosidase inhibitor acarbose reduced the risk by 32% in the STOP-NIDDM trial *(26)*, and the thiazolidinedione troglitazone reduced the risk by 56% in the TRIPOD Study *(27)*.

More recently, the investigators from the DREAM trial, a study in 5,269 adults with IGT, IFG, or both and no previous CVD were recruited from 191 sites in 21 countries and randomly assigned in a 2-by-2 factorial design to receive rosiglitazone 8 mg/day and/or ramipril 15 mg/day. There was no statistical evidence of an interaction between the ramipril and the rosiglitazone arms. After a mean follow-up of 3 years, the use of ramipril did not reduce the incidence of diabetes *(28)*, while the treatment with rosiglitazone reduced by almost 60% the incidence of T2D and increased the likelihood (+70%) of regression to normoglycemia *(29)*.

Whether diabetes prevention strategies also ultimately prevent the development of diabetic vascular complications is unknown, but cardiovascular risk factors are favorably affected *(30)*. Preventive strategies that can be implemented in routine clinical settings have been developed and evaluated. Widespread application has, however, been limited by local financial considerations, even though cost-effectiveness might be achieved at the population level.

MANAGEMENT

Prevention of Complications

Chronic poor glycemic control is associated with the development of diabetic vascular complications, including microvascular (retinopathy, neuropathy, and nephropathy) and macrovascular (coronary, cerebrovascular and peripheral vascular disease). CVD is the cause of 65% of deaths in patients with T2D *(31)*.Epidemiologic studies have shown that the risk of a myocardial infarction (MI) or CVD death in a diabetic individual with no prior history of CVD is comparable to that of an individual who has had a previous MI *(32, 33)*.

Microvascular complications can be delayed or prevented by maintaining excellent chronic glycemic control, as has been demonstrated in a number of interventional trials, including the Diabetes Control and Complications Trial (DCCT), the United Kingdom Prospective Diabetes Study (UKPDS), the Kumamoto Study, and the Stockholm Diabetes Intervention Study *(34–39)*. Further, even in acute illness, several studies have shown that intensive insulin therapy and improved glycemic control are associated with better outcomes *(40, 41)*.

Intensive glycemic control also results in reduced macrovascular compli-cations, i.e., CVD, as demonstrated in a number of epidemiological studies *(42–44)*. From the Diabetes Control and Complications Trial/Epidemiology of Diabetes Interventions and Complications (DCCT/EDIC) Study of type 1 diabetes, it is clear that intensive glycemic control prior to the onset of vascular disease has long-term beneficial effects on the risk of CVD in this population *(45)*. Patients with newly diagnosed T2D, aged 25–65 years at baseline, whose HbA1c was reduced from 7.9 to 7% in the UKPDS, did not exhibit a reduction in cardiovascular events, although a subgroup of patients treated with metformin showed a trend to a lower incidence of events *(46)*. However, 10-year follow-up data from this study showed persistence of microvascular benefits and long-term appearance of macrovascular benefits in the insulin and sulfonylurea groups despite the fact that the differences in HbA1c between the groups had disappeared *(47)*.

Three recent trials in older adults with T2D have assessed the effect of lowering blood glucose to near-normal levels on cardiovascular risk. First, patients in the Action to Control Cardiovascular Risk in Diabetes (ACCORD) trial ($n = 10,251$) had a mean age of 62.2 years at entry and 10 years of diabetes duration. Sixty-two percent were men, and 30% had prior macrovascular disease and a baseline median HbA1c level of 8.1% *(48)*. Study patients were assigned to receive intensive therapy (median HbA1c level achieved of 6.4%) or standard therapy (median HbA1c level achieved of 7.5%). After a median follow-up of 3.4 years, compared to the standard-therapy group, those in the intensive-therapy group had higher overall mor-tality (4% vs. 5%) and cardiovascular mortality (1.8% vs. 2.6%) and greater-number of hypoglycemic events (1% vs. 3.1%). Second, patients in the Action in Diabetes and Vascular Disease: Preterax and Diamicron Modi-fied Release Controlled Evaluation (ADVANCE) Study ($n = 11,140$) had a mean age of 66 years at entry and 8 years of diabetes duration. Fifty-seven percent were men and 32% had prior macrovascular disease and a baseline median HbA1c level of 7.2% *(49)*. Study patients were assigned to receive intensive therapy (median HbA1c level achieved of 6.4%) or standard therapy (median HbA1c level achieved of 7%). After a median follow-up of 5 years, compared to the standard-therapy group those in the intensive-therapy group achieved a reduction in the incidence of nephropathy (5.2% vs. 4.1%), although severe hypoglycemia was more common (1.5% vs. 2.7%). There were no differences in overall mortality (9.6% vs. 8.9%), cardiovascular mortality (5.2% vs. 4.5%), or major macrovascular events (10.6% vs. 10%). Finally, patients in the Veterans Affairs Diabetes Trial (VADT) ($n = 1,792$) had a mean age of 60.4 years at entry and 11.5 years of diabetes duration. Ninety-seven percent were men and 40% had prior macrovascular events and a baseline mean HbA1c level of 9.4% (50). They were assigned to receive intensive therapy (median HbA1c level achieved of 6.9%) or standard therapy (median HbA1c level achieved of 8.4%). After a median follow-up of 6 years, there was no significant difference in the rate of the composite primary endpoint (MI, congestive heart failure, invasive revascularization, inoperable coronary artery disease, amputation for ischemia, stroke, or cardiovascular death) between the intensive- and the standard-therapy groups (25.9% vs. 29.3%, $p = 0.12$). Fewer cardiovascular events than expected were observed in both groups, in part because of the aggressive management of blood pressure (reduction from 131/77 to 127/70 mmHg) and lipids (LDL-cholesterol and triglycerides fell from 106 and 157 mg/dl to 78 and 135 mg/dl, respectively, while HDL rose from 34 to 40 mg/dl) as well as lifestyle changes (40–57% exercised regularly, 60–68% adhered to diet, and cigarette smoking was reduced from 16% to 10%) and the increased use of antiplatelet/anticoagulants (from 76% at entry to 92% at the end of the study). Intensive therapy was associated with lower risk of the primary endpoint only in those with diabetes for less than 15 years and those who had low arterial calcium (AC) scores (AC < 100). Severe hypoglycemia requiring medical assistance was higher than expected and more frequent in the intensive than in the standard group (21.1% vs. 9.7%, $p < 0.01$). In fact, hypoglycemic events that led to impaired or loss of consciousness were independent predictors of major cardiovascular events and cardiovascular and total mortality.

Glycemic Goals

Based on results from clinical trials of glycemic control and the impact on diabetic microvascular complications, recommendations for targets of glycemic control have been put forth (1). Glycemic control is fundamental to the management of diabetes. The HbA1c is the most accepted indicator of chronic control, reflecting fasting and postprandial glucose concentrations. The goal of therapy is to achieve an HbA1c as close to normal

Table 2
Glycemic goals

HbA1c goal *for patients in general* <7%
HbA1c goal *for the frail elderly patient* <8%
Pre-prandial capillary plasma glucose* 90–130 mg/dl
Peak postprandial capillary plasma glucose* <180 mg/dl

*Capillary plasma glucose = fingerstick glucose.
Adapted from American Diabetes Association *(1)* and Brown et al. *(75)*.

as possible in the absence of hypoglycemia. Recommended glycemic goals for non-pregnant individuals are shown in Table 2. Less stringent treatment goals may be appropriate for patients with limited life expectancies and in individuals with co-morbid conditions *(51)*. Severe or frequent hypoglycemia is an indication for the modification of treatment regimens, including setting higher glycemic goals.

Nutrition and Physical Activity

Overweight and obesity are strongly linked to the development of T2D and can complicate its management. Moderate weight loss improves glycemic control and reduces CVD risk. Therefore, weight loss is an important therapeutic strategy in all overweight or obese individuals who have T2D. All patients with diabetes should be encouraged to maintain a healthy lifestyle by exercising and following an appropriate diet *(52)*. The primary approach for achieving weight loss is therapeutic lifestyle change, which includes a reduction in energy intake and an increase in physical activity.

Oral Antidiabetic Agents

A variety of antidiabetic pharmaceutical agents for the treatment of T2D are available, which target different mechanisms in the underlying pathogenesis of the disease *(53–56)* (Fig. 2). There are five categories of oral agents on the market, which can be used initially in most cases of T2D, until insulin deficiency becomes severe and insulin replacement is required. Sulfonylureas and the glitinides (repaglinide, nateglinide) are insulin secretagogues that stimulate release of insulin from the β-cells of the pancreas. Metformin, a biguanide, improves insulin sensitivity chiefly by reducing insulin resistance in the liver, thereby decreasing hepatic glucose production. The thiazolidinediones (rosiglitazone, pioglitazone) improve insulin sensitivity primarily in the muscle, thereby increasing peripheral uptake and utilization of glucose. The α-glucosidase inhibitors (acarbose) prevent the breakdown of carbohydrates to glucose in the gut, by

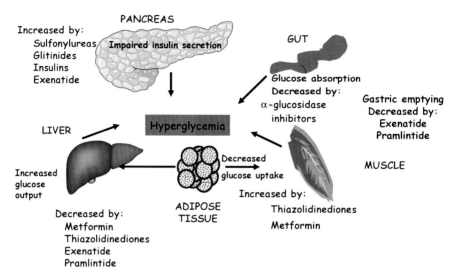

Fig. 2. Antidiabetic agents and their mechanisms of action. The variety of antidiabetic agents for the treatment of type 2 diabetes target different mechanisms in the underlying pathogenesis of the disease. Sulfonylureas and the glitinides (repaglinide, nateglinide) are insulin secretagogues that stimulate release of insulin from the pancreas. Metformin, a biguanide, improves insulin sensitivity chiefly by reducing insulin resistance in the liver, thereby decreasing hepatic glucose production. The thiazolidinediones (rosiglitazone, pioglitazone) improve insulin sensitivity primarily in the muscle, thereby increasing peripheral uptake and utilization of glucose. The α-glucosidase inhibitors (acarbose, precose) prevent the breakdown of carbohydrates to glucose in the gut, by inhibiting the enzymes that catalyze this process, thereby delaying carbohydrate absorption. Insulin and insulin analogs increase insulin levels in the presence of declining β-cell function and diminished endogenous insulin secretion. Exenatide and the synthetic amylin, pramlintide exploit novel mechanisms related to effects on glucagon secretion, gastric emptying, and satiety. (From DeFronzo *(53)*. Reprinted from Annals of Internal Medicine with permission from American College of Physicians.)

inhibiting the enzymes that catalyze this process, thereby delaying carbohydrate absorption. Sitagliptin, a dipeptidyl-peptidase (DPP)-IV inhibitor, is an agent that reduces blood glucose with less risk of hypoglycemia. Metformin is recommended as first choice for pharmacologic treatment and has good efficacy to lower HbA1c by approximately 1–1.5% as monotherapy *(57)*. However, most patients will eventually require treatment with combinations of oral medications with different mechanisms of action simultaneously in order to attain adequate glycemic control. Table 3 lists the available classes of oral antidiabetic medications, their mechanisms of action, and side effects.

Table 3
Available oral antidiabetic agents

Drug class	Mechanism of action	Major side effects
Sulfonylureas	Stimulate insulin	Weight gain
Meglitinides	secretion	Hypoglycemia
Metformin	Suppress hepatic glucose production (major)	GI side effects Lactic acidosis (rare)
	Improve insulin sensitivity in target tissues (minor)	
Thiazolidinediones	Improve insulin sensitivity in target tissues (major)	Weight gain Edema Congestive heart failure
	Suppress hepatic glucose production (minor)	
α-Glucosidase inhibitors	Delay carbohydrate absorption from the intestine	Flatulence or abdominal discomfort

Adapted and summarized from Florez et al. *(56)*.

Injectable Therapy

Injectable agents for treatment of insulin-deficient T2D include traditional insulin preparations, newer insulin analogs, amylin, and incretin mimetics (see Fig. 2). Insulin and the insulin analogs increase circulating insulin levels in the presence of declining β-cell function and diminished endogenous insulin secretion. Insulin and analogs, available in both long-acting and rapid-acting formulations, can be used in combination with oral agents in T2D or as insulin replacement therapy in long-standing, insulin-deficient T2D *(56)*. Therecent additions to the market, the incretin mimetic exenatide and the synthetic amylin, pramlintide, exploit novel mechanisms related to effects on glucagon secretion, gastric emptying, and satiety to improve glycemic control *(58, 59)*.

Other Strategies for Reduction of Comorbidities and Complications

In addition to hyperglycemia, individuals with T2D often have a constellation of other metabolic abnormalities which increase their CVD risk *(60–64)*. Risk determinants of CVD include the presence or absence of coronary heart disease (CHD), other clinical forms of atherosclerotic disease, and the major risk factors: high LDL cholesterol, cigarette smoking, hypertension, low HDL cholesterol, family history of premature CHD (defined as a relative with CHD younger than 65 years for women and 55 years for men), and age (men $\geq$ 45 years, women $\geq$ 55 years). It is important to point out that diabetes is considered to be a CHD equivalent, so the goal for LDL cholesterol is <100 mg/dl. Based on these risk determinants, the Expert Panel on Detection, Evaluation, and Treatment of High Blood Cholesterol in Adults (Adult Treatment Panel III) identifies three categories of risk that modify the goals and modalities of LDL-lowering therapy (65) (Tables 4 and 5). In very high-risk persons, an LDL-C goal of <70 mg/dl is a therapeutic option on the basis of available clinical trial evidence (66). The justification for the more aggressive LDL targets in patients with diabetes with CVD is based on three large statin-outcome trials: the Heart Protection Study (HPS), the Treating to New Targets (TNT) Study, and the Incremental Decrease in Endpoints Through Aggressive Lipid Lowering (IDEAL) Study, which also identified the diabetic subgroup as a cohort of patients with high residual risk even on statin therapy (67–69).

Table 4
ATP III classification of LDL, total, and HDL cholesterol (mg/dl).*

LDL cholesterol	
<100	Optimal
100–129	Near-optimal
130–159	Borderline high
160–189	High
$\geq$190	Very high
Total cholesterol	
<200	Optimal
200–239	Borderline high
$\geq$240	High
HDL cholesterol	
<40	Low
$\geq$60	High

*ATP indicates Adult Treatment Panel; LDL – low-density lipoprotein; HDL – high-density lipoprotein.

Adapted from Expert Panel on Detection, Evaluation, and Treatment of High Blood Cholesterol in Adults (Adult Treatment Panel III) (65).

Risk reduction strategies have been demonstrated to be highly effective in a number of studies (70). The MICRO-HOPE Study included 3,577 individuals with diabetes, with and without hypertension, and compared the cardiovascular event rates with the angiotensin-converting enzyme (ACE) inhibitor, ramipril, vs. placebo (71). The results showed that treatment with

Table 5
Three categories of risk that modify LDL cholesterol goals

Risk category	LDL goal (mg/dl)
CHD and CHD risk equivalents	<100
Multiple (2+) risk factors	<130
0–1 risk factor	<160

CHD indicates coronary heart disease. Diabetes is a CHD equivalent.
Adapted from Expert Panel on Detection, Evaluation, and Treatment of High Blood Cholesterol in Adults (Adult Treatment Panel III) *(65)*.

ramipril lowered the risk of the primary outcome of combined MI, stroke, or CVD mortality by 25%, MI by 22%, stroke by 33%, and cardiovascular death by 37%. Lowering serum cholesterol has been demonstrated in many studies to be effective at reducing CVD risks, both as primary and secondary prevention. Recent studies have questioned whether even more aggressive LDL-cholesterol lowering in high-risk individuals should be the appropriate target of such treatment *(67, 72)*.

An important study used a focused, multifactorial intervention with strict targets and individualized risk assessment in patients with T2D and microal buminuria who were at increased risk for macrovascular and microvascular complications *(73, 74)*. These data suggest that a long-term, targeted, intensive intervention involving multiple risk factors reduces the risk of both cardiovascular and microvascular events by about 50% among these patients. The advantages of a multifactorial approach to the reduction of cardiovascular risk are obvious. The challenge remains to ensure that this approach can be widely adopted.

Management of Diabetes in the Older Adult

The degree of benefit controlling blood glucose, lipids, and blood pressure in older adults with diabetes to reduce microvascular and macrovascular complications may depend on the patient's life expectancy, functional status, and comorbidities *(75)*. The heterogeneity of this population is a key consideration for clinicians developing intervention strategies and establishing clinical targets. The goals of physicians and other providers caring for the elderly diabetic patient should be to optimize glycemic control and reduce associated cardiovascular risk factors in an effort to maximize long-term quality of life. On the other hand, for frail older adults, particularly those with severe comorbidities and disabilities, aggressive management is not likely to provide benefit and may even result in harm as a consequence of frequent hypoglycemia associated with aggressive glycemic control *(56)*.

In the management of diabetes in older adults, it is necessary to assess for the presence of geriatric syndromes, a group of conditions associated with functional decline and disability that are more prevalent in the elderly. These syndromes and the different comorbidities in the elderly make the management of diabetes in this population a challenging task. Common geriatric syndromes in older adults with diabetes include depression, cognitive impairment/dementia, urinary incontinence, falls, and polypharmacy *(75)*. Diabetes is associated with depression in the elderly and mood disorders may lead to worsening of glycemic control and more diabetic complications. Hyperglycemia is associated with a greater risk for cognitive impairment, especially Alzheimer's disease (AD) and vascular dementia. It is known that the longer the duration of diabetes, the higher the prevalence of dementia and also that those treated with insulin are at higher risk. Urinary incontinence can be exacerbated because of poor glycemic control and/or because of comorbidities like heart failure and prostate disease or by medication-related side effects. All elderly diabetic patients should be screened for falls, since comorbidities, diabetic neuropathy, and medications may increase the risk of falls. Many older adults with diabetes use five or more medications (a common definition of polypharmacy), which may or may not be appropriately prescribed and may interact with other medications or with a disease process.

Psychosocial Screening

Basic assessment of psychosocial status should be included as part of the medical management of diabetes. Psychosocial screening should include patient attitudes about illness, expectations for medical care and outcomes, affect/mood, general and diabetes-related quality of life, available resources (financial, social, and emotional), and psychiatric history. It is best to incorporate psychological assessment into routine care rather than wait for identification of a specific problem or deterioration in psychological status. Opportunities for screening of psychosocial status occur at diagnosis, during regularly scheduled management visits, during hospitalizations, at discovery of complications, or at the discretion of the clinician when problems in glucose control or adherence are suspected or identified.

NEED FOR IMPROVING DIABETES CARE

Standards of care for diabetes recommended by the American Diabetes Association are revised periodically and published yearly in the journal *Diabetes Care*. The implementation of the standards of care has been suboptimal in most clinical settings. A report from the National Health and Nutrition Education Survey (NHANES) 1999–2000 and NHANES III surveys demonstrated that only 37% of US adults with diabetes achieved an HbA1c of <7%, only 36% had a blood pressure < 130/80 mmHg, and only 48% had a cholesterol < 200 mg/dl *(76)*. Only 7.3% had overall "good control," i.e., attained target goals for all vascular risk factors. Another study addressing quality of diabetes care in the United States showed that during 1988–1995 there was a gap between recommended diabetes care (HbA1c < 7%, annual dilated eye exam, annual foot exam, evaluation for urine albumin or protein excretion, achieving blood pressure and lipid goals), and the care that patients actually received *(77)*. In that study, only 28.8% of diabetics even had an HbA1c measurement, 63.3% reported a dilated eye exam, and 54.8% had had a foot exam within the previous year. Eighteen percent of these diabetic individuals had an HbA1c > 9.5%.

While many interventions to improve adherence to the recommended standards have been implemented, providing uniformly effective diabetes care remains a challenge. Education of health professionals and patients alike is one key to better success. Improved access to health care and education for all is critical. Multidisciplinary teams are ideal to provide care for people with chronic conditions like diabetes and to encourage patients to be involved in appropriate disease self-management. Cooperative efforts between health care providers, health policy experts, public health officials and patients are needed to change the climate and outcomes for individuals with diabetes and at risk for diabetes in the United States (Table 6).

Table 6
Summary of recommendations for adults with diabetes

Glycemic control	
HbA1c	<7.0%*
Preprandial capillary plasma glucose	90–130 mg/dl (5.0–7.2 mmol/l)
Peak postprandial capillary plasma glucose[+]	<180 mg/dl (<10.0 mmol/l)
Blood pressure	<130/80 mmHg
Lipids	
LDL	<100 mg/dl (<2.6 mmol/l)
Triglycerides	<150 mg/dl (<1.7 mmol/l)
HDL	>40 mg/dl (>1.1 mmol/l)[§]

*HbA1c goal for selected individual patients (those with short duration of diabetes, long life expectancy, and no significant cardiovascular disease) may be lower than the general goal if this can be achieved without significant hypoglycemia or other adverse effects of treatment. Conversely, less stringent HbA1c goal may be appropriate for patients with a history of severe hypoglycemia, limited life expectancy, advance microvascular or macrovascular complications, extensive comorbid conditions, or frail elderly patients.

HbA1c, hemoglobin A1c; LDL, low density lipoprotein; HDL, high density lipoprotein (Adapted from: American Diabetes Association) *(1)*.

REFERENCES

1. American Diabetes Association. Standards of medical care in diabetes – 2008. Diabetes Care 2008; 31:12–54.
2. Federation WHOID. Definition and diagnosis of diabetes mellitus and intermediate hyperglycemia. report of WHO/IDF consultation. http://www.who.int/diabetes/publications/en/. Accessed June 27, 2008.
3. Saudek CD, Herman WH, Sacks DB, Bergenstal RM, Edelman D, Davidson MB. A new look at screening and diagnosing diabetes mellitus. J Clin Endocrinol Metab 2008; 93(7): 2447–2453.
4. World Diabetes Foundation, & International Diabetes Federation. Diabetes Atlas. Brussels: IDF Executive Office 2006.
5. Prevention CfDCa. Fact Sheet Press Release: Number of People with Diabetes Increases to 24 million 2008; <http://www.cdc.gov/media/pressrel/2008/r080624.htm. Accessed June 27, 2008.
6. Narayan KM, Boyle JP, Thompson TJ, Sorensen SW, Williamson DF. Lifetime risk for diabetes mellitus in the United States. JAMA 2003; 290(14):1884–1890.
7. Mokdad AH, Ford ES, Bowman BA, et al. Prevalence of obesity, diabetes, and obesity-related health risk factors, 2001. JAMA 2003; 289(1):76–79.
8. Ogden CL, Carroll MD, Curtin LR, McDowell MA, Tabak CJ, Flegal KM. Prevalence of overweight and obesity in the United States, 1999–2004. JAMA 2006; 295(13):1549–1555.
9. Li C, Ford ES, McGuire LC, Mokdad AH. Increasing trends in waist circumference and abdominal obesity among US adults. Obesity (Silver Spring) 2007; 15(1):216–224.
10. Freemantle N, Holmes J, Hockey A, Kumar S. How strong is the association between abdominal obesity and the incidence of type 2 diabetes? Int J Clin Pract 2008; 62(9):1391–1396.
11. Fact Sheet Press Release: Number of People with Diabetes Increases to 24 million 2008; <http://www.cdc.gov/media/pressrel/2008/r080624.htm. Accessed June 27, 2008.
12. Wilson PW, Meigs JB, Sullivan L, Fox CS, Nathan DM, D'Agostino RB, Sr. Prediction of incident diabetes mellitus in middle-aged adults: the Framingham Offspring Study. Arch Intern Med 2007; 167(10):1068–1074.
13. Florez H. Diabetes risk engine with clinical variables. Int Diabetes Monitor 2008; 20: 119–120.
14. DeFronzo RA. Lilly lecture 1987. The triumvirate: beta-cell, muscle, liver. A collusion responsible for NIDDM. Diabetes 1988; 37(6):667–687.
15. Weyer C, Tataranni PA, Bogardus C, Pratley RE. Insulin resistance and insulin secretory dysfunction are independent predictors of worsening of glucose tolerance during each stage of type 2 diabetes development. Diabetes Care 2001; 24(1):89–94.
16. Kahn SE, Montgomery B, Howell W, et al. Importance of early phase insulin secretion to intravenous glucose tolerance in subjects with type 2 diabetes mellitus. J Clin Endocrinol Metab 2001; 86(12):5824–5829.
17. Weyer C, Bogardus C, Mott DM, Pratley RE. The natural history of insulin secretory dysfunction and insulin resistance in the pathogenesis of type 2 diabetes mellitus. J Clin Invest 1999; 104(6):787–794.
18. Mokdad AH, Ford ES, Bowman BA, et al. Diabetes trends in the U.S.: 1990–1998. Diabetes Care 2000; 23(9):1278–1283.
19. Choi BC, Shi F. Risk factors for diabetes mellitus by age and sex: results of the National Population Health Survey. Diabetologia 2001; 44(10):1221–1231.
20. Hu FB, Manson JE, Stampfer MJ, et al. Diet, lifestyle, and the risk of type 2 diabetes mellitus in women. N Engl J Med 2001; 345(11):790–797.
21. Moore AF, Florez JC. Genetic susceptibility to type 2 diabetes and implications for antidiabetic therapy. Annu Rev Med 2008; 59:95 111.
22. Cauchi S, Froguel P. TCF7L2 genetic defect and type 2 diabetes. Curr Diab Rep 2008; 8(2):149–155.

23. Pan XR, Li GW, Hu YH, et al. Effects of diet and exercise in preventing NIDDM in people with impaired glucose tolerance. The Da Qing IGT and Diabetes Study. Diabetes Care 1997; 20(4):537–544.
24. Tuomilehto J, Lindstrom J, Eriksson JG, et al. Prevention of type 2 diabetes mellitus by changes in lifestyle among subjects with impaired glucose tolerance. N Engl J Med 2001; 344(18):1343–1350.
25. Knowler WC, Barrett-Connor E, Fowler SE, et al. Reduction in the incidence of type 2 diabetes with lifestyle intervention or metformin. N Engl J Med 2002; 346(6):393–403.
26. Chiasson JL, Josse RG, Gomis R, Hanefeld M, Karasik A, Laakso M. Acarbose for prevention of type 2 diabetes mellitus: the STOP-NIDDM randomised trial. Lancet 2002; 359(9323):2072–2077.
27. Buchanan TA, Xiang AH, Peters RK, et al. Preservation of pancreatic beta-cell function and prevention of type 2 diabetes by pharmacological treatment of insulin resistance in high-risk Hispanic women. Diabetes 2002; 51(9):2796–2803.
28. Bosch J, Yusuf S, Gerstein HC, et al. Effect of ramipril on the incidence of diabetes. N Engl J Med 2006; 355(15):1551–1562.
29. Gerstein HC, Yusuf S, Bosch J, et al. Effect of rosiglitazone on the frequency of diabetes in patients with impaired glucose tolerance or impaired fasting glucose: a randomised controlled trial. Lancet 2006; 368(9541):1096–1105.
30. Crandall JP, Knowler WC, Kahn SE, et al. The prevention of type 2 diabetes. Nat Clin Pract Endocrinol Metab 2008; 4(7):382–393.
31. Geiss LS, Herman WH, Smith PJ. Mortality in non-insulin dependent diabetes. Bethesda: NIH, NIDDK; 1995.
32. Malmberg K, Yusuf S, Gerstein HC, et al. Impact of diabetes on long-term prognosis in patients with unstable angina and non-Q-wave myocardial infarction: results of the OASIS (Organization to Assess Strategies for Ischemic Syndromes) Registry. Circulation 2000; 102(9):1014–1019.
33. Haffner SM, Lehto S, Ronnemaa T, Pyorala K, Laakso M. Mortality from coronary heart disease in subjects with type 2 diabetes and in nondiabetic subjects with and without prior myocardial infarction. N Engl J Med 1998; 339(4):229–234.
34. The effect of intensive treatment of diabetes on the development and progression of long-term complications in insulin-dependent diabetes mellitus. The Diabetes Control and Complications Trial Research Group. N Engl J Med 1993; 329(14):977–986.
35. Retinopathy and nephropathy in patients with type 1 diabetes four years after a trial of intensive therapy. The Diabetes Control and Complications Trial/Epidemiology of Diabetes Interventions and Complications Research Group. N Engl J Med 2000; 342(6):381–389.
36. Effect of intensive therapy on the development and progression of diabetic nephropathy in the Diabetes Control and Complications Trial. The Diabetes Control and Complications (DCCT) Research Group. Kidney Int 1995; 47(6):1703–1720.
37. Intensive blood-glucose control with sulphonylureas or insulin compared with conventional treatment and risk of complications in patients with type 2 diabetes (UKPDS 33). UK Prospective Diabetes Study (UKPDS) Group. Lancet 1998; 352(9131):837–853.
38. Ohkubo Y, Kishikawa H, Araki E, et al. Intensive insulin therapy prevents the progression of diabetic microvascular complications in Japanese patients with non-insulin-dependent diabetes mellitus: a randomized prospective 6-year study. Diabetes Res Clin Pract 1995; 28(2):103–117.
39. Reichard P, Pihl M, Rosenqvist U, Sule J. Complications in IDDM are caused by elevated blood glucose level: the Stockholm Diabetes Intervention Study (SDIS) at 10-year follow up. Diabetologia 1996; 39(12):1483–1488.
40. Malmberg K, Ryden L, Efendic S, et al. Randomized trial of insulin-glucose infusion followed by subcutaneous insulin treatment in diabetic patients with acute myocardial infarction (DIGAMI study): effects on mortality at 1 year. J Am Coll Cardiol 1995; 26(1):57–65.
41. van den Berghe G, Wouters P, Weekers F, et al. Intensive insulin therapy in the critically ill patients. N Engl J Med 2001; 345(19):1359–1367.

42. Coutinho M, Gerstein HC, Wang Y, Yusuf S. The relationship between glucose and incident cardiovascular events. A metaregression analysis of published data from 20 studies of 95,783 individuals followed for 12.4 years. Diabetes Care 1999; 22(2):233–240.
43. Khaw KT, Wareham N, Luben R, et al. Glycated haemoglobin, diabetes, and mortality in men in Norfolk cohort of European prospective investigation of cancer and nutrition (EPIC-Norfolk). BMJ 2001; 322(7277):15–18.
44. Stratton IM, Adler AI, Neil HA, et al. Association of glycaemia with macrovascular and microvascular complications of type 2 diabetes (UKPDS 35): prospective observational study. BMJ 2000; 321(7258):405–412.
45. Nathan DM, Cleary PA, Backlund JY, et al. Intensive diabetes treatment and cardiovascular disease in patients with type 1 diabetes. N Engl J Med 2005; 353(25):2643–2653.
46. Effect of intensive blood-glucose control with metformin on complications in overweight patients with type 2 diabetes (UKPDS 34). UK Prospective Diabetes Study (UKPDS) Group. Lancet 1998; 352(9131):854–865.
47. Holman RR, Paul SK, Bethel MA, Matthews DR, Neil HAW. 10-year follow-up of intensive glucose control in type 2 diabetes. N Engl J Med 2008; 359(15):1577–1589.
48. Gerstein HC, Miller ME, Byington RP, et al. Effects of intensive glucose lowering in type 2 diabetes. N Engl J Med 2008; 358(24):2545–2559.
49. Patel A, MacMahon S, Chalmers J, et al. Intensive blood glucose control and vascular outcomes in patients with type 2 diabetes. N Engl J Med 2008; 358(24):2560–2572.
50. Kirkman MS, McCarren M, Shah J, Duckworth W, Abraira C. The association between metabolic control and prevalent macrovascular disease in Type 2 diabetes: the VA Cooperative Study in diabetes. J Diabetes Complications 2006; 20(2):75–80.
51. Huang ES, Zhang Q, Gandra N, Chin MH, Meltzer DO. The effect of comorbid illness and functional status on the expected benefits of intensive glucose control in older patients with type 2 diabetes: a decision analysis. Ann Intern Med 2008; 149(1):11–19.
52. Nathan DM. Clinical practice. Initial management of glycemia in type 2 diabetes mellitus. N Engl J Med 2002; 347(17):1342–1349.
53. DeFronzo RA. Pharmacologic therapy for type 2 diabetes mellitus. Ann Intern Med 1999; 131(4):281–303.
54. Inzucchi SE. Oral antihyperglycemic therapy for type 2 diabetes: scientific review. JAMA 2002; 287(3):360–372.
55. Kimmel B, Inzucchi SE. Oral agents for type 2 diabetes: an update. Clinical Diabetes 2005; 23:64–76.
56. Florez H, Marks J. Oral agents and insulin in care of older adults with diabetes. In: Lipsitz M, ed. In Geriatric Diabetes. New York: Informa Healthcare; 2007:283–291.
57. Nathan DM, Buse JB, Davidson MB, et al. Management of hyperglycemia in type 2 diabetes: A consensus algorithm for the initiation and adjustment of therapy: a consensus statement from the American Diabetes Association and the European Association for the Study of Diabetes. Diabetes Care 2006; 29(8):1963–1972.
58. Dungan K, Buse JB. Glucagon-like peptide-1 based therapies for type 2 diabetes: a focus on exenatide. Clinical Diabetes 2005; 23:56–62.
59. Hollander P, Maggs DG, Ruggles JA, et al. Effect of pramlintide on weight in overweight and obese insulin-treated type 2 diabetes patients. Obes Res 2004; 12(4):661–668.
60. Ginsberg HN. Insulin resistance and cardiovascular disease. J Clin Invest 2000; 106(4): 453–458.
61. Hsueh WA, Law RE. Cardiovascular risk continuum: implications of insulin resistance and diabetes. Am J Med 1998; 105(1A):4S–14S.
62. Meigs JB, Mittleman MA, Nathan DM, et al. Hyperinsulinemia, hyperglycemia, and impaired hemostasis: the Framingham Offspring Study. JAMA 2000; 283(2):221–228.
63. Cooper ME, Bonnet F, Oldfield M, Jandeleit-Dahm K. Mechanisms of diabetic vasculopathy: an overview. Am J Hypertens 2001; 14(5 Pt 1):475–486.
64. Brownlee M. Biochemistry and molecular cell biology of diabetic complications. Nature 2001; 414(6865):813–820.

65. Executive Summary of The Third Report of The National Cholesterol Education Program (NCEP) Expert Panel on Detection, Evaluation, And Treatment of High Blood Cholesterol In Adults (Adult Treatment Panel III). JAMA 2001; 285(19): 2486–2497.
66. Grundy SM, Cleeman JI, Merz CN, et al. Implications of recent clinical trials for the National Cholesterol Education Program Adult Treatment Panel III guidelines. Circulation 2004; 110(2):227–239.
67. Collins R, Armitage J, Parish S, Sleigh P, Peto R. MRC/BHF Heart Protection Study of cholesterol-lowering with simvastatin in 5963 people with diabetes: a randomised placebo-controlled trial. Lancet 2003; 361(9374):2005–2016.
68. Waters DD, Guyton JR, Herrington DM, McGowan MP, Wenger NK, Shear C. Treating to New Targets (TNT) Study: does lowering low-density lipoprotein cholesterol levels below currently recommended guidelines yield incremental clinical benefit? Am J Cardiol 2004; 93(2):154–158.
69. Pedersen TR, Faergeman O, Kastelein JJ, et al. High-dose atorvastatin vs usual-dose simvastatin for secondary prevention after myocardial infarction: the IDEAL study: a randomized controlled trial. JAMA 2005; 294(19):2437–2445.
70. Davidson MH. Global risk management in patients with type 2 diabetes mellitus. Am J Cardiol 2007; 99(4A):41B–50B.
71. Effects of ramipril on cardiovascular and microvascular outcomes in people with diabetes mellitus: results of the HOPE study and MICRO-HOPE substudy. Heart Outcomes Prevention Evaluation Study Investigators. Lancet 2000; 355(9200):253–259.
72. Cannon CP, Braunwald E, McCabe CH, et al. Intensive versus moderate lipid lowering with statins after acute coronary syndromes. N Engl J Med 2004; 350(15):1495–1504.
73. Gaede P, Vedel P, Larsen N, Jensen GV, Parving HH, Pedersen O. Multifactorial intervention and cardiovascular disease in patients with type 2 diabetes. N Engl J Med 2003; 348(5): 383–393.
74. Gaede P, Lund-Andersen H, Parving HH, Pedersen O. Effect of a multifactorial intervention on mortality in type 2 diabetes. N Engl J Med 2008; 358(6):580–591.
75. Brown AF, Mangione CM, Saliba D, Sarkisian CA. Guidelines for improving the care of the older person with diabetes mellitus. J Am Geriatr Soc 2003; 51(5 Suppl Guidelines): S265–S280.
76. Saydah SH, Fradkin J, Cowie CC. Poor control of risk factors for vascular disease among adults with previously diagnosed diabetes. JAMA 2004; 291(3):335–342.
77. Saaddine JB, Engelgau MM, Beckles GL, Gregg EW, Thompson TJ, Narayan KM. A diabetes report card for the United States: quality of care in the 1990s. Ann Intern Med 2002; 136(8):565–574.

II UPDATE ON STROKE AND DEMENTIA FOR DIABETOLOGISTS

3   Acute Ischemic Stroke

L. Jaap Kappelle and H. Bart van der Worp

CONTENTS

ABSTRACT

Stroke is the second leading cause of long-term disability in high-income countries and the second leading cause of death worldwide. In Western communities, about 80% of strokes are caused by focal cerebral ischemia secondary to arterial occlusion. Stroke incidence is highly age-dependent. The median stroke incidence in persons between 15 and 49 years of age is 10 per 100,000 per year, whereas this is 2,000 per 100,000 for persons aged 85 years or older. Established treatments of acute ischemic stroke include intravenous thrombolysis with alteplase within 4.5 h after the onset of symptoms and early administration of aspirin. In the first days after stroke onset, patients should be monitored closely for early detection and prevention of neurological and medical complications. Care is best when the patient is admitted to a specialized stroke unit. Space-occupying infarcts may be treated with early decompressive surgery. Recurrent stroke and other cardiovascular complications should be prevented by a combination of medical and – in selected patients – surgical treatment strategies.

From: *Contemporary Diabetes: Diabetes and the Brain*
Edited by: G. J. Biessels, J. A. Luchsinger (eds.), DOI 10.1007/978-1-60327-850-8_3
© Humana Press, a part of Springer Science+Business Media, LLC 2009

Key words: Stroke; Ischemic stroke; Cerebrovascular disease; Cerebral infarction; Cerebral ischemia.

EPIDEMIOLOGY

Stroke is the second leading cause of long-term disability in high-income countries and the second leading cause of death worldwide (1). In Western communities, about 80% of strokes are caused by focal cerebral ischemia, secondary to arterial occlusion, 15% by intracerebral hemorrhage, and 5% by subarachnoid hemorrhage (2). The World Health Organization has estimated that there were, worldwide, 16 million first-ever strokes and 5.7 million stroke deaths in 2005. These numbers are expected to rise to 18 million and 6.5 million, respectively, in 2015 (3).

The median annual incidence of first stroke in Western countries has been estimated to be about 200 per 100,000 for all age groups combined (2, 4). This incidence is highly age-dependent. The median stroke incidence in persons between 15 and 49 years of age is 10 per 100,000 per year, whereas this is 2,000 per 100,000 for persons aged 85 years or older (5). Most studies have shown a somewhat higher stroke incidence among men. Hispanics and African Americans have a higher risk of stroke than Caucasians; in African Americans, stroke incidence is about twice as high as in Caucasians (5). Stroke prevalence increases from about 50–100 per 100,000 in people between 25 and 34 years of age to about 10,000 per 100,000 in people of 85 years of age or older (6).

Thirty-day case fatality rates for ischemic stroke in Western communities generally range between 10 and 17% (2). Stroke outcome strongly dependsnot only on age and comorbidity, but also on the type and cause of the infarct. Early case fatality can be as low as 2.5% in patients with lacunar infarcts (7) and as high as 78% in patients with space-occupying hemispheric infarction (8).

Atherosclerosis, leading to thromboembolism or local occlusion, and cardioembolism are the leading causes of brain ischemia, but unusual causes should be considered especially if patients are younger (Table 1) (9).

PATHOPHYSIOLOGY

Ischemic brain injury results from a cascade of events running from energy depletion to necrosis or apoptosis. Intermediate factors include excitotoxicity, free radical formation, and inflammation. Initially after arterial occlusion, a central core of very low perfusion is surrounded by an area with a less severe reduction in perfusion. In this so-called ischemic penumbra,

Table 1
Common and some unusual causes of ischemic stroke

Common causes
Atherothromboembolism
Embolism from the heart
Small vessel disease

Unusual causes
Arterial dissection
Fibromuscular dysplasia
Cerebral venous thrombosis
Vasculitis
Migraine
Cocaine use
Moyamoya syndrome
Hematological disorders
CADASIL*
Mitochondrial cytopathy
Fabry disease

*CADASIL: cerebral autosomal dominant arteriopathy with subcortical infarcts and leukoencephalopathy.

there is dysfunction from metabolic and ionic disturbances, but structural integrity is still preserved. In the first minutes to hours, clinical deficits therefore do not necessarily reflect irreversible damage. Depending on residual blood flow and duration of ischemia, the penumbra will eventually be incorporated into the infarct if reperfusion is not achieved (9, 10).

DIAGNOSIS

Patients with ischemic stroke usually present with focal neurological deficit of sudden onset. Occasionally a more gradually or stepwise onset can be found, especially in patients with a hemodynamic origin of cerebral ischemia. Common deficits include dysphasia, dysarthria, hemianopia, weakness, ataxia, sensory loss, and cognitive disorders such as spatial neglect (9). Symptoms are unilateral except in some patients with posterior circulation stroke. Most patients remain alert. Mild-to-moderate headache is an accompanying symptom in about a quarter of all patients with ischemic stroke and is more common in stroke of the posterior circulation. Patients with a dissection of the carotid, vertebral, or intracranial arteries usually complain of severe headache in the early course of their illness, sometimes even for days preceding the actual stroke. By definition, signs and symptoms of stroke last for more than 24 h; deficits of shorter duration that are caused by focal cerebral ischemia are classified as transient ischemic attacks (TIAs). The distinction between ischemic stroke and TIA is useful mainly for

epidemiological purposes. Diagnostic investigations and secondary prevention should be similar. Patientswho present with symptoms within the first
24 h should be treated as a case of medical emergency, particularly when
they can be treated with intravenous thrombolysis within 4.5 h.

The accuracy of a clinical examinationby specialists in the early stage
is good, but ancillary computerized tomography (CT) or magnetic resonance imaging (MRI) of the brain is always necessary not only to distinguish with certainty between ischemic and hemorrhagic stroke, but also to
exclude other causes of the deficit, such as a subdural hematoma or a tumor.
Subtle signs of early ischemia, such as a reduced gray-white differentiation
and hemispheric sulcal effacement, as well as arterial occlusion can be identified with CT *(11)* (Fig. 1). The ischemic penumbra may be visualized with
perfusion CT *(12)*. It has been hypothesized that visualization of penumbral
tissue may be helpful for the decision whether the patient should be treated
with thrombolysis, but this remains to be proven.

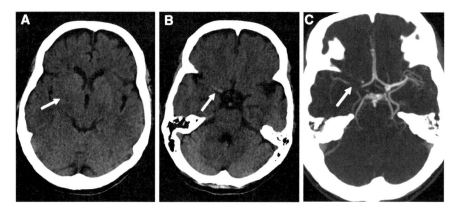

Fig. 1. A 72-year-old woman with an acute left hemiparesis, scanned within 3 h of symptom onset. The CT shows a reduced gray-white differentiation in the right basal ganglia
(**A**; *arrow*) and a hyperintense middle cerebral artery sign (**B**; *arrow*), consistent with a
proximal right middle cerebral artery occlusion found on CT angiography (**C**; *arrow*).
These findings are all suggestive of a large infarct in the territory of the right middle
cerebral artery.

MRI is better for detection of acute ischemia than CT *(13)*, but is more
expensive, less widely available, more time consuming, and often impossible in very ill or restless patients. The sensitivity and specificity of diffusion-
weighted imaging for detecting ischemic lesions within minutes after stroke
onset are about 100% *(11)* (Fig. 2). Areas with reduced or delayed perfusion can be measured with perfusion-weighted imaging. A perfusion
delay of more than 6 s as compared with the non-affected hemisphere on

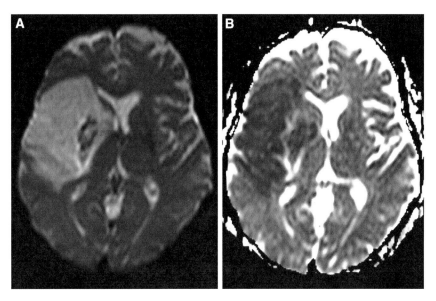

Fig. 2. MRI of the patient in Fig. 1 showing a large hyperintense lesion on diffusion-weighted imaging (DWI; **A**) and a consistent reduction of the apparent diffusion coefficient (ADC; **B**), demonstrating an acute cortical and subcortical infarct in the territory of the right middle cerebral artery.

time-to-peak maps can predict the volume of the final infarct *(14)*. Visualization of the ischemic penumbra with MRI by means of the diffusion–perfusion mismatch is much more established than with CT *(15)*, but again of unproven therapeutic value. With CT or MR angiography, all arteries can be imaged from the aortic arch to the circle of Willis in a single session to identify arterial occlusion in the acute stage (see Fig. 1) *(11)*.

ACUTE TREATMENT

Thrombolysis

Restoration of blood flow to the ischemic area by means of intravenously administered alteplase (recombinant tissue plasminogen activator [rt-PA]) should be considered the most revolutionary breakthrough in the treatment of acute ischemic stroke in history. Despitean increased risk of symptomatic intracranial hemorrhage, alteplase was demonstrated to be beneficial when administered within 3 h of stroke onset in the NINDS rt-PA study, with a number needed to treat of only seven to eight to prevent death or severe disability in a single patient *(16)*. Benefits of alteplase are sustained at 1 year *(17)*and result in significant savings in post-stroke care *(18)*.

In a pooled analysis of six randomized placebo-controlled trials of intravenous alteplase the benefit was greater the sooner patients received thrombolytic therapy, also within the time frame of 3 h *(19)*. The same analysis suggested a potential benefit beyond 3 h. This has recently been confirmed in a separate trial, in which alteplase administered between 3 and 4.5 h after stroke onset provided an absolute reduction in the risk of poor outcome of 7%, equivalent to a number to treat of 14 *(20)*.

In recent randomized trials, large intraparenchymal hemorrhage occurred in some 6% of the patients treated with intravenous rt-PA within 6 h of stroke onset and in about 1% of controls *(19)*. The risk of symptomatic intracranial hemorrhage after thrombolysis is higher with more severe strokes and higher age *(21)*. To avoid hemorrhage, clinicians should as a rule adhere to published guidelines (Table 2).

Table 2
Main contraindications to intravenous thrombolysis in patients with acute ischemic stroke

- Onset of symptoms $\geq$4.5 h before start of treatment
- Intracranial hemorrhage on CT or MRI
- Head trauma or prior stroke in previous 3 months
- Myocardial infarction in the previous 3 months
- Gastrointestinal or urinary tract hemorrhage in previous 21 days
- Major surgery in the previous 14 days
- History of previous intracranial hemorrhage
- Systolic blood pressure $\geq$185 mmHg or diastolic blood pressure $\geq$110 mmHg
- Evidence of active bleeding or acute trauma (fracture) on examination
- Use of oral anticoagulation with $\geq$INR 1.7
- Use of heparin in previous 48 h with a currently prolonged aPTT
- Platelet count <100,000 mm^{-3}
- Blood glucose concentration <50 mg/dL (2.7 mmol/L)
- Seizure with postictal residual neurological impairments

Adapted from Adams *(22)*. For a more complete overview of indications and contraindications the reader is referred to official guidelines *(22)*.

Alteplase has not been approved as a treatment for acute stroke in patients younger than 18 years of age, but there is no upper age limit *(22)*. Alteplase should probably not be withheld too rigorously in patients with mild neurological deficits *(23)* or in patients with leukoaraiosis *(24)*.

Intra-arterial thrombolysis through a microcatheter at the site of the occlusion has been studied in only prospective single phase III-randomized clinical trial *(25)*. A meta-analysis of this trial and two phase II trials has suggested that treatment with intra-arterial pro-urokinase within 6 h of onset of acute ischemic stroke caused by middle cerebral artery occlusion significantly improves clinical outcome at 90 days, despite an increased frequency of early symptomatic intracranial hemorrhage *(26)*. More studies are needed to confirm this result before intra-arterial thrombolysis can be accepted as an established treatment for acute ischemic stroke. Intra-arterial thrombolysis has been advocated for the treatment of basilar artery thrombosis, but has not yet been tested in an adequately sized randomized trial *(27, 28)*.

Intravenous thrombolysis followed by intra-arterial thrombolysis ("bridging therapy") may combine the advantage of rapid treatment and a high rate of recanalization, but requires major efforts from a stroke team and should be studied in a proper clinical trial *(29)*.

Mechanical Clot Removal

Mechanical clot disruption or removal of an occluding clot in an intracranial artery with endovascular catheters is emerging as an alternative or adjunctional therapy to thrombolysis *(29)*. Embolectomy with a Merci device has been shown to significantly restore vascular patency within 8 h of stroke onset, but has not yet been tested in a randomized clinical trial *(29, 30)*. This treatment should be performed only in highly specialized centers, preferably in the context of a clinical trial.

Antithrombotic Medication

Intravenous heparin administered within 3 h after stroke onset has been shown to be superior to normal saline in a single small trial *(31)*, but this could not be confirmed in one other small trial *(32)*. In the International Stroke Trial, administration of unfractionated heparin in a dose of 5,000 or 12,500 IU bd (twice daily) started within 48 h after stroke onset and maintained for 14 days resulted in significantly fewer recurrent ischemic strokes during the treatment period, but this was offset by a similar-sized increase in hemorrhagic strokes. Heparin was associated with a significant excess of 9 (SD 1) transfused or fatal extracranial bleeds per 1,000. Compared with 5,000 IU bd heparin, 12,500 IU bd heparin was associated with significantly more transfused or fatal extracranial bleeds, more hemorrhagic strokes, and more deaths or non-fatal strokes within 14 days. In this trial, neither heparin regimen offered any clinical advantage at 6 months (IST) *(33)*. Treatment with 300 mg or 160 mg of aspirin once daily within 48 h after stroke onset has been shown to improve functional outcome in a pooled analysis of the International Stroke Trial and the Chinese Acute Stroke Trial, probably by reducing the risk of recurrent ischemic stroke *(33, 34)*. The number needed to treat is high: 77 to avoid poor outcome in a single patient, but treatment with aspirin is cheap, simple, and safe, possible except in the first 24 h after thrombolysis.

Decompressive Surgery

Life-threatening space-occupying brain edema occurs in 1–5% of patients with a supratentorial infarct and usually manifests itself between the second and the fifth day after stroke onset *(35)*. Case fatality rates of these "malignant" middle cerebral artery infarctions have been reported as high as 78% *(8, 36)*. No medical therapy has been proven effective *(35)*.

Removal of a large part of the frontal, temporal, and parietal bones overlaying the infarcted area followed by a duraplasty reduces tissue shifts and high intracranial pressure that is caused by the edema and may save unaffected brain tissue from damage (Fig. 3). The effects on functional outcome of such decompressive surgery within two days after stroke onset in patients aged up to 60 years with space-occupying middle cerebral artery infarction have been compared with medical therapy in three European randomized controlled trials. Twelve months after stroke onset, significantly fewer patients were dead or severely disabled after surgical treatment than after conservative treatment (Fig. 4), with a number needed to treat of only four to prevent one poor outcome *(37)*.

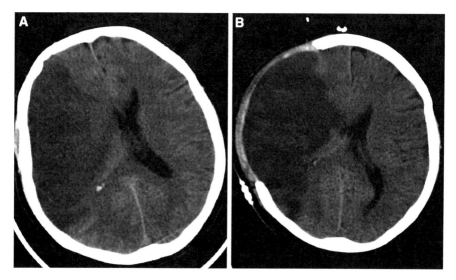

Fig. 3. A 58-year-old man with a space-occupying infarct in the territory of the right middle cerebral artery, before (**A**) and after (**B**) surgery.

More information is needed about the efficacy of decompressive surgery in patients with aphasia, patients older than 50 years of age, and patients in whom treatment is delayed until the second day after stroke onset. In the mean time, the decision to perform decompressive surgery should be made on an individual basis in every patient.

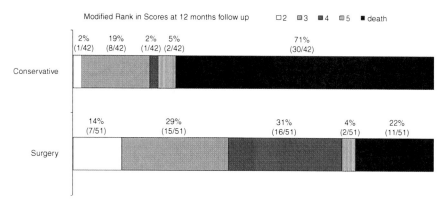

Fig. 4. Distributions of the scores on the modified Rankin scale after 12 months for patients with space-occupying middle cerebral artery infarction treated with or without decompressive surgery. (From Vahedi et al. *(37)*. Reproduced from The Lancet Neurology, with permission from Elsevier.)

Neuroprotection

In the previous 20 years, ten thousands of patients with acute ischemic stroke have participated in hundreds of clinical trials of putative neuroprotective therapies. Despite this enormous effort, there is no evidence of benefit of a single neuroprotective agent in humans, whereas over 500 have been effective in animal models *(38)*. While differences in design and methodological quality between animal studies and clinical trials may be responsible for some of this discrepancy, the failure of neuroprotective agents in the clinic may also be explained by the fact that most neuroprotectants inhibit only a single step in the broad cascade of events that lead to cell death *(9)*. Currently, there is no rationale for the use of any neuroprotective medication in patients with acute ischemic stroke.

Hypothermia

Preclinical studies have suggested that hypothermia affects a wide range of cell death mechanisms in ischemic stroke, including energy depletion, disruption of the blood–brain barrier, free radical formation, excitotoxicity, and inflammation *(39)*. The potential benefits of hypothermia have been underlined by randomized clinical trials in patients with global cerebral ischemia after cardiac arrest *(40, 41)*. In addition, a high body temperature has been associated with poor outcome after stroke *(42)*.

Cooling to temperatures below 35°C, as used in most animal studies and in clinical trials of post-anoxic encephalopathy after cardiac arrest, requires sedation, mechanical ventilation, and therefore admission to an intensive care facility. This makes this therapy less feasible in clinical practice. So far, randomized clinical trials of cooling in patients with acute ischemic stroke have been too few and too small (including a total of just 84 patients) to allow any conclusions *(43)*. Currently, active cooling in patients with acute ischemic stroke can therefore be recommended only in the context of a clinical trial.

Stroke Unit

Patients with ischemic stroke should be admitted to a specialized stroke unit. Multidisciplinary treatment of 1,000 patients in a stroke unit saves 56 patients from death or severe disability as compared to treatment on a general medical or neurological ward *(44)*. As there are no contraindications for treatment on a stroke unit, this benefit probably applies to all stroke patients who are admitted to hospital. The strength of a stroke unit is not its specific location in the hospital, but the balanced and integrated approach of a well-trained team consisting of a physician with a specific interest in stroke, a rehabilitation specialist, specialized nurses, physiotherapists, occupational therapists, speech therapists, and preferably also of a social worker, a dietician, a neuropsychologist, and a specialist in vascular medicine. This team should work according to established protocols that are based on the local situation and possibilities. Care on a stroke unit has been associated with a shorter stay in the hospital than care on a general neurological ward *(45)*.

MEDICAL COMPLICATIONS

Although the effectiveness of a stroke unit is largely based on optimal general care which largely consists of the prevention and treatment of complications, only few clinical trials have tested the effects of prevention and treatment of specific complications on patients with acute ischemic stroke.

Venous Thrombosis and Pulmonary Embolism

In an older study, deep venous thrombosis occurred in about 50% of the patients with severe stroke and was confined mainly to the paretic leg *(46)*. Severe leg weakness, a shortened activated partial thromboplastin time *(47)*, and atrial fibrillation *(48)* have been associated with an increased risk of deep venous thrombosis. The complication is feared mainly because of the risk of pulmonary embolism, which has an estimated incidence of about 1% *(49)*.

Overall, prophylactic administration of unfractionated heparin, low molecular weight heparin, or heparinoid is associated with an 81% reduction in deep venous thrombosis as detected by I^{125} fibrinogen scanning or a venogram (50).

Compression stockings are recommended for patients who cannot receive anticoagulants. Although early mobilization is not an absolute guarantee against venous thromboembolism, patients should be mobilized as early as possible.

For stroke patients with deep venous thrombosis or pulmonary embolism, the use of therapeutic anticoagulation should be weighed against the risk of intracranial hemorrhagic complications. The use of a vena cava filter may be considered in patients with absolute contraindications to anticoagulation (22).

Seizures

Between 5 and 10% of patients with ischemic stroke suffer from epileptic seizures in the first week and about 3% within the first 24 h (51, 52). Early seizures are more often partial than generalized and status epilepticus is uncommon. Most seizures occur in patients with cardioembolic stroke and in patients with cortical involvement (52). Acute seizures are associated with a higher mortality at 30 days after stroke, but seizures are not an independent risk factor of mortality at 30 days after stroke (52). Post-stroke seizures are not associated with a higher mortality or worse functional outcome. The natural history of early seizures after stroke is unknown, as most patients are promptly treated with anticonvulsants. About 1 out of every 11 patient with an early epileptic seizure develops epilepsy within 10 years after stroke onset (51).

In case of a seizure in the acute phase of stroke, administration of anticonvulsant drugs to prevent recurrent seizures has been recommended, although this is not evidence based. In case of an early seizure without recurrences the anticonvulsants can probably be stopped after the first weeks.

Hyperglycemia

In the first 12 h after stroke onset, plasma glucose concentrations are elevated in up to 68% of patients, of whom more than half are not known to have diabetes mellitus (53). An initially high blood glucose concentration in patients with acute stroke is a predictor of poor outcome (53, 54). Lowering blood glucose in the acute stage of ischemic stroke has been in only one phase III clinical trial that was terminated prematurely. This trial did not show a benefit on long-term functional outcome of early administration of insulin, but the reduction in serum glucose achieved was only small *(55)*. For more information on hyperglycemia in the acute phase of stroke, the reader is referred to *Treatment of Hyperglycemia*, Chapter 9.

Hypertension

Acute stroke is associated with a blood pressure higher than 170/110 mmHg in about two thirds of patients. Blood pressure falls spontaneously in the majority of patients during the first week after stroke. High blood pressure during the acute phase of stroke has been associated with a poor outcome *(56)*.

It is unclear how blood pressure should be managed during the acute phase of ischemic stroke. Randomized trials are needed to determine the effect of lowering blood pressure in the acute stage of stroke. Meanwhile, routine lowering of the blood pressure is not recommended in the first week after stroke, except for extremely elevated values on repeated measurements (systolic pressure >220 mmHg or diastolic pressure >120 mmHg) or in patients with cardiac ischemia, cardiac failure, or dissection of the aorta. In patients who have elevated blood pressure and are otherwise eligible for intravenous or intra-arterial thrombolysis, very careful management of blood pressure is necessary, at least during the first 24 h. If systolic blood pressure rises above 185 mmHg or if diastolic blood pressure rises above 110 mmHg, hypertension should be treated by means of intravenous labetalol or, in refractory cases, by means of intravenous sodium nitroprusside *(22)*.

Dysphagia

Swallowing difficulties have been found in 27–50% of the patients in the first days after stroke *(57)*. Although dysphagia is more common in patients with lower brain stem lesions it is found on admission in one third of conscious patients with unilateral hemispheric stroke, especially when aphasia and facial weakness are present. In most patients, dysphagia resolves spontaneously by the end of the first week, and at 1 month only a minority of survivors still has swallowing problems *(58)*. Patients with impaired swallowing have a high risk of aspiration and chest infection and a poor nutritional state. Dysphagia is associated with an increased risk of death and poor functional outcome *(57)*.

Swallowing of a small amount of water is the best early screening tool for dysphagia, but sometimes fiber optic endoscopy is necessary to assess safety of swallowing *(57)*. A Cochrane Review did not find any benefit from swallowing therapy in the acute stage of stroke *(59)*. In dysphagic stroke patients, no statistically significant effects on long-term functional outcome were observed from early tube feeding or early percutaneous endoscopic gastrostomy (PEG) feeding *(60)*.

Pressure Sores

During the first week after stroke onset, pressure sores are rare. They have been found in less than 1% of patients treated in a stroke unit *(49)*, but in 27% of stroke patients in long-term units *(61)*. Pressure sores can cause considerable pain and usually slow the patient's recovery. Immobilization is the most important cause. Previous stroke, previous trauma, and cognitive decline are also associated with an increased risk of pressure sores *(61)*. Prevention relies on an early and accurate assessment of the risk to develop pressure sores. Prevention should include regular turning of the patient, relief of bony prominences, early mobilization, and adequate nutrition *(62)*.

Bladder Dysfunction

Urinary incontinence affects up to 60% of stroke patients admitted to hospital, with 25% still having problems on hospital discharge, and around 15% remaining incontinent at 1 year. The most common cause is detrusor hyperreflexia as a direct consequence of stroke. Impaired sphincter control, preexisting bladder outflow obstruction, constipation, immobility, confusion, impaired consciousness, and urinary tract infection may also play a role *(63)*.

Data from the available trials are insufficient to guide continence care after stroke. It has been suggested that structured assessment and management of care and specialist continence nursing may reduce urinary incontinence and related symptoms after stroke *(63)*. Nursing strategies, such as scheduled voiding, intermittent catheterization, or the use of condom catheters in men, are useful first-line treatments *(64)*. Whenever possible, indwelling catheters should be avoided because of the risk of urinary tract infections. When incontinence persists, urodynamic studies are helpful in establishing the cause. After urological consultation, refractory bladder hyperreflexia can be treated with anticholinergic or antispasmodic medications and overflow incontinence with cholinergic drugs *(64)*.

Fever

Between 22 and 43% of patients develop fever or subfebrile temperatures during the first days after stroke *(42, 65)*. In most cases, pulmonary or urinary tract infections are the cause *(66)*, but fever may also exist without signs of an overt infection *(42, 65)*. Fever is more common in patients with larger infarcts *(65)*. High body temperature in the first days after stroke is associated with poor outcome *(42, 67)*. There is currently no evidence from randomized trials to support the routine lowering of body temperature above 37°C. Until data from the randomized Paracetamol (Acetaminophen) In Stroke Trial *(68)* become available, at least the source of fever should be determined and treated, and antipyretics may be given to patients with a body temperature of more than 38°C.

Mood Disorders

Up to 40% of patients develop depressive symptoms in the first 3 weeks after stroke, of which about a quarter are diagnosed as having a major depression *(69)*. There is probably no relation between the location of the stroke and the risk to develop depression. Post-stroke depression is associated with an increased risk of poor functional outcome and a reduced quality of life *(70)*.

Post-stroke depression may be treated with a serotonin reuptake inhibitor or in case of insufficient response with a tricyclic antidepressant *(71)*. Unfortunately, mood disorders are often not recognized in stroke patients and are therefore too often left untreated.

Delirium

The incidence of delirium after stroke has been reported between 13 and 48%. Delirium is more common after stroke than after myocardial ischemia, suggesting a causal relation between brain damage and the occurrence of delirium *(72)*. Specific stroke types, such as large supratentorial infarcts, may be more likely to precipitate delirium than others. In addition, case reports have suggested that delirium may be associated with specific lesions in the thalamus and caudate nucleus *(73)*. Age, pre-existing cognitive impairment or dementia, psychiatric disease, severe chronic medical illness, social isolation, previous delirium, poor vision, severe acute illness, polypharmacy, and treatment on an intensive care unit all precipitate delirium. Moreover, extensive motor impairment, neglect, and impaired vision are associated with a higher risk to develop delirium. In stroke patients, delirium is associated with a worse functional outcome, a higher mortality, a longer stay in the hospital, and an increased incidence of post-stroke dementia *(72)*.

No trials concerning treatment of delirium in acute stroke have been performed. Therefore, prevention and treatment of delirium after stroke is not evidence based and recommendations are similar to management of delirium in patients with other diseases. General management should include identification and elimination of precipitating factors. Haloperidol is the drug most frequently used, because of minor anticholinergic effects, few active metabolites, and a small chance of sedation and hypotension. Risperidone and olanzapine may be safer than haloperidol, but experience with these drugs in the treatment of delirium after stroke is limited *(72)*.

SECONDARY PREVENTION

Secondary prevention after a transient ischemic attack or ischemic stroke should be aimed at reduction of the chance of future cardiovascular complications. The main issue in secondary prevention is rigorous control of vascular risk factors such as hypertension, hyperlipidemia, smoking, and overweight. In patients with a cardiac source of embolism, coumarins should be the first choice *(74)*, whereas in other patients platelet aggregation inhibitors should be prescribed *(75)*. The combination of aspirin and dipyridamole is often used as the first-choice antiplatelet regime *(76)*, but clopidogrel recently has been demonstrated to be equally effective *(77)*. The combination of aspirin and clopidogrel should probably be avoided because of a too high risk of bleeding *(77)*. Both statins and antihypertensive agents have also been shown to reduce the risk of cardiovascular complications in a broad range of patients with TIA or non-disabling stroke of arterial origin *(78, 79)*.

Carotid surgery should be considered in case of a significant symptomatic stenosis of the internal carotid artery *(80)*. Carotid stenting should be performed in the context of a clinical trial.

REFERENCES

1. Lopez AD, Mathers CD, Ezzati M, Jamison DT, Murray CJ. Global and regional burden of disease and risk factors, 2001: systematic analysis of population health data. Lancet 2006; 367:1747–1757.
2. Feigin VL, Lawes CM, Bennett DA, Anderson CS. Stroke epidemiology: a review of population-based studies of incidence, prevalence, and case-fatality in the late 20th century. Lancet Neurol 2003; 2:43–53.
3. Strong K, Mathers C, Bonita R. Preventing stroke: saving lives around the world. Lancet Neurol 2007; 6:182–187.
4. Sudlow CL, Warlow CP. Comparable studies of the incidence of stroke and its pathological types: results from an international collaboration. International Stroke Incidence Collaboration. Stroke 1997; 28:491–499.
5. Hirtz D, Thurman DJ, Gwinn-Hardy K, Mohamed M, Chaudhuri AR, Zalutsky R. How common are the "common" neurologic disorders? Neurology 2007; 68:326–337.
6. Truelsen T, Piechowski-Jozwiak B, Bonita R, Mathers C, Bogousslavsky J, Boysen G. Stroke incidence and prevalence in Europe: a review of available data. Eur J Neurol 2006; 13: 581–598.
7. Norrving B. Long-term prognosis after lacunar infarction. Lancet Neurol 2003; 2:238–245.
8. Hacke W, Schwab S, Horn M, Spranger M, De Georgia M, von Kummer R. 'Malignant' middle cerebral artery infarction. Clinical course and prognostic signs. Arch Neurol 1996; 53:309–315.
9. Van der Worp HB, Van Gijn J. Clinical practice. Acute ischemic stroke. N Engl J Med 2007; 357:572–579.
10. Dirnagl U, Iadecola C, Moskowitz MA. Pathobiology of ischaemic stroke: an integrated view. Trends Neurosci 1999; 22:391–397.

11. Muir KW, Buchan A, von Kummer R, Rother J, Baron JC. Imaging of acute stroke. Lancet Neurol 2006; 5:755–768.

12. Wintermark M, Flanders AE, Velthuis B, et al. Perfusion-CT assessment of infarct core and penumbra: receiver operating characteristic curve analysis in 130 patients suspected of acute hemispheric stroke. Stroke 2006; 37:979–985.

13. Chalela JA, Kidwell CS, Nentwich LM, et al. Magnetic resonance imaging and computed tomography in emergency assessment of patients with suspected acute stroke: a prospective comparison. Lancet 2007; 369:293–298.

14. Seitz RJ, Meisel S, Weller P, Junghans U, Wittsack HJ, Siebler M. Initial ischemic event: perfusion-weighted MR imaging and apparent diffusion coefficient for stroke evolution. Radiology 2005; 237:1020–1028.

15. Sobesky J, Zaro WO, Lehnhardt FG, et al. Does the mismatch match the penumbra? Magnetic resonance imaging and positron emission tomography in early ischemic stroke. Stroke 2005; 36:980–985.

16. The National Institute of Neurological Disorders and Stroke rt-PA Stroke Study Group. Tissue plasminogen activator for acute ischemic stroke. N Engl J Med 1995; 333:1581–1587.

17. Kwiatkowski TG, Libman RB, Frankel M, et al. Effects of tissue plasminogen activator for acute ischemic stroke at one year. N Engl J Med 1999; 340:1781–1787.

18. Demaerschalk BM, Yip TR. Economic benefit of increasing utilization of intravenous tissue plasminogen activator for acute ischemic stroke in the United States. Stroke 2005; 36: 2500–2503.

19. Hacke W, Donnan G, Fieschi C, et al. Association of outcome with early stroke treatment: pooled analysis of ATLANTIS, ECASS, and NINDS rt-PA stroke trials. Lancet 2004; 363:768–774.

20. Hacke W, Kaste M, Bluhmki E, et al. Thrombolysis with alteplase 3 to 4.5 hours after acute ischemic stroke. N Engl J Med 2008; 359:1317–1329.

21. Khatri P, Wechsler LR, Broderick JP. Intracranial hemorrhage associated with revascularization therapies. Stroke 2007; 38:431–440.

22. Adams HP, Jr., del Zoppo G, Alberts MJ, et al. Guidelines for the early management of adults with ischemic stroke: a guideline from the American Heart Association/American Stroke Association Stroke Council, Clinical Cardiology Council, Cardiovascular Radiology and Intervention Council, and the Atherosclerotic Peripheral Vascular Disease and Quality of Care Outcomes in Research Interdisciplinary Working Groups: the American Academy of Neurology affirms the value of this guideline as an educational tool for neurologists. Stroke 2007; 38:1655–1711.

23. Smith EE, Abdullah AR, Petkovska I, Rosenthal E, Koroshetz WJ, Schwamm LH. Poor outcomes in patients who do not receive intravenous tissue plasminogen activator because of mild or improving ischemic stroke. Stroke 2005; 36:2497–2499.

24. Demchuk AM, Khan F, Hill MD, et al. Importance of leukoaraiosis on CT for tissue plasminogen activator decision making: evaluation of the NINDS rt-PA Stroke Study. Cerebrovasc Dis 2008; 26:120–125.

25. Furlan A, Higashida R, Wechsler L, et al. Intra-arterial prourokinase for acute ischemic stroke. The PROACT II Study: A randomized controlled trial. JAMA 1999; 282:2003–2011.

26. Ogawa A, Mori E, Minematsu K, et al. Randomized trial of intraarterial infusion of urokinase within 6 hours of middle cerebral artery stroke: the middle cerebral artery embolism local fibrinolytic intervention trial (MELT) Japan. Stroke 2007; 38:2633–2639.

27. Macleod MR, Davis SM, Mitchell PJ, et al. Results of a multicentre, randomised controlled trial of intra-arterial urokinase in the treatment of acute posterior circulation ischaemic stroke. Cerebrovasc Dis 2005; 20:12–17.

28. Lindsberg PJ, Mattle HP. Therapy of basilar artery occlusion: a systematic analysis comparing intra-arterial and intravenous thrombolysis. Stroke 2006; 37:922–928.

29. Sacco RL, Chong JY, Prabhakaran S, Elkind MS. Experimental treatments for acute ischaemic stroke. Lancet 2007; 369:331–341.

30. Smith WS, Sung G, Saver J, et al. Mechanical thrombectomy for acute ischemic stroke: final results of the Multi MERCI trial. Stroke 2008; 39:1205–1212.
31. Camerlingo M, Salvi P, Belloni G, Gamba T, Cesana BM, Mamoli A. Intravenous heparin started within the first 3 hours after onset of symptoms as a treatment for acute nonlacunar hemispheric cerebral infarctions. Stroke 2005; 36:2415–2420.
32. Chamorro A, Busse O, Obach V, et al. The rapid anticoagulation prevents ischemic damage study in acute stroke–final results from the writing committee. Cerebrovasc Dis 2005; 19: 402–404.
33. International Stroke Trial Collaborative Group. The International Stroke Trial (IST): a randomised trial of aspirin, subcutaneous heparin, or both, or neither among 19,435 patients with acute ischaemic stroke. Lancet 1997; 349:1569–1581.
34. CAST (Chinese Acute Stroke Trial) Collaborative Group. CAST: randomised placebo-controlled trial of early aspirin use in 20,000 patients with acute ischaemic stroke. Lancet 1997; 349:1641–169.
35. Hofmeijer J, Van der Worp HB, Kappelle LJ. Treatment of space-occupying hemispheric infarction. Crit Care Med 2003; 31:617–625.
36. Berrouschot J, Sterker M, Bettin S, Köster J, Schneider D. Mortality of space-occupying ('malignant') middle cerebral artery infarction under conservative intensive care. Intensive Care Med 1998; 24:620–623.
37. Vahedi K, Hofmeijer J, Juettler E, et al. Early decompressive surgery in malignant infarction of the middle cerebral artery: a pooled analysis of three randomised controlled trials. Lancet Neurol 2007; 6:215–222.
38. O'Collins VE, Macleod MR, Donnan GA, Horky LL, van der Worp BH, Howells DW. 1,026 experimental treatments in acute stroke. Ann Neurol 2006; 59:467–477.
39. Van der Worp HB, Sena ES, Donnan GA, Howells DW, Macleod MR. Hypothermia in animal models of acute ischaemic stroke: a systematic review and meta-analysis. Brain 2007; 130:3063–3074.
40. Bernard SA, Gray TW, Buist MD, et al. Treatment of comatose survivors of out-of-hospital cardiac arrest with induced hypothermia. N Engl J Med 2002; 346:557–563.
41. Hypothermia after Cardiac Arrest Study Group. Mild therapeutic hypothermia to improve the neurologic outcome after cardiac arrest. N Engl J Med 2002; 346:549–556.
42. den HH, van der WB, van GM, Dippel D. Therapeutic hypothermia in acute ischemic stroke. Expert Rev Neurother 2007; 7:155–164.
43. den Hertog MH, Van der Worp HB, Tseng M, Dippel DWJ. Cooling therapy for acute stroke. Cochrane Database Syst Rev 2008.
44. Stroke Unit Trialists' Collaboration. Organised inpatient (stroke unit) care for stroke. Cochrane Database Syst Rev 2002;(1):CD000197.
45. Indredavik B, Fjaertoft H, Ekeberg G, Loge AD, Morch B. Benefit of an extended stroke unit service with early supported discharge: A randomized, controlled trial. Stroke 2000; 31: 2989–2994.
46. Warlow C, Ogston D, Douglas AS. Deep venous thrombosis of the legs after strokes. B M J 1976; 1:1178–1183.
47. Landi G, D'Angelo A, Boccardi E, et al. Venous thromboembolism in acute stroke. Prognostic importance of hypercoagulability. Arch Neurol 1992; 49:279–283.
48. Noel P, Gregoire F, Capon A, Lehert P. Atrial fibrillation as a risk factor for deep venous thrombosis and pulmonary emboli in stroke patients. Stroke 1991; 22:760–762.
49. Indredavik B, Rohweder G, Naalsund E, Lydersen S. Medical complications in a comprehensive stroke unit and an early supported discharge service. Stroke 2008; 39: 414–420.
50. Sandercock PAG, van den Belt AGM, Lindley RI, Slattery J. Antithrombotic therapy in acute ischaemic stroke: an overview of the completed randomised trials. J Neurol Neurosurg Psychiatry 1993; 56:17–25.
51. So EL, Annegers JF, Hauser WA, O'Brien PC, Whisnant JP. Population-based study of seizure disorders after cerebral infarction. Neurology 1996; 46:350–355.

52. Szaflarski JP, Rackley AY, Kleindorfer DO, et al. Incidence of seizures in the acute phase of stroke: a population-based study. Epilepsia 2008; 49:974–981.
53. Toni D, Sacchetti ML, Argentino C, et al. Does hyperglycaemia play a role on the outcome of acute ischaemic stroke patients? J Neurol 1992; 239:382–386.
54. McCormick MT, Muir KW, Gray CS, Walters MR. Management of hyperglycemia in acute stroke: how, when, and for whom? Stroke 2008; 39:2177–2185.
55. Gray CS, Hildreth AJ, Sandercock PA, et al. Glucose-potassium-insulin infusions in the management of post-stroke hyperglycaemia: the UK Glucose Insulin in Stroke Trial (GIST-UK). Lancet Neurol 2007; 6:397–406.
56. Willmot M, Leonardi-Bee J, Bath PM. High blood pressure in acute stroke and subsequent outcome: a systematic review. Hypertension 2004; 43:18–24.
57. Carnaby G, Hankey GJ, Pizzi J. Behavioural intervention for dysphagia in acute stroke: a randomised controlled trial. Lancet Neurol 2006; 5:31–37.
58. Ramsey DJ, Smithard DG, Kalra L. Early assessments of dysphagia and aspiration risk in acute stroke patients. Stroke 2003; 34:1252–1257.
59. Bath PM, Bath FJ, Smithard DG. Interventions for dysphagia in acute stroke. Cochrane Database Syst Rev 2000;(2):CD000323.
60. Dennis MS, Lewis SC, Warlow C. Effect of timing and method of enteral tube feeding for dysphagic stroke patients (FOOD): a multicentre randomised controlled trial. Lancet 2005; 365:764–772.
61. Capon A, Pavoni N, Mastromattei A, Di Lallo D. Pressure ulcer risk in long-term units: prevalence and associated factors. J Adv Nurs 2007; 58:263–272.
62. Capon A, Lehert P, Opsomer L. Naftidrofuryl in the treatment of subacute stroke. J Cardiovasc Pharmacol 1990; 16(Suppl 3):S62–S66.
63. Thomas LH, Cross S, Barrett J, et al. Treatment of urinary incontinence after stroke in adults. Cochrane Database Syst Rev 2008;(1):CD004462.
64. Nakayama H, Jorgensen HS, Pedersen PM, Raaschou HO, Olsen TS. Prevalence and risk factors of incontinence after stroke. The Copenhagen Stroke Study. Stroke 1997; 28:58–62.
65. Azzimondi G, Bassein L, Nonino F, et al. Fever in acute stroke worsens prognosis. A prospective study. Stroke 1995; 26:2040–2043.
66. Emsley HC, Hopkins SJ. Acute ischaemic stroke and infection: recent and emerging concepts. Lancet Neurol 2008; 7:341–353.
67. Reith J, Jørgensen S, Pedersen PM, et al. Body temperature in acute stroke: relation to stroke severity, infarct size, mortality, and outcome. Lancet 1996; 347:422–425.
68. van Breda EJ, Van der Worp HB, van Gemert HM, et al. PAIS: paracetamol (acetaminophen) in stroke; protocol for a randomized, double blind clinical trial [ISCRTN 74418480]. BMC Cardiovasc Disord 2005; 5:24.
69. Nys GM, van Zandvoort MJ, Van der Worp HB, de Haan EH, de Kort PL, Kappelle LJ. Early depressive symptoms after stroke: neuropsychological correlates and lesion characteristics. J Neurol Sci 2005; 228:27–33.
70. Gabaldon L, Fuentes B, Frank-Garcia A, ez-Tejedor E. Poststroke depression: importance of its detection and treatment. Cerebrovasc Dis 2007; 24(Suppl 1):181–188.
71. Jorge RE, Robinson RG, Arndt S, Starkstein S. Mortality and poststroke depression: a placebo-controlled trial of antidepressants. Am J Psychiatry 2003; 160:1823–1829.
72. Oldenbeuving AW, de Kort PLM, Jansen BPW, Roks G, Kappelle LJ. Delirium in acute stroke: a review. Int J Stroke 2007; 2:270–275.
73. Henon H, Lebert F, Durieu I, et al. Confusional state in stroke: relation to preexisting dementia, patient characteristics, and outcome. Stroke 1999; 30:773–779.
74. EAFT (European Atrial Fibrillation Trial) Study Group. Secondary prevention in nonrheumatic atrial fibrillation after transient ischaemic attack or minor stroke. Lancet 1993; 342:1255–1262.
75. Sacco RL, Adams R, Albers G, et al. Guidelines for prevention of stroke in patients with ischemic stroke or transient ischemic attack: a statement for healthcare professionals from the American Heart Association/American Stroke Association Council on Stroke: co-sponsored

by the Council on Cardiovascular Radiology and Intervention: the American Academy of Neurology affirms the value of this guideline. Stroke 2006; 37:577–617.

76. Halkes PH, Van Gijn J, Kappelle LJ, Koudstaal PJ, Algra A. Aspirin plus dipyridamole versus aspirin alone after cerebral ischaemia of arterial origin (ESPRIT): randomised controlled trial. Lancet 2006; 367:1665–1673.

77. Sacco RL, Diener HC, Yusuf S, et al. Aspirin and extended-release dipyridamole versus clopidogrel for recurrent stroke. N Engl J Med 2008; 359:1238–1251.

78. Heart Protection Study Collaborative Group. MRC/BHF Heart Protection Study of cholesterol lowering with simvastatin in 20536 high-risk individuals: a randomised placebo-controlled trial. Lancet 2002; 360:7–22.

79. PROGRESS Collaborative Group. Randomised trial of a perindopril-based blood-pressure-lowering regimen among 6,105 individuals with previous stroke or transient ischaemic attack. Lancet 2001; 358:1033–1041.

80. Rothwell PM, Eliasziw M, Gutnikov SA, et al. Analysis of pooled data from the randomised controlled trials of endarterectomy for symptomatic carotid stenosis. Lancet 2003; 361: 107–116.

4

Neuropsychological Assessment

Roy P.C. Kessels and Augustina M.A. Brands

CONTENTS

ABSTRACT

In this chapter, methodological aspects of neuropsychological assessment will be discussed. First, a brief theoretical neuropsychological framework is presented related to the study of brain–behavior interactions. We will focus on the use of global screening tests, specific neuropsychological tests, computerized assessment, and the development of a test battery that is optimized for use in young and older diabetes patients. The important cognitive domains will be introduced in relation to their assessment: intelligence, executive function, learning and memory, attention and working memory, perception, language, and information-processing speed. The chapter will address psychometric aspects, such as validity and reliability, as well as sensitivity, which are important for the interpretation of test results. Other psychological constructs that are potential confounders for cognitive performance in diabetes patients are discussed, such as coping, personality, motivation, and mood. Finally, the chapter will discuss the clinical significance of statistically significant differences between cases and controls, both with respect to clinical decision-making in individual patients and on group level.

From: *Contemporary Diabetes: Diabetes and the Brain*
Edited by: G. J. Biessels, J. A. Luchsinger (eds.), DOI 10.1007/978-1-60327-850-8_4
© Humana Press, a part of Springer Science+Business Media, LLC 2009

Key words: Neuropsychology; Assessment; Psychological Test; Cognition; Dementia; Aging; Personality.

INTRODUCTION

Neuropsychology as a research field examines the interplay between brain function and dysfunction and behavior and cognition. In short, neuropsychologists study the cognitive processes that are involved in thinking, planning, remembering, talking, walking, seeing, and feeling and their neural correlates. These cognitive processes can be impaired following brain disease or dysfunction, and these deficits may have great impact on everyday function of patients. Moreover, these deficits also provide further insight into theoretical aspects of human information processing and the workings of the human brain in relation to pathophysiological processes. To study brain–behavior interactions, the measurement of cognition is crucial. Complex theories exist on the processes that are involved in, for example, memory and language, but these individual processes can rarely be assessed with specific tests or tasks.

Tests that are used in clinical neuropsychology in most cases examine one or more aspects of cognitive domains, which are theoretical constructs in which a multitude of cognitive processes are involved. For example, a memory test in which a series of words has to be remembered aims to assess verbal memory function, as part of the cognitive domain memory. While such a test typically involves attention, encoding, consolidation, storage and retrieval of information, it also relies on auditory perception and speech. Furthermore, some cognitive domains are clearly not a unitary construct, but can be subdivided into multiple cognitive functions. For instance, the cognitive domain executive functioning refers to the goal setting, generation, planning, monitoring, inhibition, and shifting of behavior. By definition, a subdivision in cognitive domains is arbitrary, and many different classifications exist. We will use the following classification of cognitive domains: intelligence, long-term memory and learning, working memory, executive function, attention and speed of information processing, praxis and motor function, language, and perception *(1)*.

ASSESSMENT OF COGNITIVE FUNCTION

In assessing cognitive deficits, two important questions must be answered. Firstly, the question is whether an individual patient, or a patient group, has cognitive dysfunction compared to a reference group. Secondly, we need to look at the pattern of impairment: whether selective deficits of one or more cognitive processes – or domains – exist. By establishing this pattern of cognitive deficits, we can subsequently relate this information to cerebral dysfunction in general or specific brain lesions. Although neuropsychological assessment in isolation can neither determine whether patients have "organic" lesions or not, nor accurately identify the side or site of the lesion, it provides information about cognitive function that can be interpreted in conjunction with other variables, such as neuroimaging findings or clinical history. For example, a person who performs poorly on a memory test does not necessarily have a memory disorder, since other non-cognitive factors may contribute to the task performance as well, such as motivation, or impairments in other cognitive domains, such as an attention deficit. However, if we know that this person is over 75 years, has had diabetes type 2 for over 15 years, shows a decline that has been progressive since approximately 2 years and that interferes with everyday functioning, and shows profound medial temporal lobe atrophy as visible on MRI, it is likely that this patient indeed has a memory disorder and can be classified as having dementia. However, if we know this person is a 43-year-old woman who has had diabetes type 1 since childhood, has recently been divorced, and shows signs of major depression, it is likely that other factors determine the low performance on this memory test that just the memory function or cerebral dysfunction.

This chapter will focus on ways to measure cognitive function. First, we will discuss the major cognitive domains and focus on neuropsychological tests that can be applied to measure these specific cognitive domains. Furthermore, we provide information about test batteries that have been developed to assess multiple cognitive functions, often in a computerized way. Next, we will discuss screening instruments that can be used to determine whether there is evidence for cognitive decline in individuals. Finally, we discuss the most important confounding factors in neuropsychological assessment of diabetes-related cognitive decline and we will illustrate the issue of clinical relevance.

Neuropsychological Tests

Since "cognition" is not a unitary construct, specific tests have been developed that can be used to assess the different cognitive domains in a wide range of neuropsychological syndromes. Most tests have been designed for application in patients and healthy adults of a broad age range. Neuropsychological function tests are aimed at the assessment of the extent of the cognitive deficit, irrespective of the patient's medical diagnosis, rather than aimed at identifying and classifying people using a strict cut-off score. This makes it possible to measure even mild cognitive decrements and reliably examine performance differences in longitudinal designs using the same tasks. However, for a test to be recommended, several criteria must be met. First, a test must have adequate reliability: the test must yield similar outcomes when applied over multiple test sessions, i.e., have good test–retest reliability. A potential problem in this respect can be the occurrence of practice effects. A test performance can be higher at a second administration compared to the first, because the participant may simply remember specific items from the previous session (e.g., the to be remembered words) or is generally more familiar with the examination procedure (i.e., he or she knows what can be expected during the examination and may consequently be less nervous). Furthermore, the interobserver reliability is important, in that the test must have a standardized assessment procedure and is scored in the same manner by different examiners.

Second, the test must have adequate validity. Here, different forms of validity are important. Content validity is established by expert raters with respect to item formulation, item selection, etc. Construct validity refers to the underlying theoretical construct that the test is assumed to measure. To assess construct validity, both convergent and divergent validities are important. Convergent validity refers to the amount of agreement between a given test and other tests that measure the same function. In turn, a test with a good divergent validity correlates minimally with tests that measure other cognitive functions. Moreover, predictive validity (or criterion validity) is related to the degree of correlation between the test score and an external criterion, for example, the correlation between a cognitive test and functional status.

One major problem in selecting neuropsychological tests is that numerous tests meet the above-mentioned criteria (1, 2). While neuropsychologists are often criticized for their lack of consensus on which tests to use in clinical assessment, this situation is no different from radiologists using different brands and types of MR scanners or even measuring the height of an object with different spring rules. Each specific test has its own strengths and weaknesses, but similar test paradigms measure similar cognitive processes. It is not the aim of the current chapter to provide a comprehensive overview of neuropsychological tests. Rather, we briefly introduce different paradigms that are generally accepted to assess specific cognitive domains.

Intelligence

Intelligence is a theoretically ill-defined construct. In general, it refers to the ability to think in an abstract manner and solve new problems. Typically, two forms of intelligence are distinguished, crystallized intelligence (academic skills and knowledge that one has acquired during schooling) and fluid intelligence (the ability to solve new problems). Crystallized intelligence is better preserved in patients with brain disease than fluid intelligence *(3)*. Intelligence tests have formed the basis of modern psychometrics. In the late nineteenth century, psychologists were interested in individual differences of mental ability resulting from the then-upcoming Darwinist view on human function. Intelligence tests are often extensive test batteries comprised of many different tasks measuring a broad range of mental functions, such as arithmetic, memory, information-processing speed, abstract reasoning, verbal skills, and visuospatial functions. The performance on the different subtests is transformed into a deviation intelligence quotient (IQ) that provides information on the individual's intelligence level in relation to the general population. Examples of widely used intelligence tests are the Wechsler Adult Intelligence Scale (WAIS; currently in its fourth edition) Test *(4)* and the Kaufman Adult Intelligence Test (KAIT) *(5)*. From a neuropsychological viewpoint, the concept of intelligence as a unitary construct (often referred to as *g-factor*) does not provide valuable information, since deficits in specific cognitive functions may be averaged out in the total IQ score. Thus, in most neuropsychological studies, intelligence tests are included because of specific subtests that are assumed to measure specific cognitive functions, and the performance profile is analyzed rather than considering the IQ measure as a compound score in isolation.

Since intelligence test batteries generally take a long time to administer (1 2 h), in many situations the intelligence level must be estimated. This can be done in different manners. Educational background, vocation, general functioning, and demographic variables may not always provide valid information about an individual's premorbid intellectual function. Therefore, tests have been developed that estimate the level of premorbid intelligence by assessing crystallized intellectual functions, such as a person's vocabulary. An example of a widely used test to measure premorbid intelligence level is the National Adult Reading Test (NART) *(6)*. Premorbid intelligence level can also be used to match patient and control groups. Current fluid intelligence is often assessed by non-verbal tests that measure problem solving, such as the Raven Progressive Matrices *(7)*.

Long-Term Memory and Learning

Memory refers to the ability to encode, store, and retrieve information. Episodic memory is related to memory for personal events and facts, which are closely linked to the context in which the information was acquired. This may entail autobiographical memories, such as remembering a wedding day, or memory for recently acquired information, such as words on a list or pictures presented in a test session. Semantic memory is related to facts or knowledge that are not related to one's personal experience, but are shared by most people within a given cultural system and of which the context of acquisition is lost, such as knowing that Rome is the capital of Italy, that grass is green or that Roosevelt was an American president. Both episodic memory and semantic memory are forms of declarative long-term memory: information is encoded and stored for conscious retrieval at a later point in time (that can be either 1 min later or five decades). Non-declarative forms of long-term memory can refer to procedural knowledge, such as knowing how to ride a bike, which has become automatic and do not require conscious control. Neuropsychological testing in most cases focuses on declarative memory.

Episodic memory is examined by presenting information in one or more trials that has to be remembered as accurately as possible, such as word list, short stories, pictures, or spatial locations. This information has to be either recalled freely (naming as many items as possible that were previously presented) or recognized among distracter items (requiring only a yes/no response). The latter is typically less effortful and easier. Presenting information over subsequent trials makes it possible to determine a learning curve, reflecting the ability to acquire new information, and inclusion of a delayed recall test makes it possible to measure memory decay – the amount of forgetting over time compared to immediate recall. Recognition performance compared to free recall gives information about the ability to retrieve previously stored information. Furthermore, autobiographical memory tests also assess the ability to retrieve previously stored information about one's past. Paired-associate learning measures the ability to form new associations and to use cues to retrieve these associations. Semantic memory is often measured by having participant name as many items of a semantic category as possible, such as animals or professions. Also, tests that require individuals to provide the similarity between two concrete or abstract items rely on semantic memory. The California Verbal Learning Test (CVLT), the Hopkins Verbal Learning Test (HVLT), and the Rey Auditory Verbal Learning Test (RAVLT) are common verbal episodic memory tests (8, 9). The Benton Visual Retention Test (10) and Location Learning Test (11) are examples of non-verbal episodic memory tests. The Wechsler Memory Scale (WMS-IV) is an extensive test battery that assesses most aspects of memory function (12).

Working Memory

Not all information that we encounter must be stored into long-term memory for later retrieval. For example, if we rehearse a telephone number and subsequently dial it on a phone, we often can forget the number as soon as the connection is established. The online maintenance and manipulation of information in the here-and-now is referred to as working memory. Working memory refers to a passive store (often referred to as short-term memory) and processes needed to actively manipulate information held in this passive store. In Baddeley's model of working memory, the active processing component is the central executive that can be distinguished from store systems for verbal and visuospatial information *(13)*. Note that the short-term aspect of working memory refers to the brief period of time that information is maintained and not to memory for recent events (since these are part of long-term memory). Theoretically, working memory is also related to the concept of executive functions: manipulation of the briefly held information requires active control. Moreover, working-memory function is related to information-processing capacity, which is by definition limited.

To measure working-memory processing, tasks are used that are in a span-like format. For example, the digit span task requires the subject to repeat strings of digits of increasing length in the same order as presented. In general, the performance on this task is approximately 7 plus or minus 2 digits, often referred to as the "attention span." To enhance the working-memory load, span tasks often include a more cognitively demanding condition, in which again information is presented, but the participant has to reproduce the information in reverse order. The performance on the backward span is then compared to the forward reproduction to provide an estimate of the executive aspect of working memory next to the passive store capacity. As an alternative for the digit span, spatial span tasks are widely used, which in most cases consist of a board with nine or ten blocks at different positions. Here, the experimenter taps block sequences of increasing length that have to be reproduced by the participant in the same or reverse order (see Fig. 1), in analog of the digit span task.

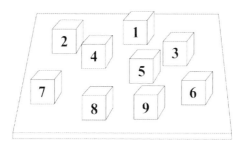

Fig. 1. The Corsi-Block Tapping Task that can be used to determine the spatial span as part of working-memory function *(14)*. The experimenter taps block sequences of gradually increasing length that have to be repeated by the patient in the same order.

Generally, the difference between forward and backward condition on a spatial span task is smaller than on digit span tasks that in most cases result in better forward than backward reproduction *(14)*. Furthermore, several computer tasks exist that also can be applied to assess working-memory capacity, such as the Spatial Working Memory subtest of the CANTAB test battery *(15)*.

Executive Functions

The ability to plan our behavior, set and monitor goals, generate, shift, and inhibit responses is referred to as executive functioning *(16)*. Not a cognitive domain in the strict sense, executive functioning is comprised of various cognitive processes that are crucial for everyday functioning. As a result, executive functioning is difficult to assess with a single test. In turn, executive function tests often address various processes that are important in this domain. For example, the Wisconsin Card Sorting Test aims to measure the planning, shifting, and inhibition of behavior. The participant has to detect a sorting principle for cards that are presented sequentially, using either color, form, or number of stimuli printed on the cards, based on feedback whether a response is correct or not *(17)*. Other executive tests emphasize the ability to generate different types of responses, for example, in fluency tasks or planning and problem-solving behavior, such as the Tower of London Test (see Fig. 2) where a number of balls of different colors have to be transferred according to a set of rules *(18)*. Other tasks assess mental flexibility, i.e., the ability to shift a response according to the task instruction, such as the Trail Making Test (see Fig. 3) *(19)*. Reacting impulsively during testing or showing perseverative responses may also be the result of executive dysfunction. Historically, executive deficits have been linked to prefrontal dysfunction, even to a degree that executive function tests were often regarded as "frontal

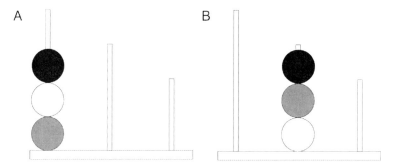

Fig. 2. Example of a trial of the Tower of London Test as a test for planning. (A) Shows the initial situation, (B) the end situation that has to be accomplished by a set of rules: the participants are only allowed to move one ball at a time and the balls must always be moved to another stick.

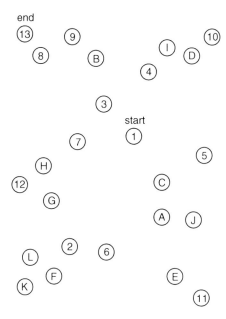

Fig. 3. The Trail Making Test (Part B) as a measure of cognitive flexibility: the participant has to connect numbers and letters in an alternating way using a pencil as fast as possible, i.e., 1-A-2-B-3-C.

tests," but it has become clear that other cortical and subcortical brain areas are equally important for executive behavior. If behavioral disturbances are prominent next to severe executive deficits, patient may be classified as having the "dysexecutive syndrome," but in most patients executive deficits are more subtle.

Executive control processes are also crucial for other cognitive domains. For example, working-memory function is determined by executive function, i.e., the ability to manipulate information online. Also, attention is a domain that is closely related to executive function, for example, in the ability to divide attention over multiple tasks, focus attention, or select information from our environment and the ability to structure and organize information. Furthermore, concepts such as mental effort relate to the ability to generate and control responses. Executive function tests are often highly susceptible to intellectual function and education level, and thus many tests rely on functions that are also included in intelligence batteries, such as working memory, abstract reasoning, and problem solving. Test batteries exist that include different aspects of executive functioning, such as the Behavioral Assessment of the Dysexecutive Syndrome (BADS) battery *(20)*. This test battery also includes the Dysexecutive Questionnaire (DEX) that can be administered to the patient and a significant other, providing information about the patient's ability to monitor his own behavior, which is a crucial aspect of executive function, and provides a measure of insight.

Attention, Speed of Information Processing, and Concentration

Attention is a concept that in general relates to the selection of relevant information from our environment and the suppression of irrelevant information (selective or "focused" attention), the ability to shift attention between tasks (divided attention), and to maintain a state of alertness to incoming stimuli over longer periods of time (concentration and vigilance). Many different structures in the human brain are involved in attentional processing and, consequently, disorders in attention occur frequently after brain disease or damage *(21)*. Related concepts are speed of information processing and alertness.

Selective attention is measured using tests such as the Stroop Color Word Test *(22)* or computer paradigms. For example, the Go/NoGo task is a computerized paradigm in which participants have to respond depending on the type of stimulus that is presented (e.g., button press if a digit is presented and no button press if a letter is shown). The suppression of irrelevant information is closely related to the inhibition process as part of executive function, but the actual lower-level *selection* of relevant (visual) information depends on a parietal network *(23)*. Disorders of the selection stage may include hemispatial neglect, in which patients with right parietal lesions typically ignore stimuli in their left visual field. Neglect can be quantified using cancellation tasks, such as crossing out all "O's" presented on a sheet between distracter letters. Also, specialized test batteries exist, notable the Behavioral Inattention Test (BIT) *(24)*.

Divided attention is typically assessed using dual tasks: participants perform a primary task while doing a secondary task at the same time. For instance, in the Paced Auditory Serial Addition Task (PASAT) a series of digits is presented serially at a fixed rate, and the participant has to add the last two presented digits and say the outcome out loud *(25)*. Thus, the participant is engaged in both performing a mathematical operation (adding) and remembering the last two digits (tapping working-memory function). Dual-tasks performance reflects information-processing capacity, which deteriorates with age. Consequently, dual-task research is also used to assess the automaticity of functions. Divided attention is a process that also engages executive function, specifically the monitoring and shifting of behavior.

The ability to maintain a state of alertness over time (i.e., minutes to even hours) is referred to as concentration or sustained attention. Tests that measure concentration require the participant to continuously perform a repetitive task, for example, crossing out every *d* " between distracter items that are presented in lines on a paper sheet as fast as possible in the d2 Test *(26)*. Vigilance is a concept related to concentration, only here a sustained level of alertness is required to detect *in*frequent events, e.g., which is required when driving in a car and reacting to a child crossing the street. Vigilance is often tested using a Continuous Performance Task, a computerized paradigm in which stimuli (e.g., letters) are presented serially on a computer screen during a longer period of time and the participant is required to only react by button press if one specific stimulus appears on the screen (e.g., the letter "X").

Speed of information processing is a prerequisite for optimal cognitive function. Speed of information processing is not a localized cognitive function, but depends greatly on the integrity of the cerebral network as a whole, the subcortical white matter and the interhemispheric and intrahemispheric connections. It is one of the cognitive functions that clearly declines with age and it is highly susceptible to brain disease or dysfunction of any kind. "Mental slowness," often classified among impairments of attention, can seriously hamper functioning in other cognitive domains, such as (working) memory and executive function. Different aspects of speed of information processing can be studied using reaction-time tasks. To measure alertness, patients have to respond using a button box as quickly as possible to stimuli that appear on a computer screen (simple reaction times or phasic alertness) or have to make multiple responses (e.g., left button press if a digit is shown, right button press if a letter is shown, a so-called choice reaction-time test). Reaction-time tasks are potentially very sensitive to brain dysfunction, but an optimal response also requires good vision that can be impaired by retinopathy, intact basic motor functions (that can be hampered by neuropathy).

Speed of information processing can also be assessed using timed paper-and-pencil tasks. For example, in the Digit Symbol Substitution Test from the WAIS-IV, the participant has to place as many symbols that match certain digits on a paper sheets as possible in a 2-min period. Also, tests such as the Trail Making Test Part A, or the Stroop Color Word Test Part I, provide a gross index of information-processing speed.

Praxis and Motor Function

The planning and performance of goal-directed and purposeful movement is also an important neuropsychological domain. Whereas physical therapists and medical doctors primarily focus on aspects of motor functions such as strength and coordination and occupational therapists study the basic and complex activities of daily living, neuropsychologists do not examine the motor function or the action themselves, but the cognitive processes needed to plan and perform an action. In most cases, these actions refer to movement of the hands and range from fine-motor function, such as mounting pegs on a board as quickly as possible, to symbolic actions (for example, waving goodbye) and behavior that consist of multiple actions, for instance making coffee. Different ways of classifying disorders of praxis, or apraxia, have been described that can be either based on the type of movement or the body part affected. A typical distinction that is made is between ideomotor apraxia and ideational apraxia *(27)*. Ideomotor apraxia is the inability to make movements based on verbal instructions, whereas ideational apraxia is an impairment in making movement sequences, where the movements themselves are unimpaired. Ideomotor apraxia is often assessed by having the patients mirror movements that the examiner makes, ideational apraxia is measured by asking the patient to mime an action (e.g., "pretend that you hold a tooth brush and brush your teeth," "please salute like soldiers do"). A third form of apraxia is visuoconstructive apraxia, in which a patient is unable to make or copy drawings or make a puzzle.

Pegboards can be used to measure psychomotor function, i.e., the ability to perform fine-grained actions, where typically a series of pegs have to be mounted on a board as quickly as possible. The assessment of praxis in a neuropsychological examination also requires the study of executive and visuospatial functions, since impairments in planning and performing (a series of) actions may also be the result of executive deficits, notably impaired planning, or visuospatial dysfunction, such as neglect.

Language

The ability to express ourselves and communicate in a verbal manner is one of the cognitive functions that distinguishes man from other primates. Clinically, a distinction is often made between the expression of language and language comprehension, based on clinical observation of patients with language impairment after stroke that has ultimately led to the distinction between Broca's and Wernicke's aphasia. In a test situation, the expression of language is often measured using fluency tasks (generate as many possible animals or words beginning with "F"), naming tasks, or clinical observation during spontaneous speech. Pathological characteristics of speech may include phonemic paraphasias, i.e., errors that are due to incorrect phonemic processing (such as BLANT instead of PLANT), or semantic paraphasias that are due to semantic confusion (TREE instead of FLOWER). Word finding can be measured using naming tests that require the participant to name pictures of objects or scenes that differ in complexity. Note that language function closely relates to aspects of memory, especially semantic memory, since verbal expression requires adequate access to our semantic knowledge and phonemic lexicon. The comprehension of language can be measured with tests that require the participant to perform written or orally presented instructions. For example, in the Token Test, participants have to perform several tasks using a series of colored tokens (circles and squares), such as "pick up the red circle and place it under the blue square"*(28)*. More extensive language tests exist that address various language functions in great detail, such as the Boston Diagnostic Aphasia Examination *(29)*. Since many language tests have been developed for the diagnosis of aphasia after stroke, performance on these tests in people without aphasia may result in a ceiling performance.

Perception

Perception is a domain that encompasses the ability to process information coming from our senses, which can be visual, auditory, tactile, or chemical (smell and taste). In neuropsychological assessment procedures, testing is in most cases limited to visual and sometimes auditory perception. Visual perception can be measured at different levels of processing. For example, color blindness at a retinal level can be assessed using the Ishihara stimulus cards *(30)*. The Cortical Vision Screening Test (CORVIST) is a test that consists of subtests to measure various aspects of visual perception that can be impaired after cortical lesions, such as acuity, shape and size perception, hue discrimination, spatial perception, and face perception *(31)*. Higher-order perception also involves the ability to address meaning to what we see, e.g., after seeing a cup we immediately recognize it as such (even if we have not seen this particular cup ever before), we can say it is a cup and we know where it is for and how to use it. This requires the integration of visual features to a semantic concept. Perceptual deficits at this level, such as agnosia, can be detected using tests such as the Visual Object and Space Perception battery (VOSP) *(32)* or the Benton Test of Facial Matching *(10)*. Visual-field defects, such as hemianopia, can be detected using the confrontation method or by means of perimetry.

Neuropsychological Test Batteries

Most aforementioned tests aim to address one single cognitive domain or specific processes within that cognitive domain. However, cognitive function can also be assessed using extensive test batteries that have been validated to measure a wide range of cognitive functions. For example, the Halstead–Reitan battery consists of eight tests that assess reasoning, mental flexibility, motor function, perception, and language *(1)*. However, this battery does not include a specific memory test, which has to be added to form a complete neuropsychological battery. Several index scores can then be computed that supposedly provide evidence for brain impairment, lateralization, and localization. However, it should be stressed that cognitive tests alone cannot be used as ultimate proof for organic brain damage, but should be used in combination with more direct measures of cerebral abnormalities, such as neuroimaging.

Some test batteries have been developed for the diagnosis of specific disorders. For example, the US-based Consortium to Establish a Registry for Alzheimer's Disease (CERAD) has developed a test battery for diagnosing Alzheimer's dementia, consisting of neuropsychological tests of memory, language, and praxis, in addition to the MMSE *(33)*. However, this battery has been criticized since it does not include measures of executive function that limits its use outside the field of Alzheimer assessment. Furthermore, thorough assessment of Alzheimer-type cognitive profile also requires additional tests *(34)*. A more extensive test battery is the Repeatable Battery for the Assessment of Neuropsychological Status (RBANS) that was originally also developed for the assessment of dementia *(35)*, but that has gained wider applicability over recent years. A strength of the RBANS is that it makes repeated assessment possible, taking possible learning effects into account.

Most individual tests and test batteries are paper and pencil tasks, but an increasing number of computerized assessment procedures has been developed over the years. While computerized assessment has certain advantages, such as standardized presentation of stimuli, automated response registration, and instant computation of standard scores, there are also important disadvantages. First, there is increasing evidence that computer tasks and paper and pencil tests differ with respect to a number of crucial aspects, such as response mode, stimulus presentation, and possibility for corrections. For example, the performance on three computerized variants of the Wisconsin Card Sorting Test has been compared to the performance on the standard paper and pencil version, showing that the computerized versions were not equivalent with the original paper and pencil test, resulting in differences in test performance within participants *(36)*. The same was found for Raven's Progressive Matrices, in which participants obtained higher IQs in the paper and pencil task than in a computerized version using the same stimuli *(37)*.

When using computer tasks, care must be taken regarding the user interface, since many older people or participants with lower education levels may not be familiar with using an automated test setup. To overcome most disadvantages, a touch-sensitive screen or a button box can be applied to register the responses. With respect to the test scores, many computerized test batteries offer (semi-)automated reporting, with cut-off scores presented for clinical decision-making. However, it should be noted that normative data for computer tests are often of inferior quality compared to paper and pencil tests, often acquired in small samples with little or no attention to the distribution of education level, ethnicity, or confounding factors such as history of neurological or psychiatric illness *(1)*. Still, computerized tests may be a valuable addition to a paper and pencil test battery, but both researchers and clinicians should make sure that a qualitative analysis of the results always provides additional information, not only for clinical differential diagnosis, but also on the quality of the data that are acquired.

Screening Instruments

While extensive neuropsychological testing can be considered as the "gold standard" to assess cognition, detailed assessment of every cognitive domain in all patients is not always feasible in clinical practice. Therefore, brief assessment procedures have been developed over the years that are not optimized for quantifying the performance in cognitive domains, but can be used as initial screen. Most screening instruments are (relatively) short and easy to administer and have been developed for a specific population or neurological condition. Ideally, screening instruments have both a high sensitivity and specificity, not only maximizing the probability of identifying individuals with cognitive decline, but also minimizing the probability of incorrectly classifying an individual as cognitively impaired. The Mini-Mental State Examination (MMSE) is a screening instrument that has been developed to determine whether older adults have cognitive impairments that are in agreement with the clinical criteria for Alzheimer's dementia *(38)*. It consists of a range of items assessing orientation, memory for words, drawing, backward counting, and semantic knowledge, with a maximum score of 30. Cut-off scores have been described that can be used to classify patients as cognitively impaired or having dementia. The MMSE has also been used in research of cognition in diabetes, in most cases showing a relation between MMSE score and biomedical variables *(39, 40)*. However, numerous studies have shown that the MMSE has poor sensitivity and specificity, as well as a low-test–retest reliability *(41–43)*. Furthermore, the MMSE has been developed to determine cognitive decline that is typical for Alzheimer's dementia, but has been found less useful in determining cognitive decline in non-demented patients *(44)* or in patients with other forms of dementia. This is important since odds ratios for both vascular dementia and Alzheimer's dementia are increased in diabetes *(45)*. Notwithstanding this increased risk, most patients with diabetes have subtle cognitive deficits *(46, 47)* that may easily go undetected using gross screening instruments such as the MMSE. For research in diabetes a high sensitivity is thus especially important. Additionally, the MMSE does not tap all cognitive domains; executive function, language, and perception are only minimally screened.

Consequently, new screening instruments have been developed to overcome these disadvantages. For example, the Cambridge Cognitive Examination (CAMCOG) is a screening instrument that examines cognition more reliably, for example, by including items that rely on executive function and reasoning, and has been more successful in determining dementia-related cognitive decline *(48)*. Other screening instruments, such as the Mattis Dementia Rating Scale also provide valuable information about cognitive decline in relation to dementia diagnosis *(49)*. However, although a vast improvement over the MMSE, new screening instruments also primarily target cognitive decline that is indicative of dementia. Also, normative data have been collected exclusively in older people, who are generally more at risk for developing dementia, and clear ceiling effects are found when using these tests in younger adults. Moreover, cognitive deficits in single domains or mild overall cognitive impairments are often as clinically relevant as severe deterioration, but may be easily missed with insensitive screening instruments. While short cognitive screening instruments may appear useful at first glance, overall validity and reliability are poor making these not the most sensitive outcome measure in diabetes-related research on cognition. In addition, data on the reliability and validity of the performance on the different subdomains assessed using screening tests are lacking.

Assessment of Other Psychological Concepts

Poor test performances on cognitive tests are not necessarily the result of brain disease. For example, a depressed mood may impair attention and consequently memory performance, in the absence of evidence for organic lesions. Also, patients who participate in neuropsychological assessment procedures may not always perform at their optimal performance level due to lack of motivation, psychiatric disease, or even malingering. Furthermore, it should be stressed that neuropsychological tests measure neurocognitive *impairments*, i.e., deficits at the level of a specific cognitive function, for example, an encoding deficit in memory, but do not assess *disabilities* that reflect the impact on everyday activities of the patient (e.g., the inability to read a book) or *participation problems* in societal functioning. Moreover, cognitive impairment measured on tests does not necessarily relate to the subjective performance of the patient. For example, an older patient who occasionally forgets things and who is consequently extremely worried that she has Alzheimer's disease may rate her memory function as very poor, even if test scores show an age-appropriate performance. In contrast, a patient with dysexecutive syndrome who shows severe behavioral deficits, personality changes, and executive deficits may show lack of insight into his deficits, rating his cognitive function as normal, despite gross impairments on tests. Also, personality characteristics and coping skills are often relevant in the interpretation of test findings.

A wide range of instruments is available for the assessment of mood, subjective complaints, personality, coping style, behavioral changes, and everyday functioning. Depressive mood is in most cases measured using (self-report) questionnaires, such as the Beck Depression Inventory (BDI-II) *(50)*. Some of these questionnaires are somewhat biased for use in hospitalized patients, in that they often contain somatic items indicative for depression that, however, also may be present in patients without mood disorders but with somatic conditions. Instruments have been developed that take this explicitly into account, such as the Hospital Anxiety and Depression Scale (HADS) *(51)* or the Geriatric Depression Scale (GDS) *(52)*. Also, questionnaires have been developed that measure a broader range of subjective complaints next to depressive symptoms, such as cognitive deficits or feelings of anxiety, for example, the Symptom Checklist (SCL-90-R) *(53)*. The Cognitive Failures Questionnaire (CFQ) is a more specific measure for the assessment of cognitive complaints *(54)*. Although these measures provide insight into the subjective complaints, they do not necessarily correlate with objective test performance as noted above *(55, 56)*. While subjective complaints can be considered as state variables that may be subject to change due to, for example, improvement in medical condition or the occurrence of psychological stressors, factors such as personality or coping skills may represent more stable factors. Personality is a construct originating from research on individual differences, commonly regarded as a more or less stable set of characteristics. Most models of personality are derived from factor analysis, such as the Big Five model that consists of five broad factors of personality Extraversion, Openness, Agreeableness, Conscientiousness, and Neuroticism *(57)*. The Revised NEO Personality Inventory (NEO-PI-R) is an example of a personality test to measure these dimensions *(58)*. Coping skills refer to the ability to cope with challenges one encounters in life; a coping style refers to someone's typical way to address these problems, e.g., by actively trying to solve them or avoiding. Tests to measure coping styles are self-report measures, designed for use in specific diseases *(59)*. A questionnaire that can be used to assess the emotional and psychological impact of diabetes on everyday life is the Problem Areas in Diabetes Scale (PAID) *(60)*.

CLASSIFICATION OF TEST RESULTS IN INDIVIDUALS AND GROUPS

Neuropsychological assessment is more than just administering a number of tests in a patient. Although each test is presented and scored in a standardized manner, raw test results do not have any meaning. Only few tests measure functions at a ceiling level, allowing immediate interpretation. However, ceiling effects in test performance often result in a lack of sensitivity. Subtle impairments are easily missed, resulting in a high proportion of false-negative cases (people classified as cognitively unimpaired where in fact they are). Hence, good neuropsychological tests are sensitive to a range of functioning, both at very low levels of cognitive functioning as well as in people with above-average cognitive abilities. In addition, test results are always affected by confounding factors such as age, intelligence, education level, sex, cultural background, and native language. Consequently, the performance on neuropsychological test cannot be classified as impaired using a simple cut-off score, but normative data are required that adjust for these confounding factors. Extensive normative datasets are available for the widely used neuropsychological tests, either published in test manuals or in comprehensive textbooks *(1, 2, 61)*. Basically, two types of norm sets exist, *stratified norms* and *regression-based norms*. In stratified norm sets, an individual test score is compared to the mean performance of a matched norm group, for example, people of comparable age and education level. In contrast, in regression-based norms the individual's expected score is computed based on a number of potentially confounding variables, such as age, IQ, and gender, by means of a regression formula. The difference between the individual's expected and actual score (the residue score) is then compared to a frequency table to determine the probability that this residue score is found in a normal population.

Both stratified and regression-based norms convert the raw score that an individual obtains on a specific task to a standard score that is corrected for factors, such as age, education level, intelligence, and sex. This standard score can subsequently be interpreted using the normal distribution, often referred to as the bell curve (see Fig. 4), which indicates the probability that a given performance is to occur in a normal population. For example, z-scores have a mean of 0 and a standard deviation (SD) of 1, which means that a performance that equals a z-score of -1.5 is 1.5 standard deviations below the normative mean. Figure 4 shows that this equals the 7th percentile, indicating that 7% of the normative group (which represents the normal population) obtains this (or a lower) score. Clinically, the cut-off point that is used for determining whether a given performance is "impaired" depends on this percentile range. There is, however, not a strict rule for which cut-off point should be used. In most cases, a performance over 2 SDs below the mean is used, which equals a percentile of 2.3 *(1)* but less conservative cut-off points are also widely used, such as 1.5 SD or 1.65 SD *(62)*, the latter being the generally accepted probability of incorrectly rejecting a statistical hypothesis (equaling a percentile range of 5). Test scores that fall below 1 SD of the normative mean, but above the cut-off score for an impaired

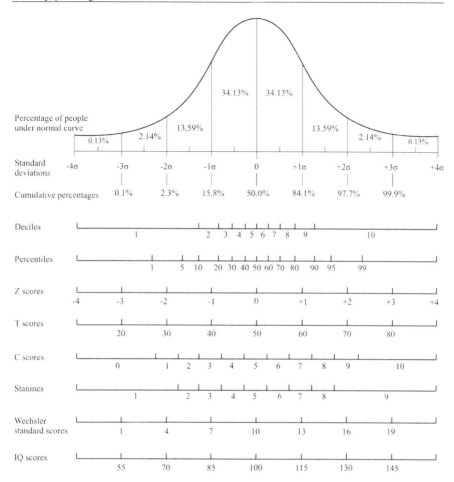

Fig. 4. The normal distribution in relation to standard scores that can be used to interpret neuropsychological test results

performance are typically classified as below average (but not impaired). Whether below-average performances have a clinical significance cannot be determined only on the basis of statistical analyses. As a rule of thumb applied by most clinical neuropsychologists, below-average test scores have a clinical significance if they (1) represent a consistent pattern (e.g., below-average scores on various memory tests and average scores on other tests or a below-average performance on one executive function test and impaired scores on other tests of executive functioning), (2) have a relation with the subjective complaints by either the patient or his/her significant other(s) (e.g., below-average performance on tests of speed of information processing in a patient who experiences a decline in mental speed), (3) can be linked to typical neuropsychological findings in patients with a specific disease or syndrome (e.g., a below-average performance on attention tests in a patient with multiple sclerosis or a below-average performance on executive functioning in an older patient with type 2 diabetes). In addition, the premorbid performance level of a patient also provides information about a possible decline in cognitive function, which can be estimated using crystallized intelligence tests, such as the NART, or education level, professional history, and socioeconomic background.

Apart from using test results to classify a patient at an individual level, group differences can also be measured. Where statistical testing is performed to indicate whether two-sample means significantly differ, a statistically significant finding does not immediately mean that such a between-group difference is clinically meaningful. The size of the group differences is relevant here: the larger the effect, the more relevant it will be for clinical practice. However, given the variety between the various neuropsychological tests and the variables that are used (e.g., reaction times, number correct, % incorrect), raw test scores are not suitable to assess the magnitude of an effect. For the interpretation of a difference between two groups, a standardized effect size (d) is mostly used, expressed as the differences between the two means divided by the pooled standard deviation. In practice, a somewhat arbitrary classification is used, in which effect sizes are considered small if $d = 0.2$, medium if d is about 0.5, and large if d is approximately 0.8 (63). Consequently, small effect sizes would probably not be clinically significant, in that it is unlikely that many individuals in the group would be classified as "impaired" at an individual level, whereas large effect sizes would indicate clinically meaningful differences, i.e., resulting in an "impaired" performance in many of the individuals.

INTERPRETATION OF TEST RESULTS

Both in clinical practice and in research settings, neuropsychological assessment typically has two aims; the first is to contribute to the differential diagnosis of diseases or syndromes, the second is to provide information about cognitive strengths or weaknesses that can be used for decision-making with respect to treatment or care or educate the patient or his caregivers or significant others about neurocognitive changes that may be present. For making a reliable medical diagnosis, however, neuropsychological testing rarely contributes uniquely. While a low score on the MMSE is indicative for cognitive decline typically seen in Alzheimer dementia, a low performance may also be due to vascular cognitive impairments, Parkinson's disease, or even to problems in hearing. If cognitive tests or screening instruments are used for establishing medical diagnoses, information about the test's sensitivity and specificity should be available. To prevent the occurrence of missed diagnoses or false-positive test results, a good instrument should have a good sensitivity and an adequate sensitivity. Neuropsychological tests generally lack this combination, simply because cognitive impairments can be the results of a wide range of medical conditions and low test scores may also occur in healthy people. Related to this, many older neuropsychological tests had been originally developed as tests for organicity (as opposed to functional complaints or psychiatric disease), but more recent studies combining neuropsychological test results and measures of cerebral dysfunction, such as MRI, PET, or EEG, indicate that when these tests are used in isolation they are invalid for this purpose. Also, function localization on the basis of test outcome has been found to lack validity, not only because of inadequate test characteristics but also because original theories on lateralization (e.g., the left hemisphere mediates verbal cognitive functions and the right hemisphere is specialized in spatial function) have been found to be inaccurate or even completely incorrect. Nowadays, advanced neuroimaging techniques, such as SPECT and MRI, outperform behavioral tests with respect to lesion localization. Still, combining imaging data and neuropsychological test results provide valuable insight into the working of the brain and impairments in patients with cerebral dysfunction.

MEASURING COGNITION IN DIABETES

The present chapter does not summarize the cognitive findings typical for diabetes type 1 and type 2. Nevertheless, we wish to address issues that need to be considered in order to design an optimal test battery for the assessment of diabetes-associated cognitive decline. Firstly, when patients with diabetes are compared with non-diabetic controls, effect sizes for the differences in performance between the groups are generally small (Chapters 10–12). This indicates that an optimal test battery should be very sensitive to be able to detect small changes in cognitive function and should not suffer from ceiling effects. Cognitive domains that are generally sensitive to brain dysfunction are speed of information processing and executive function, both requiring either fast or effortful processing. Furthermore, the impact of confounding factors should be kept to a minimum. In diabetes, potentially confounding factors are peripheral complications, such as neuropathy which may result in slowing of reactions in reaction-time paradigms and retinopathy that may cause visual impairment that becomes disturbing in tests using visually presented stimuli. Other confounding factors include lack of motivation, the effects of having a chronic illness that may depress the patient's mood, and individual differences, such as coping style and personality traits.

Moreover, diabetes patients with cognitive complaints are more likely to be older, so tests should be selected that have been designed for use in older participants. Since type 2 diabetes (and possibly the occurrence of complications in type 1 diabetes) is also related to socioeconomic status, low education (or even illiteracy), as well as cultural and ethnic diversity are also factors that should be considered. Since diabetes is also associated with a higher risk of developing dementia in older patients (Chapter 13), a test battery should also be sensitive to the pattern of deterioration that is typical for dementia. Thus, it should include measures of episodic memory, since memory impairment is prominent in Alzheimer's disease, and measures of speed of information processing and executive function which may be impaired in vascular dementia. If a screening instrument for dementia is considered, researchers and clinicians should consider the test's sensitivity and specificity.

Table 1 summarizes domains and tests that could be considered for the assessment of patients with diabetes, but it should be noted that no strict guidelines can be given and no fixed battery can be recommended. In general, tests should be cognitively demanding to avoid ceiling effects in

Table 1
Summary of cognitive domains, psychological functions, and examples of tests that can be used for the assessment of patients with diabetes

Domain or function	Brief description	Example of tests
Intelligence	Premorbid academic functioning (crystallized intelligence) and actual problem-solving ability (fluid intelligence)	WAIS-IV; KAIT; Raven's Progressive Matrices; NART
Long-term memory and learning	The ability to acquire new information or to retrieve previously stored information, either related to personal memories (episodic) or general knowledge (semantic)	RAVLT; CVLT; HVLT; Benton Visual Retention Test; Location Learning Test; WMS-IV
Working memory	The capacity to actively maintain and manipulate information for a brief period of time (seconds to minutes), includes short-term memory	Digit span; Corsi-Block Tapping Task

Table 1
(continued)

Domain or function	Brief description	Example of tests
Executive function	The planning, monitoring, initiation, shifting, and inhibition of behavior	Trail Making Test; Tower of London test; Wisconsin Card Sorting Test; BADS
Attention, concentration, and speed of information processing	Selection of relevant information, dual tasking, sustaining a state of alertness, and the "mental speed" with which information is processed	Reaction-time tests; Digit Symbol Substitution Test; PASAT; d2 Test; Continuous Performance Task
Praxis and motor function	Cognitive processes that underlie basic motor functions and complex actions	Pegboard tests; behavioral testing
Language	Communication skills, understanding others, and verbal expressing	Boston Diagnostic Aphasia Battery; Token Test; Verbal Fluency Tests
Perception	Both low-level and higher-order processing of visual, auditory, and tactile stimuli	Ishihara Test for Color Blindness; CORVIST; VOSP; Benton Test of Facial Matching
Overall cognition	Screening for cognitive decline regardless of cognitive domains	MMSE; CAMCOG-R; Mattis DRS-2
Mood	Symptoms of depression	BDI-II; HADS; GDS
Psychological complaints and coping	Complaints related to psychological distress as experienced by the patient and style of dealing with these	SCL-90-R; CFQ; PAID
Personality	Stable characteristics or traits that vary between individuals	NEO-PI-R

Note: see text for abbreviations.

patients with mild cognitive dysfunction. Related to this, some cognitive domains are more sensitive to cognitive decline than others. Consequently, sensitive domains such as speed of information processing, (working) memory, attention, and executive function should be examined thoroughly in diabetes patients, whereas other domains such as language, motor function, and perception are less likely to be affected. Intelligence should always be taken into account, and confounding factors such as mood, emotional distress, and coping are crucial for the interpretation of the neuropsychological test results. Only by relating cognitive function to other disease-related variables can researchers and clinicians disentangle the crucial aspects of cognitive decline in diabetes.

REFERENCES

1. Lezak MD, Howieson DB, Loring DW eds. *Neuropsychological Assessment*, 4th ed. New York: Oxford University Press, 2004.
2. Strauss E, Sherman EMS, Spreen O eds. *A Compendium of Neuropsychological Tests: Administration, Norms, and Commentary*, 3rd ed. New York: Oxford University Press, 2006.
3. Beauducel A, Brocke B, Liepmann D. Perspectives on fluid and crystallized intelligence: facets for verbal, numerical, and figural intelligence *Pers Indiv Diff* 2001; 30:977–994.
4. Wechsler D. *WAIS-IV Administration and Scoring Manual*. San Antonio, TX: Psychological Corporation, 2008.
5. Kaufman AS, Kaufman NL. *Kaufman Adolescent and Adult Intelligence Test* (KAIT). Circle Pines, MN: American Guidance Service, 1993.
6. Nelson HE, O'Connell A. Dementia: the estimation of premorbid intelligence levels using the National Adult Reading Test. *Cortex* 1978; 14:234–244.
7. Carpenter PA, Just MA, Shell P. What one intelligence test measures: a theoretical account of the processing in the Raven Progressive Matrices Test. *Psychol Rev* 1990; 97:404–431.
8. Lacritz LH, Cullum CM. The Hopkins Verbal Learning Test and CVLT: Implications for the assessment of memory disorders *Arch Clin Neuropsychol* 1998; 13:623–628.
9. Van der Elst W, van Boxtel MP, van Breukelen GJ, Jolles J. Rey's verbal learning test: normative data for 1855 healthy participants aged 24–81 years and the influence of age, sex, education, and mode of presentation. *J Int Neuropsychol Soc* 2005; 11:290–302.
10. Benton AL, Sivan AB, deS Hamsher K, Varney NR, Spreen, O eds. *Contributions to Neuropsychological Assessment: A Clinical Manual*. New York: Oxford University Press; 1994.
11. Bucks RS, Willison JR. Development and validation of the Location Learning Test (LLT): a test of visuo-spatial learning designed for use with older adults and in dementia *Clin Neuropsychol* 1997:11; 273–286.
12. Wechsler D, ed. *Wechsler Memory Scale-Fourth edition (WMS-IV)* San Antonio, TX: Harcourt Assessment, 2008.
13. Baddeley A. *Working Memory, Thought, and Action*. New York: Oxford University Press, 2007.
14. Kessels RPC, van den Berg E, Ruis C, Brands AMA. The backward span of the Corsi Block-Tapping Task and its association with the WAIS-III Digit Span. *Assessment* 2008; 15: 426–434.
15. Robbins TW, James M, Owen AM, Sahakian BJ, McInnes L, Rabbitt, P. Cambridge Neuropsychological Test Automated Battery (CANTAB): a factor analytic study of a large sample of normal elderly volunteers. *Dementia* 1994; 5:266–281.
16. Shallice T. *From Neuropsychology to Mental Structure*. Cambridge: Cambridge University Press, 1988.

17. Milner B. Effects of different brain lesions on card sorting. *Arch Neurol* 1963; 9:100–110.
18. Shallice T. Specific impairments of planning. *Philos Trans R Soc Lond B* 1982; 298: 199–209.
19. Bowie CR, Harvey PD. Administration and interpretation of the Trail Making Test. *Nat Protoc* 2006; 1:2277–2281.
20. Wilson BA, Alderman N, Burgess PW, Emslie H, Evans JJ eds. *Behavioural Assessment of the Dysexecutive Syndrome (BADS)*. Bury St. Edmunds, UK: Thames Valley Test Company, 1996.
21. De Haan E, Kessels R. Disorders of attention. In Johnson A, Proctor RW, eds. *Attention: Theory and Practice*. London, UK: Sage; 2004:367–395.
22. Stroop JE. (1935). Studies of interference in serial verbal reactions. *J Exp Psychol* 1935; 18:643–662.
23. Posner MI, Dehaene S. Attentional networks. *Trends Neurosci* 1994; 17:75–79.
24. Wilson B, Cockburn J, Halligan P. *The Behavioural Inattention Test*. Suffolk, UK: Thames Valley Test Co, 1987.
25. Gronwall DM. Paced auditory serial-addition task: a measure of recovery from concussion. *Percept Mot Skills* 1977; 44:367–373.
26. Bates ME, Lemay Jr. EP. (2004) The d2 Test of attention: construct validity and extensions in scoring techniques *J Int Neuropsychol Soc* 2004; 10:392–400.
27. Liepmann H. Apraxie. In Brugsch T, ed. *Ergebnisse der gesamten Medizin*. Berlin: Urban & Schwarzenberg; 1920:516–543.
28. De Renzi E, Vignolo LA. The Token Test: a sensitive test to detect disturbances in aphasics. *Brain* 1962; 85:665–678.
29. Goodglass H, Kaplan E. *The Assessment of Aphasia and Related Disorders*, 2nd ed. Philadelphia: Lea & Febiger, 1983.
30. Ishihara S. *Tests for Colour Blindness*. Tokyo: Handaya Company, 1917.
31. James M, Plant GT, Warrington EK. *CORVIST: Cortical Vision Screening Test.* Oxford: Thames Valley Test Company, 2001.
32. Rapport LJ, Millis SR, Bonello PJ. Validation of the Warrington theory of visual processing and the Visual Object and Space Perception Battery. *J Clin Exp Neuropsychol* 1998; 20: 211–220.
33. Morris JC, Mohs RC, Rogers H, Fillenbaum G, Heyman A. Consortium to establish a registry for Alzheimer's disease (CERAD) clinical and neuropsychological assessment of Alzheimer's disease. *Psychopharmacol Bull* 1988; 24:641–652.
34. Strauss ME, Fritsch T. Factor structure of the CERAD neuropsychological battery *J Int Neuropsychol Soc* 2004; 10:559–565.
35. Randolph C, Tierney MC, Mohr E, Chase TN. The Repeatable Battery for the Assessment of Neuropsychological Status (RBANS): preliminary clinical validity. *J Clin Exp Neuropsychol* 1998; 20:310–319.
36. Feldstein SN, Keller FR, Portman RE, Durham RL, Klebe KJ, Davis HP. A comparison of computerized and standard versions of the Wisconsin Card Sorting Test. *Clin Neuropsychol* 1999; 13:303–313.
37. French CC, Beaumont JG. A clinical study of the automated assessment of intelligence by the Mill Hill Vocabulary test and the Standard Progressive Matrices test. *J Clin Psychol* 1990; 46:129–140.
38. Folstein M, Folstein SE, McHugh PR. Mini-Mental State: a practical method for grading the cognitive state of patients for the clinician. *J Psychiatric Res* 1975; 12:189–198.
39. Niwa H, Koumoto C, Shiga T, et al. Clinical analysis of cognitive function in diabetic patients by MMSE and SPECT. *Diabetes Res Clin Pract* 2006; 72:142–147.
40. Umegaki H, Iimuro S, Kaneko T, et al. Factors associated with lower Mini Mental State Examination scores in elderly Japanese diabetes mellitus patients. *Neurobiol Aging* 2007; 29(7):1022–1026.
41. Olin JT, Zelinski EM. The 12-month reliability of the Mini-Mental State Examination. *Psychological Assessment* 1991; 3:427–432.

42. Wind AW, Schellevis FG, Van Staveren G, Scholten RP, Jonker C, Van Eijk JT. Limitations of the Mini-Mental State Examination in diagnosing dementia in general practice. *Int J Geriatr Psychiatry* 1997; 12:101–108.

43. Kilada S, Gamaldo A, Grant EA, Moghekar A, Morris JC, O'Brien RJ. Brief screening tests for the diagnosis of dementia: comparison with the mini-mental state exam. *Alzheimer Dis Assoc Disord* 2005; 19: 8–16.

44. Nys GMS, van Zandvoort MJE, de Kort PLM, Jansen BPW, Kappelle LJ, De Haan EHF. Restrictions of the Mini-Mental State Examination in acute stroke. *Arch Clin Neuropsychol* 2005; 20:623–629.

45. Biessels GJ, Staekenborg S, Brunner E, Brayne C, Scheltens P. Risk of dementia in diabetes mellitus: a systematic review. *Lancet Neurol* 2006; 5:64–74.

46. Areosa SA, Grimley EV. Effect of the treatment of Type II diabetes mellitus on the development of cognitive impairment and dementia. *Cochrane Database Syst Rev* 2002; 4: CD003804.

47. Brands AMA, Biessels GJ, De Haan EHF, Kappelle LJ, Kessels RPC. The effects of type 1 diabetes on cognitive performance: a meta-analysis *Diab Care* 2005; 28:726–735.

48. Lindeboom J, Ter Horst R, Hooyer C, Dinkgreve M, Jonker C. Some psychometric properties of the CAMCOG. *Psychol Med* 1993; 23:213–219.

49. Smith GE, Ivnik RJ, Malec JF, Kokmen E, Tangalos E, Petersen RC. Psychometric properties of the Mattis dementia rating scale. *Assessment* 1994; 1:123–132.

50. Beck AT, Steer RA, Brown GK eds. *Beck Depression Inventory–Second Edition: Manual*. San Antonio, TX: Psychological Corporation, 1996.

51. Zigmond AS, Snaith RP. The hospital anxiety and depression scale. *Acta Psychiatr Scand* 1983; 67:361–370.

52. Yesavage JA, Brink TL, Rose TL, et al. Development and validation of a geriatric depression screening scale: a preliminary report. *J Psychiatric Res* 1983; 17:37–49.

53. Derogatis LR. *Symptom Checklist-90-R: Administrative Scoring and Procedures Manual*. Minneapolis, MN: NCS Pearson, 1994.

54. Broadbent DE, Cooper PF, FitzGerald P, Parkes KR. The Cognitive Failures Questionnaire (CFQ) and its correlates *Br J Clin Psychol* 1982; 21:1–16.

55. Antikainen R, Hanninen T, Honkalampi K, et al. Mood improvement reduces memory complaints in depressed patients. *Eur Arch Psychiatry Clin Neurosci* 2001; 251:6–11.

56. Wessels AM, Pouwer F, Geelhoed-Duijvestijn PH, et al. No evidence for increased self-reported cognitive failure in Type 1 and Type 2 diabetes: a cross-sectional study. *Diabet Med* 2007; 24:735–740.

57. Hofstee WK, de Raad B, Goldberg LR. Integration of the big-five and circumplex approaches to trait structure *J Pers Soc Psychol* 1992; 63:146–163.

58. Costa PT, McCrae RR. *Revised NEO Personality Inventory (NEO-PI-R) and NEO Five-Factor Inventory (NEO-FFI) Professional Manual*. Odessa, FL: Psychological Assessment Resources, 1992.

59. Nomura M, Fujimoto K, Higashino A, et al. Stress and coping behavior in patients with diabetes mellitus *Acta Diabetol* 2000; 37:61–64.

60. Welch GW, Jacobson AM, Polonsky WH. The Problem Areas in Diabetes Scale: An evaluation of its clinical utility *Diab Care* 1997; 20:760–766.

61. Mitrushina MN, Boone KB, Razani J, D'Elia LF, eds. *Handbook of Normative Data for Neuropsychological Assessment*. New York: Oxford University Press, 2005.

62. Van den Berg E, Kessels RPC, De Haan EHF, Kappelle LJ, Biessels GJ. Mild impairments in cognition in patients with type 2 diabetes mellitus: the use of the concepts MCI and CIND. *J Neurol Neurosurg Psychiatry* 2005; 76:1466–1467.

63. Cohen J. *Statistical Power Analysis for the Behavioral Sciences*, 2nd ed. Hillsdale, NJ: Lawrence Earlbaum, 1988.

5

Clinical Evaluation and Treatment of Cognitive Dysfunction and Dementia

Laura A. van de Pol, Wiesje M. van der Flier, and Philip Scheltens

CONTENTS

ABSTRACT

It is estimated that within the next 50 years the number of patients with dementia in Europe will rise to over 16 million, due to increasing life expectancy in Western society. Besides the physical, social and psychological burden on carers of patients with dementia, the financial burden on society will grow exponentially too. Dementia is defined as an acquired impairment of cognitive function in at least two cognitive domains, including memory, which interferes with normal social or occupational performance. Dementia can be caused by various underlying diseases, the most common of which is Alzheimer's disease. The first part of this chapter will discuss the clinical signs and symptoms and neuropathological findings of the most important types of dementia. An accurate diagnosis of a certain type of dementia is crucial for therapy and counselling of the patient and his family. Therefore, the second part of this chapter will review history and physical examination and the contribution of ancillary investigations, such

From: *Contemporary Diabetes: Diabetes and the Brain*
Edited by: G. J. Biessels, J. A. Luchsinger (eds.), DOI 10.1007/978-1-60327-850-8_5
© Humana Press, a part of Springer Science+Business Media, LLC 2009

as MRI, cerebrospinal fluid markers, PET and EEG in diagnosing dementia. Finally, therapeutic options will be reviewed.

Key words: Dementia; Diagnosis; Signs and symptoms; MRI; CSF; PET.

INTRODUCTION

Dementia is one of the most widely feared age-related neurological diseases, and together with stroke, it is the only neurological disease listed in the ten most important causes of disease burden in developed countries *(1)*. The life-time risk of any dementia has been estimated to be more than 1 in 5 for women and 1 in 6 for men *(2)*. Worldwide, about 24 million people have dementia, with 4.6 million new cases of dementia every year *(3)*.

The term dementia encompasses the spectrum of clinical diseases characterized by progressive deterioration of cognitive functions, leading to interference with social and occupational performance *(4, 5)*. Behavioural and psychological problems occur more frequently as the disease becomes more severe. Eventually, patients become dependent on others and often have to be cared for in a nursing home.

Dementia can be caused by various underlying diseases, the most common of which is Alzheimer's disease (AD) accounting for roughly 70% of cases in the elderly. The second most common cause of dementia is vascular dementia (VaD), accounting for 16% of cases. Other, less common, causes include dementia with Lewy bodies (DLB) and frontotemporal lobar degeneration (FTLD). Below the age of 65 years dementia is far less common, and the distribution of the different types of dementia differs from that observed in the elderly. AD remains the most common cause, but its relative prevalence is reduced to one third of cases, with VaD accounting for 18% approximately *(6)*. In clinical practice, patients who fulfil the clinical diagnostic criteria for AD, often show co-existing cerebrovascular pathology, especially with increasing age. There is evidence that these two pathologies interact.

An accurate diagnosis of the specific type of the dementia is of great importance in terms of therapeutic possibilities and counselling of the patient and his family. In the absence of neuropathological confirmation, the aetiological diagnosis is primarily based on clinical criteria, in combination with ancillary investigations.

In the first part of this chapter we will discuss the clinical signs and symptoms and neuropathological features of the most important types of dementia. The second part will be dedicated to the diagnostic process, including ancillary investigations such as neuroimaging and laboratory tools that can be used. Finally, therapeutic options will be discussed.

TYPES OF DEMENTIA

Alzheimer's Disease

The most frequently used clinical criteria for AD are those proposed by the National Institute of Neurological and Communicating Disorders and Stroke and the Alzheimer's Disease and Related Disorders Association (NINCDS–ADRDA) Work Group (Table 1) *(7)*.

Table 1
NINCDS–ADRDA criteria for the diagnosis for probable Alzheimer's disease

1. Dementia established by clinical examination and confirmed by neuropsychological tests
2. Deficits in two or more areas of cognition, including memory impairment
3. Progressive worsening of memory and other cognitive functions
4. No disturbances of consciousness
5. Onset between ages 40 and 90
6. Absence of systemic disorders or other brain disease that in and of themselves could account for the progressive deficits in memory and cognition

Adapted from McKhann et al. *(7)*.

Typically, AD is characterized by an insidious onset of cognitive decline, starting with deficits in episodic memory. Patients and their family complain, for example, of forgetting recent personal and family events, losing items around the house, and repetitive questioning. As the disease progresses, deficits in other cognitive domains, such as aphasia, apraxia, agnosia, visuospatial difficulties and executive dysfunction, arise gradually. Psychological and behavioural problems such as mood disorders, psychosis, agitation and sleep disorders, occur more frequently as the disease becomes more severe. The patient becomes increasingly dependent on others. The average survival in AD is typically about 7 years from the onset of symptoms to death *(8)*.

Besides the typical neuropsychological profile of AD presenting with early memory deficits, there is evidence from clinico-neuropathological studies that AD patients can present with different neuropsychological profiles *(9)*. Well described are first the posterior cortical atrophy, presenting either as a Balint-like syndrome (optic ataxia, simultanagnosia, optic apraxia) or an apperceptive visual agnosia; second the fluent or non-fluent aphasia; and third the biparietal variant presenting with apraxia, visual disorientation and navigation problems. These atypical variants of AD suggest that the distribution of neuropathological changes, rather than the nature of the disease, is reflected in the clinical syndrome and that in clinical practice AD should be considered as diagnosis in a broad range of focal cognitive syndromes.

The cause of AD is still not fully understood, except for the familial autosomal dominant inherited cases with early onset, associated with mutations in the amyloid precursor protein (APP) and presenilin genes (*PS1* and *PS2*), discovered in the early 1990s *(10)*. However, the familial form of AD is extremely rare, with a prevalence below 0.1% *(11)*. The far more common, sporadic form of AD is genetically associated with the apolipoprotein E4 allele (APOEe4), although APOEe4 is neither necessary nor sufficient to cause AD. It has been shown that the APOEe4 allele increases the risk of the disease by 3 times in heterozygotes and by 15 times in homozygotes *(12)*. Apart from genetic risk factors, the most important risk factor for AD is age. It is estimated that both the incidence and the prevalence double with every 5-year increase in age. Other risk factors for AD include female sex and vascular risk factors, such as diabetes, hypercholesterolaemia and hypertension *(13)*. Whether these vascular risk factors are causally related to the neuropathological process of AD or whether they induce cerebrovascular damage that coincides with or adds to Alzheimer-type neuropathology remains to be established. This is an important issue with regard to potential preventive measures.

A definitive diagnosis of AD can only be made by pathological examination of the brain at autopsy or by brain biopsy in exceptional cases. The characteristic lesions at the microscopic level are extracellular neuritic plaques, consisting of beta-amyloid (Aβ), and intracellular neurofibrillary tangles consisting of hyperphosphorylated tau protein. The staging system developed by Braak and Braak describes the extent, location and sequence of accumulating neurofibrillary tangle pathology, which in AD progresses in a typical fashion, starting in the transentorhinal and entorhinal areas, before spreading to the hippocampus, the association cortices, and the rest of the cortex (Fig. 1) *(14)*.

Current histological criteria for the diagnosis of AD are based on both the density of neuritic plaques and neurofibrillary tangles in the neocortex and limbic areas *(15)*. The histopathological diagnosis is still considered the gold standard, and considerable discrepancies between pathological diagnoses at post-mortem and the clinical diagnoses during life-time exist. A prospective, population-based study on the prevalence of AD in people over 85 years found that 55% of the individuals who met the neuropathological criteria for AD were either not demented during life-time or classified as vascular dementia. Conversely, they also found that 35% of those with clinical AD did not fulfil the pathological criteria *(16)*. Furthermore, there is evidence that,

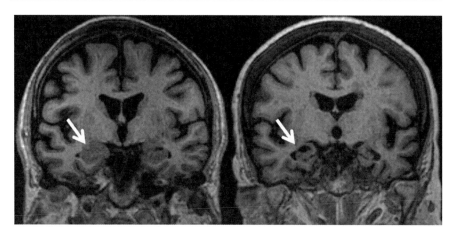

Fig. 1. Coronal T1-weighted MRI scans of control (*left*) and patient with AD (*right*). Both subjects are 70 years old. The patient with AD shows clear atrophy of the hippocampus, compared do the control subject (as indicated by arrows).

besides Alzheimer-type neuropathology, cerebrovascular pathology plays a role in AD. The majority of subjects with clinical, late-onset AD show coexisting vascular pathology at post-mortem (*17*), and previous studies have suggested that the two pathologies interact (*18, 19*).

Mild Cognitive Impairment

Mild cognitive impairment (MCI) is a concept designed to identify subjects who experience cognitive decline not yet severe enough to fulfil diagnostic criteria for dementia, but who are at increased risk to develop dementia in the future. Several clinical definitions for this intermediate phase exist, of which the criteria for amnestic MCI developed by Petersen et al. are most frequently used (Table 2) (*20, 21*).

Table 2
Criteria for amnestic MCI by Petersen et al. (1, 20)

1. Memory complaint, preferably corroborated by an informant
2. Objective memory impairment of age and education, at neuropsychological testing
3. Normal general cognition
4. Preserved activities of daily living
5. No dementia

Subjects who fulfil criteria for amnestic MCI are at increased risk of developing clinical AD at a rate of about 12–15% per year, as compared to 1–2% per year in the age-matched general population *(20)*. However, not all subjects with MCI will develop AD, some will develop other types of dementia, whereas others will remain stable or even improve *(22, 23)*. The neuropathological outcome of patients dying with dementia, who had a prior diagnosis of amnestic MCI, has been shown to be heterogeneous, often consisting of two or more distinct pathological entities *(24)*. Therefore ancillary investigations, such as neuroimaging and laboratory investigations that may give clues to the type of neuropathology, can be useful especially in early disease stages.

Vascular Dementia

VaD is the second most common type of dementia. Clinically, this type of dementia is often characterized by deficits in executive functioning; the patient is typically slow, and apathetic, but symptoms can be highly variable, depending on the location and type of underlying vascular lesions. In contrast with AD, progression of cognitive deficits is mostly stepwise and with an acute or subacute onset. The most frequently used criteria for a clinical diagnosis of VaD are the National Institute of Neurological Disorders and Stroke (NINDS)–Association pour la Recherche et l'Enseignement et Neurosciences (AIREN) criteria (Table 3). Criteria are fulfilled when there is a dementia and cerebrovascular disease and the two are presumed to be related *(25)*.

Table 3
NINDS–AIREN criteria for the diagnosis of vascular dementia

I. Dementia established by clinical examination and confirmed by neuropsychological tests
II. Cerebrovascular disease defined as a combination of
  1. Focal signs on neurological examination
  2. Vascular lesion on CT or MRI, including multiple large vessel infarcts or single strategically placed infarct (angular gyrus, thalamus, basal forebrain, arteria cerebri anterior or posterior territories) or multiple basal ganglia and white matter lacunes or extensive periventricular white matter lesions or combinations thereof
III. A. relationship between the above two disorders manifested or inferred by the presence of one of the following
  1. Onset of dementia within 3 months after a recognized stroke
  2. Abrupt deterioration in cognitive functions
  3. Fluctuating, stepwise progression of cognitive deficits

Adapted from Roman *(25)*.

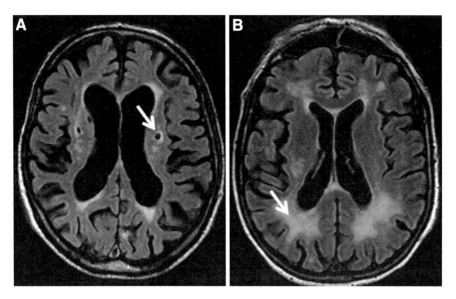

Fig. 2. Cerebrovascular pathology on axial fluid-attenuated inversion recovery (FLAIR) MRI scans. The arrows indicate: (**a**) Lacunar infarcts. (**b**) Confluent white matter hyperintensities.

The NINDS–AIREN criteria are the only criteria for VaD that include radiological criteria in addition to clinical criteria (Fig. 2). Various other definitions for VaD exist, resulting in different prevalence estimates and identifying different groups of patients. The lack of comparability between the different definitions forms a barrier to clinical care and research. Furthermore, it can be difficult to determine to which degree cerebrovascular lesions on neuroimaging contribute to the cognitive deficits. Cerebrovascular pathology is common, in pathological series 29–41% of dementia cases from population-based cohorts show some vascular pathology, whilst pure vascular pathology accounted for dementia in only about 10% *(26)*. Especially, when cerebrovascular accidents remained unnoticed ('silent brain infarcts', but also white matter hyperintensities), the obligatory relationship with time may be difficult to demonstrate. Another challenge is the lack of neuropathological consensus on the definition of vascular dementia postmortem *(27)*. Despite all methodological difficulties, it is clear that cerebrovascular disease is one of the major causes of cognitive decline. Vascular risk factors such as diabetes mellitus and hypertension have been recognized as risk factors for VaD *(28, 29)*, which are potential targets for preventive measures.

Frontotemporal Lobar Degeneration

Individuals with FTLD present with alterations in personality and cognitive dysfunction. Symptoms usually emerge before the age of 65 years. The widely used clinical diagnostic criteria of Neary recognize three subtypes of FTLD, a behavioural variant: frontotemporal dementia (FTD), and two language variants: semantic dementia and progressive non-fluent aphasia *(30)*. FTD is characterized by profound changes in character and behaviour, often resulting in emotional bluntness and social inappropriateness. Cognitive deterioration, in particular in the domains of executive function, language and memory, can be less prominent at presentation, but inevitably leads to dementia in the course of the disease. In semantic dementia and progressive non-fluent aphasia, language deficits are more prominent than change in character. Semantic dementia is characterized by a severe loss of semantic knowledge. Semantic paraphasias occur, while spontaneous speech remains fluent. In contrast, progressive non-fluent aphasia presents with an effortful, non-fluent speech characterized by word finding difficulties and grammatical errors. Eventually, as the disease spreads, deficits in other cognitive domains arise.

The minority of FTLD cases are familial *(31)*. Mutations in the tau and more recently in the progranulin gene, both located on chromosome 17, have been identified *(32, 33)*. The majority of FTLD cases, however, is sporadic. Risk factors for FTLD have not been found yet. At post-mortem examination, FTLD is characterized by focal frontal and/or temporal atrophy associated with a number of histopathological features, including tau positive or ubiquitin positive inclusions; alternatively they may lack distinguishing hallmarks. Clinico-pathological studies have shown that there is no strong relation between the type of neuropathology and clinical phenotype *(34)*.

Dementia with Lewy Bodies

Clinically, DLB is a dementia with prominent visuoperceptual and executive dysfunction, accompanied by three core features; visual hallucinations, attentional fluctuation and parkinsonism *(35)*. Together with Parkinson's disease with dementia, DLB forms a continuum referred to as Lewy body disease. If dementia has preceded the motor symptoms, or if the dementia has developed within 1 year after the onset of motor symptoms, the term DLB is used. In contrast, if the motor symptoms preceded cognitive symptoms by more than 1 year, the diagnosis of Parkinson's disease with dementia is made. Discussion exists whether this distinction is clinically relevant. Neuropathologically, Lewy bodies, containing alpha-synuclein, are found, especially in the hypothalamus, basal forebrain, amygdala and temporal cortex.

Corticobasal Degeneration

Corticobasal degeneration (CBD) is a rare neurodegenerative disease presenting with asymmetrical motor symptoms in combination with dementia. Usually, the disease becomes manifest between the sixth and eighth decades of life *(36)*. Clinically, asymmetrical extrapyramidal signs, such as bradykinesia, rigidity and dystonia, myoclonus and cortical sensory loss occur *(36)*. Most commonly, the patient becomes aware of a stiff, clumsy arm. The patient complains that the hand does not behave itself or that it feels as if it belongs to somebody else ('alien hand') *(37)*. The dementia is characterized by severe apraxia and executive function deficits. Behaviour disturbances and non-fluent dysphasia occur later in the disease. The underlying pathology consists of strikingly asymmetrical degeneration of posterior frontal, inferior parietal and superior temporal cortices, the thalamus, substantia nigra, and cerebellar dentate nuclei. Swollen, achromatic, tau-positive neurons are found at the microscopic level *(37)*. Currently this disorder is classified as belonging to the spectrum of tauopathies (FTLD), as is progressive supranuclear palsy (see below).

Progressive Supranuclear Palsy

Progressive supranuclear palsy (PSP or syndrome of Steele–Richardson Olszweski) is characterized by a supranuclear gaze palsy with hypometric or slow saccades, particularly on downgaze in combination with parkinsonism and dementia. PSP is diagnosed using the NINDS–SPSP criteria *(38)*. Typically, the first symptoms occur between the ages of 60 and 65 years. The patient complains of problems going downstairs or looking at his watch. Furthermore, axial rigidity and early gait disturbance with falls (particularly backwards) occur. The dementia is characterized by profound slowness, personality change and executive dysfunction. Patients may show utilization behaviour. Typically, PSP is subdivided into Richardson's syndrome with mainly the fronto-executive symptoms and gaze palsy and the extrapyramidal syndrome in which extrapyramidal features dominate. In contrast to what is often said the typical gaze palsy occurs late in the disease course leading to long patient–doctor delays. Pathologically, PSP is characterized by the destruction of several subcortical structures, including the substantia nigra, globus pallidus, subthalamic nucleus and midbrain and pontine reticular formation. Histopathologically, insoluble aggregates of tau protein are found *(39)*.

Creutzfeldt–Jakob Disease

Four forms of Creutzfeldt–Jakob disease (CJD) exist, of which sporadic CJD (sCJD) is the most common, although still very rare, with an annual incidence of 1–2 cases per million. The onset of sCJD is usually between 60 and 75 years of age *(40)*. Clinically, the early symptoms are variable, most frequently changes in behaviour, emotional response and cognition occur, followed by ataxia and abnormalities in vision. The early stages are characterized by confusion, hallucinations and agitation. The disease is very rapidly progressive; patients deteriorate in weeks or even days. Myoclonic contractions and pyramidal and extrapyramidal symptoms may be observed in some patients. In the end stages of the disease there is a mute state leading to coma and death, usually within 1 year from disease onset. In 1996, a new form of CJD, variant CJD (vCJD) with a different neuropathological profile was recognized in the UK *(41)*. vCJD is characterized by a younger onset of the disease, around 30 years of age. Clinically, vCJD presents with psychiatric symptoms, such as psychosis or depression, and non-specific sensory complaints, such as paraesthesia *(40)*. Later in the disease cerebellar signs and involuntary movements may occur. Death occurs after a median survival of about 14 months. Roughly 5–15% of CJD cases are recognized as a familial, autosomal dominant disorder, with mutations in the prion protein gene. Clinically, the familial form is comparable with sporadic CJD, however, the age of onset is often younger, between 50 and 60 years, and disease duration may be longer. Increasingly rare is the iatrogenic form of CJD, caused by injection of human growth hormone or gonadotropins or by neurosurgical procedures.

The infectious agent causing CJD is a prion protein that catalyzes the conversion of a normal cellular protein PrPc to an abnormal isoform PrPSc. Associated with depositions of PrPSc protein in the brain are the characteristic, diffuse neuropathological changes including extensive astroglial proliferation, intraneuronal vacuolation and neuronal loss. In vCJD it has been shown that the prion strain is identical to the one from affected cattle, possibly transmitted through the ingestion of infected meat.

DIAGNOSIS AND ANCILLARY INVESTIGATIONS

A diagnosis of dementia is preferentially made in a multidisciplinary setting, based on clinical criteria *(4, 5)*. These criteria include the presence of multiple cognitive deficits leading to a significant impairment in social and occupational functioning and a significant decline from a previous level of functioning. The clinical challenge is to define the aetiological diagnosis in an early phase, based on criteria such as those reviewed on the previous pages. This is crucial with regard to early initiation of therapy and optimal counselling of the patient and his family, especially when realizing that significant accumulation of neuropathology has taken place many years, even decades, before the first symptoms arise *(42)*.

History and Physical Examination

When exploring cognitive complaints, a careful history is the basis for a good examination. A reliable informant is essential in this process, since the patient is often unaware of his own deficits. Important issues to assess in detail are premorbid functioning, the onset, time course and nature of cognitive complaints. Was the onset acute or insidious? What were the first observed problems? The first complaints may often prove to be of great diagnostic relevance *(43)*. Cognitive domains to be explored are memory, language, executive function, praxis and visuospatial ability. In AD, memory deficits are often the first symptoms. When assessing memory complaints it is useful to divide memory into episodic memory and semantic memory. Episodic memory comprises anterograde memory and retrograde memory. Anterograde memory is the recall of new episodic information, for example, recalling messages and news facts; does the patient need lists? Has he become repetitive? Examples of retrograde memory deficits are the recall of past personal events, such as holidays, past homes and recall of public events. Semantic memory deficits include loss of vocabulary, names and general factual knowledge *(43, 44)*. Patients with semantic dementia and primary progressive aphasia present with language deficits, which can be observed during history taking, in particular problems with fluency, prosody and grammatical errors are noticeable. Patients with vascular dementia can present with problems in executive functioning, which can present as apathy, and problems with planning. Attention should be given to mood disturbances and behavioural changes. Furthermore, the impact of the cognitive complaints on activities of daily living, occupational and social functioning should be explored, as this is critical information in fulfilling dementia criteria. A family history and risk factors, such as vascular risk factors, are relevant, as well as concomitant disease and use of medication. In the consulting room a short cognitive assessment can allow a differential diagnosis to be reached. During the history taking the patient should be observed, and a general impression of cognitive functioning can be obtained, including cooperation, level of alertness, attention and insight. A 'head-turning sign', when the patient looks at his partner for help when asked a question, can be a clue to dementia. The history and clinical impression determine the direction of further examination. A quick screening test is the mini-mental state examination (MMSE) *(45)*. The score ranges from 0 to 30, with broad cut-offs of >25: no impairment; >20 but <25: mild dementia; >12 but <20: moderate dementia and <12 severe dementia (see previous chapter). The standard diagnostic work-up of dementia should include a general neurological examination, with specific attention for extrapyramidal signs, associated with DLB, CBD and PSP, focal neurological deficits, associated with

vascular dementia, or the alien limb in CBD (for overview of dementia associated neurological features (see Kipps and Hodges *(43)*). Besides the neurological examination a general physical examination is warranted in every
patient, with attention to blood pressure measurement and signs of hypothyroidism.

Neuropsychological Examination

A more formal approach to the quantification of cognitive deficits is the
use of standard neuropsychological tests (Fig. 3). Such tests have been validated in the population to produce normal ranges, and thus assessments
using a well-selected battery of tests can determine the extent and pattern
of an individual's degree of cognitive impairment compared to that expected
for age. Although neither 100% sensitive nor specific for a given disease, the
pattern of cognitive impairment demonstrated using neuropsychology may
give useful clues to the underlying disease process (see previous chapter for
detailed discussion).

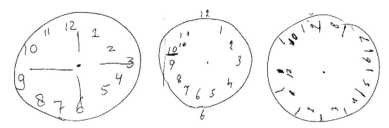

Fig. 3. Clock drawings by patients with AD. In the clock-drawing test, the patient is
asked to draw a clock and set the time at 10 past 11.

Laboratory Testing

Routine laboratory investigations are recommended to exclude possible
reversible causes of cognitive impairment. The practice parameter of the
American Academy of Neurology (AAN) states that vitamin B12 deficiency
and hypothyroidism should be ruled out, as these are comorbidities that
are likely to appear in the elderly and in patients with suspected dementia
in particular *(26)*. Unless the patient has some specific risk factor or evidence of prior syphilitic infection, screening for neurosyphilis is not recommended *(26)*. Additionally, blood sedimentation rate, complete blood cell
count, electrolytes, glucose, renal and liver function tests can be tested to
evaluate possible comorbidities at first evaluation.

Neuroimaging

Structural neuroimaging is recommended in the routine evaluation of patients with dementia *(26)*. Traditionally, imaging was used to exclude other abnormalities that needed intervention such as tumour, hydrocephalus or subdural haematoma. A meta-analysis assessing the use of routine CT scanning in patients with dementia showed that in about 4% theoretically treatable causes were present *(46)*. Although detection of such a lesion is rare, the possibility of a treatable cause must always be considered before the diagnosis of a degenerative dementia is made. Both CT and MRI are generally sufficient to demonstrate such lesions. Whilst current guidelines do not recommend the use of imaging in the positive diagnosis of dementia *(26)*, in the correct setting neuroimaging may be useful in this respect. Especially, MRI scanning is increasingly being used to add support to a clinical diagnosis of AD and other neurodegenerative dementias. In vascular dementia, imaging already forms a mandatory part of some clinical criteria.

The microscopic histological changes in the neurodegenerative diseases are inevitably associated with progressive regional and global brain atrophies, which may be assessed in vivo using MRI. In AD, focal atrophy in the medial temporal region, including the hippocampus, has been the focus of extensive study. It reflects the typical pattern of progression of neuropathology, spreading from the entorhinal cortex and hippocampus to the association cortices, as described by Braak and Braak *(14)*. Neuropathological studies have shown that hippocampal volumes, as measured using MRI, correlate well with the neuropathological burden at post-mortem *(47, 48)*. Many studies initially using CT and later MRI have assessed the diagnostic value of hippocampal atrophy for AD. (For overview, see *(49, 50)*). In a meta-analysis of studies using visual and linear measurements of medial temporal lobe atrophy (MTA) on MRI, the overall sensitivity and specificity for detection of AD compared with controls were estimated to be 85 and 88%, respectively *(50)*. In clinical practice simple visual rating scales estimating hippocampal atrophy are useful. A widely used, well-validated visual rating scale is the five-point scale of Scheltens et al. (Table 4 and Fig. 4) *(51)*. This scale provides a measure for global atrophy of the medial temporal lobe and is based on visually scoring the height of the hippocampus and the width of the surrounding cerebrospinal fluid. The severity of MTA is scored from 0 (no atrophy) to 4 (most severe atrophy), on each side of the brain on a coronal T1-weighted MRI sequence.

Studies in MCI have shown that hippocampal atrophy is detectable on MRI before subjects are clinically demented. The presence of hippocampal

Table 4
Medial temporal lobe atrophy visual rating scale

Score	Width of choroid fissure	Width of temporal horn	Height of the hippocampus
0	Normal	Normal	Normal
1	↑	Normal	Normal
2	↑↑	↑	↓
3	↑↑↑	↑↑	↓↓
4	↑↑↑	↑↑↑	↓↓↓

A score of 0–4 is given separately for the left and right side. (↑) = increase; (↓) = decrease.

Adapted from Scheltens et al. *(51)*.

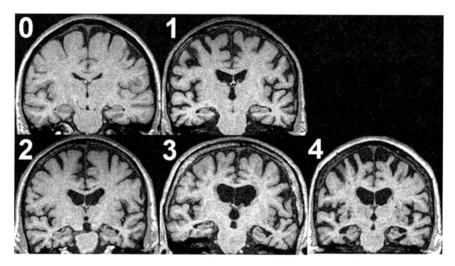

Fig. 4. Examples of scores on medial temporal lobe atrophy visual rating scale on coronal T1-weighted coronal MRI scans.

atrophy in subjects with amnestic MCI is associated with a diagnosis of dementia at follow-up *(48, 52)*.

In the differential diagnosis between different types of dementia, the presence of hippocampal atrophy on neuroimaging is less useful, as hippocampal atrophy has been shown to be present in other types of dementia, such as FTLD, DLB and vascular dementia, as well *(53–55)*.

In clinical practice, evaluation of the pattern of atrophy of the entire brain should be taken into account, rather than an isolated evaluation of the medial temporal lobe. Usually, AD is characterized by global atrophy with prominent atrophy of the medial temporal lobe. However, atypical forms of AD

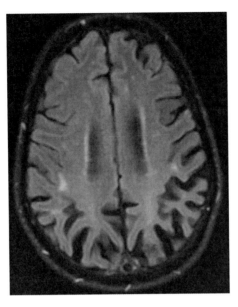

Fig. 5. Posterior cortical atrophy on axial T1-weighted MRI scan.

have been described with prominent posterior atrophy, especially prevalent among younger AD patients (Fig. 5).

Frontal and temporal localized atrophy is suggestive of FTLD, although a normal MRI scan is not uncommon in this disorder *(30)*. Semantic dementia is characterized by left-sided anterior, temporal lobe atrophy, and progressive non-fluent aphasia by left-sided perisylvian atrophy *(30, 53)*.

Some types of dementia show pathognomonic imaging features on MRI such as the characteristic marked hyperintensity of the caudate head and putamen that is seen in 70–80% of cases with sporadic CJD *(56, 57)* and the hyperintensity in the pulvinar in new variant CJD *(57)*. PSP is associated with midbrain atrophy on midsagittal MRI, referred to as the 'hummingbird sign' (Fig. 6).

Besides atrophy, cerebrovascular neuropathology has been associated with cognitive deficits. The radiological NINDS–AIREN criteria for vascular dementia include large and small vessel diseases *(25)*. Large vessel disease includes large territorial or strategic infarcts. Small vessel disease encompasses white matter hyperintensities (WMH), lacunar infarcts (lacunes) and microbleeds. Evidence of small vessel disease is commonly present on MRI of patients throughout the cognitive spectrum *(58, 59)*. Although pure vascular dementia is rare, cerebrovascular pathology is frequently observed on MRI and in pathological studies of patients clinically diagnosed with AD *(17, 19)*. The clinical significance of WMH remains

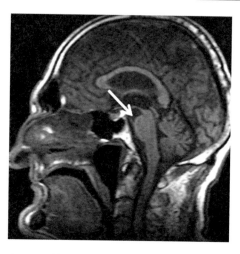

Fig. 6. Midbrain atrophy on midsagittal T1-weighted MRI scan in PSP.

unclear, in both AD and normal ageing. WMH have been associated with subtle cognitive deficits, especially in executive function and psychomotor speed. Evidence exists that AD and cerebrovascular pathology act synergistically *(60)*. In MCI with concomitant WMH, an increased risk of AD has been reported *(61)*, and although a recent study could not confirm this finding, an association between increasing amounts of white matter

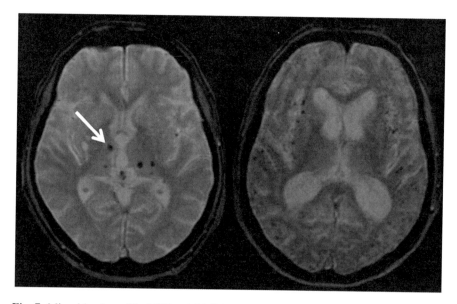

Fig. 7. Microbleeds on Flash/2D axial MRI scan.

hyperintensities and progression to mixed type and vascular dementia was demonstrated *(62)*. Microbleeds are another expression of cerebrovascular pathology that have been associated not only with amyloid angiopathy, but also with other conditions (Fig. 7) *(63)*.

Positron Emission Tomography

Brain metabolism can be studied using positron emission tomography (PET). Changes in brain metabolism may precede structural brain changes. Glucose metabolism can be visualized using the metabolic tracer [18F] fluorodeoxyglucose (FDG). In AD temporal and parietal hypometabolism is found, discriminating AD patients from controls with good discriminatory power (sensitivity and specificity in the range of 85–90%). However, in routine clinical practice PET is not used, since the added value over clinical diagnosis and structural imaging has not been demonstrated. In the diagnosis of FTLD, especially in cases without evidence of atrophy on structural imaging, PET may be useful, demonstrating regional metabolic change *(64)*.

An exciting novel application of PET is the in vivo imaging of amyloid. The amyloid β protein is considered essential to the pathogenesis of AD, as it is the main constituent of neuritic plaques – one of the neuropathological hallmarks of AD. After years of preclinical research, several PET tracers have been developed for this purpose. The Pittsburgh compound-B (carbon-11-labelled PIB) ($[^{11}C]$PIB) *(65)* is the most widely studied amyloid tracer in AD patients. The future development of fluorine-18-labelled PIB with a slower radioactive decay will greatly facilitate clinical implementation of amyloid imaging, which is currently restricted to centres with a cyclotron for on-site production of the tracer. In vivo amyloid imaging may considerably add to our understanding of the underlying pathophysiological mechanisms of AD. Furthermore, imaging of amyloid may prove to be a sensitive diagnostic marker and enable prognoses in the earliest stages of formation of neuropathology. Finally, it may prove valuable as a surrogate marker of disease in studies of antiamyloid drugs.

Cerebrospinal Fluid Markers

Because cerebrospinal fluid (CSF) is in contact with the extracellular space of the brain, biochemical changes in the brain are thought to be reflected in the CSF. Most research regarding CSF in dementia has focussed on the following three biomarkers: amyloid-beta 1-42 (Aβ42), total tau and phosphorylated tau (p-tau).

Decreased levels of Aβ42, to about 40–50% of controls, have been consistently found in the CSF of AD patients *(66, 67)*. The reduced level of Aβ42 is hypothesized to be caused by deposition of Aβ42 in the neuritic plaques, with lower levels diffusing to the CSF. Reported sensitivities and specificities for distinguishing patients with AD from normal elderly controls are 78–92% and 81–83%, respectively (66–68). Moreover, it has been shown that even in the early MCI stage a reduced level of Aβ42 can be demonstrated (69), predicting dementia at follow-up (70). However, decreased levels of Aβ42 have also been shown in other types of dementia, such as FTLD, DLB and vascular dementia (71–73).

Increased levels of CSF total tau in AD patients have been found in numerous studies, to about threefold levels compared to control subjects. CSF total tau levels have been shown to differentiate AD from normal controls with a sensitivity of 80–97% and a specificity of 86–95% (66, 67, 74, 75). It is thought that the level of CSF total tau reflects neuronal damage. In acute conditions, such as stroke or head trauma there is a marked transient increase in total tau levels (76). The level of CSF total tau is highest in the disorders with the highest rate of neuronal degeneration such as CJD (77).

In AD increased levels of phosphorylated tau (p-tau) have been demonstrated in CSF (73, 78). In contrast with total tau, as a marker of neuronal degeneration in general, p-tau may be expected to be more specific to AD, since neurofibrillary tangles are abundant of abnormally phosphorylated tau. Indeed normal levels of p-tau have been reported in the majority of patients with FTD, VaD, DLB and CJD (72, 73, 79, 80).

The diagnostic value of CSF markers may be improved by combination of the different CSF biomarkers, with at least two out of three biomarkers positive for AD (81). Although examination of CSF biomarkers is currently not recommended in the guidelines for routine practice in the work-up of patients with cognitive complaints, it may be considered in difficult diagnostic cases and especially in young (<65 years) patients, because of the broader differential diagnosis in these patients.

When there is a high clinical suspicion of sporadic CJD, measurement of CSF 14-3-3 protein level is recommended, which has a sensitivity and specificity above 90% (26). The 14-3-3 protein is a marker for rapid neuronal degeneration, besides CJD it can be increased in acute stroke, brain tumour or encephalitis (82, 83).

Electroencephalography

In AD generalized slowing of the background rhythm on electroencephalography (EEG) is found frequently. These abnormalities correlate with the severity of the disease. However, this pattern is not very specific for AD, since the same abnormalities can be found in other encephalopathies, such as DLB. In case of doubt, an abnormal EEG substantially raises the chance of AD, however, a normal EEG has relatively little meaning. In MCI, the EEG has not been shown to reliably predict progression to AD *(84)*. The EEG in FTLD may be entirely normal, even in advanced disease stages *(85)*. In contrast, in patients with CJD very specific EEG changes consisting of 'periodic sharp wave complexes' are often present *(86)*. Epilepsy rarely causes memory deficits. Even in patients without evident clinical epileptic signs, but with evidence of epileptic activity on the EEG, treatment with antiepileptic medication should be considered *(87)*.

TREATMENT

At present there is no curative treatment for AD or any of the other neurodegenerative types of dementia. Therefore one of the hallmarks in the management of dementia patients is providing care and information to the patient and his family in several stages of the disease. Since vascular risk factors have been associated with VaD as well as AD attention should be paid to management of hypertension, hyperlipidaemia, diabetes mellitus and smoking in dementia patients. Several options of symptomatic treatment are available, however, to the clinician in the management of patients with dementia.

Cholinesterase Inhibitors

Multiple, randomized, placebo-controlled clinical trials have shown that the cholinesterase inhibitors, galantamine, rivastigmine and donepezil, have a positive effect on cognition and on activities of daily living in patients with mild-to-moderate AD (MMSE score: 10–26) *(88)*. The rationale behind these agents is the cholinergic hypothesis, based on the finding of loss of cholinergic neurons in the basal forebrain in post-mortem examination of brains of patients with AD, resulting in a substantial presynaptic cholinergic deficit*(89)*. Although it is now widely acknowledged that loss of cholinergic transmission alone cannot account for the whole clinico-pathological picture of AD, treatment with cholinesterase inhibitors is still the standard therapy in AD treatment nowadays. However, the effect of cholinesterase inhibitors in the symptomatic treatment of AD is modest, and side-effects are not uncommon. Stabilization of cognitive decline over a period of 6 months can be considered as a successful response to therapy. Clinical trials of cholinesterase inhibitors in MCI failed to show a decreased progression of MCI to AD *(90)*. In about 20% of patients, side-effects such as gastro-intestinal complaints (diarrhoea, nausea and vomiting), loss of appetite, weight loss, headache, dizziness occur.

Memantine

For patients with moderate-to-severe dementia (MMSE <14) memantine, an N-methyl-D-aspartate-receptor antagonist, can be considered. Glutamate plays a role in the neural pathways associated with learning and memory, abnormal levels of glutamate may be responsible for neuronal cell dysfunction and eventual cell death in AD (91). In a Cochrane analysis, it was concluded that memantine has a modest, positive effect on activities of daily living in these patients (92). Memantine has relatively few side-effects, in about 5% of patients dizziness, tiredness and headache occur.

Treatment of Other Types of Dementia

There is evidence that cholinesterase inhibitors may be indicated for patients with mild-to-moderate VaD and DLB. No large, randomized, controlled trials exist in other types of degenerative dementias, such as FTLD, PSP or CBD (5).

Antipsychotic Medication

In later stages of AD, and other types of dementia, neuropsychiatric symptoms such as psychosis may occur. Haloperidol is often the drug of choice in these cases. Randomized trials show that haloperidol is only more effective than a placebo in case of agitation with aggression (93). Side-effects, such as extrapyramidal symptoms, frequently occur. In DLB, haloperidol is contraindicated since it often has a contrary effect. Atypical antipsychotic medication such as olanzapine and risperidone are no longer indicated in patients with dementia, due to serious side-effects.

New Developments

New developments in AD therapy aim at targeting the disease process itself rather than its symptoms. The amyloid hypothesis is one of the most used hypotheses explaining the pathophysiology of AD (94). Cerebral accumulation of $A\beta42$ is thought to play a major role in the pathogenesis of AD, which gives opportunity for secondary prevention of AD. Promising new therapies include antiamyloid therapies and vaccination.

$A\beta42$ is generated by the proteolytic processing of amyloid precursor protein (APP), encoded by a gene on chromosome 21. The insoluble form of $A\beta42$, which is associated with AD, is formed under the influence of the enzymes gamma-secretase and beta-secretase that cleave APP. To prevent the formation of $A\beta42$, much research is focussed on the development of gamma-secretase and beta-secretase inhibitors (95). Another way to prevent Aβ42 production is to stimulate the alternative cleavage route via alpha-secretase. Alternatively, immunization of patient with antibodies is tested in several trials in an attempt to clear Aβ42 from the brain. Although, a phase IIa clinical trial had to be stopped when 17 of 360 patients developed meningoencephalitis clinically, a substantial reduction of Aβ plaques in comparison to control AD brains was found at post-mortem examination of these patients *(96)*. Several trials using active and passive immunization in Aβ42 are currently being carried out.

REFERENCES

1. World Health Organization. Word Health Report 2003 – Shaping the future. Geneva. WHO 2003; 2008.
2. Seshadri S, Wolf PA. Lifetime risk of stroke and dementia: current concepts, and estimates from the Framingham Study. Lancet Neurol 2007; 6:1106–1114.
3. Ferri CP, et al. Global prevalence of dementia: a Delphi consensus study. Lancet 2005; 366:2112–2117.
4. APA. Diagnostic and statistical manual of mental disorders (DSM IV) IV ed., 1994.
5. Waldemar G, et al. Recommendations for the diagnosis and management of Alzheimer's disease and other disorders associated with dementia: EFNS guideline. Eur J Neurol 2007;14:e1–e26.
6. Harvey RJ, Skelton-Robinson M, Rossor MN. The prevalence and causes of dementia in people under the age of 65 years. J Neurol Neurosurg Psychiatry 2003;74:1206–1209.
7. McKhann G, et al. Clinical diagnosis of Alzheimer's disease: report of the NINCDS-ADRDA Work Group under the auspices of Department of Health and Human Services Task Force on Alzheimer's Disease. Neurology 1984; 34:939–944.
8. Ganguli M, et al. Apolipoprotein E polymorphism and Alzheimer disease: The Indo-US Cross-National Dementia Study. Arch Neurol 2000; 57:824–830.
9. Galton CJ, Patterson K, Xuereb JH, Hodges JR. Atypical and typical presentations of Alzheimer's disease: a clinical, neuropsychological, neuroimaging and pathological study of 13 cases. Brain 2000; 123 (Pt 3):484–498.
10. Hardy J. Amyloid, the presenilins and Alzheimer's disease. Trends Neurosci 1997; 20:154–159.
11. Harvey RJ, Skelton-Robinson M, Rossor MN. The prevalence and causes of dementia in people under the age of 65 years. J Neurol Neurosurg Psychiatry 2003; 74:1206–1209.
12. Farrer LA, et al. Effects of age, sex, and ethnicity on the association between apolipoprotein E genotype and Alzheimer disease. A meta-analysis. APOE and Alzheimer Disease Meta Analysis Consortium. JAMA 1997; 278:1349–1356.
13. Mayeux R. Epidemiology of neurodegeneration. Annu Rev Neurosci 2003; 26:81–104.
14. Braak H, Braak E. Neuropathological stageing of Alzheimer-related changes. Acta Neuropathol 1991;82: 239–259.
15. Consensus recommendations for the postmortem diagnosis of Alzheimer's disease. The National Institute on Aging, and Reagan Institute Working Group on Diagnostic Criteria for the Neuropathological Assessment of Alzheimer's Disease. Neurobiol Aging 1997; 18:S1–S2.
16. Polvikoski T, et al. Prevalence of Alzheimer's disease in very elderly people: a prospective neuropathological study. Neurology 2001; 56:1690–1696.
17. Pathological correlates of late-onset dementia in a multicentre, community-based population in England and Wales. Neuropathology Group of the Medical Research Council Cognitive Function and Ageing Study (MRC CFAS). Lancet 2001; 357:169–175.

18. Nagy Z, et al. The effects of additional pathology on the cognitive deficit in Alzheimer disease. J Neuropathol Exp Neurol 1997; 56:165–170.
19. Snowdon DA, et al. Brain infarction and the clinical expression of Alzheimer disease. The Nun Study. JAMA 1997; 277:813–817.
20. Petersen RC, et al. Mild cognitive impairment: clinical characterization and outcome. Arch Neurol 1999; 56:303–308.
21. Petersen RC, et al. Current concepts in mild cognitive impairment. Arch Neurol 2001; 58:1985–1992.
22. Bennett DA, et al. Natural history of mild cognitive impairment in older persons. Neurology 2002; 59:198–1205.
23. Visser PJ, Kester A, Jolles J, Verhey F. Ten-year risk of dementia in subjects with mild cognitive impairment. Neurology 2006; 67:1201–1207.
24. Jicha GA, et al. Neuropathologic outcome of mild cognitive impairment following progression to clinical dementia. Arch Neurol 2006; 63:674–681.
25. Roman GC, et al. Vascular dementia: diagnostic criteria for research studies. Report of the NINDS-AIREN International Workshop. Neurology 1993; 43:250–260.
26. Knopman DS, et al. Practice parameter: diagnosis of dementia (an evidence-based review). Report of the Quality Standards Subcommittee of the American Academy of Neurology. Neurology 2001; 56:1143–1153.
27. Murray ME, Knopman DS, Dickson DW. Vascular dementia: clinical, neuroradiologic and neuropathologic aspects. Panminerva Med 2007; 49:197–207.
28. Curb JD, et al. Longitudinal association of vascular and Alzheimer's dementias, diabetes, and glucose tolerance. Neurology 1999; 52:971–975.
29. Hebert R, et al. Vascular dementia: incidence and risk factors in the Canadian study of health and aging. Stroke 2000;31:1487–1493.
30. Neary D, et al. Frontoteporal lobar degeneration: a consensus on clinical diagnostic criteria. Neurology 1998; 51:1546–1554.
31. Chow TW, Miller BL, Hayashi VN, Geschwind DH. Inheritance of frontotemporal dementia. Arch Neurol 1999; 56:817–822.
32. Cruts M, et al. Null mutations in progranulin cause ubiquitin-positive frontotemporal dementia linked to chromosome 17q21. Nature 2006; 442:920–924.
33. Stevens M, et al. Familial aggregation in frontotemporal dementia. Neurology 1998; 50:1541–1545.
34. Hodges JR, et al. Clinicopathological correlates in frontotemporal dementia. Ann Neurol 2004; 56:399–406.
35. McKeith IG, et al. Consensus guidelines for the clinical and pathologic diagnosis of dementia with Lewy bodies (DLB): report of the consortium on DLB international workshop. Neurology 1996; 47:1113–1124.
36. Mahapatra RK, Edwards MJ, Schott JM, Bhatia KP. Corticobasal degeneration. Lancet Neurol 2004; 3:736–743.
37. Brooks DJ. Diagnosis and management of atypical parkinsonian syndromes. J Neurol Neurosurg Psychiatry 2002; 72 (Suppl 1):I10–I16.
38. Litvan I, et al. Clinical research criteria for the diagnosis of progressive supranuclear palsy (Steele-Richardson-Olszewski syndrome): report of the NINDS-SPSP international workshop. Neurology 1996; 47:1–9.
39. O'Sullivan, S.S. et al. Clinical outcomes of progressive supranuclear palsy and multiple system atrophy. Brain 2008; 131:1362–1372.
40. Donald C. Creutzfeldt-Jacob Disease. Practical Neurol Jun 2002; 2:186–172.
41. Will, R.G. et al. A new variant of Creutzfeldt-Jakob disease in the UK. Lancet 347, 921–925 (1996).
42. Davies L., et al. A4 amyloid protein deposition and the diagnosis of Alzheimer's disease: prevalence in aged brains determined by immunocytochemistry compared with conventional neuropathologic techniques. Neurology 1988; 38:1688–1693.

43. Kipps CM, Hodges JR. Cognitive assessment for clinicians. J Neurol Neurosurg Psychiatry 2005; 76 (Suppl 1): i22–i30.
44. Hodges JR. Cognitive assessment for clinicians. Oxford Medical Publications. Oxford: Oxford University Press, 1994.
45. Folstein MF, Folstein SE, McHugh PR. "Mini-mental state". A practical method for grading the cognitive state of patients for the clinician. J Psychiatr Res 1975; 12:189–198.
46. Foster GR, Scott DA, Payne S. The use of CT scanning in dementia. A systematic review. Int J Technol Assess Health Care 1999; 15:406–423.
47. Gosche KM, Mortimer JA, Smith CD, Markesbery WR, Snowdon DA. Hippocampal volume as an index of Alzheimer neuropathology: findings from the Nun Study. Neurology 2002; 58:1476–1482.
48. Jack CR, Jr., et al. Prediction of AD with MRI-based hippocampal volume in mild cognitive impairment. Neurology 1999; 52:1397–1403.
49. Bosscher L, Scheltens P. MRI of the temporal lobe. In: Qizilbash N SL, Chui H, eds. Evidence based dementia. Oxford: Blackwell Publishing; 2008.
50. Scheltens P, Fox N, Barkhof F, De CC. Structural magnetic resonance imaging in the practical assessment of dementia: beyond exclusion. Lancet Neurol. 2002; 1:13–21.
51. Scheltens P, et al. Atrophy of medial temporal lobes on MRI in "probable" Alzheimer's disease and normal ageing: diagnostic value and neuropsychological correlates. J Neurol Neurosurg Psychiatry 1992; 55:967–972.
52. Korf ES, Wahlund LO, Visser PJ, Scheltens P. Medial temporal lobe atrophy on MRI predicts dementia in patients with mild cognitive impairment. Neurology 2004; 63:94–100.
53. Chan D, et al. Patterns of temporal lobe atrophy in semantic dementia and Alzheimer's disease. Ann Neurol 2001; 49:433–442.
54. Kril JJ, Patel S, Harding AJ, Halliday GM. Patients with vascular dementia due to microvascular pathology have significant hippocampal neuronal loss. J Neurol Neurosurg Psychiatry 2002; 72:747–751.
55. Laakso MP, et al. Hippocampal volumes in Alzheimer's disease, Parkinson's disease with and without dementia, and in vascular dementia: An MRI study. Neurology 1996; 46:678–681.
56. Finkenstaedt M, et al. MR imaging of Creutzfeldt-Jakob disease. Radiology 1996; 199:793–798.
57. Schroter A, et al. Magnetic resonance imaging in the clinical diagnosis of Creutzfeldt-Jakob disease. Arch Neurol 2000; 57:1751–1757.
58. Burns JM, et al. White matter lesions are prevalent but differentially related with cognition in aging and early Alzheimer disease. Arch Neurol 2005; 62:1870–1876.
59. de Leeuw FE, et al. Prevalence of cerebral white matter lesions in elderly people: a population based magnetic resonance imaging study. The Rotterdam Scan Study. J Neurol Neurosurg Psychiatry 2001; 70:9–14.
60. van der Flier WM, et al. Medial temporal lobe atrophy and white matter hyperintensities are associated with mild cognitive deficits in non-disabled elderly people: the LADIS study. J Neurol Neurosurg Psychiatry 2005; 76:1497–1500.
61. Wolf H, Ecke GM, Bettin S, Dietrich J. Gertz HJ. Do white matter changes contribute to the subsequent development of dementia in patients with mild cognitive impairment? A longitudinal study. Int J Geriatr Psychiatry 2000; 15:803–812.
62. Bombois S, et al. Vascular subcortical hyperintensities predict conversion to vascular and mixed dementia in MCI patients. Stroke 2008; 39:2046–2051.
63. Cordonnier C, Al-Shahi SR, Wardlaw J. Spontaneous brain microbleeds: systematic review, subgroup analyses and standards for study design and reporting. Brain 2007; 130:1988–2003.
64. Santens P, et al. Differential regional cerebral uptake of (18)F-fluoro-2-deoxy-D-glucose in Alzheimer's disease and frontotemporal dementia at initial diagnosis. Eur Neurol 2001; 45:19–27.
65. Klunk WE, et al. Imaging brain amyloid in Alzheimer's disease with Pittsburgh Compound-B. Ann Neurol 2004; 55:306–319.

66. Blennow K, Hampel H. CSF markers for incipient Alzheimer's disease. Lancet Neurol 2003;2:605–613.

67. Galasko D, et al. High cerebrospinal fluid tau and low amyloid beta42 levels in the clinical diagnosis of Alzheimer disease and relation to apolipoprotein E genotype. Arch Neurol 1998; 55:937–945.

68. Hulstaert F, et al. Improved discrimination of AD patients using beta-amyloid(1-42) and tau levels in CSF. Neurology 1999; 52:1555–1562.

69. Hampel H, et al. Value of CSF beta-amyloid1-42 and tau as predictors of Alzheimer's disease in patients with mild cognitive impairment. Mol Psychiatry 2004; 9:705–710.

70. Bouwman FH, et al. CSF biomarkers and medial temporal lobe atrophy predict dementia in mild cognitive impairment. Neurobiol Aging 2007; 28:1070–1074.

71. Kanemaru K, Kameda N, Yamanouchi H. Decreased CSF amyloid beta42 and normal tau levels in dementia with Lewy bodies. Neurology 2000; 54:1875–1876.

72. Nagga K, Gottfries J, 1Blennow K, Marcusson J. Cerebrospinal fluid phospho-tau, total tau and beta-amyloid(1-42) in the differentiation between Alzheimer's disease and vascular dementia. Dement Geriatr Cogn Disord 2002; 14:183–190.

73. Schoonenboom NS, et al. Amyloid beta(1-42) and phosphorylated tau in CSF as markers for early-onset alzheimer disease. Neurology 2004; 62:1580–1584.

74. Andreasen N, et al. Sensitivity, specificity, and stability of CSF-tau in AD in a community-based patient sample. Neurology 1999; 53:1488–1494.

75. Blennow K, Vanmechelen E, Hampel H. CSF total tau, Abeta42 and phosphorylated tau protein as biomarkers for Alzheimer's disease. Mol Neurobiol 2001; 24:87–97.

76. Hesse C, et al. Transient increase in total tau but not phospho-tau in human cerebrospinal fluid after acute stroke. Neurosci Lett 2001; 297:187–190.

77. Otto M, et al. Elevated levels of tau-protein in cerebrospinal fluid of patients with Creutzfeldt-Jakob disease. Neurosci Lett 1997; 225:210–212.

78. Buerger K, et al. Differential diagnosis of Alzheimer disease with cerebrospinal fluid levels of tau protein phosphorylated at threonine 231. Arch Neurol 2002; 59:1267–1272.

79. Parnetti L, et al. CSF phosphorylated tau is a possible marker for discriminating Alzheimer's disease from dementia with Lewy bodies. Phospho-Tau International Study Group. Neurol Sci 2001; 22:77–78.

80. Riemenschneider M, et al. Phospho-tau/total tau ratio in cerebrospinal fluid discriminates Creutzfeldt-Jakob disease from other dementias. Mol Psychiatry 2003; 8:343–347.

81. Zetterberg H, Wahlund LO, Blennow K. Cerebrospinal fluid markers for prediction of Alzheimer's disease. Neurosci Lett 2003; 352:67–69.

82. Hsich G, Kenney K, Gibbs CJ, Lee KH, Harrington MG. The 14-3-3 brain protein in cerebrospinal fluid as a marker for transmissible spongiform encephalopathies. N Engl J Med 1996; 335:924–930.

83. Zerr I, et al. Detection of 14-3-3 protein in the cerebrospinal fluid supports the diagnosis of Creutzfeldt-Jakob disease. Ann Neurol 1998; 43:32–40.

84. Jelic V, et al. Quantitative electroencephalography in mild cognitive impairment: longitudinal changes and possible prediction of Alzheimer's disease. Neurobiol Aging 2000; 21: 533–540.

85. Chan D, et al. Rates of global and regional cerebral atrophy in AD and frontotemporal dementia. Neurology 2001; 57:1756–1763.

86. Steinhoff BJ, et al. Accuracy and reliability of periodic sharp wave complexes in Creutzfeldt-Jakob disease. Arch Neurol 1996; 53:162–166.

87. Hogh P, et al. Epilepsy presenting as AD: neuroimaging, electroclinical features, and response to treatment. Neurology 2002; 58:298–301.

88. Birks J. Cholinesterase inhibitors for Alzheimer's disease. Cochrane. Database Syst Rev 2006:CD005593.

89. Mesulam MM, Geula C. Nucleus basalis (Ch4) and cortical cholinergic innervation in the human brain: observations based on the distribution of acetylcholinesterase and choline acetyltransferase. J Comp Neurol 1988; 275:216–240.

90. Loy C, Schneider L. Galantamine for Alzheimer's disease and mild cognitive impairment. Cochrane Database Syst Rev 2006:CD001747.
91. van Marum RJ. Current and future therapy in Alzheimer's disease. Fundam Clin Pharmacol 2008; 22:265–274.
92. McShane R, Areosa SA, Minakaran N. Memantine for dementia. Cochrane Database Syst Rev 2006:CD003154.
93. Ballard C, Waite J. The effectiveness of atypical antipsychotics for the treatment of aggression and psychosis in Alzheimer's disease. Cochrane Database Syst Rev 2006:CD003476.
94. Hardy JA, Higgins GA. Alzheimer's disease: the amyloid cascade hypothesis. Science 1992; 256:184–185.
95. Risner ME, et al. Efficacy of rosiglitazone in a genetically defined population with mild-to-moderate Alzheimer's disease. Pharmacogenomics J 2006; 6:246–254.
96. Schenk D. Hopes remain for an Alzheimer's vaccine. Nature 2004; 431:398.

III ACUTE CEREBRAL DISTURBANCES IN DIABETES

6 Hypoglycemia

Brian M. Frier, *MD, FRCP (Edin)*

CONTENTS

ABSTRACT

Hypoglycemia is a common side-effect of insulin therapy for diabetes and is the major factor that limits the maintenance of strict glycemic control. It can be caused by too much insulin, insufficient carbohydrate, or strenuous exercise.

The brain depends on a continuous supply of glucose and rapidly malfunctions if deprived. Failure to reverse the falling blood glucose allows coma to supervene. Several mechanisms have evolved to protect the brain from neuroglycopenia. Counterregulatory hormones, glucagon and epinephrine (adrenaline), are secreted while sympathoadrenal activation generates autonomic warning symptoms along with those associated with cognitive dysfunction. Responses to hypoglycemia occur at different blood glucose thresholds; they can be modified by strict glycemic control and recurrent exposure to hypoglycemia.

In type 1 diabetes the annual prevalence of severe hypoglycemia (requiring help for recovery) is 30–40% while the annual incidence varies depending on the duration of diabetes. In insulin-treated type 2 diabetes, the frequency is lower but increases with duration of insulin therapy. Nocturnal hypoglycemia is common with all insulin regimens. Severe episodes are associated with serious morbidity, causing coma, seizures, injuries, and accidents. Recurrent hypoglycemia can induce acquired syndromes, which include counterregulatory hormonal

From: *Contemporary Diabetes: Diabetes and the Brain*
Edited by: G. J. Biessels, J. A. Luchsinger (eds.), DOI 10.1007/978-1-60327-850-8_6
© Humana Press, a part of Springer Science+Business Media, LLC 2009

deficiencies and impaired awareness of hypoglycemia, which increase the risk of severe hypoglycemia.

Key words: Hypoglycemia; Glucose counterregulation; Hypoglycemia symptoms; Cognitive dysfunction; Nocturnal hypoglycemia; Impaired awareness of hypoglycemia; Hypoglycemia-associated autonomic failure; Hypoglycemia and driving.

INTRODUCTION

Since the discovery of insulin in the early 1920s, the treatment of diabetes has made encouraging advances with the development of a wide range of insulin formulations and regimens, the emergence of effective monitoring with home blood glucose testing and glycated hemoglobin concentrations, and the impetus to seek strict glycemic control to prevent the long-term complications of this disorder. This progress has increased the life expectancy and improved the quality of life of people with diabetes. However, one troublesome and potentially dangerous side-effect of insulin therapy has remained immutable – the ever present threat of hypoglycemia. This problem is also associated with insulin secretagogue drugs (principally the sulfonylureas), but hypoglycemia is predominantly a complication of treatment with insulin and remains the greatest single barrier to achieving and maintaining good glycemic control. The serious morbidity that may result from hypoglycemia and the profound and detrimental impact that it can have on everyday life explain why it is greatly feared by people treated with insulin and is a continual source of concern to their relatives. The frequent development of acquired syndromes of hypoglycemia, such as impaired awareness of hypoglycemia (IAH), detracts from the success of modern treatment of diabetes in diminishing the frequency and severity of the vascular complications of diabetes. These hypoglycemia-induced complications present different, but equally difficult, problems for the person living with insulin-treated diabetes.

In the context of treating diabetes, the biochemical definition of hypoglycemia differs markedly from that used to designate pathological (spontaneous) hypoglycemia occurring in the non-diabetic person, for which there may be many potential causes. In most endocrine textbooks spontaneous hypoglycemia is defined as a blood glucose of 2.2 mmol/l (40 mg/dl) or lower. However, in people with diabetes, a decline in capillary blood glucose below 3.5 mmol/l (63 mg/dl) can have significant consequences, and any value below this level is usually considered to be clinically relevant. The American Diabetes Association has proposed a higher threshold to represent hypoglycemia of 3.9 mmol/l (70 mg/dl) (1), but many specialists consider this level to be too high, as it encompasses blood glucose values between 3.5

and 3.9 mmol/l (63–70 mg/dl) that seldom appear to have any clinical consequence for the individual. It is important to distinguish between measurements made in arterialized venous blood in experimentally induced hypoglycemia, which yield higher values for glucose than the capillary blood or whole venous blood samples that are commonly used in clinical practice. The glycemic thresholds that have been identified experimentally for the generation of symptoms and the onset of cognitive dysfunction are widely quoted as the usual values in the non-diabetic state. However, they are derived from measurements made from arterialized blood in experimental settings that are higher than would be observed using conventional methods of blood glucose monitoring. Although small incursions into the hypoglycemic range may be relevant to the induction of the acquired syndromes of hypoglycemia, serious morbidity is usually a consequence of severe hypoglycemia and exposure to significant neuronal glucose deprivation (neuroglycopenia).

In clinical practice, hypoglycemia is defined by the capacity of the affected individual to self-treat: *mild* events are self-treated (irrespective of the intensity or nature of the symptoms that are experienced) while *severe* hypoglycemia is any episode that requires external assistance to induce recovery; loss of consciousness (coma) is not a pre-requisite. When significant neuroglycopenia develops, the affected person is unable to self-treat hypoglycemia, although this definition cannot be used in young children who need assistance to treat all forms of hypoglycemia. These definitions were used in the Diabetes Control and Complications Trial (DCCT) *(2)* and have been widely adopted for clinical use. They are simple and practical to apply, and neither specifies a blood glucose threshold to define the severity, nor relies on the method that is used to treat the hypoglycemia. A robust but more restrictive clinical definition of severe hypoglycemia is confined to an episode of coma or one that requires parenteral therapy with either intravenous (i.v.) glucose or intramuscular (i.m.) glucagon. Inevitably the frequency using this definition is much lower. In some therapeutic trials "major," "moderate," and "minor" hypoglycemic events have been described, but often the definitions used have been idiosyncratic or vague, and they are not used clinically.

HYPOGLYCEMIA IN THE NON-DIABETIC STATE

Physiological Changes in Response to Hypoglycemia

In normal health, blood glucose is maintained within a very narrow range and many homeostatic mechanisms have evolved to preserve normoglycemia. This protects the normal functioning of the brain, which is almost entirely dependent on glucose as its principal fuel and source of energy. The functioning of the brain is optimal within this range; cognitive function rapidly becomes impaired when the blood glucose falls below 3.0 mmol/l (54 mg/dl) (3). Similarly, but much less dramatically, cognitive function deteriorates when the brain is exposed to high glucose concentrations (4). The rate-limiting step in the supply of glucose to the brain is its transport across the blood–brain barrier, which is performed by a glucose transporter, and this process cannot be up-regulated quickly in response to a glucose deficit. Modest fluctuations in blood glucose within the physiological range are detected by glucose sensors in the portal venous system, which activate mechanisms to modulate insulin secretion, but if blood glucose falls below normal, this is quickly sensed within the human brain, which activates a hierarchy of counterregulatory mechanisms to restore normoglycemia. The nature and the location of these central glucose sensors await elucidation in humans.

When exogenous insulin is injected into a non-diabetic adult human, peripheral tissues such as skeletal muscle and adipose tissue rapidly take up glucose, while hepatic glucose output is suppressed. This causes blood glucose to fall and triggers a series of counterregulatory events to counteract the actions of insulin; this prevents a progressive decline in blood glucose and subsequently reverses the hypoglycemia. In people with insulin-treated diabetes, many of the homeostatic mechanisms that regulate blood glucose are either absent or deficient.

Counterregulation: The initial endocrine response to a fall in blood glucose in non-diabetic humans is the suppression of endogenous insulin secretion. This is followed by the secretion of the principal counterregulatory hormones, glucagon and epinephrine (adrenaline) (5). Cortisol and growth hormone also contribute, but have greater importance in promoting recovery during exposure to prolonged hypoglycemia. These hormones are released through simultaneous activation of the hypothalamo-pituitary–adrenal axis and central autonomic centers within the brain, which stimulates the peripheral autonomic nervous system, particularly the sympathoadrenal system. Activation of the peripheral sympathetic nervous system and the adrenal glands provokes the release of a copious quantity of catecholamines, epinephrine, and norepinephrine, which have potent effects in mobilising 3-carbon precursors for glucose synthesis from peripheral tissues (skeletal muscle and adipose tissue) and also convert hepatic glycogen to glucose. Glucagon is secreted from the alpha cells of the pancreatic islets, apparently in response to localized neuroglycopenia and independent of central neural control. Glucagon acts solely in the liver to stimulate glycogenolysis and gluconeogenesis, the net effect being to rapidly release glucose into the systemic circulation for immediate transport to the brain.

The large amounts of catecholamines that are secreted in response to hypoglycemia exert other powerful physiological effects that are unrelated to counterregulation. These include major hemodynamic actions with direct effects on the heart and blood pressure. Myocardial contractility and cardiac output are increased and peripheral vascular resistance and central blood pressure fall (6). Electrophysiological changes occur in the heart, which include QT prolongation. In response to autonomic stimulation and catecholamine secretion, regional blood flow changes occur during hypoglycemia that encourages the transport of substrates to the liver for gluconeogenesis and simultaneously of glucose to the brain. Organs that have no role in the response to acute stress, such as the spleen and kidneys, are temporarily under-perfused. The mobilisation and activation of white blood cells are accompanied by hemorheological effects, promoting increased viscosity, coagulation, and fibrinolysis and may influence endothelial function (6). In normal health these acute physiological changes probably exert no harmful effects, but may acquire pathological significance in people with diabetes of long duration.

Symptomatic response: If blood glucose continues to fall despite counterregulation, the autonomic stimulation and the effects of neuroglycopenia on cognitive function generate typical symptoms of hypoglycemia, usually when blood glucose falls to a specific level or glycemic threshold. The sudden onset of sympathoadrenal activation used to be called the "autonomic reaction," a term that unfortunately has fallen into disuse, although it succinctly describes the intense explosion of autonomic activity that occurs in response to acute hypoglycemia. The effects of autonomic stimulation of end-organs such as the heart and sweat glands underlie the typical autonomic symptoms of hypoglycemia such as pounding heart and sweating (Fig. 1). When these are perceived via sensory feedback to the brain, the person with previous experience of low blood glucose recognizes the onset of hypoglycemia and will take appropriate action to counteract the symptoms (by ingesting glucose).

The neuroglycopenic symptoms of hypoglycemia are manifestations of cognitive dysfunction, such as difficulty in concentrating, drowsiness, and altered speech, and are equally useful in detecting the early onset of hypoglycemia (3, 7). Common symptoms of hypoglycemia in young adults, and how they are classified, are shown in Table 1. However, symptoms are idiosyncratic and age-specific. Behavioral symptoms are prominent in young children, while elderly people exhibit a cluster of neurological symptoms including visual disturbance and motor incoordination (3, 7). In clinical research, it is important to apply a symptom scoring system that is appropriate to the age group under study, and patient education about hypoglycemia should also acknowledge these age-related differences in symptom profiles.

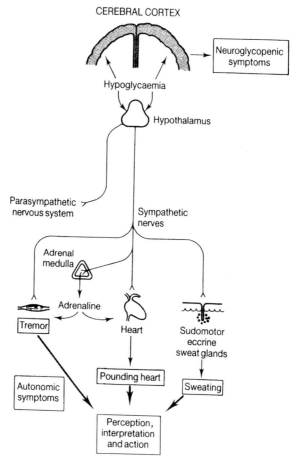

Fig. 1. Generation of neuroglycopenic and autonomic symptoms in response to hypoglycemia. Activation of the autonomic system, particularly the sympathoadrenal system, stimulates end-organs and provokes typical symptoms of hypoglycemia. (From Frier *(11)*. Reprinted with permission from Blackwell Publishing, John Wiley and Sons.)

Mood changes: In addition to the generation of warning symptoms, changes in mood occur during hypoglycemia, which are predominantly negative. These vary between individuals and comprise feelings of tense-tiredness (anxious tension), low energy, irritability, unhappiness, anger, and general pessimism. The effects of hypoglycemia on emotions are unpleasant but important, yet are frequently ignored by clinicians.

Cognitive impairment: Cognitive functions, which include several forms of mental activity, start to become impaired at around the same blood glucose level as the emergence of the autonomic response to hypoglycemia. The more complex and attention-demanding cognitive tasks, and those that

Table 1
Classification of common symptoms of insulin-induced hypoglycemia, as observed in young adults with type 1 diabetes

Autonomic	Neuroglycopenic	Malaise/non-specific
Sweating	Confusion	Headache
Pounding heart	Drowsiness	Nausea
Hunger	Difficulty in	
Tremor	speaking	
	Odd behavior	
	Incoordination	

Adapted from Deary *(3)*, with permission from John Wiley & Sons Ltd (Publishers) Ltd

require speeded responses are more affected by hypoglycemia than simple tasks or those that do not require any time restraint *(3)*. The overall speed of response of the brain in making decisions is slowed, yet for many tasks, accuracy is preserved at the expense of speed *(8, 9)*. Many aspects of mental performance become impaired when blood glucose falls below 3.0 mmol/l (54 mg/dl), but individual differences exist in the levels at which impairment commences and in the magnitude of dysfunction that occurs. Recovery of cognitive function does not occur immediately after the blood glucose returns to normal, but in some cognitive domains may be delayed for 60 min or more *(3)*, which is of practical importance to the performance of tasks that require complex cognitive functions, such as driving.

Glycemic thresholds: These major changes that occur during hypoglycemia – counterregulatory hormone secretion, symptom generation, and cognitive dysfunction – occur as components of a hierarchy of responses, each being triggered as the blood glucose falls to its glycemic threshold. The sequence of these physiological responses is shown in Fig. 2. In nondiabetic individuals, the glycemic thresholds are fixed and reproducible *(10)*, but in people with diabetes, these thresholds are dynamic and plastic, and can be modified by external factors such as glycemic control or exposure to preceding (antecedent) hypoglycemia *(11)*. Changes in the glycemic thresholds for the responses to hypoglycemia underlie the effects of the acquired hypoglycemia syndromes that can develop in people with insulin-treated diabetes, as described below. The glycemic thresholds are often quoted as being 3.8 mmol/l (68 mg/dl) for counterregulatory hormones, 3.0 mmol/l (54 mg/dl) for the onset of symptoms, and around 2.7 mmol/l (48 mg/dl) for cognitive impairment *(10, 11)*, but, as noted previously, these were measured in *arterialized* venous blood in experimental studies using glucose clamp techniques and are higher than the capillary or venous blood measurements that are employed in everyday clinical practice.

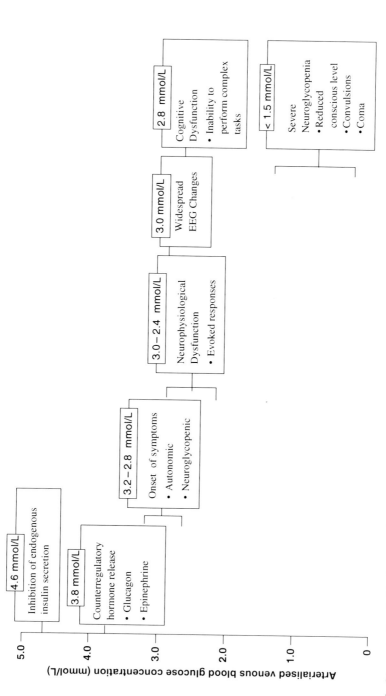

Fig. 2. Glycemic thresholds for secretion of counterregulatory hormones and onset of physiological, symptomatic and cognitive changes in response to hypoglycemia in the non-diabetic human. Reproduced from Frier BM and Fisher BM[8]. In: *Hypoglycaemia in Clinical Diabetes.* (eds Frier BM, Fisher BM), 1999. Reproduced with permission of John Wiley and Sons, Chichester.

HYPOGLYCEMIA IN PEOPLE WITH DIABETES

Epidemiology

Most data on the frequency of hypoglycemia have been collected retrospectively in people with type 1 diabetes and predominantly focus on severe events, which are relatively robust to measure as they can be recalled with accuracy for up to 1 year in people with normal symptomatic awareness *(12)*. Total amnesia of severe hypoglycemia is common, and obtaining an accurate estimate is often difficult in people who have impaired awareness of hypoglycemia; relatives and friends may provide a more reliable history than the patient. Mild (self-treated) episodes are quickly forgotten and can be recalled by individuals for only about a week *(12)*. However, prospective studies in Denmark and England that were performed 20 years apart, during which time insulin formulations and regimens changed considerably, have shown that the average incidence of mild hypoglycemia has remained unchanged at around two episodes per week *(12, 13)*. Prospective recording of hypoglycemic events over a defined period of time is much more accurate when measuring the prevalence or incidence of mild and severe hypoglycemia, but discrepancies between studies are often related to differences in definition of hypoglycemia, heterogeneity of the populations studied, and accuracy of ascertainment of events, and may be affected by factors such as the quality of glycemic control.

The comprehensive prospective study of the DCCT is widely cited as demonstrating the most accurate frequency of severe hypoglycemia in type 1 diabetes, and certainly the annual prevalence of severe hypoglycemia of 36% *(2, 14)* is entirely consistent with that reported in many other large studies, of between 30 and 40% *(12, 15–18)*. The incidence of severe hypoglycemia in the DCCT was reported as 0.6 episodes per patient-year in the intensively treated group with strict glycemic control (mean HbA1c 7%), which was three times greater than in the conventionally treated group with less strict control (mean HbA1c 9%) *(2, 14)*. While the threefold difference in incidence (Fig. 3) is a valuable clinical observation of direct relevance to the consequences of tightening glycemic control, the overall incidences reported in the DCCT are deceptively low. This is because at recruitment for the DCCT anyone who had a history of severe hypoglycemia was excluded *(19)* (therefore omitting people with impaired awareness of hypoglycemia), and the participants were young, healthy with few complications, had diabetes of short duration, and received a level of clinical support during the course of the trial that was the envy of most diabetes clinics. Thus, the DCCT cohort was highly selected and atypical, and although severe hypoglycemia was relatively common, the incidence even in the intensively treated group was much lower than those reported in unselected cohorts of people with

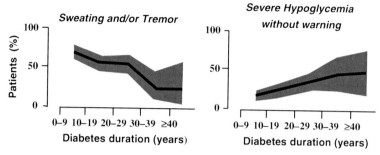

Fig. 3. Comparisons between the duration of diabetes and the percentages of 411 type 1 diabetic patients reporting changes in symptoms of sweating and/or tremor as two of the cardinal autonomic symptoms of hypoglycemia (*left panel*) and severe hypoglycemic events without warning symptoms (*right panel*). Values are medians; shaded areas show 95% confidence limits. (From Pramming et al. *(12)*. Reprinted with permission of Blackwell Publishing, John Wiley & Sons, Ltd.)

Table 2
Epidemiology of severe hypoglycemia in type 1 diabetes

Study	Severe hypoglycemia: prevalence (%)	Severe hypoglycemia: incidence (episodes per patient-year)
Pramming et al. *(12)*	30.0%	1.4
Pedersen-Bjergaard et al. *(13)*	36.7%	1.3
MacLeod et al. *(16)*	29.2%	1.6
ter Braak et al. *(17)*	40.5%	1.5
DCCT Research Group *(14)*	35% men 31% women	0.19–0.62
UK Hypoglycaemia Study Group *(18)*	22% (<5 years duration) 46% (>15 years duration)	1.1 (<5 years duration) 3.2 (>15 years duration)

type 1 diabetes that include people who are at high risk of hypoglycemia (Table 2).

The incidence of severe hypoglycemia in unselected groups with type 1 diabetes was more than double that reported in the DCCT and in those who have good glycemic control (mean HbA1c 7.6%) and type 1 diabetes for more than 15 years, it was several fold higher *(18)*. The distribution of severe events is skewed, with a relatively small proportion of patients experiencing multiple episodes *(13)*. Fewer data are available for people with type 2 diabetes, and a common misperception is that severe hypoglycemia is relatively uncommon in insulin-treated type 2 diabetes *(20)*. However, a number of studies have indicated that while the frequency of severe hypoglycemia is lower than in type 1 diabetes *(21–23)*, it becomes progressively more common the longer the patients are treated with insulin *(24)*. When people with type 1 diabetes and insulin-treated type 2 diabetes were matched for duration of insulin therapy, the frequency was similar *(25)*.

The UK Hypoglycaemia Study Group *(18)*, a large multicenter, prospective study group in the UK, confirmed that the incidence of severe hypoglycemia in people with insulin-treated type 2 diabetes increases steadily with duration of insulin therapy (Table 3), as pancreatic beta-cell failure develops. The under-recognized risk of severe hypoglycemia in insulin-treated type 2 diabetes is of great practical importance as this group is numerically much larger than people with type 1 diabetes and encompasses many older, and some very elderly, people who may be exposed to much greater danger because they often have co-morbidities such as macrovascular disease, osteoporosis, and general frailty.

Table 3
Epidemiology of severe hypoglycemia in type 2 diabetes

Study	Severe hypoglycemia: prevalence (%)	Severe hypoglycemia: incidence (episodes per patient-year)
VACSDM *(21)*	n/a	0.02
Henderson et al. *(24)*	15%	0.28
Leese et al. *(22)*	0.8% (oral agents)	0.009 (SU Rx)
	7.3% (insulin)	0.005 (metformin Rx)
		0.12 (insulin)
Donnelly et al. *(23)*	3%	0.35
UK Hypoglycaemia	7% (oral agents)	0.1 (oral agents)
Study Group *(18)*	7% (<2 years duration)	0.1 (<2 years duration)
	25% (>5 years duration)	0.7 (>5 years duration)

Nocturnal hypoglycemia is common with all insulin regimens, is usually asymptomatic, and is often unidentified as symptoms are absent during sleep and because blood glucose is rarely measured routinely during the night *(26)*. Surveys have demonstrated biochemical hypoglycemia in up to 50% of overnight blood glucose profiles in adults and in nearly 80% of children with insulin-treated diabetes; this has been confirmed by the use of continuous blood glucose monitoring *(27)*. Nocturnal hypoglycemia is often prolonged, sometimes lasting for up to 6 h. The timing of nocturnal hypoglycemia varies with different insulin regimens and times of maximum vulnerability vary. Symptomatic clues to the occurrence of nocturnal hypoglycemia are often subtle, such as vivid dreams or nightmares, morning headache or "hangover" (without preceding alcohol consumption), chronic fatigue, poor quality of sleep, and mood change, including depression.

Causes and Risk Factors

Causation of hypoglycemia is often multifactorial and in many severe episodes no definite cause can be identified. Causes of hypoglycemia (Table 4) should be distinguished from risk factors, which increase the

Table 4
Causes of hypoglycemia in insulin-treated diabetes

Causes

Change in insulin sensitivity/bioavailability

- Acute remission in newly diagnosed diabetes following treatment
- Post-delivery in diabetic pregnancy
- Menstruation (variable)
- Renal impairment/failure
- Effects of exercise

Change in insulin pharmacokinetics

- Change of insulin formulation
- Change of insulin injection site
- Effects of temperature (e.g., hot bath, sauna)

Inadequate dietary carbohydrate

- Unexpected physical exertion
- Social: sport, training, travel, change of occupation
- Dieting (in extreme cases – anorexia nervosa)
- Breast feeding
- Malabsorption (celiac disease)
- Gastroparesis (autonomic neuropathy)

Other related conditions

- Endocrine failure (Addison's disease, hypopituitarism, hypothyroidism)
- Psychological disorders (factitious)

Adapted from Tattersall RB. Frequency and causes of hypoglycaemia. In: *Hypoglycaemia and Diabetes: Clinical and Physiological Aspects*, Editors Frier, B. M. and Fisher, B. M. (1993), pp. 176–189, Edward Arnold, London)

Table 5
Risk factors for severe hypoglycemia in type 1 diabetes and in insulin-treated type 2 diabetes

Risk factors

Duration of diabetes (type 1 diabetes)
Duration of insulin therapy (type 2 diabetes)
Age
Strict glycemic control
Impaired awareness of hypoglycemia
History of previous severe hypoglycemia
Sleep
C-peptide negativity
Social class

propensity to develop hypoglycemia (Table 5). Hypoglycemia occurs when a mismatch develops between the plasma concentrations of glucose and insulin, particularly when the latter is inappropriately high, which is common during the night. Hypoglycemia can result when too much insulin is injected relative to oral intake of carbohydrate or when a meal is missed or delayed after insulin has been administered. Strenuous exercise can precipitate hypoglycemia through accelerated absorption of insulin and depletion of muscle glycogen stores. Alcohol enhances the risk of prolonged hypoglycemia by inhibiting hepatic gluconeogenesis, but the hypoglycemia may be delayed for several hours.

Errors of dosage or timing of insulin administration are common, and there are few conditions where the efficacy of the treatment can be influenced by so many extraneous factors. The time–action profiles of different insulins can be modified by factors such as the ambient temperature or the site and depth of injection and the person with diabetes has to constantly try to balance insulin requirement with diet and exercise. It is therefore not surprising that hypoglycemia occurs so frequently. Other causes of an increased propensity to hypoglycemia include the covert development of other autoimmune disorders such as Addison's disease and celiac disease (gluten enteropathy). Gastroparesis, secondary to autonomic neuropathy, frequently provokes severe hypoglycemia because of delayed absorption of glucose from the upper gastrointestinal tract. Renal impairment reduces the clearance of insulin and prolongs its biological activity, also promoting hypoglycemia. These are all direct causes of hypoglycemia and should not be confused with risk factors for hypoglycemia (Table 5).

Risk factors include strict glycemic control, as was noted earlier in the DCCT with a threefold difference in the incidence of severe hypoglycemia between the intensively treated and conventionally treated groups *(2, 14)*. The lower the median blood glucose during the day, the greater the frequency of symptomatic and biochemical hypoglycemia; if the median blood glucose is 5.0 mmol/l (90 mg/dl), blood glucose will be below 3.0 mmol/l (54 mg/dl) around 10% of the time *(28)*, a sobering statistic that should be carefully considered when demanding that patients strive to maintain very stringent levels of control. Strict glycemic control can also induce the acquired hypoglycemia syndromes, impaired awareness of hypoglycemia (a major risk factor for severe hypoglycemia), and counterregulatory hormonal deficiencies (which interfere with blood glucose recovery). These are described in more detail below. Severe hypoglycemia is more common at the extremes of age – in very young children and in elderly people. A history of previous severe hypoglycemia is associated with a greater risk of subsequent events, and the DCCT showed that warning symptoms were absent in a third (36%) of events during waking hours *(29)*. Sympathoadrenal activation is diminished during sleep *(30)*, which may contribute to the promotion of severe nocturnal hypoglycemia – 55% of all events in the DCCT *(29)*. In type 1 diabetes the frequency of severe hypoglycemia increases with duration of diabetes *(12)*, while in type 2 diabetes it is associated with increasing duration of insulin treatment *(18)*. Some people may have a genetic predisposition to severe hypoglycemia, with attention being focused on the genotype associated with angiotensin-converting enzyme (ACE) activity – high serum ACE concentrations were reported to be associated with an increased risk of severe hypoglycemia in Danish patients with type 1 diabetes *(31)*. However, others have observed only a weak relationship *(32)*, and the value of this measurement as an index of risk of severe hypoglycemia is unclear.

Management of Hypoglycemia

The key to successful treatment of hypoglycemia is early detection by the affected individual of the fall in blood glucose to allow prompt self-treatment and so prevent progression to more severe hypoglycemia. This may not rely solely on the perception of the initial symptoms, but may utilize frequent blood glucose testing to demonstrate biochemical hypoglycemia and draw upon experience acquired over many years of diabetes self-management to anticipate when hypoglycemia may be a potential problem in relation to meals and exercise. Any proposed guidelines for the self-treatment of mild hypoglycemia are arbitrary in nature and in some instances may be considered to be too prescriptive. Hypoglycemia stimulates the intake of calories to replace energy stores and encourages the consumption of foods that are high in fat *(33)*. These food choices generally have a low glycemic index and may be relatively inadequate at treating and preventing the recurrence of further hypoglycemia.

Most treatment guidelines recommend the initial consumption of 10–15 g of refined (monosaccharide) carbohydrate (e.g., 3–5 glucose tablets), followed by some form of unrefined (starch) carbohydrate to prevent hypoglycemia recurring (34). A quantity of 15 g of oral fast-acting carbohydrate causes blood glucose to rise by 2.1 mmol/l (38 mg/dl) within 20 min (34). It is not possible to relieve the symptoms of hypoglycemia with oral glucose within 10 min, no matter what type of rapidly absorbed glucose is used to treat an acute episode, and while waiting for this delayed response the sufferer often experiences an intense drive to ingest more carbohydrate (33). Overtreatment of hypoglycemia should be avoided whenever possible, as it leads to rebound hyperglycemia and promotes weight gain. The latter can also result when "defensive eating" is used as a strategy to prevent hypoglycemia. With experience, most people learn how much carbohydrate they need to consume to treat mild hypoglycemia. The application of glucose gel, honey, or a fruit conserve containing sugar such as jam to the buccal mucosa is an alternative to swallowing orange juice or other glucose-containing beverages, but is absorbed more slowly (35). When a patient is receiving continuous subcutaneous insulin infusion (CSII) therapy, rapid-acting carbohydrate alone is required to treat hypoglycemia, because the insulin infusion can be temporarily discontinued and further ingestion of oral complex carbohydrate is not required.

In 10% of episodes of severe hypoglycemia affecting people with type 1 diabetes and around 30% of those in people with insulin-treated type 2 diabetes, the assistance of the emergency medical services is required (23). However, most episodes (both mild and severe) are treated in the community, and few people require admission to hospital. An algorithm summarising the treatment of acute hypoglycemia is shown in Table 6 (36). In severe hypoglycemia, the nature of the treatment that is required will depend on the conscious state of the individual. If the person is fully conscious and can swallow without difficulty, oral carbohydrate can be given, but when people are confused and cognitively impaired, this treatment may be refused; in semi-conscious individuals there is a risk of aspiration and parenteral treatment is necessary. Glucagon is administered either intramuscularly or subcutaneously in a dose of 1 mg (0.5 mg in young children), and relatives can be trained to give this treatment. It acts by stimulating hepatic glycogenolysis and releasing glucose from the liver. Nausea (and occasionally vomiting) is common. Alternatively, intravenous dextrose can be given. An injection of 25 g of dextrose (50 ml of 50% dextrose) is generally recommended, but because 50% dextrose has a very irritant effect on veins, most physicians now use 20% dextrose. In the case of prolonged

Table 6
The therapeutic spectrum of hypoglycemia

		Duration of hypoglycemia		
Minutes				*Hours*
By patient	*By family*	*Primary/ paramedical care*	*Emergency department*	*In-hospital (ITU – cerebral edema)*
Oral carbohydrate (>20 g)	Oral carbohydrate (liquid/ solid) or 1 mg glucagon plus oral carbohydrate 20–40 g when fully conscious	1 mg glucagon IM or IV or 25 g dextrose IV	25 g dextrose IV or 1 mg glucagon IV plus oral carbohydrate when fully conscious	Mannitol (20% solution, 200 ml) Dexamethasone (16–24 mg/ day) plus High flow oxygen Anticonvulsants Sedation Dextrose/insulin infusion Potassium infusion

Adapted from MacCuish *(36), with permission of Edward Arnold (Publishers)*

hypoglycemia, a continuous intravenous infusion of dextrose and frequent oral feeding will be required. When hypoglycemic coma does not respond to intravenous dextrose, neuroimaging must be performed urgently to look for cerebral edema, a recognized complication of severe hypoglycemia that is associated with a high mortality, and to exclude other intracranial pathology. Treatment of cerebral edema includes intravenous mannitol and high dose corticosteroids in addition to supportive measures such as high flow oxygen, sedation, and if indicated, anticonvulsant therapy *(36)*. It may take several days to recover from profound hypoglycemic coma.

The practical management of hypoglycemia (particularly when severe) should also include some retrospective analysis of why the episode had occurred and how it can be avoided in future. Prevention of hypoglycemia is an important aspect of management because fear of hypoglycemia interferes with the long-term maintenance of glycemic control.

Morbidity of Hypoglycemia

Severe hypoglycemia is potentially dangerous and has a significant mortality and morbidity, particularly in older people with insulin-treated diabetes who often have premature macrovascular disease. The hemo-dynamic effects of autonomic stimulation may provoke acute vascular events such as myocardial ischemia and infarction, cardiac failure, cerebral ischemia, and stroke *(6)*. In clinical practice the cardiovascular and cerebrovascular consequences of hypoglycemia are frequently overlooked because the role of hypoglycemia in precipitating the vascular event is missed. The VADT *(37)* and the ACCORD study *(38)* have demonstrated the risks of very strict glycemic control in a population at risk of vascular events. These studies examined the effects of glycemic control in people with type 2 diabetes who had several vascular risk factors or had overt cardiovascular disease. The group with very strict glycemic control had greater exposure to severe hypoglycemia, which inevitably has been implicated as the cause of increased mortality, although a direct causal association cannot be proven. Unfortunately, the inherent difficulty of demonstrating a causal relationship between a severe hypoglycemic event and a serious vascular outcome has obscured this putative association, and clinical evidence for the vascular consequences of hypoglycemia is mainly anecdotal *(6)*.

The profuse secretion of catecholamines in response to hypoglycemia provokes a fall in plasma potassium and causes electrocardiographic (ECG) changes, which in some individuals may provoke a cardiac arrhythmia, several of which have been described *(39)*. A possible mechanism that has been observed with ECG recordings during hypoglycemia is prolongation of the QT interval, which is associated with an increased risk of cardiac conduction defects and dangerous ventricular arrhythmias *(39)*. Hypoglycemia-induced arrhythmias during sleep have been implicated as the cause of the "dead in bed" syndrome that is recognized in young people with type 1 diabetes *(40)*.

Total cerebral blood flow is increased during acute hypoglycemia while regional blood flow within the brain is altered acutely. Blood flow increases in the frontal cortex, presumably as a protective compensatory mechanism to enhance the supply of available glucose to the most vulnerable part of the brain. These regional vascular changes become permanent in people who are exposed to recurrent severe hypoglycemia and in those with impaired awareness of hypoglycemia, and are then present during normoglycemia *(41)*. This probably represents an adaptive response of the brain to recurrent exposure to neuroglycopenia. However, these permanent hypoglycemia-induced changes in regional cerebral blood flow may encourage localized neuronal ischemia, particularly if the cerebral circulation is already compromised by the development of cerebrovascular disease associated with diabetes. This may increase the risk of localized cerebral ischemia when the individual is exposed to other forms of hemodynamic stress that affect the cerebrovascular circulation. Transient ischemic attacks and hemiplegia are recognized manifestations of hypoglycemia and in the elderly may be misdiagnosed as evidence of cerebrovascular disease.

The main neurological consequences of severe hypoglycemia are coma and seizures, which exposes the affected patient to potentially serious morbidity, including fracture-dislocations, soft tissue injuries, and head injury. Around one quarter of all episodes of severe hypoglycemia result in coma *(42)*. When electroencephalography (EEG) has been performed during hypoglycemia in awake resting subjects, a decrease in alpha waves, an increase in theta waves, and increased bursts of delta waves are observed, occurring diffusely over the cerebral cortex, but the EEG changes are more pronounced over the anterior part of the brain. Studies in adolescents with type 1 diabetes have demonstrated more pronounced abnormalities than in non-diabetic controls, with a greater tendency to epileptiform activity, and theta wave changes persist after blood glucose has recovered *(43)*. Hypoglycemia-induced EEG changes can persist for days or become permanent, particularly after recurrent severe hypoglycemia, and this may interfere with investigations to exclude idiopathic epilepsy.

Focal neurological lesions as a consequence of acute hypoglycemia are rare, as is severe brain damage, which probably requires several hours of exposure to profound hypoglycemia. These isolated events are usually associated with deliberate insulin overdose or excessive alcohol consumption. However, transient and reversible neurological deficits have increasingly been demonstrated in individual cases with sophisticated neuroimaging techniques *(44, 45)*, indicating that functional changes within the brain may be commonplace, without leaving a permanent structural abnormality. Structural abnormalities of the brain that are observed in the survivors of exposure to profound hypoglycemia include cortical and hippocampal atrophies and ventricular dilatation. Such individuals either exist in a vegetative state or have evidence of profound cognitive damage. In patients with profound and protracted hypoglycemic coma, prognosis can be difficult to determine, but if serum markers of brain damage, neurone-specific enolase and the protein S-100, become elevated within 24–48 h of the onset of the coma, this usually indicates a poor outcome *(46)*.

Hypoglycemia increases the risk of falls in the elderly, many of whom are frail and have osteoporosis, which increases their vulnerability to hypoglycemia-induced injury and bony fractures. In addition to the effects of trauma, when hypoglycemia occurs during driving it can cause road traffic accidents, with resultant morbidity.

Mortality of Hypoglycemia

The frequency of fatal episodes of hypoglycemia is difficult to determine because of the problem of determining whether low blood glucose was

present before death and is compounded by the inaccuracy of death certifica-
tion. As alluded to earlier, many fatal cases in elderly patients are attributed
to a cardiovascular or cerebrovascular event, and the precipitating effect of
acute hypoglycemia is not identified.

Most studies in populations with type 1 diabetes suggest that the proportion of deaths caused by hypoglycemia is between 2 and 6%, which is lower
than the mortality associated with ketoacidosis. Death may result suddenly
from a cardiac arrhythmia or more slowly from profound neuroglycopenia
causing severe cerebral damage. In the large British Diabetic Association
Cohort Study of people who had developed type 1 diabetes before the age of
30, acute metabolic complications of diabetes were the greatest single cause
of excess death under the age of 30; hypoglycemia was the cause of death in
18% of males and 6% of females in the 20–49 age group (47).

Acquired Hypoglycemia Syndromes

Chronic exposure to hyperglycemia has long been recognized to be the
major cause of vascular disease in diabetes and the severity of microangiopathic complications is directly related to the quality of glycemic control
(14). Conversely, recurrent exposure to hypoglycemia of any severity causes
syndromes that are both hypoglycemia-related and impair the capacity of the
individual to respond to this metabolic stress, further increasing the risk of
severe hypoglycemia and effectively creating a vicious circle that is difficult
to break. These syndromes of counterregulatory hormonal deficiencies and
impaired awareness of hypoglycemia (IAH) develop over a period of years
and ultimately affect a substantial proportion of people with type 1 diabetes
and a lesser number with insulin-treated type 2 diabetes. They are considered
to be components of hypoglycemia-associated autonomic failure (HAAF),
through down-regulation of the central mechanisms within the brain that
would normally activate glucoregulatory responses to hypoglycemia, including the release of counterregulatory hormones and the generation of warning
symptoms (48).

Counterregulatory deficiencies: The glucagon secretory response to
hypoglycemia becomes diminished or absent within a few years of the onset
of insulin-deficient diabetes. With glucagon deficiency alone, blood glucose
recovery from hypoglycemia is not noticeably affected because the secretion
of epinephrine maintains counterregulation. However, almost half of those
who have type 1 diabetes of 20 years duration have evidence of impairment of both glucagon and epinephrine in response to hypoglycemia (49);
this seriously delays blood glucose recovery and allows progression to more
severe and prolonged hypoglycemia when exposed to low blood glucose.
People with type 1 diabetes who have these combined counterregulatory

hormonal deficiencies have a 25-fold higher risk of experiencing severe hypoglycemia if they are subjected to intensive insulin therapy compared with those who have lost their glucagon response but have retained epinephrine secretion (50, 51). In people with type 1 diabetes, counterregulatory deficiencies co-segregate with IAH (52), suggesting that they share a common pathogenetic mechanism within the brain.

Impaired awareness of hypoglycemia (IAH): The awareness of hypoglycemia can be defined as the perception of the initial symptoms of falling blood glucose (11). This may become diminished or blunted in people with insulin-treated diabetes, particularly with type 1 diabetes, and is thought to result from diminished sympathoadrenal activation producing a resultant reduction in the autonomic symptom response to a given level of hypoglycemia (11). Impaired awareness is not an "all or none" phenomenon. "Partial" impairment of awareness may develop, with the individual being aware of some episodes of hypoglycemia but not others (53). Alternatively, the intensity or number of symptoms may be reduced, and neuroglycopenic symptoms predominate. This gradually progresses to loss of awareness where the patient is no longer aware of the onset of hypoglycemia, although total absence of any symptoms, albeit subtle, is very uncommon, a fact that underpins the use of "Blood Glucose Awareness Training" that has been devised to help people with IAH (54).

Several mechanisms have been proposed as the cause of IAH, including chronic exposure to low blood glucose as in strict glycemic control (similar to the effects of insulinoma in non-diabetic patients), the effects of antecedent hypoglycemia, and HAAF (11). The glycemic thresholds for generation of symptoms, counterregulatory hormone secretion, and cognitive impairment are all re-set at lower blood glucose levels, as a manifestation of cerebral adaptation to repeated low blood glucose. Although affected individuals are able to function normally at low blood glucose levels, the window of opportunity to identify hypoglycemia and take avoiding action becomes very narrow, and severe neuroglycopenia can rapidly ensue (11).

IAH affects 20–25% of patients with type 1 diabetes (11, 55) and less than 10% with type 2 diabetes (24), becomes more prevalent with increasing duration of diabetes (12) (see Fig. 3), and predisposes the patient to a sixfold higher risk of severe hypoglycemia than people who retain normal awareness (56). When IAH is associated with strict glycemic control during intensive insulin therapy or has followed episodes of recurrent severe hypoglycemia, it may be reversible by relaxing glycemic control or by avoiding further hypoglycemia (11), but in many patients with type 1 diabetes of long duration, it appears to be a permanent defect.

Central autonomic failure: Because counterregulatory deficiencies and IAH usually co-exist and are associated with an increased frequency of severe hypoglycemia, the concept of a "hypoglycemia-associated autonomic failure" (HAAF) (Fig. 4) was developed by Cryer (48), who argued that recurrent severe hypoglycemia is the primary problem which provokes these acquired abnormal responses, through cerebral adaptation to recurrent or chronic exposure to low blood glucose concentrations. It is reasoned that antecedent hypoglycemia in people with type 1 diabetes (48) and those with type 2 diabetes who have progressed to pancreatic beta-cell failure (57) causes defective glucose counterregulation in the absence of glucagon secretion because the epinephrine response is then markedly attenuated during exposure to subsequent hypoglycemia, while IAH develops through blunting of the sympathoadrenal response and reduced generation of autonomic symptoms (58).

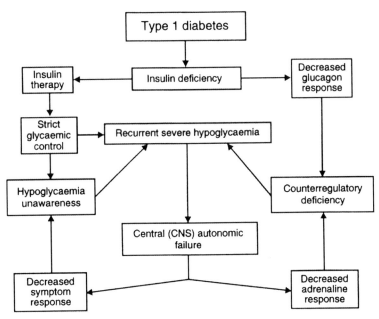

Fig. 4. Schematic diagram of the concept of hypoglycemia-associated autonomic failure, based on Cryer (48). (From Frier (11). Reprinted with permission from Blackwell Publishing, John Wiley and Sons.)

Effects of Hypoglycemia on Everyday Life

For the person with insulin-treated diabetes, hypoglycemia is a fact of life and is indisputably the greatest barrier to maintaining good glycemic control. Because it is common, unpredictable, and potentially dangerous, it impinges on every aspect of daily existence and provokes fear and apprehension in those with diabetes and in their relatives. Fear of hypoglycemia causes anxiety and psychological distress and is so great in some people that it provokes behavioral change and may negatively influence their approach to self-management (59). This may underlie the resistance shown by some patients to therapeutic recommendations to intensify treatment to achieve strict glycemic control. Hypoglycemia can affect personal relationships (sometimes causing marital tension), employment prospects, driving, recreational activities including exercise and sport, travel, and holidays, and acceptance for insurance. Detailed accounts of the everyday problems of living with hypoglycemia, and how these may be addressed, are available elsewhere (60, 61).

Driving is a very common everyday activity that requires complex psychomotor abilities, which are particularly vulnerable to the effects of acute neuroglycopenia and merits further comment. Driving simulators have been used to examine the effects of hypoglycemia on the driving performance of people with type 1 diabetes and have shown that driving performance becomes impaired when arterialized blood glucose is lowered below 3.8 mmol/l (68 mg/dl) (62). Two thirds of the subjects did not recognize that their blood glucose was low while driving so took no corrective treatment, and fewer than 25% of participants were aware that their driving performance was impaired during hypoglycemia, typical manifestations of which were speeding and inappropriate braking, driving off the road or crossing the midline, ignoring "Stop" signs, and an increased number of "crashes."

Insulin-treated drivers should be informed about how to avoid hypoglycemia when driving, and what to do if this occurs. Typical recommendations are shown in Table 7, yet many drivers persistently ignore this advice. In a specialist diabetes center where information and education about driving and hypoglycemia are provided routinely to drivers when they commence treatment with insulin, a survey of 202 drivers with insulin-treated diabetes showed that around half never tested their blood glucose before driving, and only 14% did this with any regularity (mostly people with IAH) (63). Other deficiencies in safe practice for driving included not carrying carbohydrate for emergency use in the vehicle, not stopping the car if hypoglycemia developed, and believing that blood glucose values below 3.0 mmol/l (54 mg/dl) were safe for driving (63). A major education problem exists to persuade drivers to implement these simple practical measures for safe driving, and regular reinforcement is necessary.

The occurrence of hypoglycemia while driving is a recognized cause of road traffic accidents, although the frequency is difficult to determine. Diabetologists are often required to provide medical reports about the likelihood of hypoglycemia having caused or contributed to a motor accident for legal and insurance purposes. Evidence is often circumstantial and it may be

Table 7
Driving and insulin-treated diabetes: precautions to avoid and treat hypoglycemia

Prevention of hypoglycemia

- Test blood glucose before driving and every 2 h during long journeys
- Take regular snacks/meals
- Take regular breaks or rest periods
- Avoid drinking alcohol
- Keep an accessible emergency supply of fast-acting carbohydrate and a supply of food in the vehicle

If hypoglycemia occurs

- Stop the vehicle in a safe location
- Consume fast-acting carbohydrate, followed by a snack
- Defer driving for at least 45 min to allow cognitive recovery

difficult to prove a causal relationship between suspected hypoglycemia and a driving accident. Taking a careful history, particularly of events preceding the incident, is essential when assessing the potential role of hypoglycemia in any individual case.

Prevention of Hypoglycemia

The modern management of diabetes strives to achieve strict glycemic control using intensive therapy to avoid or minimize the long-term complications of diabetes; this strategy tends to increase the risk of hypoglycemia and promotes development of the acquired hypoglycemia syndromes. Prevention of hypoglycemia therefore requires education of patients (and their relatives) when they commence treatment with insulin (and also those using sulfonylureas) and regular review and reinforcement about its avoidance and treatment, with reference to various activities and circumstances. This includes setting realistic targets for blood glucose in individual patients, which, for pragmatic reasons, may have to be in a higher range in some groups of patient such as the very young, the elderly, and those with advanced complications or other co-morbidities such as ischemic heart disease, as suggested by recent trials (38, 37). A higher than desirable frequency of hypoglycemia may have to be tolerated in certain situations, such as pregnancy, where strict glycemic control is essential for fetal well-being.

Frequent monitoring of blood glucose is necessary to identify asymptomatic biochemical hypoglycemia, particularly when median blood glucose is within a normoglycemic range (28) and when patients have developed impaired awareness of hypoglycemia. There is a pressing need for an effective glucose sensor with an alarm system to detect (nocturnal) hypoglycemia during sleep *(26)*. In addition, a long-acting or slowly absorbed carbohydrate supplement would be valuable, which can be ingested at bedtime and will act throughout the night. To be effective this would have to counteract nocturnal hyperinsulinemia and prevent a fall in blood glucose without compromising glycemic control or encouraging weight gain. Hypoglycemia that recurs at a particular time of day may be eradicated by changing the insulin regimen or the timing and dose of a particular insulin – such as changing the timing of the long-acting (basal) insulin to lower the risk of nocturnal hypoglycemia *(26, 27)*. Claims that insulin analogs (rapid-acting and long-acting) have substantially lowered the risk of hypoglycemia (other than at night) have not withstood critical scrutiny *(64)*, and hypoglycemia remains just as great a risk today with modern, multiple injection insulin regimens, as it was in the past. The increasing use of continuous subcutaneous insulin delivery with insulin pumps (which may be associated with a lower risk of severe hypoglycemia *(65)*) and real-time continuous glucose monitoring systems should improve hypoglycemia detection as glucose-sensing technology improves; more frequent information about prevailing blood glucose would then be available than can be provided by intermittent single-point monitoring *(66)*.

REFERENCES

1. American Diabetes Association Workgroup on Hypoglycemia. Defining and reporting hypoglycemia in diabetes. Diabetes Care 2005; 28:1245–1249.
2. The Diabetes Control and Complications Trial Research Group. Hypoglycemia in the Diabetes Control and Complications Trial. Diabetes 1997; 46:271–286.
3. Deary IJ. Symptoms of hypoglycaemia and effects on mental performance and emotions. In: Hypoglycaemia in Clinical Diabetes, (Second edition). Frier BM, Fisher M, eds. Chichester: John Wiley & Sons; 2007:25–48.
4. Sommerfield AJ, Deary IJ, Frier BM. Acute hyperglycemia alters mood state and impairs cognitive performance in people with Type 2 diabetes. Diabetes Care 2004; 27:2335–2340.
5. Cryer PE. Glucose counterregulation in man. Diabetes 1981; 30:261–264.
6. Wright R, Frier BM. Vascular disease and diabetes: is hypoglycaemia an aggravating factor? Diab/Metab Res Revs 2008; 24:353–63.
7. McAulay V, Deary IJ, Frier BM. Symptoms of hypoglycaemia in people with diabetes. Diabet Med 2001; 18: 690–705.
8. Tallroth G, Lindgren M, Stenberg G, Rosen I, Agardh CD. Neurophysiological changes during insulin-induced hypoglycaemia and in the recovery period following glucose infusion in type 1 (insulin-dependent) diabetes mellitus and in normal man. Diabetologia 1990; 33:319–323.
9. Lindgren M, Eckert B, Stenberg G, Agardh CD. Restitution of neurophysiological functions, performance, and subjective symptoms after moderate insulin-induced hypoglycaemia in non-diabetic men. Diabet Med 1996; 13:218–225.
10. Vea H, Jorde R, Sager G, Vaaler S, Sundsfjord J. Reproducibility of glycaemic thresholds for activation of counterregulatory hormones and hypoglycaemic symptoms in healthy subjects. Diabetologia 1992; 35:958–961.

11. Frier BM. Impaired awareness of hypoglycaemia. In: Hypoglycaemia in Clinical Diabetes, (Second edition). Frier BM, Fisher M, eds. Chichester: John Wiley & Sons; 2007:141–170.
12. Pramming S, Thorsteinsson B, Bendtson I, Binder C. Symptomatic hypoglycaemia in 411 type 1 diabetic patients. Diabet Med 1991; 8:217–222.
13. Pedersen-Bjergaard U, Pramming S, Heller SR, et al. Severe hypoglycaemia in 1076 adult patients with type 1 diabetes: influence of risk markers and selection. Diabetes Metab Res Rev 2004; 20:479–486.
14. The Diabetes Control and Complications Trial Research Group. The effect of intensive insulin treatment of diabetes on the development and progression of long term complications in insulin-dependent diabetes mellitus. N Engl J Med 1993; 329:977–986.
15. The EURODIAB IDDM Complications Study Group. Microvascular and acute complications in IDDM patients: the EURODIAB IDDM Complications Study. Diabetologia 1994; 37:278–285.
16. MacLeod KM, Hepburn DA, Frier BM. Frequency and morbidity of severe hypoglycaemia in insulin-treated diabetic patients. Diabet Med 1993; 10:238–245.
17. ter Braak EWMT, Appelman AMMF, Van de Laak MF, Stolk RP, Van Haeften TW, Erkelens DW. Clinical characteristics of type 1 diabetic patients with and without severe hypoglycemia. Diabetes Care 2000; 23:1467–1471.
18. UK Hypoglycaemia Study Group. Risk of hypoglycaemia in types 1 and type 2 diabetes: effects of treatment modalities and their duration. Diabetologia 2007; 50:1140–1147.
19. The Diabetes Control and Complications Trial Research Group. Diabetes Control and Complications Trial (DCCT): results of feasibility study. Diabetes Care 1987; 10:1–19.
20. Zammitt NN, Frier BM. Hypoglycemia in type 2 diabetes: pathophysiology, frequency, and effects of different treatment modalities. Diabetes Care 2005; 28:2948–2961.
21. Abraira C, Colwell JA, Nuttall FQ, et al. Veterans Affairs Cooperative Study on glycemic control and complications in type II diabetes (VACSDM): results of the feasibility trial. Diabetes Care 1995; 18:1113–1123.
22. Leese GP, Wang J, Broomhall J, et al. (for the DARTS/MEMO Collaboration). Frequency of severe hypoglycemia requiring emergency treatment in type 1 and type 2 diabetes: a population-based study of health service resource use. Diabetes Care 2003; 26:1176–1180.
23. Donnelly LA, Morris AD, Frier BM, et al. (for the DARTS/MEMO Collaboration). Frequency and predictors of hypoglycaemia in type 1 and insulin-treated type 2 diabetes: a population-based study. Diabet Med 2005; 22:449–455.
24. Henderson JN, Allen KV, Deary IJ, Frier BM. Hypoglycaemia in insulin-treated Type 2 diabetes: frequency, symptoms and impaired awareness. Diabet Med 2003; 20:1016–1021.
25. Hepburn DA, MacLeod KM, Pell ACH, Scougal IJ, Frier BM. Frequency and symptoms of hypoglycaemia experienced by patients with Type 2 diabetes treated with insulin. Diabet Med 1993; 10:231–237.
26. Allen KV, Frier BM. Nocturnal hypoglycaemia: clinical manifestations and therapeutic strategies toward prevention. Endocrine Practice 2003; 9:530–543.
27. Heller SR. Nocturnal hypoglycaemia. In: Hypoglycaemia in Clinical Diabetes, (Second edition). Frier, B.M., Fisher, M, eds. Chichester: John Wiley & Sons; 2007:83–99.
28. Thorsteinsson B, Pramming S, Lauritzen T, Binder C. Frequency of daytime biochemical hypoglycaemia in insulin-treated diabetic patients: relation to daily median blood glucose concentrations. Diabet Med 1986; 3:147–151.
29. The DCCT Research Group. Epidemiology of severe hypoglycemia in the Diabetes Control and Complications Trial. Am J Med 1991; 90:450–459.
30. Jones TW, Porter P, Sherwin RS, et al. Decreased epinephrine responses to hypoglycemia during sleep. N Engl J Med 1998; 338:1657–1662.
31. Pedersen-Bjergaard U, Agerholm-Larsen B, Pramming S, Hougaard P, Thorsteinsson B. Prediction of severe hypoglycaemia by angiotensin-converting enzyme activity and genotype in type 1 diabetes. Diabetologia 2003; 46:89–96.
32. Zammitt NN, Geddes J, Warren RE, Marioni R, Ashby JP, Frier BM. Serum angiotensin-converting enzyme and frequency of severe hypoglycaemia in Type 1 diabetes: does a relationship exist? Diabet Med 2007; 24:449–454.

33. Dewan S, Gillett A, Mugarza JA, Dovey TM, Halford JCG, Wilding JPH. Effects of insulin-induced hypoglycaemia on energy intake and food choice at a subsequent test meal. Diab Metab Res Revs 2004; 20:405–410.

34. Brodows RG, Williams C, Amatruda JM. Treatment of insulin reactions in diabetics. J Am Med Assoc 1984; 252:3378–381.

35. Slama G, Traynard PY, Desplanque N, et al. The search for an optimised treatment of hypoglycemia. Carbohydrates in tablets, solution, or gel for the correction of insulin reactions. Arch Intern Med 1990; 150:589–593.

36. MacCuish AC. Treatment of hypoglycaemia. In: Hypoglycaemia and Diabetes: Clinical and Physiological Aspects. Frier BM, Fisher BM, eds. London: Edward Arnold, 1993:212–221.

37. Duckworth W, Abraira C, Moritz T, et al. Glucose control and vascular complications in veterans with type 2 diabetes. N Engl J Med 2008; 360:129–139.

38. The Action to Control Cardiovascular Risk in Diabetes Study Group. Effects of intensive glucose lowering in type 2 diabetes. New Engl J Med 2008; 358:2545–2559.

39. Fisher M, Heller S. Mortality, cardiovascular morbidity and possible effects of hypoglycaemia on diabetic complications. In: Hypoglycaemia in Clinical Diabetes, (Second edition). Frier BM, Fisher M, eds. Chichester: John Wiley & Sons; 2007:265–283.

40. Tattersall RB, Gill GV. Unexplained deaths of type 1 diabetic patients. Diabet Med 1991; 8:49–58.

41. MacLeod KM, Hepburn DA, Deary IJ, Goodwin GM, Dougall N, Ebmeier KP, Frier BM. Regional cerebral blood flow in IDDM patients: effects of diabetes and of recurrent severe hypoglycaemia. Diabetologia 1994; 37:257–263.

42. Strachan MWJ. Frequency, causes and risk factors for hypoglycaemia in type 1 diabetes. In: Hypoglycaemia in Clinical Diabetes, (Second edition). Frier BM, Fisher M, eds. Chichester: John Wiley & Sons, 2007:49–81.

43. Bjorgaas M, Sand T, Vik T, Jorde R. Quantitative EEG during controlled hypoglycaemia in diabetic and non-diabetic children. Diabet Med 1998; 15:30–37.

44. Bottcher J, Kunze A, Kurrat C, et al. Localized reversible reduction of apparent diffusion coefficient in transient hypoglycemia-induced hemiparesis. Stroke 2005; 36:e20–e22.

45. Cordonnier C, Oppenheim C, Lamy C, Meder JF, Mas JL. Serial diffusion and perfusion-weighted MR in transient hypoglycemia. Neurology 2005; 65:175.

46. Strachan MWJ, Abraha HD, Sherwood RA, Lammie GA, Deary IJ, Ewing FME, Perros, P, Frier BM. Evaluation of serum markers of neuronal damage following severe hypoglycaemia in adults with insulin-treated diabetes mellitus. Diab/Metab Res Revs 1999; 15:5–12.

47. Laing SP, Swerdlow AJ, Slater SD, et al. The British Diabetic Association Cohort Study, II: cause-specific mortality in patients with insulin-treated diabetes mellitus. Diabet Med 1999; 16:466–471.

48. Cryer PE. Hypoglycaemia: the limiting factor in the management of Type 1 and Type 2 diabetes. Diabetologia 2002; 45:937–948.

49. Gerich JE, Bolli GB. Counterregulatory failure. In: Hypoglycaemia and Diabetes: Clinical and Physiological Aspects. Frier BM, Fisher BM, eds. London: Edward Arnold; 1993:253–267.

50. White NH, Skor DA, Cryer PE, Levandoski LA, Bier DM, Santiago JV. Identification of type 1 diabetic patients at increased risk for hypoglycemia during intensive therapy. New Engl J Med 1983; 308:485–491.

51. Bolli GB, Tsalikian E, Haymond MW, Cryer PE, Gerich JE. Defective glucose counterregulation after subcutaneous insulin in non-insulin-dependent diabetes mellitus. J Clin Invest 1984; 73:1532–1541.

52. Ryder RE, Owens DR, Hayes TM, Ghatei MA, Bloom SR. Unawareness of hypoglycaemia and inadequate hypoglycaemic counterregulation: no causal relation with diabetic autonomic neuropathy. Br Med J 1990; 301:783–787.

53. Hepburn DA, Patrick AW, Eadington DW, Ewing DJ, Frier BM. Unawareness of hypoglycaemia in insulin-treated diabetic patients: prevalence and relationship to autonomic neuropathy. Diabet Med 1990; 7:711–717.

54. Cox D.J, Gonder-Frederick L, Polonsky W, Schlundt D, Kovatchev B, Clarke W. Blood glucose awareness training (BGAT-2). Long term benefits. Diabetes Care 2001; 24:637–642.

55 Geddes J, Schopman JE, Zammitt NN, Frier BM. Prevalence of impaired awareness of hypoglycaemia in adults with Type 1 diabetes. Diabet Med 2008; 25:501–504.

56. Gold AE, MacLeod KM, Frier BM. Frequency of severe hypoglycemia in patients with impaired awareness of hypoglycemia. Diabetes Care 1994; 17:697–703.

57. Segel SA, Paramore DA, Cryer PE. Hypoglycemia-associated autonomic failure in advanced type 2 diabetes. Diabetes 2002; 51:724–733.

58. Cryer PE. Diverse causes of hypoglycemia-associated autonomic failure in diabetes. N Engl J Med 2004; 350:2272–2279.

59. Wild D, von Maltzahn R, Brohan E, Christensen T, Clauson P, Gonder-Frederick L. A critical review of the literature on fear of hypoglycemia in diabetes: implications for diabetes management and patient education. Patient Education and Counseling 2007; 68:10–15.

60. Frier BM. Living with hypoglycaemia. In: Hypoglycaemia in Clinical Diabetes, (Second edition). Frier BM, Fisher M, eds. Chichester: John Wiley & Sons; 2007:309–332.

61. Frier BM. How hypoglycaemia can affect the life of a person with diabetes. Diab Metab Res Revs 2008; 24:87–92.

62. Cox DJ, Gonder-Frederick LA, Kovatchev B, Julian DM, Clarke WL. Progressive hypoglycemia's impact on driving simulation performance. Occurrence, awareness and correction. Diabetes Care 2000; 23:163–170.

63. Graveling AJ, Warren RE, Frier BM. Hypoglycaemia and driving in people with insulin-treated diabetes: adherence to recommendations for avoidance. Diabet Med 2004; 21:1014–1019.

64. Siebenhofer A, Plank J, Berghold A, et al. Meta-analysis of short-acting insulin analogues in adult patients with type 1 diabetes: continuous subcutaneous insulin infusion versus injection therapy. Diabetologia 2004; 47:1895–1905.

65. Pickup JC, Sutton A.J. Severe hypoglycaemia and glycaemic control in type 1 diabetes: meta-analysis of multiple daily insulin injections compared with continuous subcutaneous insulin infusion. Diabet Med 2008; 25:765–774.

66. Klonoff DC. Continuous glucose monitoring. Roadmap for 21st century diabetes therapy. Diabetes Care 2005; 28:1231–1239.

7

Ketoacidosis and Hyperglycemic Hyperosmolar State

Matthew Freeby and Susana Ebner

CONTENTS

From: *Contemporary Diabetes: Diabetes and the Brain*
Edited by: G. J. Biessels, J. A. Luchsinger (eds.), DOI 10.1007/978-1-60327-850-8_7
© Humana Press, a part of Springer Science+Business Media, LLC 2009

ABSTRACT

A review of the two classical acute hyperglycemic syndromes in type 1 and type 2 diabetes, ketoacidosis and hyperglycemic hyperosmolar state, with particular emphasis on cerebral complications.

Key words: Type 1 and type 2 diabetes; Hyperglycemia; Diabetic ketoacidosis; Cerebral edema.

DIABETIC KETOACIDOSIS: DEFINITION AND EPIDEMIOLOGY

In the absence of insulin, diabetic ketoacidosis (DKA) complicates type 1 diabetes mellitus (T1DM). DKA is defined by a triad of hyperglycemia, ketosis, and acidemia and occurs in the absolute or near-absolute absence of insulin. Acidosis is defined as venous pH <7.3 or serum bicarbonate concentrations <18 mmol/l. Glucosuria, ketonuria, and ketonemia are typically present. Serum glucose concentrations are typically >13.8 mmol/l (250 mg/dl), but may be normal in select cases of partial treatment or pregnancy (1). DKA predominantly affects those with T1DM, but can occur in type 2 diabetes mellitus (T2DM), especially in African-Americans and other minorities who are newly diagnosed (2–4).

DKA accounts for the bulk of morbidity and mortality in children with T1DM. National population-based studies estimate DKA mortality at 0.15% in the United States (4), 0.18–0.25% in Canada (4, 5), and 0.31% in the United Kingdom (6). Rates are higher in adults of age 65 years and older (7)as well as in children with DKA-related cerebral edema (4).

DKA can present in newly diagnosed or pre-existing T1DM. Rates reach 25–67% in those who are newly diagnosed (4, 8, 9). The rates are higher in younger children (<5 years of age) and in children with little access to medical care (4). The risk of DKA among patients with pre-existing diabetes is 1–10% annual per person (10, 11). The American Diabetes Association estimates that 5–25% of children with newly diagnosed T2DM have DKA (12).

ETIOLOGY AND PRECIPITATING FACTORS

Insulin deficiency and increased counter-regulatory hormone secretion (i.e., glucagon, growth hormone, catecholamines, and cortisol) underlie the basic mechanism leading to DKA in patients with diabetes. If insulin is present, lipolysis and the development of ketoacidosis are prevented. The most common precipitants of DKA are infections (such as pneumonia and urinary tract infection) and insulin omission or under-treatment (13). Other precipitant factors associated with DKA include cardiovascular events, pancreatitis, medications (i.e., thiazides, corticosteroids, sympathomimetics, and atypical anti-psychotics), and use of illicit drugs (i.e., cocaine) *(14)*.

PATHOGENESIS

There are multiple factors that promote disturbances in carbohydrate, protein, and lipid metabolism that ultimately lead to hyperglycemia and ketosis, the hallmark of DKA. In the absence of insulin, hepatic glucose production increases while glucose utilization in muscle and adipose tissue decreases. Increased counter-regulatory hormone concentrations promote further hepatic gluconeogenesis and glycogenolysis. These metabolic processes combined lead to hyperglycemia. Hyperglycemia saturates the renal threshold for glucose reabsorption, causing glucosuria which causes osmotic diuresis, leading to dehydration and electrolyte loss. Hyperosmolarity and impaired renal function (pre-renal failure) may sometimes occur. Insulin deficiency and increased counter-regulatory hormones promote lipolysis, resulting in free fatty acid and glycerol production. Glycerol is used as precursor for glucose production in the process of gluconeogenesis, whereas free fatty acids are used for ketone production (ketogenesis).

A high glucagon-to-insulin ratio results in decreased malonyl co-enzyme A (CoA) concentrations, an intermediary product in the synthesis of long-chain fatty acids. Carnitine palmitoyl acetyltransferase (CPT1), a key enzyme in ketogenesis, is stimulated by low levels of malonyl CoA leading to enhanced production of ketone bodies by the liver *(15–17)*. Ketone bodies, which include acetoacetate and β-hydroxybutyrate, are weak acids; as bicarbonate buffers these acids, the alkali reserves dwindle and ketone body accumulation results in ketoacidosis. Since these acids are unmeasured anions, this type of acidosis is called an "anion-gap acidosis." Figure 1 illustrates the pathogenesis of DKA and the hyperglycemic hyperosmolar state (HHS). HHS will be reviewed in a later section.

PRESENTATION

Clinical Characteristics

DKA can present with mild-to-severe symptoms. Patients may complain of symptoms related to hyperglycemia and glucosuria such as polyuria and polydipsia. As a consequence of the increased urinary water loss, patients may present with signs of dehydration, such as tachycardia and dry mucus membranes. In severe cases, hypotension, due to volume depletion may occur. Vomiting, abdominal pain, malaise, and weight loss are common presenting symptoms in ketoacidosis. Signs related to the ketoacidotic

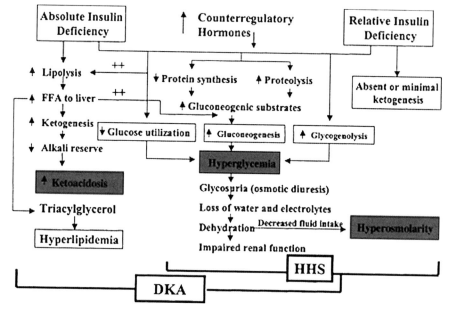

Fig. 1. DKA and HHS pathogenesis. (Copyright ©*American Diabetes Association Diabetes Care* ®, Vol. 29, 2006; 2739–2748. Reprinted with permission from The American Diabetes Association.)

state include hyperventilation with deep breathing (Kussmaul's respiration) which is a compensatory respiratory response to an underlying metabolic acidosis. Acetonemia may cause a fruity odor to the breath. Diffuse abdominal tenderness on palpation is often elicited on physical exam; if the abdominal tenderness is localized, one should consider a focal abdominal process *(18)*.

Laboratory Abnormalities

The American Diabetes Association's criteria for DKA include *(18)*

- Blood glucose > 13.8 mmol/l (250 mg/dl)
- pH < 7.30
- Serum bicarbonate < 18 mmol/l
- Anion gap > 10
- Serum ketones

Elevated glucose levels are almost always present; however, euglycemic DKA has been described *(19)*. Anion-gap metabolic acidosis is the hallmark of this condition and is caused by elevated ketone bodies. Ketone bodies include acetoacetate, β-hydroxybutyrate, and acetone. β-Hydroxybutyrate is the main ketone body found in DKA; however, when measuring serum ketones, most laboratories test for acetoacetate by a nitroprusside dip-stick test. Direct measurements of β-hydroxybutyrate can be performed. Decreased serum bicarbonate levels correlate with the degree of acido-sis. Renal losses of electrolytes, such as potassium, magnesium, and phos-phate, occur following osmotic diuresis. Increased intravascular osmotic pressure due to hyperglycemia causes a shift in water from the intracellular to intravascular spaces resulting in dilutional hyponatremia. Increased white blood cells can be found in patients with DKA, even in the absence of infec-tion. Additionally, elevated lipase and amylase levels from non-pancreatic sources may be observed (20).

COMPLICATIONS: CEREBRAL DYSFUNCTION IN DKA

Cerebral abnormalities may occur in the setting of hyperglycemia and ketoacidosis. When compared to those with T1DM and normoglycemia, patients with diabetic ketoacidosis demonstrate increased levels of trypto-phan and 5-hydroxyindoleacetic acid in the cerebrospinal fluid (CSF) (21). Plasma tyrosine and CSF tyrosine and homovanillic acid concentrations are typically normal. Similar findings are demonstrated in those with uremia and hepatic encephalopathy, as well as in rodents with diabetes and DKA secondary to streptozotocin administration. Magnetic resonance (MR) spec-troscopy studies in children with DKA have demonstrated possible neuronal injury and/or dysfunction. In one study, 29 children underwent MR spec-troscopy and were evaluated with brain ratios of N-acetylaspartate (NAA) to creatinine (Cr) during therapy and after recovery from DKA (22). NAA/Cr levels were significantly lower during DKA therapy in the basal ganglia sug-gesting compromised neuronal function.

In the presence of DKA, confusion and headache may occur. Patients with new or pre-existing T1DM and acute ketoacidosis may have abnormal elec-troencephalograms (EEG). In a study of 39 patients aged from 11 months to 16 years who underwent serial EEGs at 1, 12, 24 h, and 5 days after initia-tion of treatment for DKA, 30 patients were found to have abnormal studies initially (23). EEG severity correlated with serum glucose, osmolality, bicar-bonate, β-hydroxybutyrate and acetoacetate levels, but did not correlate with pH and glycosylated hemoglobin. Abnormal EEG findings were resolved in 20 of 30 patients in 5 days. EEGs were repeated 2–5 months after treatment; five of seven patients undergoing repeat EEG had persistent abnormalities despite DKA resolution.

Neuropsychological testing profiles have yielded mixed results in patients with diabetes with and without DKA. In one study, chronically elevated glucose without ketoacidosis portended negative changes in neuropsycho-logical profiles (24). While a second study found no correlation between negative neuropsychological profiles and variables such as age at diabetes onset, poor chronic control, or major metabolic crises such as hypoglycemia and ketoacidosis *(25)*.

CEREBRAL EDEMA

Clinically significant cerebral edema occurs in approximately 1% of patients with diabetic ketoacidosis *(26)*, and there is a higher incidence in patients presenting with an initial diagnosis of T1DM. In one report, DKA-related cerebral edema occurs in 0.23% of patients with established T1DM *(26)*and in 3.3% of patients with newly diagnosed T1DM. More recent data suggest that subclinical cerebral edema may be even more common *(27)*. Narrowing of the frontal horns of the lateral ventricles by MRI was present in 22 of 41 (54%) children admitted for DKA treatment. More alarming, data obtained by MR spectroscopy suggest that subtle cerebral injury occurs with subclinical cerebral edema *(22)*. Ultimately, DKA-related cerebral edema may represent a continuum. Mild forms resulting in subtle edema may result in modest mental status abnormalities whereas the most severe manifestations result in overt cerebral injury.

At this time, there are no prospective randomized trials evaluating treatment options; current knowledge is based mostly on case series and case–control studies. The etiology, risk factors, and treatment of cerebral edema are still under study and will require continued research in order to reduce the devastating complications.

CEREBRAL EDEMA IN DKA: PRESENTATION

Cerebral edema typically presents 4–12 h after the treatment for DKA is started *(28, 29)*, but can occur at any time. In up to 5% of cases, cerebral edema may present prior to initiation of DKA therapy *(6, 28–30)*. Signs and symptoms are variable but include headache, mental status deterioration, inappropriately slowed heart rate, and increases in blood pressure *(31, 32)*. Subclinical presentation of cerebral edema is more common *(33, 34)* and may be associated with smaller third and lateral ventricles during therapy *(33)*. Glaser and colleagues measured intercaudate widths of the frontal horns of lateral ventricles in 41 children and found narrowing in 54% just after initiation of DKA therapy as compared to after recovery *(27)*. Children with narrowing were more likely to have Glasgow Coma Scale (GCS) scores below 15 during therapy ($p = 0.03$), but did not exhibit neurological abnormalities sufficient for diagnosis of symptomatic cerebral edema.

CEREBRAL EDEMA IN DKA: RISK FACTORS

Epidemiologic studies have identified several risk factors for cerebral edema in DKA. Younger age *(31)* and newly diagnosed diabetes both potentially increase risk of cerebral edema in DKA *(6, 31, 35)*. Additionally, patients presenting with longer duration of symptoms are at increased risk *(26)*, which may be related to severity of DKA *(28)*. Other risk factors have been identified in retrospective case-controlled studies. A complete list of risk factors associated with cerebral edema in DKA is shown in Table 1.

Table 1
**Risk factors associated with cerebral
edema in diabetic ketoacidosis**

DKA-related cerebral edema
Risk factors
New-onset T1DM *(6, 31, 35)*
Young age *(31)*
Longer duration of symptoms *(26)*
Acidosis *(36, 37)*
Low P_aCO_2 *(27, 28, 36–38)*
Hyperkalemia *(37)*
Uremia *(28, 37, 38)*
Bicarbonate therapy *(28)*
Increased insulin dose *(37)*
High i.v. fluid volumes *(36, 37)*

Low partial pressure of arterial carbon dioxide (pCO_2) levels may be a marker of cerebral edema. A large multicenter study by Glaser et al. reported 61 cases of cerebral edema among 6,977 children with DKA *(28)*. Cerebral edema was associated with lower pCO_2 prior to treatment (for every decrease in 7.8 mmHg, RR 3.4, 95% CI: 1.9–6.3). In a second study, hypercapnia and low pCO_2 levels were risk factors for the development of cerebral edema in 9 of 153 children admitted for one or more episodes of DKA *(36)*. In patients with asymptomatic cerebral edema, low initial pCO_2 and bicarbonate levels have also been associated with asymptomatic cerebral edema *(27)*.

Hyponatremia, hyperkalemia, and uremia have also been associated with cerebral edema in DKA *(37)*. Uremia and hyperkalemia may be reflective of longer illness duration, severity of insulin deficiency, and pre-renal failure states. Glaser et al. found an association with higher initial serum urea nitrogen levels (for each increase of 9 mg/dl, RR 1.7, 95% CI: 1.2–2.5) and cerebral edema *(28)*. There was no association with the degree of hyperglycemia.

Mahoney et al. and Edge et al. also found no association with degree of hyperglycemia *(36, 37)*. In a recently published study, MR diffusion-weight imaging was used to quantify cerebral edema *(38)*. The apparent diffusion coefficients (ADCs) of brain water during and after DKA treatment were compared in 26 children and correlated with clinical and biochemical variables. Serum urea nitrogen levels and initial respiratory rates were elevated. ADC was not correlated with initial serum glucose or sodium abnormalities. Although initial reports suggested that changes in effective osmolality increased cerebral edema risk *(39, 40)*, ADC did not correlate with initial osmolality *(38)*.

It is unknown if certain therapies increase the risk for DKA-related cerebral edema. Edge and colleagues found cerebral edema associated with early insulin administration *(37)*. Patients treated with insulin in the first hours were at higher risk for cerebral edema (OR 12.7, $p = 0.02$). Higher volumes of fluid administered over the first 4 h (OR 6.55, $p = 0.01$) *(37)*also increased the risk for cerebral edema. A second study also found higher initial intravenous fluid volumes (>50 ml/kg in the first 2–4 h) to be a risk factor *(36)*. Although there is no definitive mechanism that characterizes cerebral edema, insulin activates the sodium/proton pump and allows for influx of sodium into brain cells *(41)*. Insulin may also be involved in cerebral volume regulation via potassium and chloride influx *(42)*. Therefore, early administration of both insulin and fluids may cause an influx of various electrolytes within the cell and increase cellular brain volumes *(37)*. Dilute fluids have also been associated with higher odds ratios for cerebral edema, but the study by Edge et al. was not properly powered for significance *(37)*. Although bicarbonate administration was not associated with an increased rate in cerebral edema in the study by Edge *(37)*, Glaser et al. found an increased risk of cerebral edema with bicarbonate therapy *(28)*.

CEREBRAL EDEMA IN DKA: PATHOPHYSIOLOGY

Potential causes of DKA-related cerebral edema include (1) generation of inflammatory mediators *(43, 44)*; (2) disruption of cell membrane ion transport and aquaporin channels *(45–47)*; (3) generation of intracellular organic osmolytes and subsequent osmotic imbalance *(48)*; and (4) changes in cerebral blood flow *(49)*.

Inflammatory Mediators

Inflammatory mediators may cause cerebral edema. Studies have demonstrated that inflammatory mediators can disrupt endothelial cells of the blood–brain barrier (BBB) *(43)*. Routes for penetration include the paracellular tight junctional pathways and vesicular mechanisms. Many inflammatory agents increase endothelial permeability and vessel diameter, causing significant leaks and cerebral edema formation. Such inflammatory agents include bradykinin, serotonin, and histamine. cGMP signaling may be involved in bradykinin and histamine BBB disruption (44).

Aquaporin Channels

Aquaporin channels may also play a role in cerebral edema formation. Aquaporins are small membrane proteins that provide pathways for water transport and can be found in cells of the kidney, lung, and other tissues. In the brain, several types have been described and they participate in production and reabsorption of brain fluid (47). Aquaporin-4 (AQP4) is a glial membrane water channel and likely plays a significant role in brain water transport. Mice deficient in AQP4 have improved survival in models of acute water intoxication and demonstrate reduced brain tissue water content and swelling of pericapillary astrocytic foot processes (47).

Osmotic Imbalance

Intracellular organic osmolytes (i.e., taurine, myoinositol, choline, and glucose) have been implicated in the creation of cerebral edema. One group evaluated streptozotocin-induced non-ketotic and ketotic diabetes in normonatremic rats (50). Animals were sacrificed before or after treatment with hypotonic saline and insulin. Brain analysis of water, electrolyte, and organic osmolyte content prior to treatment demonstrated 2% reduction in brain water despite a 12% increase in plasma osmolality. When cerebral edema occurred, there was decreased brain sodium content and no change in total major brain organic osmolytes. However, there were significant increases in glutamine and taurine after treatment. Other studies have also found increases in taurine in the brains of ketotic animals (51, 52).

In humans, MRI and MR spectroscopy have been used to evaluate regional cerebral abnormalities in DKA (53). Eight hyperglycemic children with or without DKA all demonstrated abnormal signal changes in the frontal regions on fluid-attenuated inversion recovery (FLAIR) MR imaging, suggestive of mild cerebral edema. MR spectroscopy abnormalities included increased levels of taurine, myoinositol, and glucose in DKA as compared to children without DKA. Taurine concentrations were greater in the frontal than occipital regions. The authors of the study proposed that increased levels of taurine, an osmotically active amino acid, may pose an increase in vulnerability to cerebral edema during episodes of DKA.

However, larger epidemiologic trials have not provided a definitive link between osmolality and risk for cerebral edema in DKA (37, 38). When cerebral edema is present before DKA therapy, there is no definitive correlation with levels of sodium, glucose, and osmolality *(54)*. Additionally, therapies that include insulin and intravenous fluids cause shifts in osmotic balances, but have not been definitively linked with cerebral edema *(27, 28, 37)*.

Changes in Cerebral Blood Flow

Cerebral hypoperfusion may also play a dominant role. Animal models of DKA suggest reduced cerebral blood flow and dehydration prior to cerebral edema formation *(54, 55)*. The Na–K–Cl co-transporter in brain microvascular endothelial cells (blood–brain barrier endothelial cells) may play a role in edema formation via perfusion changes *(54)*. In conditions of cerebral ischemia (i.e., stroke) the Na–K–Cl co-transporter is stimulated in astrocytes and blood–brain barrier (BBB) endothelial cells increasing sodium chloride and water transport across the BBB from blood to brain. The ketoacids, acetoacetate and β-hydroxybutyrate, have also been found to stimulate Na–K–Cl co-transporter activity *(54, 56)*. In a study by Lam et al., streptozotocin-induced diabetic rats with DKA underwent MR diffusion-weighted imaging and demonstrated cerebral edema by apparent diffusion coefficient (ADC) values *(54)*. When rats received bumetanide, an inhibitor of the Na–K–Cl co-transporter, prior to DKA treatment, cerebral edema formation was reduced; however, no reduction of cerebral edema was observed in rats given bumetanide after insulin and intravenous fluids. More recently, Yuen et al. provided more clear evidence of reduced cerebral blood flow in rats with untreated DKA *(55)*. In this study, cerebral blood flow was responsive to pCO₂ and is consistent with previous studies correlating hypocapnia with cerebral hypoperfusion in humans *(28, 37)*. Cerebral blood flow and ADC were negatively correlated with blood urea nitrogen concentrations suggesting that dehydration may contribute to cerebral hypoperfusion.

Some studies in humans also suggest that cerebral hypoperfusion may be associated with increased risk for cerebral edema-related DKA *(28, 37, 38)*. Patients with DKA with higher serum urea nitrogen levels (a marker of dehydration) are at increased risk for cerebral edema. Hypocapnia, present in DKA, results from hyperventilation and can cause cerebral vasoconstriction. DKA-related cerebral hypoperfusion prior to treatment may lead to subsequent vasogenic edema with reperfusion *(38)*.

THERAPEUTIC INTERVENTIONS IN DKA-RELATED CEREBRAL EDEMA

Children should be monitored closely including hourly vitals, capillary blood glucose monitoring, and frequent neurological observations *(1)*. Laboratory testing every 2–4 h should include electrolytes, urea, hematocrit, blood glucose, and blood gases *(1)*. In more severe cases, electrolytes and glucose may need to be monitored more closely.

If cerebral edema is suspected, treatment should begin immediately by reducing intravenous fluid administration *(1, 57)* and by providing supportive care. Mannitol may be administered intravenously as 0.25–1.0 g/kg over 20 min in impending respiratory failure, while hypertonic saline (3%, 5–10 ml/kg over 30 min) may be used as an alternative. In cases of respiratory failure or alterations in sensorium, intubation and ventilation may be necessary. Assisted hyperventilation has resulted in poor outcomes in children with DKA-related cerebral edema *(58)*. Although a detailed review of DKA treatment is beyond the scope of this chapter, Fig. 2 illustrates general guidelines.

DKA-RELATED CEREBRAL EDEMA: PROGNOSIS

Increased intracranial pressure with cerebral edema has been recognized as the leading cause of morbidity and mortality in pediatric patients with DKA *(59)*. Mortality from DKA-related cerebral edema in children is high, up to 90% *(26, 31, 33, 35, 60)* and accounts for 60–90% of the mortality seen in DKA *(28, 31, 35)*. DKA-related cerebral edema also accounts for a

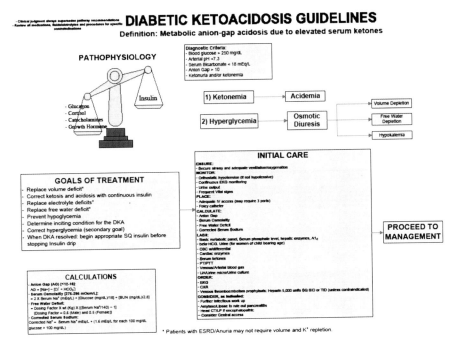

Fig. 2. Treatment guidelines for DKA.

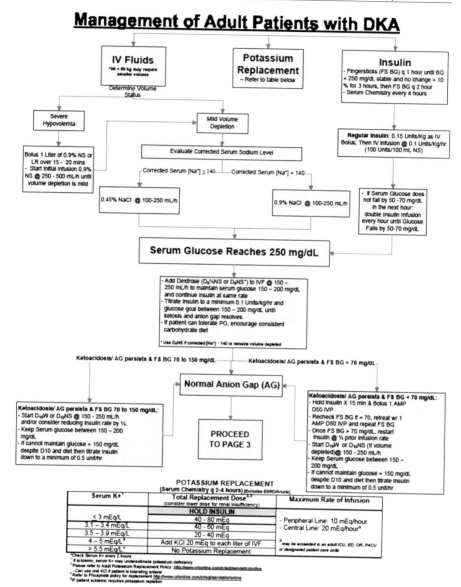

Fig. 2. (continued)

high percentage of morbidity since many patients are left with major neurological deficits (28, 31, 35). In a large retrospective series published in 1990, cerebral edema was associated with a 64% case fatality rate, 9% survival with minor disabilities, and 13% survival with severe disability or vegetative state (31).

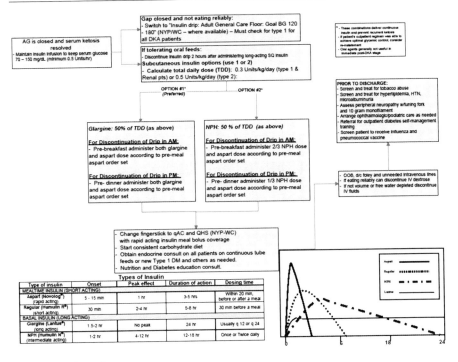

Fig. 2. (continued)

HYPERGLYCEMIC HYPEROSMOLAR STATE

Definition and Epidemiology

The hyperosmolar hyperglycemic state (HHS) is also an acute complication that may occur in patients with diabetes mellitus. It is seen primarily in patients with T2DM and has previously been referred to as "hyperglycemic hyperosmolar non-ketotic coma" or "hyperglycemic hyperosmolar non-ketotic state" (13). HHS is marked by profound dehydration and hyperglycemia and often by some degree of neurological impairment.

The term hyperglycemic hyperosmolar state is used because (1) ketosis may be present and (2) there may be varying degrees of altered sensorium besides coma (13). Like DKA, the basic underlying disorder is inadequate circulating insulin, but there is often enough insulin to inhibit free fatty acid mobilization and ketoacidosis. Figure 2 illustrates the differences in the underlying abnormalities seen in DKA and HHS.

Up to 20% of patients diagnosed with HHS do not have a previous history of diabetes mellitus (14). Population studies are lacking and therefore HHS incidence is difficult to determine. Kitabchi et al. estimated the rate of hospital admissions due to HHS to be lower than DKA, accounting for less than 1% of all primary diabetic admissions *(13)*. Yet, HHS causes significant morbidity and mortality. Mortality rates near 15% *(13, 61)* and are even higher in patients who are substantially older or have concomitant life-threatening illnesses *(13)*.

ETIOLOGY AND PRECIPITATING FACTORS

Glucose levels rise in the setting of relative insulin deficiency. The low levels of circulating insulin prevent lipolysis, ketogenesis, and ketoacidosis *(62)* but are unable to suppress hyperglycemia, glucosuria, and water losses. Levels of counter-regulatory hormones such as glucagon, catecholamines, cortisol, and growth hormone are elevated, increasing gluconeogenic substrates, gluconeogenesis, and glycogenolysis. Meanwhile, glucose utilization is decreased. Glucose levels rise, leading to glucosuria, osmotic diuresis, and dehydration *(14)*. Those patients who are unable to maintain an adequate fluid intake to compensate for the urinary losses, for example, elderly patients, will develop marked hyperglycemia and a hyperosmolar state. Mental status changes are more common in HHS than in DKA because of the greater degrees of hyperosmolarity in HHS *(63)*.

HHS typically presents with one or more precipitating factors, similar to DKA. Precipitating factors may include infection, cardiovascular events, trauma, drugs, or other illnesses *(14)*. Acute infections include pneumonia, urinary tract infections, and sepsis, which account for approximately 32–50% of precipitating causes *(13)*. Other less common precipitating factors include intestinal obstruction, acute pancreatitis, renal failure, hypothermia, severe burns, thyrotoxicosis, Cushing's syndrome, and acromegaly. Drug use and therapy may exacerbate hyperglycemia and stimulate ketoacid production. These include β-adrenergic blocker, calcium-channel blockers, chlorpromazine, cimetidine, diazoxide, diuretics, ethacrynic acid, immunosuppressive agents, l-asparaginase, loxapine, phenytoin, propranolol, and steroids *(13)*.

DIAGNOSIS

Clinical Presentation

HHS develops subacutely in time over days to weeks. Hyperglycemia increases glucosuria and water losses which further impair the ability to excrete excess serum glucose. Patients often complain of polyuria, polydipsia, lethargy, and weight loss. The classic presentation is altered sensorium, but patients also demonstrate signs of dehydration, weakness, tachycardia, and hypotension. A comparison of the varying abnormalities seen in DKA and HHS is listed in Table 2.

Table 2
Diagnostic criteria delineating DKA and HHS.

	DKA			HHS
	Mild	*Moderate*	*Severe*	
Plasma glucose (mg/dl)	>250	>250	>250	>600
Arterial pH	7.25–7.30	7.00–<7.24	<7.00	>7.30
Serum bicarbonate (mEq/l)	15–18	10–<15	<10	>15
Urine ketones	Positive	Positive	Positive	Small
Serum ketones	Positive	Positive	Positive	Small
Effective serum osmolality (mOsm/kg)	Variable	Variable	Variable	>320
Anion gap	>10	>12	>12	<12
Alteration in sensoria or mental obtundation	Alert	Alert/drowsy	Stupor/coma	Stupor/Coma

Laboratory Abnormalities

The American Diabetes Association' diagnostic criteria for HHS include *(18)*

- Blood glucose > 33.3 mmol/l (600 mg/dl)
- pH > 7.30
- Serum bicarbonate > 15 mmol/l
- Serum osmolality > 320
- A small amount of ketones may be present

Although the criteria for HHS and DKA diagnoses are at two ends of the spectrum, there is often significant overlap, including duration of symptoms, co-existing medical conditions, precipitants, and laboratory abnormalities *(14)*. In a review of 123 patients admitted for DKA, 37% of patients demonstrated increased serum osmolality *(14)*.

NEUROLOGICAL COMPLICATIONS IN HHS

Neurological complications in the hyperglycemic hyperosmolar state present as a spectrum of abnormalities and can range from lucidity to confusion or lethargy to complete coma. Other neurological manifestations, including hemiparesis, hemianopsia, chorea, and partial motor or generalized seizure activity, have also been described *(14, 64)*.

Altered Sensorium and Coma

The most common and classic clinical presentation in the hyperglycemic hyperosmolar state is an altered sensorium (14). Varying degrees of mental status alterations can be observed. Early in the process, patients can present with weakness and visual disturbances (65). As the process worsens with increasing hyperosmolarity and dehydration, lethargy, confusion, and coma may develop.

Those with higher degrees of hyperosmolarity are at increased risk of mental obtundation and coma (13, 63, 66). Neurological deterioration can occur after plasma osmolality climbs higher than 320–330 mOsmol/kg (14, 66). It is also important to note that the stuporous patient with an effective osmolality less than 320 mOsmol/Kg should be evaluated for other causes of altered mental status (14).

Hyperosmolarity may cause dehydration of brain tissue leading to diffuse cortical abnormalities. Yet, post-mortem studies suggest no evidence of dehydration in cerebral tissue (67). In laboratory animals, cerebral dehydration and death occur within 60–90 min if plasma glucose is elevated rapidly (68). However, if plasma glucose is elevated at slower rates, brain water content is initially lost but regained in 4–6 h. In these studies, water was ultimately retained in brain cells because of osmotic equilibrium between the brain osmole content increased to that of the plasma. The compensation by glucose, lactate, sorbitol, myoinositol, urea, sodium, potassium, and chloride only partially accounts for the rise and therefore unidentified "idiogenic osmoles" likely exist (67). Glucose levels likely play less of a role in altered sensorium. Despite glucose levels in excess of 600 mg/dl, coma rarely occurs if the plasma osmolality is near-normal (69). Although brain edema is common in patients with DKA, it is rare in those with non-ketotic coma (67).

Hemiparesis/Hemiplegia

The hyperglycemic hyperosmolar state can present as a stroke-like picture with hemiparesis or hemiplegia. There may be some difficulty in determining the cause or effect (i.e., stroke precipitating HHS or HHS precipitating hemiparesis). In fact, stroke was the most common admitting diagnosis in patients with HHS in the 1960s (67). Although hemiparesis may occur independently in HHS, it is more often related to post-ictal activity after a seizure (70). As per one report, hemiparesis is temporary and relieved within days after treatment of the underlying hyperglycemic hyperosmolar state (70).

Hemianopsia

Transient homonymous hemianopsia has been reported as a reversible complication of the hyperglycemic hyperosmolar state (64). There have been at least 12 cases of homonymous hemianopsia reported in patients with hyperosmolar hyperglycemia (64, 71–75). In addition to hemianopsia, these patients have noted other visual disturbances including blurred or fragmented vision, visual-field hallucinations, and flashing lights (64, 74). MRI findings such as decreased T2 signal of the white matter, subtle gyral swelling, and enhancement of the overlying meninges have been observed in these patients (64). Other studies have reported transient hemianopsia without MRI changes (74). Case reports range from mild improvement to total resolution in visual disturbances after treatment of the underlying hyperglycemic state (64, 74). In cases of hemianopsia, it is important to consider HHS as the cause when no lesion is detected on MRI. Other visual phenomena reported in patients with HHS include polyopia, flashing and flickering lights, hallucinations, and a persistence and transposition of objects in the visual fields (74).

CHOREIFORM MOVEMENTS

Chorea or ballismus has been observed in the hyperosmolar hyperglycemic state (76). In a report of HHS patients presenting with chorea, the mean age was 71.1 years and had a 2:1 ratio of women to men (76). In patients with HHS, choreiform movements are often but not always unilateral and occur concurrent with or shortly after the episode of hyperglycemia (77). Diabetes is usually newly diagnosed in these patients and develops subacutely over days to months (77).

In states of hyperglycemia, potential pathological causes of choreiform movements include decreased GABA–enkephalin inhibitory neurons, intracellular acidosis, accumulation of extracellular glutamate, brain edema formation, disruption of the blood–brain barrier, and global decrease in cerebral blood flow (78, 79). Resolution of hyperglycemia and increases in GABA levels do not always reverse chorea (77, 78). Chronic arteriolar disease and lacunar infarctions have been proposed as a mechanism, but subacute development of disease, generalized distribution of chorea in certain cases, and new-onset diabetes argue against these etiologies. Autoimmune attack, possibly via anti-GAD65 antibodies with opening of the blood–brain barrier has been proposed. Yet, anti-GAD65 antibodies were absent in the majority of patients in one study of HHS and chorea (77). MRI findings in patients with HHS and chorea may be abnormal and involve contralateral striatal hyperintensities on T1-weighted MR imaging, uniformly present in the putamen and usually involving the caudate (77, 78). In a rat model of transient focal ischemia, T1 striatal hyperintensities were present and histology revealed no hemorrhage or infarct, but did show diffuse and selective neuronal death and proliferation of astrocytes (80). These findings were similar to biopsies of the striatum in a human suffering with chorea, but not HHS *(81)*. The metabolic derangements present in hyperglycemia may render the striatum vulnerable to partial neuronal death and dysfunction and ultimately cause transient or permanent choreiform movement.

Blood glucose control, neuroleptics, and benzodiazepines are the main-stays of therapy for this neurological complication. Ventral thalamotomy has been used successfully in one case *(76)*. Abnormal movements usu-ally resolve or improve after hyperglycemia treatment in the majority of patients *(76)*.

Seizure Activity

Seizures can present in up to 25% of patients with HHS *(82)*. The major-ity are partial *(83, 84)*, but generalized tonic clonic seizures can also occur or may present secondarily. Epilepsia partialis continua (EPC), a rare simple partial motor seizure restricted to one part of the body *(85)* is a common form of seizure activity in HHS, observed in 14 of 21 patients in one study *(83)*. Movement-induced or kinesigenic and gaze-evoked visual seizures have also been reported *(72, 86)*. Brick et al. described reflex epilepsy in five patients with HHS who repeatedly induced focal seizures by limb movement *(87)*. Non-motor seizures may also occur and may be less recognized as symp-toms include apnea, speech arrest, aphasia, somatosensory symptoms, visual disturbances, and cardiac arrhythmias *(64)*.

Potential mechanisms for increasing risk in HHS may include hyper-glycemia, hyperosmolarity, low levels of GABA, and focal ischemia *(83)*. GABA is an inhibitory transmitter that lowers the seizure threshold. GABA is decreased in HHS secondary to increased metabolism *(85)*. Addition-ally, seizure activity is rarely witnessed in DKA where GABA levels are increased secondary to increased activity of glutamic acid decarboxylase and acidosis *(71, 85)*. Others have postulated that pre-existing areas of focal ischemia in cortical lesions may foster epileptogenic foci in periods of altered metabolic conditions *(85)*. Other studies suggest that hyperglycemia can result in reversible focal ischemia without structural damage by decreas-ing blood flow in specific cerebral areas *(88)*.

Although MR imaging is typically unremarkable *(85, 89–91)*, various studies have reported abnormal findings. In case reports, patients with partial status epilepticus and HHS showed transient subcortical T2 MRI hypointen-sities near the epileptic focus *(75, 91)* that correlated well with EEG as well as striatal T2 hyperintensities *(91)*. Abnormalities are typically reversed on repeat imaging weeks to years later. Other studies have also reported tran-sient focal lesions on computed tomography *(82)*.

Seizure activity in HHS is treated by insulin and rehydration reducing hyperglycemia and hyperosmolarity. Seizure activity stops immediately after the treatment of hyperglycemia by insulin *(82, 83, 86)* and can recur if glucose is not controlled *(86)*. Seizures are often refractory to anti-epileptic medications *(64, 82, 86, 92)*.

Other Neurological Manifestations

Other neurological manifestations of the hyperglycemic hyperosmolar state have been reported. Hallucinations, which may precede stupor or coma are usually visual and may range from simple to complex images or scenarios *(70)*. Other neurological abnormalities described include tonic eye deviation, nystagmus, abnormal papillary reflexes, aphasia, hemisensory defects, unilateral hyperreflexia, Babinski signs, abnormal body tone, hyperpnea, and meningeal signs *(67, 70)*. Meningeal signs include nuchal rigidity, positive Kernig's sign, and photophobia. The cerebrospinal fluid demonstrates no evidence of infection, but high glucose levels increased osmolality, and hyperchloremia may be present *(70)*. These changes suggest diffuse cortical or subcortical damage, which is usually reversible with correction of the underlying metabolic abnormalities *(67)*.

THERAPEUTIC INTERVENTIONS

HHS is marked by severe dehydration, insulin deficiency, and electrolyte abnormalities. Critical factors in reversing the underlying state include (1) vigorous fluid replacement, (2) electrolyte replacement, (3) insulin therapy, and (4) treatment of any underlying precipitant. A detailed review of treatment is beyond the scope of this chapter.

PROGNOSIS

The mortality rates for HHS vary between 10 and 20% *(14, 93)*. Mortality is usually related to the underlying precipitating illness *(14, 94–97)*, age *(93)*, degree of dehydration *(93)*, hemodynamic instability *(96)*, degree of consciousness *(94)*, and higher serum osmolality *(93)*. It is important to encourage patients with T2DM adherence to blood glucose monitoring and compliance with medications to prevent HHS. Adequate access to fluids and proper intake is especially important to prevent hyperosmolar states. There are a number of neurological abnormalities that manifest with HHS, which may or may not abate. Therefore, prevention of the hyperglycemic hyperosmolar state is of utmost importance.

REFERENCES

1. Dunger DB, Sperling MA, Acerini CL, et al. European Society for Paediatric Endocrinology/Lawson Wilkins Pediatric Endocrine Society consensus statement on diabetic ketoacidosis in children and adolescents. Pediatrics 2004; 113(2):e133–e140.
2. Umpierrez GE, Woo W, Hagopian WA, et al. Immunogenetic analysis suggests different pathogenesis for obese and lean African-Americans with diabetic ketoacidosis. Diabetes care 1999; 22(9):1517–1523.
3. Balasubramanyam A, Zern JW, Hyman DJ, Pavlik V. New profiles of diabetic ketoacidosis: type 1 vs type 2 diabetes and the effect of ethnicity. Arch Int Med 1999; 159(19):2317–2322.
4. Rosenbloom AL. Hyperglycemic comas in children: new insights into pathophysiology and management. Rev Endocr Metab Disord 2005; 6(4):297–306.
5. Curtis JR, To T, Muirhead S, Cummings E, Daneman D. Recent trends in hospitalization for diabetic ketoacidosis in Ontario children. Diabetes care 2002; 25(9):1591–1596.
6. Edge JA, Ford-Adams ME, Dunger DB. Causes of death in children with insulin dependent diabetes 1990–1996. Arch Dis Child 1999; 81(4):318–323.
7. Malone ML, Gennis V, Goodwin JS. Characteristics of diabetic ketoacidosis in older versus younger adults. J Am Geriatrics Soc 1992; 40(11):1100–1104.
8. Pinkey JH, Bingley PJ, Sawtell PA, Dunger DB, Gale EA. Presentation and progress of childhood diabetes mellitus: a prospective population-based study. The Bart's-Oxford Study Group. Diabetologia 1994; 37(1):70–74.
9. Faich GA, Fishbein HA, Ellis SE. The epidemiology of diabetic acidosis: a population-based study. Am J Epidemiol 1983; 117(5):551–558.
10. Johnson DD, Palumbo PJ, Chu CP. Diabetic ketoacidosis in a community-based population. Mayo Clin Proc 1980; 55(2):83–88.
11. Microvascular and acute complications in IDDM patients: the EURODIAB IDDM Complications Study. Diabetologia 1994; 37(3):278–285.
12. Type 2 diabetes in children and adolescents. American Diabetes Association. Diabetes Care 2000; 23(3):381–389.
13. Kitabchi AE, Umpierrez GE, Murphy MB, et al. Management of hyperglycemic crises in patients with diabetes. Diabetes Care 2001; 24(1):131–153.
14. Kitabchi AE, Umpierrez GE, Murphy MB, Kreisberg RA. Hyperglycemic crises in adult patients with diabetes: a consensus statement from the American Diabetes Association. Diabetes Care 2006; 29(12):2739–2748.
15. McGarry JD, Mannaerts GP, Foster DW. A possible role for malonyl-CoA in the regulation of hepatic fatty acid oxidation and ketogenesis. J Clin Invest 1977; 60(1):265–270.
16. Declercq PE, Falck JR, Kuwajima M, Tyminski H, Foster DW, McGarry JD. Characterization of the mitochondrial carnitine palmitoyltransferase enzyme system. I. Use of inhibitors. J Biol Chem 1987; 262(20):9812–9821.
17. McGarry JD, Woeltje KF, Kuwajima M, Foster DW. Regulation of ketogenesis and the renaissance of carnitine palmitoyltransferase. Diabetes Metab Rev 1989; 5(3):271–284.
18. Kitabchi AE, Umpierrez GE, Murphy MB, et al. Hyperglycemic crises in diabetes. Diabetes Care 2004; 27(Suppl 1):S94–S102.
19. Burge MR, Hardy KJ, Schade DS. Short-term fasting is a mechanism for the development of euglycemic ketoacidosis during periods of insulin deficiency. J Clin Endocrinol Metabolism 1993; 76(5):1192–1208.
20. Haddad NG, Croffie JM, Eugster EA. Pancreatic enzyme elevations in children with diabetic ketoacidosis. J Pediatr 2004; 145(1):122–124.
21. Curzon G, Kantamaneni BD, Callaghan N, Sullivan PA. Brain transmitter precursors and metabolites in diabetic ketoacidosis. J Neurol Neurosurgery Psychiatry 1982; 45(6):489–493.
22. Wootton-Gorges SL, Buonocore MH, Kuppermann N, et al. Cerebral proton magnetic resonance spectroscopy in children with diabetic ketoacidosis. AJNR 2007; 28(5):895–899.
23. Tsalikian E, Becker DJ, Crumrine PK, Daneman D, Drash AL. Electroencephalographic changes in diabetic ketosis in children with newly and previously diagnosed insulin-dependent diabetes mellitus. J Pediatr 1981; 99(3):355–359.

24. Northam EA, Anderson PJ, Werther GA, Warne GL, Andrewes D. Predictors of change in the neuropsychological profiles of children with type 1 diabetes 2 years after disease onset. Diabetes Care 1999; 22(9):1438–1444.

25. Northam E, Bowden S, Anderson V, Court J. Neuropsychological functioning in adolescents with diabetes. J Clin Exp Neuropsychol 1992; 14(6):884–900.

26. Bello FA, Sotos JF. Cerebral oedema in diabetic ketoacidosis in children. Lancet 1990; 336(8706):64.

27. Glaser NS, Wootton-Gorges SL, Buonocore MH, et al. Frequency of sub-clinical cerebral edema in children with diabetic ketoacidosis. Pediatr Diabetes 2006; 7(2):75–80.

28. Glaser N, Barnett P, McCaslin I, et al. Risk factors for cerebral edema in children with diabetic ketoacidosis. The Pediatric Emergency Medicine Collaborative Research Committee of the American Academy of Pediatrics. NE J Med 2001; 344(4):264–269.

29. Edge JA. Cerebral oedema during treatment of diabetic ketoacidosis: are we any nearer finding a cause? Diabetes Metabol Res Rev 2000; 16(5):316–324.

30. Glasgow AM. Devastating cerebral edema in diabetic ketoacidosis before therapy. Diabetes Care 1991; 14(1):77–78.

31. Rosenbloom AL. Intracerebral crises during treatment of diabetic ketoacidosis. Diabetes Care 1990; 13(1):22–33.

32. Rosenbloom AL, Schatz DA, Krischer JP, et al. Therapeutic controversy: prevention and treatment of diabetes in children. J Clin Endocrinol Metabol 2000; 85(2):494–522.

33. Krane EJ, Rockoff MA, Wallman JK, Wolfsdorf JI. Subclinical brain swelling in children during treatment of diabetic ketoacidosis. NE J Med 1985; 312(18):1147–1151.

34. Hoffman WH, Steinhart CM, el Gammal T, Steele S, Cuadrado AR, Morse PK. Cranial CT in children and adolescents with diabetic ketoacidosis. AJNR 1988; 9(4):733–739.

35. Edge JA, Hawkins MM, Winter DL, Dunger DB. The risk and outcome of cerebral oedema developing during diabetic ketoacidosis. Arch Dis Child 2001; 85(1):16–22.

36. Mahoney CP, Vlcek BW, DelAguila M. Risk factors for developing brain herniation during diabetic ketoacidosis. Pediatr Neurol 1999; 21(4):721–727.

37. Edge JA, Jakes RW, Roy Y, et al. The UK case-control study of cerebral oedema complicating diabetic ketoacidosis in children. Diabetologia 2006; 49(9):2002–2009.

38. Glaser NS, Marcin JP, Wootton-Gorges SL, et al. Correlation of Clinical and Biochemical Findings with Diabetic Ketoacidosis-Related Cerebral Edema in Children Using Magnetic Resonance Diffusion-Weighted Imaging. J Pediatr 2008.

39. Carlotti AP, Bohn D, Halperin ML. Importance of timing of risk factors for cerebral oedema during therapy for diabetic ketoacidosis. Arch Disease Child 2003; 88(2):170–173.

40. Arieff AI, Kleeman CR. Cerebral edema in diabetic comas. II. Effects of hyperosmolality, hyperglycemia and insulin in diabetic rabbits. J Clin Endocrinol Metabol 1974; 38(6):1057–1067.

41. van der Meulen JA, Klip A, Grinstein S. Possible mechanism for cerebral oedema in diabetic ketoacidosis. Lancet 1987; 2(8554):306–308.

42. Pollock AS, Arieff AI. Abnormalities of cell volume regulation and their functional consequences. Am J Physiol 1980; 239(3):F195–F205.

43. Abbott NJ. Inflammatory mediators and modulation of blood-brain barrier permeability. Cell Molecular Neurobiol 2000; 20(2):131–147.

44. Sarker MH, Fraser PA. The role of guanylyl cyclases in the permeability response to inflammatory mediators in pial venular capillaries in the rat. J Physiol 2002; 540(Pt 1):209–218.

45. O'Donnell ME, Martinez A, Sun D. Cerebral microvascular endothelial cell Na-K-Cl cotransport: regulation by astrocyte-conditioned medium. Am J Physiol 1995; 268(3 Pt 1):C747–C754.

46. Kimelberg HK, Rutledge E, Goderie S, Charniga C. Astrocytic swelling due to hypotonic or high K+ medium causes inhibition of glutamate and aspartate uptake and increases their release. J Cereb Blood Flow Metab 1995; 15(3):409–416.

47. Manley GT, Fujimura M, Ma T, et al. Aquaporin-4 deletion in mice reduces brain edema after acute water intoxication and ischemic stroke. Nature Med 2000; 6(2):159–163.

48. McManus ML, Churchwell KB, Strange K. Regulation of cell volume in health and disease. NE J Med 1995; 333(19):1260–1266.
49. Yang GY, Betz AL. Reperfusion-induced injury to the blood-brain barrier after middle cerebral artery occlusion in rats. Stroke 1994; 25(8):1658–1664; discussion 1664–1665.
50. Silver SM, Clark EC, Schroeder BM, Sterns RH. Pathogenesis of cerebral edema after treatment of diabetic ketoacidosis. Kidney Int 1997; 51(4):1237–1244.
51. Harris GD, Lohr JW, Fiordalisi I, Acara M. Brain osmoregulation during extreme and moderate dehydration in a rat model of severe DKA. Life Sci 1993; 53(3):185–191.
52. Rose SJ, Bushi M, Nagra I, Davies WE. Taurine fluxes in insulin dependent diabetes mellitus and rehydration in streptozotocin treated rats. Adv Exp Med Biol 2000; 483: 497–501.
53. Cameron FJ, Kean MJ, Wellard RM, Werther GA, Neil JJ, Inder TE. Insights into the acute cerebral metabolic changes associated with childhood diabetes. Diabet Med 2005; 22(5):648–653.
54. Lam TI, Anderson SE, Glaser N, O'Donnell ME. Bumetanide reduces cerebral edema formation in rats with diabetic ketoacidosis. Diabetes 2005; 54(2):510–516.
55. Yuen N, Anderson SE, Glaser N, Tancredi DJ, O'Donnell ME. Cerebral blood flow and cerebral edema in rats with diabetic ketoacidosis. Diabetes 2008; 57(10):2588–2594.
56. Isales CM, Min L, Hoffman WH. Acetoacetate and beta-hydroxybutyrate differentially regulate endothelin-1 and vascular endothelial growth factor in mouse brain microvascular endothelial cells. J Diabetes Complications 1999; 13(2):91–97.
57. Dunger DB, Sperling MA, Acerini CL, et al. ESPE/LWPES consensus statement on diabetic ketoacidosis in children and adolescents. Arch Dis Child 2004; 89(2):188–194.
58. Marcin JP, Glaser N, Barnett P, et al. Factors associated with adverse outcomes in children with diabetic ketoacidosis-related cerebral edema. J Pediatr 2002; 141(6):793–797.
59. Fiordalisi I, Novotny WE, Holbert D, Finberg L, Harris GD. An 18-yr prospective study of pediatric diabetic ketoacidosis: an approach to minimizing the risk of brain herniation during treatment. Pediatr Diabetes 2007; 8(3):142–149.
60. Duck SC, Wyatt DT. Factors associated with brain herniation in the treatment of diabetic ketoacidosis. J Pediatr 1988; 113(1 Pt 1):10–14.
61. Hamblin PS, Topliss DJ, Chosich N, Lording DW, Stockigt JR. Deaths associated with diabetic ketoacidosis and hyperosmolar coma. 1973–1988. Med J Aust 1989; 151(8):439, 441–432, 444.
62. Chupin M, Charbonnel B, Chupin F. C-peptide blood levels in keto-acidosis and in hyperosmolar non-ketotic diabetic coma. Acta Diabetol Lat 1981; 18(2):123–128.
63. Lorber D. Nonketotic hypertonicity in diabetes mellitus. Med Clin North Am 1995; 79(1):39–52.
64. Lavin PJ. Hyperglycemic hemianopia: a reversible complication of non-ketotic hyperglycemia. Neurol 2005; 65(4):616–619.
65. Stoner GD. Hyperosmolar hyperglycemic state. Am Fam Physician 2005; 71(9):1723–1730.
66. Fulop M, Tannenbaum H, Dreyer N. Ketotic hyperosmolar coma. Lancet 1973;2(7830):635–639.
67. Guisado R, Arieff AI. Neurologic manifestations of diabetic comas: correlation with biochemical alterations in the brain. Metabolism 1975; 24(5):665–679.
68. Van Harreveld A, Hooper NK, Cusick JT. Brain electrolytes and cortical impedance. Am J Physiol 1961; 201:139–143.
69. Gerich JE, Martin MM, Recant L. Clinical and metabolic characteristics of hyperosmolar nonketotic coma. Diabetes 1971; 20(4):228–238.
70. Maccario M. Neurological dysfunction associated with nonketotic hyperglycemia. Arch Neurol 1968; 19(5):525–534.
71. Harden CL, Rosenbaum DH, Daras M. Hyperglycemia presenting with occipital seizures. Epilepsia 1991; 32(2):215–220.
72. Duncan MB, Jabbari B, Rosenberg ML. Gaze-evoked visual seizures in nonketotic hyperglycemia. Epilepsia 1991; 32(2):221–224.

73. Brazis PW, Lee AG, Graff-Radford N, Desai NP, Eggenberger ER. Homonymous visual field defects in patients without corresponding structural lesions on neuroimaging. J Neurooph-thalmol 2000; 20(2):92–96.

74. Freedman KA, Polepalle S. Transient homonymous hemianopia and positive visual phenom-ena in nonketotic hyperglycemic patients. Am J Ophthalmol 2004; 137(6):1122–1124.

75. Seo DW, Na DG, Na DL, Moon SY, Hong SB. Subcortical hypointensity in partial sta-tus epilepticus associated with nonketotic hyperglycemia. J Neuroimaging 2003; 13(3):259–263.

76. Oh SH, Lee KY, Im JH, Lee MS. Chorea associated with non-ketotic hyperglycemia and hyperintensity basal ganglia lesion on T1-weighted brain MRI study: a meta-analysis of 53 cases including four present cases. J Neurol Sci 2002; 200(1–2):57–62.

77. Ahlskog JE, Nishino H, Evidente VG, et al. Persistent chorea triggered by hyperglycemic crisis in diabetics. Mov Disord 2001; 16(5):890–898.

78. Chu K, Kang DW, Kim DE, Park SH, Roh JK. Diffusion-weighted and gradient echo magnetic resonance findings of hemichorea-hemiballismus associated with diabetic hyperglycemia: a hyperviscosity syndrome? Arch Neurol 2002; 59(3):448–452.

79. Iwata A, Koike F, Arasaki K, Tamaki M. Blood brain barrier destruction in hyperglycemic chorea in a patient with poorly controlled diabetes. J Neurol Sci 1999; 163(1):90–93.

80. Fujioka M, Taoka T, Hiramatsu KI, Sakaguchi S, Sakaki T. Delayed ischemic hyperintensity on T1-weighted MRI in the caudoputamen and cerebral cortex of humans after spectacular shrinking deficit. Stroke 1999; 30(5):1038–1042.

81. Shan DE, Ho DM, Chang C, Pan HC, Teng MM. Hemichorea-hemiballism: an explanation for MR signal changes. AJNR 1998; 19(5):863–870.

82. Cochin JP, Hannequin D, Delangre T, Guegan-Massardier E, Augustin P. [Continuous partial epilepsy disclosing diabetes mellitus]. Rev Neurol (Paris) 1994; 150(3):239–241.

83. Tiamkao S, Pratipanawatr T, Nitinavakarn B, Chotmongkol V, Jitpimolmard S. Seizures in nonketotic hyperglycaemia. Seizure 2003; 12(6):409–410.

84. Stahlman GC, Auerbach PS, Strickland WG. Neurologic manifestations of non-ketotic hyper-glycemia. J Tenn Med Assoc 1988; 81(2):77–80.

85. Cokar O, Aydin B, Ozer F. Non-ketotic hyperglycaemia presenting as epilepsia partialis con-tinua. Seizure 2004; 13(4):264–269.

86. Hennis A, Corbin D, Fraser H. Focal seizures and non-ketotic hyperglycaemia. J Neurol Neu-rosurg Psychiatry 1992; 55(3):195–197.

87. Brick JF, Gutrecht JA, Ringel RA. Reflex epilepsy and nonketotic hyperglycemia in the elderly: a specific neuroendocrine syndrome. Neurology 1989; 39(3):394–399.

88. Duckrow RB, Beard DC, Brennan RW. Regional cerebral blood flow decreases during hyper-glycemia. Ann Neurol 1985; 17(3):267–272.

89. Lammouchi T, Zoghlami F, Ben Slamia L, Grira M, Harzallah MS, Benammou S. [Epileptic seizures in non-ketotic hyperglycemia]. Neurophysiol Clin 2004; 34(3–4):183–187.

90. Ozer F, Mutlu A, Ozkayran T. Reflex epilepsy and non-ketotic hyperglycemia. Epileptic Dis-ord 2003; 5(3):165–168.

91. Raghavendra S, Ashalatha R, Thomas SV, Kesavadas C. Focal neuronal loss, reversible sub-cortical focal T2 hypointensity in seizures with a nonketotic hyperglycemic hyperosmolar state. Neuroradiol 2007; 49(4):299–305.

92. Singh BM, Strobos RJ. Epilepsia partialis continua associated with nonketotic hyperglycemia: clinical and biochemical profile of 21 patients. Ann Neurol 1980; 8(2):155–160.

93. MacIsaac RJ, Lee LY, McNeil KJ, Tsalamandris C, Jerums G. Influence of age on the pre-sentation and outcome of acidotic and hyperosmolar diabetic emergencies. Int Med J 2002; 32(8):379–385.

94. Chu CH, Lee JK, Lam HC, Lu CC. Prognostic factors of hyperglycemic hyperosmolar non-ketotic state. Chang Gung Med J 2001; 24(6):345–351.

95. Zouvanis M, Pieterse AC, Seftel HC, Joffe BI. Clinical characteristics and outcome of hyperglycaemic emergencies in Johannesburg Africans. Diabet Med 1997; 14(7):603–606.

96. Pinies JA, Cairo G, Gaztambide S, Vazquez JA. Course and prognosis of 132 patients with diabetic non ketotic hyperosmolar state. Diabetes Metabol 1994; 20(1):43–48.
97. Rolfe M, Ephraim GG, Lincoln DC, Huddle KR. Hyperosmolar non-ketotic diabetic coma as a cause of emergency hyperglycaemic admission to Baragwanath Hospital. South African medical journal = Suid-Afrikaanse tydskrif vir geneeskunde 1995; 85(3):173–176.

8   Stroke and Diabetes Mellitus

Boris N. Mankovsky

Contents

Abstract

This chapter discusses the key findings from the literature regarding stroke incidence in patients with diabetes (DM), DM-specific and non-specific risk factors of stroke in the diabetic population, course and outcome of stroke in subjects with DM, and the peculiarities of type, site, and size of stroke in diabetic patients. The results of major clinical trials aimed at correcting hyperglycemia, hypertension, and dyslipidemia to prevent stroke in people with DM are also reviewed.

DM has been consistently shown to represent a strong independent risk factor of ischemic stroke. The same applies to the full cluster of the insulin resistance syndrome. The contribution of hyperglycemia to increased stroke risk is not proven. The association of diabetes with the risk of hemorrhagic stroke remains controversial. The course of stroke in patients with DM is characterized by higher mortality, more severe disability, and higher recurrence rate compared to non-diabetic subjects. Aggressive control of arterial hypertension and dyslipidemia allows to substantially decrease the risk of stroke in diabetic

From: *Contemporary Diabetes: Diabetes and the Brain*
Edited by: G. J. Biessels, J. A. Luchsinger (eds.), DOI 10.1007/978-1-60327-850-8_8
© Humana Press, a part of Springer Science+Business Media, LLC 2009

patients, while the importance of glucose control for stroke prevention remains unproven.

Key words: Diabetes mellitus; Hyperglycemia; Stroke; Cerebral infarction; Cerebral ischemia; Stroke prevention.

INTRODUCTION

This chapter discusses the key findings from the literature regarding stroke incidence in patients with DM, DM-specific and non-specific risk factors of stroke in the diabetic population, course and outcome of stroke in subjects with DM, and the peculiarities of type, site, and size of stroke in diabetic patients. The results of major clinical trials aimed at correcting hyperglycemia, hypertension, and dyslipidemia to prevent stroke in people with DM are also reviewed.

EPIDEMIOLOGY OF STROKE IN PATIENTS WITH DIABETES

Stroke is the third leading cause of death in Western society affecting more than 600,000 persons per year in the USA *(1, 2)*. Many epidemiological studies have convincingly shown that DM is one of the leading risk factors for stroke. Several large prospective studies report a population risks of stroke attributable to DM (proportion of cases which potentially could be prevented by eliminating DM) ranging from 2 to 42%, depending on the race–ethnicity of the population studied, type of stroke suffered, and gender *(3–6)*. Fifteen percent of total costs of cerebrovascular disease is related to DM *(7)*. Moreover, the association between DM and stroke is on the rise – from 1996/1997 to 2005/2006 the numbers of admissions with DM and stroke recorded rose almost twofold – from 6.2 to 11.3% for stroke *(8)*.

The results of major prospective studies addressing the impact of DM on stroke risk are summarized in Table 1. It is now well accepted that the risk of stroke in individuals with DM is equal to that of individuals with a history of myocardial infarction or stroke, but no DM *(24–26)*. This was confirmed in a recently published large retrospective study which enrolled all inhabitants of Denmark (more than 3 million people out of whom 71,802 patients with DM) and were followed-up for 5 years. In men without DM the incidence of stroke was 2.5 in those without and 7.8% in those with prior myocardial infarction, whereas in patients with DM it was 9.6 in those without and 27.4% in those with history of myocardial infarction. In women the numbers were 2.5, 9.0, 10.0, and 14.2%, respectively *(22)*.

Table 1
The risk of stroke in patients with diabetes mellitus

Authors	Study population	Follow-up, years	Relative risk
Stegmayr and Asplund (3)	Sweden, 241,000, 35–74 years old	8	Men – 4.1 Women – 5.8
Kannel and McGee (9)	Framingham Study, 5,209 people, 30–62 years old	20	Men – 2.5 Women – 3.6
Abbott et al. (10)	Honolulu Heart Program, 690 patients with and 6,908 without diabetes, 45–70 years old	12	2.0
Lehto et al. (11)	Finland, 1,059 patients with and 1,373 without diabetes, 45–64 years old	7	Men – 3.3 Women – 5.4
Niskanen et al. (12)	133 middle-aged patients with newly diagnosed type 2 diabetes and 144 controls, 45–64 years old	15	Men – 2.4 Women – 6.8
Folsom et al. (4)	Atherosclerosis Risk in Communities Study, 15,792 persons, 45–64 years old	6–8	Those diagnosed as having fasting glucose >140 mg/dl – 3.7 Those diagnosed as having fasting glucose >126 mg/dl – 3.23
Wannamethee et al. (13)	UK, 7,735 men, 40–59 years old	16.8	2.07 (for those with diabetes at baseline) 2.27 (for those diagnosed within the study period)
Abu-Lebdeh et al. (14)	Olmsted County, Minnesota, 9,936 (449 with diabetes), 40–70 years old	15	3.5
Kuusisto et al. (15)	Finland, 1,298 (229 diabetics), 65–74 years old	3.5	Men – 1.36 Women – 2.25

(continued)

Table 1
(continued)

Authors	Study population	Follow-up, years	Relative risk
Hart et al. *(16)*	Renfrew/Paisley, Scotland, 7,052 men, 8,354 women, 45–64 years old	20	Men – 1.52 Women – 2.83
Manson et al. *(17)*	USA, Nurse Study, 116,177 women, 30–55 years old	8	5.4
Aronow and Ahn *(18)*	USA, Hispanics, 201 men, 302 women, 70–90 years old	3.5	Men – 3.5 Women – 5.0
Mulnier et al. *(19)*	UK, general practice, 41,799 patients with type 2 diabetes, 202,733 without diabetes aged 35–89 years old	7.5	Men – 2.08 Women – 2.32
Almdal et al. *(20)*	Denmark, Copenhagen, 13,105 subjects	20	Men – 1.5–2 Women – 2–6.5 (the relative risk of the first incident and admission for stroke were assessed)
Ottenbacher et al. *(21)*	USA, Mexican-Americans, 3,050 subjects, 690 with diabetes, older than 65 years old	7	1.8
Schramm et al. *(22)*	Denmark, all population (more than 3 million), 71,802 patients with diabetes	5	Men – 2.51 Women – 2.45
Jeerakathil et al. *(23)*	Saskatchewan, Canada, 12,272 patients with newly diagnosed type 2 diabetes mellitus	5	From 1.8 in persons >75 years to 5.6 in those 30- to 44-year-old

The impact of DM on stroke risk and mortality varies depending on the economical development of the country and race. The number of deaths from stroke attributable to DM is highest in low-and-middle-income countries in South Asia and East Asia and Pacific (27, 28).

The risk of stroke associated with DM is observed across all age groups, although the relative risk conveyed by DM is greater in younger subjects (23, 29–31), possibly because the relative contribution of DM to stroke risk is greater in young individuals without additional risk factors than in older individuals with other co-morbid conditions.

It is not well known whether type 1 or type 2 DM affects stroke risk differently. Most studies addressing the association between DM and stroke recruited middle-aged or elderly subjects, who mainly had type 2 DM. In the WHO Multinational Study of Vascular Disease in DM (WHO MSVDD) the event rates of stroke were similar in type 1 and type 2 patients (32). In the large cohort of women enrolled in the Nurses' Health Study (116,316 women followed for up to 26 years) it was shown that the incidence of total stroke was fourfold higher in women with type 1 DM and twofold higher among women with type 2 DM than for non-diabetic women (33).

The impact of DM duration as a stroke risk factor has not been clearly defined. Some studies find no obvious relation between DM duration and stroke risk (23, 34), while several other studies do report such a relation (11, 15, 35). In this context it is important to note that the actual duration of type 2 DM is difficult to determine precisely.

RISK FACTORS FOR STROKE IN DIABETIC SUBJECTS

Traditional risk factors for stroke such as arterial hypertension, dyslipidemia, atrial fibrillation, heart failure, and previous myocardial infarction are more common in people with DM (3, 36). However, the impact of DM on stroke is not just due to the higher prevalence of these risk factors, as the risk of mortality and morbidity remains over twofold increased after correcting for these factors (4, 37). Risk factors for stroke in diabetic patients identified in previous studies are summarized in Table 2. It is informative to distinguish between factors that are non-specific and specific to DM. DM-specific factors, including chronic hyperglycemia, DM duration, DM type and complications, and insulin resistance, may contribute to an elevated stroke risk either by amplification of the harmful effect of other "classical" non-specific risk factors, such as hypertension, or by acting independently.

Table 2
Risk factors of stroke in patients with diabetes

Authors	Risk factors
Davis et al. *(38)*	Age, male sex, arterial hypertension, atrial fibrillation
Lehto et al. *(11)*	Prior cerebrovascular disorders, arterial hypertension, smoking, elevated cholesterol and triglyceride levels, low HDL cholesterol, hyperglycemia, duration of diabetes
Sasaki et al. *(39)*	Age, arterial hypertension, ischemic change on ECG, microvascular complications, therapeutic regimen
Abu-Lebdeh et al. *(14)*	Age, arterial hypertension, smoking, baseline glucose levels
Yoshinari et al. *(40)*	Total cholesterol, male gender
Fuller et al. *(32)*	Systolic blood pressure, duration of disease (only in women with type 2 diabetes), smoking (in men with type 2 diabetes), probable ECG changes (type 1 diabetic men), possible ECG changes (type 2 diabetics)
Yang et al. 2007 *(41)*	Age, hemoglobin A1C, spot urine albumin-to-creatinine ratio, and history of coronary heart disease
Giorda et al. 2007 *(42)*	Age and history of stroke
Mulnier et al. 2006 *(19)*	Younger age, females, duration of diabetes, smoking, obesity, atrial fibrillation, and hypertension

DM-Specific Risk Factors

As hyperglycemia is the typical metabolic abnormality in patients with DM it is important to address the association between the elevated glucose levels and the risk of stroke in diabetic patients. A casual and linear relationship between hyperglycemia and the risk of microvascular complications of DM has been proven by many epidemiological and interventional studies. In contrast, for macrovascular complications the relation with high glucose levels remains controversial. Hyperglycemia was shown to be a significant predictor of the risk of fatal or non-fatal stroke in subjects with DM in a substantial number of studies *(11–15, 43, 44)*. Some studies suggest that this relation may be more evident in type 2 than type 1 DM *(32)*. In a meta-analysis of three studies addressing the relationship between HbA1c levels and the risk of cardiovascular disease in type 2 diabetic patients the pooled relative risk for stroke was 1.17 for each 1-percentage point increase in HbA1c level *(45)*.

The recently published data from the Northern Manhattan Study suggested that inappropriate glycemic control, rather than the presence of DM itself, was associated with an increased risk of stroke. It was shown that diabetic subjects with elevated fasting blood glucose were at increased risk of stroke with the hazard ratio of 2.7, but those with target fasting glucose levels were not (46). In the same study it was revealed that an association between risk of stroke and fasting glycemia exists in African-Americans only while being non-significant in subjects of other ethnic origin (47).

Age seems to modify the role of hyperglycemia as a stroke risk factor. A linear increase in stroke morbidity and mortality for each 1% increment of HbA1c was found in older diabetic patients with onset of disease at an age older than 30 years, while there was no such association in younger subjects (48, 49).

The UKPDS showed that the odds of stroke being fatal was 1.37 per 1% HbA1c (50), but did not confirm the importance of hyperglycemia in stroke incidence (51). The estimated decrease in risk of stroke for a 1% reduction in HbA1c was 4% ($p = 0.44$) (52).

The controversy on the relation between blood glucose levels and the risk of stroke extends beyond studies in individuals with DM. While several studies report relations between different indices of glucose metabolism and the risk of stroke in non-diabetic individuals (53–55), other studies do not confirm such associations (56–58).

We may conclude that the relationship between hyperglycemia and stroke remains subject of debate. In this respect, the association between hyperglycemia and cerebrovascular disease is established less strongly than the association between hyperglycemia and coronary heart disease. Nevertheless, better understanding of the impact of hyperglycemia on increased stroke risk is important to establish effective guidelines for stroke prevention. The results of clinical trials addressing the possibility of decreasing the risk of macrovascular complications by achieving normoglycemia could provide the deeper insight into the role of hyperglycemia as the stroke risk factor in diabetic patients (see below).

Other DM-specific stroke risk factors are microvascular complications and diabetic neuropathy. Patients with retinopathy are at increased risk of predominantly lacunar stroke (59, 60) [but see (61)], and post-stroke mortality is increased (62–64). The relation between stroke and retinopathy is more evident in type 2 than type 1 DM (32), but this may be due to the age of the patients who were studied. Proteinuria may also be an independent risk factor for stroke (65, 66), but the relation between the degree of proteinuria (microalbuminuria or macroalbuminuria) and the level of the risk of stroke is not yet clear (32, 66, 67), and some studies failed to reveal a significant association between albuminuria and the risk of stroke or stroke mortality

(38, 68, 69). Diabetic autonomic neuropathy represents another risk factor for stroke *(70, 71)*. The presence of orthostatic drop of blood pressure of 10 mmHg, for example, doubled the risk of stroke associated with sympathetic autonomic neuropathy *(71)*.

The presence of the diabetic foot syndrome also increases the risk of stroke *(72)*, although this association may be attributed to the underlying generalized vascular damage or severe neuropathy.

Metabolic Syndrome (MS) as Stroke Risk Factor

The term "metabolic syndrome" (MS) refers to a cluster of risk factors, including hypertension, dyslipidemia, obesity, and abnormalities in glucose metabolism that are closely associated with DM (in particular type 2 DM) and with cardiovascular disease, including stroke. Although the fact that these risk factors often co-occur is not debated, it is yet uncertain if the whole concept of the MS entails more than its individual components. The clustering of risk factors complicates the assessment of the contribution of individual components to the risk of vascular events, as well as assessment of synergistic or interacting effects. In addition, there is no general agreement on the actual definition of the syndrome (NCEP, 2001, 2005; WHO, 1999; IDF, 2005), and it is yet unclear if the presence of the MS has a higher predictive value for cardiovascular disease than widely used prediction scores such as Framingham, PROCAM, and SCORE *(73–75)*. In the context of DM and stroke, the main relevance of the MS is that the majority of individuals with DM2 can be classified as having the MS. Moreover, the MS may precede the actual onset of type 2 DM by many years. Consequently, the MS, or its individual components, could represent key factors in the increased stroke risk in individuals with type 2 DM.

Indeed, the presence of the MS is associated with an approximately two- to threefold increased stroke risk, depending on the population studied and the MS definition used *(76–78)*. In the recently published results of the prospective study of 7,853 subjects the HR for ischemic stroke in men were 1.59, 1.52, 1.16, and 1.27, respectively, for the WHO, NCEP, NCEP revised, and IDF definitions of MS, and in women – 2.20, 2.68, 2.31, and 1.91, respectively. None of the definitions of MS predicted hemorrhagic stroke *(79)*. In the Framingham Offspring Study it was found that relative risk of stroke in persons with both DM and MS was 3.3 and was higher than that for either condition alone; 2.1 – for MS alone, 2.5 – for DM alone. The population-attributable risk, owing to its greater prevalence, was greater for the MS alone than for DM alone (19% vs. 7%), particularly in women (27% vs. 5%) *(80)*. In a prospective study of more than 14 thousand patients with pre-existing atherosclerotic vascular disease, subjects with the MS without DM exhibited a 1.5-fold increased odds for ischemic stroke or TIA, whereas those with frank DM had a 2.3-fold increased odds. The relative odds for ischemic stroke or TIA, associated with presence of the MS per se, were 1.4 in men but 2.1 in women (81). However, in a recently published prospective study of 594 diabetic patients followed-up for more than 10 years neither MS nor the combinations of its components predicted the development of ischemic stroke (82). Possibly, the relative impact of MS on increased stroke risk differs in patients with normal or impaired glucose tolerance or overt DM.

Insulin resistance is considered to be the central pathogenetic mechanism of the MS. There are some studies which addressed an association between insulin resistance and the risk of stroke. In the analysis of the data from the Third National Health and Nutrition Survey (1988–1994), it was found that patients with stroke had lower insulin sensitivity as assessed by HOMA index than participants without stroke and HOMA was independently associated with stroke (83). However, in another study, although the HOMA beta-cell index was inversely related to the stroke risk, there was no relation between the HOMA insulin resistance index and stroke risk, suggesting that insulin deficiency is a more important risk factor for stroke than insulin resistance (84). Also, in the landmark UKPDS, insulin sensitivity as measured by HOMA was not associated with subsequent stroke and estimation of insulin sensitivity provided no additional useful information with respect to the risk of the first occurrence of stroke in patients with newly diagnosed type 2 DM (85).

Hyperinsulinemia indicating insulin resistance was found in some groups of patients with stroke although these results were not consistent in different studies (86–88). Prospective studies addressing the role of hyperinsulinemia as a risk factor for stroke did not provide conclusive answers. An association between higher insulin levels and increase in incidence of either thromboembolic or hemorrhagic stroke was revealed in the Honolulu Heart Study (89). There was a J-shaped relationship between non-fasting serum insulin levels and the risk of stroke in non-diabetic men and this risk was higher in the first and fourth or higher quintiles compared to the second quintile (13). However, although hyperinsulinemia was associated with an increased risk for stroke morbidity and mortality in some studies this association became statistically non-significant after adjustment for obesity and other confounding variables (90–92). While the fasting insulin level was found to be a significant predictor of stroke in elderly non-diabetic subjects, there was no such an association in diabetic patients (15). In the recently published results of the prospective study of 1,151 elderly men increased fasting intact proinsulin level and decreased insulin sensitivity revealed by clamp predicted subsequent fatal and non-fatal stroke/TIA, independently of DM whereas fasting insulin did not *(93)*. Hyperinsulinemia was not a stroke predictor in the UKPDS *(38)*.

TYPE OF STROKE IN DIABETIC SUBJECTS

Most studies have consistently shown that DM is an important risk factor for ischemic stroke, while the incidence of hemorrhagic stroke in subjects with DM does not seem to be increased. Consequently, the ratio of ischemic to hemorrhagic stroke is higher in patients with DM than in those stroke patients without DM *(10, 31, 94–97)*, also in post-mortem studies *(98–100)*.

The data regarding an association between DM and the risk of hemorrhagic stroke are quite conflicting. In the most series no increased risk of cerebral hemorrhage was found *(10, 101)*, and in the Copenhagen Stroke Registry, hemorrhagic stroke was even six times less frequent in diabetic patients than in non-diabetic subjects *(102)*. The severity of fibrinoid necrosis of small cerebral arteriole walls, which is usually associated with intracerebral hemorrhage, was less pronounced in patients with DM and arterial hypertension compared to those with arterial hypertension alone *(100)*. It is plausible to speculate that such vascular characteristics could underlie the less frequent occurrence of hemorrhagic stroke in diabetic patients.

However, in another prospective population-based study DM was associated with an increased risk of primary intracerebral hemorrhage *(103)*. Stegmayr and Asplund *(3)* found a two times higher incidence of intracerebral hemorrhage in diabetic subjects compared to non-diabetic subjects. The significance of DM as a risk factor of hemorrhagic stroke could differ depending on ethnicity of subjects or type of DM. In the large Nurses' Health Study type 1 DM increased the risk of hemorrhagic stroke by 3.8 times while type 2 DM did not increase such a risk *(96)*. In the Honolulu Heart Study, DM was not associated with an increased risk of hemorrhagic stroke in Japanese-American men, while in the Framingham study there was a 4.5-fold excess risk of this type of stroke in white men with DM *(104)*.

It is yet unclear if DM predominantly predisposes to either large or small vessel ischemic stroke. Nevertheless, lacunar stroke (small, less than 15 mm in diameter infarction, cyst-like, frequently multiple) is considered to be the typical type of stroke in diabetic subjects *(105–107)*, and DM may be present in up to 28–43% of patients with cerebral lacunar infarction *(108–110)*. In the ARIS, the population-attributable fraction for DM was 26.3% for lacunar vs. 11.3% for non-lacunar stroke *(111)*. Other studies, however, indicate that the increased risk of ischemic stroke in DM does not predominantly involve lacunes *(112, 113)*. In the Nurses' Health Study, the risk for large-artery infarction and lacunar infarction in diabetic patients was similarly increased compared to non-diabetic population *(96)*. In a systematic review of studies addressing the risk factors for lacunar infarction, Jackson and Sudlow *(114)* revealed that while hypertension and DM appeared commoner among patients with lacunar vs. non-lacunar infarction, DM was not independently associated with an increased risk of lacunar infarction. In other studies addressing the prevalence of DM among subjects with different subtypes of cerebral infarction the prevalence of DM was found to be higher in subjects with either lacunar and thromboembolic stroke *(115, 116)* or similar compared to other subtypes of cerebral infarction *(117)*.

COURSE AND OUTCOME OF STROKE IN PATIENTS WITH DM

DM is an independent risk factor of death from stroke (Table 3). Tuomilehto et al. *(35)* calculated that 16% of all stroke mortality in men and 33% in women could be directly attributed to DM. Patients with DM have higher hospital and long-term stroke mortality, more pronounced residual neurological deficits, and more severe disability after acute cerebrovascular accidents *(120–126)*. The 1-year mortality rate, for example, was twofold higher in diabetic patients compared to non-diabetic subjects (50% vs. 25%) *(127)*. Only 20% of people with DM survive over 5 years after the first stroke and half of these patients die within the first year *(36, 128)*. Worse outcome in ischemic stroke involves all major stroke subtypes, including brainstem and cerebellar *(129)* or lacunar infarctions *(130)*. While earlier studies did not reveal any association between DM and the outcome of hemorrhagic stroke (intracerebral or subarachnoidal) or TIA *(131–133)*, it was later shown that DM was a major independent determinant of death in patients with intracerebral hemorrhage *(126, 134)*. Moreover, among subjects who had TIA or minor stroke, DM was predictive of further stroke, myocardial infarction, and vascular death *(135–137)*.

The mechanisms underlying the worse outcome of stroke in diabetic subjects are not fully understood. One possibility could be the higher prevalence of atrial fibrillation, arterial hypertension, heart failure, and prior myocardial infarctions in diabetic stroke patients compared to non-diabetic subjects with stroke *(3, 36, 138)*. However, DM was associated with worse outcome of stroke independently of other risk factors *(139)*.

Table 3
Risk of stroke mortality in patients with diabetes mellitus

Authors	Study	Age of subjects, years	Relative risk of stroke mortality
Tuomilehto et al. *(35)*	East Finland Men – 8,077 Women – 8,572 Follow-up – 16.4 years	30–59	Men – 3.4 Women – 4.9
Fuller et al. *(32)*	Whitehall, UK 18,403 men Follow-up – 10 years	40–64	Men – 3.9
Hart et al. *(16)*	Renfrew/Paisley, Scotland 7,052 men and 8,354 women Follow-up – 20 years	45–64	Men – 2.42 Women – 3.86
Tanne et al. *(118)*	Israel 9,374 men Follow-up – 21 years	>42	Men – 1.86
Neaton et al. *(95)*	USA 353,340 men Follow-up – 11.6 years	35–57	Non-hemorrhagic stroke – 3.8 Subarachnoid hemorrhage – 1.12 Intracranial hemorrhage – 1.49
Rastenyte et al. *(56)*	Kaunas, Lithuania 2,295 men Follow-up – 17.5 years	45–59	4.17
Stegmayr and Asplund *(3)*	Northern Sweden 241,000 Follow-up – 8 years	35–74	Men – 4.4 Women – 5.1
Haheim et al. *(119)*	Oslo, Norway 16,209 men Follow-up – 18 years	40–49	Men – 7.87
De Marco et al. *(34)*	Verona, Italy 7,148 patients with type 2 diabetes Follow-up – 5 years	35–85	1.48 Men – 1.35 Women – 1.57
Laing et al. *(31)*	United Kingdom 23,751 patients with type 1 diabetes Follow-up – 17 years	<30	Men – 3.1 Women – 4.4

(continued)

Table 3

(continued)

Authors	Study	Age of subjects, years	Relative risk of stroke mortality
Hu et al. *(25)*	Finland 25,155 men and 26,423 women Follow-up – 18.9 years	25–74	Men – 5.26 Women – 7.29
Ottenbacher et al. *(21)*	USA, Mexican-Americans 3050 subjects, 690 with diabetes, Follow-up – 7 years	Older than 65 years old	2.02

DM is associated with an increased incidence of recurrent cerebrovascular events in the majority of studies *(140, 141)* [but see *(142, 143)*]. The rate of early stroke recurrence (within 30 days) was 4.9 and 2.7% in patients with and without DM, respectively *(140)*. Moreover, this trend was maintained over 2 years of follow-up after the first stroke with a recurrence rate 19.8% in diabetic patients as compared with 12.3% in non-diabetic subjects *(141)*.

DM is an independent risk factor for post-stroke dementia with some racial differences – among African-Americans and Hispanics approximately one third of stroke-associated dementia was attributed to DM compared to 17% in Whites *(144–146)*.

The independent impact of hyperglycemia on the course and outcome of stroke either in diabetic or non-diabetic subjects remains subject of intense debate. Hyperglycemia in people with stroke could result from previously known or newly manifesting DM or could be "transitory" in subjects with otherwise preserved glucose tolerance. Alternatively, hyperglycemia may independently affect and worsen the outcome of stroke or merely reflect the severity, type, site, and size of stroke, being an epiphenomenon not influencing course of stroke itself. The role of hyperglycemia in stroke outcome is covered in detail in the following chapter.

One of the possible explanations for the worse outcome of stroke in patients with DM could be the difference in site and size of cerebral infarction. Earlier autopsy studies showed a relatively high prevalence of infratentorial (brainstem and cerebellar) infarctions and —three to four times higher prevalence of lesions in the areas of the pons and diencephalon in people with DM *(100, 147, 148)*. Infratentorial infarcts ≥5 mm in diameter were more frequent in diabetic patients older than 65 years while the prevalence of supratentorial infarcts was not different, which could reflect a higher vulnerability of vertebrobasilar circulation in diabetic patients (149).

Studies on the relation between DM and infarct size show inconsistent results (150–155). Potential factors that may have affected the differential observations of the available studies are the timing of the infarct volume assessment and differences in glucose and HbA1c levels between studies. The data regarding the epidemiology of stroke in patients with DM are summarized in Table 4.

Table 4
Epidemiology of stroke in diabetes: summary

Evidence	Fact
Strong evidence for	Increased risk of ischemic stroke in patients with DM compared to general population
	This increased risk is independent of other risk factors associated with DM
	The metabolic syndrome is associated with an increased risk of stroke
	In patients with DM outcome after stroke is worse, mortality is higher, and recurrent stroke is more frequent
Weaker evidence for	The significance of microvascular complications of DM (retinopathy, nephropathy), autonomic neuropathy as stroke risk factor
	The significance of obesity, central obesity, insulin resistance, hyperinsulinemia as stroke risk factors in patients with DM
	Lacunar infarction is the typical type of stroke for patients with DM
Controversies regarding	The significance of hyperglycemia as stroke risk factor
	The significance of DM duration as stroke risk factor
	The significance of DM type as stroke risk factor
	The risk of primary intracerebral hemorrhage and subarachnoid hemorrhage in patients with DM
	The size of cerebral infarction in patients with DM
	The origin of hyperglycemia during acute stroke

PREVENTION OF STROKE IN PATIENTS WITH DM

The results of large-scale randomized controlled clinical trials provide important leads for the prevention of stroke in high-risk populations including people with DM. A large number of diabetic patients were enrolled in most trials, thereby allowing post hoc analyses specific for DM.

Regarding prevention of stroke in patients with DM, it may be less relevant than in non-DM subjects to distinguish between primary and secondary prevention as all patients with DM are considered to be high-risk subjects regardless of the history of cerebrovascular accidents or the presence of clinical and subclinical vascular lesions. However, the aggressiveness of the preventive measures should be most pronounced in those who have DM and history of stroke or TIA. Obvious targets for the prevention of stroke in patients with DM are the correction of DM-specific risk factors, mainly hyperglycemia, and other diabetes non-specific factors, such as arterial hypertension or dyslipidemia. While in most trials addressing the correction of these latter factors the relative risk reduction was similar between patients with or without DM, the absolute risk reduction of stroke was usually higher in those with DM due to significantly higher risk in this subgroup of subjects.

Glycemic Control

In the long-term 17 years follow-up of type 1 DM patients who received intensive or standard insulin treatment in the Diabetes Control and Complications Trial, the combined risk of stroke, myocardial infarction, and cardiovascular death was 57% lower in those treated intensively *(156)*, but the data did not allow to draw conclusions regarding the long-term treatment effect on stroke as a single end-point *(156)*. It is interesting to note that the difference in the risk of cardiovascular disease between the two treatment arms appeared long after the end of the randomized treatment period which suggests the presence of the "metabolic memory" and emphasizes the need of active treatment from the early stages of the disease.

In contrast, the UKPDS did not support the hypothesis that control of glycemia could prevent stroke in type 2 DM patients. Conversely, an 11% statistically non-significant increase in stroke incidence was found in the intensively treated diabetic patients compared to the conventionally treated diabetic patients *(157)*. Recently the results of three large clinical trials (ADVANCE, ACCORD, VADT) that aimed to prevent cardiovascular disease in patients with DM through strict glycemic control have been presented. None of them was able to demonstrate a reduction of the risk of cardiovascular disease in patients intensively treated to achieve good glycemic control *(158, 159)*. Furthermore, in ACCORD trial, in the group of intensively treated subjects who achieved mean HbA1c levels of 6.4% a significant increase of cardiovascular mortality compared to standard-treated group was observed while the rate of non-fatal stroke was similar between the groups *(159)*.

The influence of the mode of antihyperglycemic treatment on the risk of stroke is uncertain. Mortality from cerebrovascular disease increased to a similar extent in patients treated by oral hypoglycemic medications or insulin compared to those on diet only *(160)*. Although the incidence of stroke was higher in diabetic subjects treated with insulin than in those receiving oral medications or diet this difference disappeared after adjustment for other confounding factors *(11)*. Stroke incidence did not differ in patients treated with chlorpromamide, glibenclamide, or insulin in the UKPDS. However, in overweight diabetic patients, intensive therapy with metformin was more effective in preventing stroke compared to other intensive treatment modalities, achieving a stroke reduction by 42% compared to the conventionally treated group *(161)*. Although in the UKPDS an early addition of metformin in sulfonylurea-treated patients did not lead to an increased stroke incidence *(161)*, another study showed a 2.3-fold increased mortality from stroke in patients treated with both medications compared to those treated with sulfonylurea alone *(162)*. However, it is not known whether such a harmful effect of this combined treatment reflects adverse interactions of both medications or more severe DM requiring the prescription of both drugs to achieve optimal metabolic control.

The PROACTIVE trial showed that pioglitazone was able to decrease the risk of recurrent stroke in patients with DM by 47%, while there was no effect on the prevention of a first stroke *(163)*. One of the possible underlying mechanisms of such protective action could be the slowing of the progression of carotid artery intima–media thickness shown for pioglitazone compared to glimepiride in CHICAGO trial *(164)*. However, the risks associated with the use of medications of this class (thiazolidinediones) such as increased risk of heart failure, myocardial infarction, edema, bone fractures, and weight gain probably do not allow recommending their wide use for stroke prevention.

Earlier it was suggested that oral sulfonylurea medications could adversely influence the outcome of ischemic events. However, sulfonylurea medications were not independent predictors for increased mortality, deterioration of stroke, or stroke severity and even could have beneficial effect of the outcome of non-lacunar stroke in diabetic subjects *(165, 166)*.

Treatment of Hypertension

There are no doubts that there is a linear relation between elevated systolic blood pressure and the risk of stroke, both in people with or without DM. Recently, at the Asia Pacific Cohort Study Cooperation, it was calculated that each 10 mmHg increase in systolic blood pressure was associated with 29% higher risk of ischemic stroke and 56% of hemorrhagic stroke among those with DM *(167)*. Although DM and arterial hypertension represent significant independent risk factors for stroke if they co-occur in the same patient the risk increases dramatically. A prospective study of almost 50 thousand subjects in Finland followed up for 19 years revealed that the hazard ratio for stroke incidence was 1.4, 2.0, 2.5, 3.5, and 4.5 and for stroke mortality was 1.5, 2.6, 3.1, 5.6, and 9.3, respectively, in subjects with an isolated modestly elevated blood pressure (systolic 140–159/diastolic 90–94 mmHg), isolated more severe hypertension (systolic >159 mmHg, diastolic >94 mmHg, or use of antihypertensive drugs), with isolated DM only, with both DM and modestly elevated blood pressure, and with both DM and more severe hypertension, relative to subjects without either of the risk factors *(168)*.

Correction of arterial hypertension effectively prevents stroke. The results of trials comparing active antihypertensive treatment and placebo addressing the incidence of stroke in patients with DM are summarized in Table 5. Control of arterial hypertension as the approach to decrease of stroke incidence is at least as or in some trials even more effective in diabetic patients than in the general population *(170, 171)*. Moreover, while in the placebo arms of these trials the risk for stroke in diabetic patients was increased, it became indistinguishable from non-diabetic subjects in actively treated hypertensive diabetic patients suggesting that effective antihypertensive treatment was able to eliminate the excess cardiovascular risk in people with DM *(170–172)*. The incidence of ischemic stroke was similar in treated hypertensive and normotensive diabetic patients, whereas it was significantly higher in those with untreated hypertension *(40)*. Guidelines addressing the treatment of arterial hypertension agree that the goal for blood pressure in patients with DM should be less than 130/80 mmHg *(177, 178)* although it has to be noted that these recommendations are based on the results of the epidemiological observations and are not yet supported by clinical trials which generally failed to achieve this tight control of blood pressure.

In diabetic patients, the efficacy of antihypertensive treatment in the UKPDS trial was higher than expected based on the data from epidemiological analysis. The calculation made based on epidemiological data indicated that 10 mmHg reduction of mean systolic blood pressure would be

Table 5
Reduction of stroke risk by antihypertensive treatment in patients with diabetes

Trial	Treatment	Number of diabetic/non-diabetic subjects	Reduction of blood pressure, mmHg	Medium follow-up, years	Reduction of stroke compared to placebo group (%)
UKPDS (169)	ACE inhibitor or beta blocker	1,148/0	Systolic – 10 Diastolic – 5	8.4	44
Syst-Eur (170)	Calcium antagonist with addition of enalapril or hydrochlorothiazide	492/4,203	Systolic – 8.6 Diastolic – 3.9	2	73
Syst-China (171)	Calcium antagonist with addition of captopril and/or hydrochlorothiazide	98/2,296	Systolic – 6.0 Diastolic – 4.7	2	45
SHEP (172)	Diuretic (chlorthalidone) with addition of atenolol or reserpine	583/4,149	Systolic – 9.8 Diastolic – 2.2	5	22
HOT (173)	Calcium antagonist	1,501/17,289	Diastolic ≤80 compared to ≤90	3.8	30
HOPE (174, 175)	ACE inhibitor	3,577/5,962	Systolic – 3.8 Diastolic – 2.8	4.5	33
ADVANCE (176)	ACE inhibitor + diuretic	11,140/0	Systolic – 5.86 Diastolic – 2.2	4.3	6

associated with a decrease in stroke risk by 19%, while as in the trial the same blood pressure reduction (by ACE-inhibitor captopril or beta-blocker atenolol) led to much greater actual decrease in stroke incidence – by 44% (179). These results suggest the possibility of some protective action of these agents beyond their antihypertensive efficacy. This assumption is supported by the results of the HOPE trial, which showed a greater than antici-pated reduction of stroke incidence following treatment with ACE inhibitor ramipril (174).

Nevertheless, it remains unclear whether some classes of antihyperten-sive agents provide a stronger protection against stroke in diabetic patients than others. There was no difference in the reduction of stroke incidence between groups of subjects who were treated with captopril or atenolol in the UKPDS (180). In two trials directly comparing the efficacy of different antihypertensive medications on the incidence of cardiovascu-lar events in patients with DM [ABCD – amlodipine vs. enalapril (181) and FACET – felodipine vs. fosinopril (182)], no significant difference in the stroke rate was noted. Similarly, no significant difference in the inci-dence of cerebrovascular events was observed in diabetic patients treated with the calcium-channel blocker diltiazem or captopril, on one side, or a diuretic and beta blocker, on the other side in the NORDIL and CAPPP trials, respectively (183–185). Moreover, a similar incidence of stroke in three groups of patients treated with newer medications (ACE inhibitors or calcium antagonists) or older ones (beta blockers and diuretics) was reported in the STOP-Hypertension-2 trial (186, 187). In a meta-analysis of three trials (ABCD, FACET, STOP-2) no significant difference in stroke incidence was found between ACE inhibitors or calcium channel block-ers in patients with DM (188). No difference in stroke incidence between groups of patients with arterial hypertension assigned either to amlodip-ine, chlorthalidone or lisinopril treatment was noted in 13,101 patients with DM and 1,399 subjects with IFG in the largest hypertension trial ALLHAT although in those without DM stroke was more common in those treated with lisinopril compared to chlorthalidone (189). In the meta-analysis of 14 trials addressing the efficacy of calcium channel blockers in patients with DM and arterial hypertension, it was shown that compared with the conventional therapy, calcium antagonists may have reduced the risk of stroke by 13% and had the similar effect on stroke prevention compared to blockers of the renin–angiotensin system (190). In the LIFE trial reduc-tion of stroke risk by 21.2% was reported in patients with DM treated with the angiotensin-receptor (AT1) blocker losartan compared to those treated with the beta-blocker atenolol. However, this difference did not reach the level of statistical significance, possibly due to inadequate statistical power (191). Recently, no benefits in stroke reduction were found for telmisartan or its combination with ramipril compared to ramipril alone in the large ONTARGET trial which enrolled more than 9 thousand patients with DM *(192)*.

However, in the subgroup of 5,137 diabetic patients enrolled into ASCOT trial the treatment with amlodipine combined with perindopril if necessary led to the reduction of the stroke incidence by 25% compared to treatment with beta-blocker atenolol combined with diuretic bendroflumethiazide in the total group of patients studied. Moreover, the amlodopine–perindopril regimen was associated with a 30% reduction of the risk of new cases of DM *(193)*.

In summary, effective antihypertensive treatment is highly beneficial for reduction of stroke risk in diabetic patients, but the advantages of any particular class of antihypertensive medications are not substantially proven.

Treatment of Dyslipidemia

High cholesterol levels are associated with an increased risk of stroke regardless of the presence of DM. In the Asia Pacific Cohort Studies Collaboration each 1 mmol/l increase of total cholesterol was associated with a 23% increased risk of ischemic stroke in subjects with DM and 31% in those without *(194)*. A significant reduction of the risk of stroke was observed in the CARDS trial which enrolled 2,838 patients with DM randomized to receive atorvastatin 10 mg daily or placebo. After only 3.9 years of follow-up, atorvastatin treatment was associated with a 50% reduction in non-hemorrhagic stroke and a 48% reduction for all strokes combined *(195)*. In the cohort of 2,532 patients with DM followed for 3.3 years, who were enrolled in ASCOT-LLA trial, the administration of atorvastatin in a dose of 10 mg daily resulted in the reduction of LDL by 1 mmol/l and a reduction of the risk of stroke by 33% which was not, however, statistically significant, probably due to low absolute number of events that occurred *(196)*. Pravastatin, 40 mg/day, reduced the risk of stroke by 39% in 1,077 diabetic patients and by 42% in 944 subjects with IFG in the LIPID trial which lasted for 6 years *(197)*. In the CARE trial, which included 586 diabetic subjects, treatment with pravastatin over a 5-year period led to a decrease in the relative risk of stroke by 14% in diabetic and by 37% in non-diabetic people *(198)*. In the 4S trial including 202 diabetic patients treatment with simvastatin over 5.4 years resulted in a reduction of cerebrovascular events in the diabetic cohort by 62% and by 23% in people without DM *(199)*. In the Heart Protection Study, which enrolled almost 6,000 patients with DM, a 24% reduction of the risk of stroke was found in diabetic cohort *(200)*. It seems that the beneficial effect of statins is dose-dependent. The lower the LDL level that is achieved the stronger the cardiovascular protection. In the cohort of 1,501 diabetic patients with coronary heart disease enrolled in

TNT trial the prescription of atorvastatin in a dose of 80 mg daily resulted in a reduction of the risk of cerebrovascular accidents by 31% compared to those who were treated with atorvastatin in doses of 10 mg daily (201). Recently, the results of the meta-analysis of 14 randomized trials of statins in 18,686 patients with DM had been published. It was calculated that statins use in diabetic patients can result in a 21% reduction of the risk of any stroke per 1 mmol/l reduction of LDL achieved which was not significantly different from 16% reduction observed in non-diabetics (202). This reduction was irrespective from prior history of vascular disease and other baseline characteristics.

There is no evidence from trials that supports efficacy of fibrates for stroke prevention in diabetic patients. In the large FIELD trial which enrolled 9,795 patients with type 2 DM use of fenofibrate did not result in significant reduction of the risk either of total or non-hemorrhagic stroke (203). No reduction of stroke risk by fibrates was shown also in a meta-analysis of eight trials enrolled 12,249 patients with type 2 DM (204).

Antiplatelet Therapy

Significant reductions in stroke risk in diabetic patients receiving antiplatelet therapy were found in large-scale controlled trials (205). It appears that based on the high incidence of stroke and prevalence of stroke risk factors in the diabetic population the benefits of routine aspirin use for primary and secondary stroke prevention outweigh its potential risk of hemorrhagic stroke especially in patients older than 30 years having at least one additional risk factor (206). However, the HOT trial did not show any beneficial effect of aspirin treatment on stroke incidence despite confirmed efficacy in preventing myocardial infarction in diabetic patients (173). Nevertheless, both guidelines issued by the AHA/ADA or the ESC/EASD on the prevention of cardiovascular disease in patients with DM support the use of aspirin in a dose of 50–325 mg daily for the primary prevention of stroke in subjects older than 40 years of age and additional risk factors, such as DM (207, 208). The use of aspirin in those younger than 40 years old without additional risk factor should not be advocated as the tool for primary stroke prevention.

The newer antiplatelet agent, clopidogrel, was more efficacious in prevention of ischemic stroke than aspirin with greater risk reduction in the diabetic cohort especially in those treated with insulin compared to non-diabetics in CAPRIE trial (209). However, the combination of aspirin and clopidogrel does not appear to be more efficacious and safe compared to clopidogrel or aspirin alone based on the results of MATCH and CHARISMA programs (210–212). The combined treatment with aspirin and dipyridamole was associated with a decreased incidence of recurrent stroke, but this reduction was not statistically significant in the subgroup of diabetic subjects (213).

The advantage of the combination of aspirin and dipyridamole over aspirin alone for the prevention of vascular events in patients with ischemic stroke was shown in ESPRIT trial *(214)*. In the recently published meta-analysis of five trials that enrolled 7,612 patients the combination of aspirin and dipyridamole was more effective than aspirin alone in patients with TIA or ischemic stroke of presumed arterial origin in the secondary prevention of stroke and other vascular events in all subgroups including patients with DM *(215)*.

Multifactorial Treatment

Gaede et al. *(216)* have shown in the Steno 2 study that intensive multifactorial intervention aimed at correction of hyperglycemia, hypertension, dyslipidemia, and microalbuminuria along with aspirin use resulted in a reduction of cardiovascular morbidity including non-fatal stroke (20 vs. 3 cases in conventionally and intensively treated patients, respectively). Moreover, recently the results of the extended 13.3 years follow-up of this study were presented and the reduction of cardiovascular mortality by 57% and morbidity by 59% along with the reduction of the number of non-fatal stroke (6 vs. 30 events) in intensively treated group was convincingly demonstrated *(217)*.

Antihypertensive, hypolipidemic treatment, use of aspirin should thus be recommended as either primary or secondary prevention of stroke for patients with DM. The adoption of a healthy life style has proven to be beneficial in preventing cardiovascular disease in diabetic patients. Moderate-to-vigorous physical activity was inversely related to the risk of ischemic stroke in women with DM in the Nurses' Health Study *(218)*.

Such an aggressive approach to the stroke prevention explains probably the decrease in incidence in first and recurrent stroke in women with DM (but not in men) recently revealed over 19-year period in the Northern Sweden MONICA Project Stroke registry and this decrease was significantly greater than in non-diabetic women *(219)*.

Treatment of Carotid Stenosis

Available results regarding the efficacy of carotid endarterectomy as a stroke preventive measure in patients with high-grade asymptomatic carotid stenosis are inconclusive, highly dependent on surgical risk, and have not been specifically assessed in patients with DM. In general, the Stroke Council of American Heart Association recommended that endarterectomy might be considered in patients with high-grade asymptomatic carotid stenosis performed by a surgeon, with <3% morbidity/mortality rate *(220)*. The risk of carotid endarterectomy could be an issue especially in patients with DM as the 30-day and 1-year mortality after such treatment was significantly higher in diabetics mainly due to cardiac complications, while post-operative morbidity did not differ (221). DM was also associated with increased risk of ipsilateral stroke following carotid endarterectomy (222). However, other studies have demonstrated that carotid endarterectomy could be performed in diabetic subjects with favorable perioperative morbidity and mortality rates and stroke-free and survival rates were not different from non-diabetic populations (223, 224).

Carotid endarterectomy should be considered in symptomatic patients – those who have stenosis of more than 50% and suffered from TIA or stroke on the side of the stenosis. In the large meta-analysis by Rothwell et al. (225), which included 974 patients with diabetes, it was revealed that such intervention was the most effective in reducing the risk of stroke in males, in those older than 75 years, and in patients operated within first 2 weeks after the last ischemic episode while there was no significant difference in the efficacy of the operation between patients with and without DM. The interventions to prevent stroke and their efficacy in patients with DM are summarized in Table 6.

Table 6
Prevention of stroke in diabetic patients: summary

Evidence	Intervention
Strong evidence for	Correction of arterial hypertension aiming at blood pressure below 130/80 mmHg (level of evidence A)
	Correction of dyslipidemia using statins with the goal of LDL below 100 mg/dl (2.6 mM/l) as primary prevention or 70 mg/dl (1.8 mM/l) as the secondary prevention (level of evidence A)
	Use of antiplatelet medications (secondary prevention) (level of evidence A)
	Carotid endarterectomy for symptomatic stenosis ≥70% (level of evidence A)
	Cessation of smoking (level of evidence A)
Weaker evidence for	Normalization of body mass (level of evidence C)
	Physical exercise (level of evidence C)
	Carotid endarterectomy for symptomatic stenosis 50–69% (level of evidence B)
	Use of antiplatelet medications (primary prevention) (level of evidence B)

(continued)

Table 6
(continued)

Evidence	Intervention
Controversies regarding	Correction of hyperglycemia aiming at HbA1c levels below 7.0 or 6.5% (level of evidence U)
	Correction of insulin resistance (level of evidence U)
	Is control of blood pressure more important for stroke prevention than the choice of antihypertensive agent used?
	Do any antihypertensive medications have benefits beyond their antihypertensive action?
	Is combination of statins with fibrates or other hypolipidemic medications safe and efficacious for stroke prevention in diabetic patients?
	Is it any specific dose of aspirin to prescribe for stroke prevention?
	Is it any threshold of HbA1c level associated with an increased stroke risk?
	Should we aim at achieving normoglycemia in all diabetic patients?
	Are any hypoglycemic medications more effective for stroke prevention in patients with DM?

Levels of evidence:

A – Established as effective, ineffective, or harmful for the given condition in the specified population. (Level A rating requires at least two consistent Class I studies.)

B – Probably effective, ineffective, or harmful for the given condition in the specified population. (Level B rating requires at least one Class I study or at least two consistent Class II studies.)

C – Possibly effective, ineffective, or harmful for the given condition in the specified population. (Level C rating requires at least one Class II study or two consistent Class III studies.)

U – Data inadequate or conflicting given current knowledge, treatment is unproven.

REFERENCES

1. Rosamond WD, Folsom AR, Chambless LE, et al. Stroke incidence and survival among middle-aged adults: 9-year follow-up of the Atherosclerosis Risk in Communities (ARIC) cohort. Stroke 1999; 30:736–743.
2. Lloyd-Jones D, Adams R, Carnethon M, et al. Heart disease and stroke statistics—2009 Update: A Report From the American Heart Association Statistics Committee and Stroke Statistics Subcommittee. Circulation 2009; 119: e21–e181
3. Stegmayr B, Asplund K. Diabetes as a risk factor for stroke. A population perspective. Diabetologia 1995; 38:1061–1068.

4. Folsom AR, Rasmussen ML, Chambless ME, et al. Prospective associations of fasting insulin, body fat distribution, and diabetes with risk of ischemic stroke. The Atherosclerosis Risk in Communities (ARIC) Study Investigators. Diabetes Care 1999; 22:1077–1083.
5. Kissela BM, Khoury J, Kleindorfer D, et al. Epidemiology of ischemic stroke in patients with diabetes: the greater Cincinnati/Northern Kentucky Stroke Study. Diabetes Care 2005; 28:355–359.
6. Lee CM, Huxley RR, Lam TH, et al. Prevalence of diabetes mellitus and population attributable fractions for coronary heart disease and stroke mortality in the WHO South-East Asia and Western Pacific regions. Asia Pac J Clin Nutr 2007; 16:87–92.
7. Currie CJ, Morgan CL, Gill L, Scott NC, Peters JR. Epidemiology and costs of acute hospital care for cerebrovascular disease in diabetic and nondiabetic populations. Stroke 1997; 28:1142–1146.
8. Bottle A, Millett C, Khunti K, Majeed A. Trends in cardiovascular admissions and procedures for people with and without diabetes in England, 1996–2005. Diabetologia 2009; 52:74–80.
9. Kannel WB, McGee DL. Diabetes and cardiovascular disease. The Framingam study. JAMA 1979; 241:2035–2038.
10. Abbott RD, Donahue RO, MacMahon SW, Reed DM, Yano K. Diabetes and the risk of stroke. The Honolulu Heart Program. JAMA 1987; 257:949–952.
11. Lehto S, Rönnemaa T, Pyörälä K, Laakso M. Predictors of stroke in middle-aged patients with non–insulin-dependent diabetes. Stroke 1996; 27:63–68.
12. Niskanen L, Turpeinen A, Penttila I, Uusitupa MI. Hyperglycemia and compositional lipoprotein abnormalities as predictors of cardiovascular mortality in type 2 diabetes: a 15-year follow-up from the time of diagnosis. Diabetes Care 1998; 21:1861–1869.
13. Wannamethee SG, Perry IJ, Shaper AG. Nonfasting serum glucose and insulin concentrations and the risk of stroke. Stroke 1999; 30:780–786.
14. Abu-Lebdeh HS, Hodge DO, Nguyen TT. Predictors of macrovascular disease in patients with type 2 diabetes mellitus. Mayo Clin Proc 2001; 76:707–712.
15. Kuusisto J, Mykkanen L, Pyorala K, Laakso M. Non-insulin-dependent diabetes and its metabolic control are important predictors of stroke in elderly patients. Stroke 1994; 25:1157–1164.
16. Hart CL, Hole DJ, Smith GD. Comparison of risk factors for stroke incidence and stroke mortality in 20 years of follow-up in men and women in the Renfrew/Paisley Study in Scotland. Stroke 2000; 31:1893–1896.
17. Manson JE, Colditz GA, Stampfer MJ, et al. A prospective study of maturity-onset diabetes mellitus and risk of coronary heart disease and stroke in women. Arch Intern Med 1991; 151:1141–1147.
18. Aronow WC, Ahn C. Risk factors for new atherothrombotic brain infarction in older Hispanic men and women. J Gerontol A Biol Sci Med Sci 2002; 57:M61–M63.
19. Mulnier HE, Seaman HE, Raleigh VS, et al. Risk of stroke in people with type 2 diabetes in the UK: a study using the General Practice Research Database. Diabetologia 2006; 49: 2859–2865.
20. Almdal T, Scharling H, Jensen JS, Vestergaard H. The independent effect of type 2 diabetes mellitus on ischemic heart disease, stroke, and death: a population-based study of 13,000 men and women with 20 years of follow-up. Arch Intern Med 2004; 164:1422–1426.
21. Ottenbacher KJ, Ostir GV, Peek MK, Markides KS. Diabetes mellitus as a risk factor for stroke incidence and mortality in Mexican American older adults. J Gerontol A Biol Sci Med Sci 2004; 59:640–645.
22. Schramm TK, Gislason GH, Køber L, et al. Diabetes patients requiring glucose-lowering therapy and nondiabetics with a prior myocardial infarction carry the same cardiovascular risk: a population study of 3.3 million people. Circulation 2008; 117:1945–1954.
23. Jeerakathil T, Johnson JA, Simpson SH, Majumdar SR. Short-term risk for stroke is doubled in persons with newly treated type 2 diabetes compared with persons without diabetes: a population-based cohort study. Stroke 2007; 38:1739–1743.

24. Ho JE, Paultre F, Mosca L, for the Women's Pooling Project. Is diabetes mellitus a cardio-vascular disease risk equivalent for fatal stroke in women? Data from the Women's Pooling Project. Stroke 2003; 34:2812–2816.
25. Hu G, Jousilahti P, Sarti C, Antikainen R, Tuomilehto J. The effect of diabetes and stroke at baseline and during follow-up on stroke mortality. Diabetologia 2006; 49:2309–2316.
26. Lee CD, Folsom AR, Pankow JS, Brancati FL, Atherosclerosis Risk in Communities (ARIC) Study Investigators. Cardiovascular events in diabetic and nondiabetic adults with or without history of myocardial infarction. Circulation 2004; 109:855–860.
27. Danaei G, Lawes CM, van der Hoorn S, Murray CJ, Ezzati M. Global and regional mortality from ischaemic heart disease and stroke attributable to higher-than-optimum blood glucose concentration: comparative risk assessment. Lancet 2006; 368:1651–1659.
28. Sacco RL, Boden-Albala B, Abel G, et al. Race-ethnic disparities in the impact of stroke risk factors: the Northern Manhattan Stroke Study. Stroke 2001; 32: 1725–1731.
29. Noto D, Barbagallo M, Cavera G, et al. Leukocyte count, diabetes mellitus and age are strong predictors of stroke in a rural population in southern Italy: an 8-year follow-up. Atherosclerosis 2001; 157:225–231.
30. Lin M, Chen Y, Sigal RJ. Stroke associated with diabetes among Canadians: sex and age differences. Neuroepidemiology 2007; 28:46–49.
31. Laing SP, Swerdlow AJ, Carpenter LM, et al. Mortality from cerebrovascular disease in a cohort of 23 000 patients with insulin-treated diabetes. Stroke 2003; 34:418–421.
32. Fuller JH, Stevens LK, Wang SL, the WHO Multinational Study Group Risk factors for cardiovascular mortality and morbidity: The WHO multinational study of vascular disease in diabetes. Diabetologia 2001; 44:S54–S64.
33. Janghorbani M, Hu FB, Willett WC, et al. Prospective study of type 1 and type 2 diabetes and risk of stroke subtypes: the Nurses' Health Study. Diabetes Care 2007; 30: 1730–1735.
34. De Marco R, Locatelli F, Zoppini G, Verlato G, Bonora E, Muggeo M. Cause-specific mortality in type 2 diabetes. The Verona Diabetes Study. Diabetes Care 1999; 22:756–761.
35. Tuomilehto J, Rastenyte D, Jousilahti P, Sarti C, Vartiainen E. Diabetes mellitus as a risk factor for death from stroke. Prospective study of the middle-aged Finnish population. Stroke 1996; 27:210–215.
36. Olsson T, Vitanen M, Asplund K, Eriksson S, Hagg E. Prognosis after stroke in diabetic patients. A controlled prospective study. Diabetologia 1990; 33:244–249.
37. Barrett-Connor E, Khaw KT. Diabetes mellitus: an independent risk factor for stroke? Am J Epidemiol 1988; 128:116–123.
38. Davis TM., Millns H, Stratton IM, Holman RR, Turner RC. Risk factors for stroke in type 2 diabetes mellitus: United Kingdom Prospective Diabetes Study (UKPDS) 29. Arch Intern Med 1999; 159:1097–1103.
39. Sasaki A, Horiuchi N, Hasegawa K, Uehara M. Mortality from coronary heart disease and cerebrovascular disease and associated risk factors in diabetic patients in Osaka District, Japan. Diab Res Clin Pract 1995; 27:77–83.
40. Yoshinari M, Kaku R, Iwase M, et al. Development of ischemic stroke in normotensive and hypertensive diabetic patients with or without antihypertensive treatment: an 8-year follow up study. J Diabetes Complications 1997; 11:9–14.
41. Yang X, Kong AP, So WY, et al. Effects of chronic hyperglycaemia on incident stroke in Hong Kong Chinese patients with type 2 diabetes. Diabetes Metab Res Rev 2007; 23: 220–226.
42. Giorda CB, Avogaro A, Maggini M, et al. Incidence and risk factors for stroke in type 2 diabetic patients: the DAI study. Stroke 2007; 38:1154–1160.
43. Selvin E, Coresh J, Shahar E, Zhang L, Steffes M, Sharrett AR. Glycaemia (haemoglobin A1c) and incident ischaemic stroke: the Atherosclerosis Risk in Communities (ARIC) Study. Lancet Neurol 2005; 4:821–826.

44. Elley CR, Kenealy T, Robinson E, Drury PL. Glycated haemoglobin and cardiovascular outcomes in people with Type 2 diabetes: a large prospective cohort study. Diabet Med 2008; 25:1295–1301.
45. Selvin E, Marinopoulos S, Berkenblit G, et al. Meta-analysis: glycosylated hemoglobin and cardiovascular disease in diabetes mellitus. Ann Intern Med 2004; 141:421–431.
46. Boden-Albala B, Cammack S, Chong J, et al. Diabetes, fasting glucose levels, and risk of ischemic stroke and vascular events: findings from the Northern Manhattan Study (NOMAS). Diabetes Care 2008; 31:1132–1137.
47. Eguchi K, Boden-Albala B, Jin Z, et al. Usefulness of fasting blood glucose to predict vascular outcomes among individuals without diabetes mellitus (from the Northern Manhattan Study). Am J Cardiol 2007; 100:1404–1409.
48. Moss SE, Klein R, Klein BEK, Meuer SM. The association of glycemia and cause-specific mortality in diabetic population. Arch Intern Med 1994; 154:2473–2479.
49. Lowe LP, Liu K, Greenland P, Metzger BE, Dyer AR, Stamler J. Diabetes, asymptomatic hyperglycemia, and 22-year mortality in black and white men. The Chicago Heart Association Detection Project in Industry Study. Diabetes Care 1997; 20:163–169.
50. Stevens RJ, Coleman RL, Adler AI, Stratton IM, Matthews DR, Holman RR. Risk factors for myocardial infarction case fatality and stroke case fatality in type 2 diabetes: UKPDS 66. Diabetes Care 2004; 27:201–207.
51. Colagiuri S, Cull CA, Holman RR. Are lower fasting plasma glucose levels at diagnosis of type 2 diabetes associated with improved outcomes? U.K. Prospective diabetes study 61. Diabetes Care 2002; 25:1410–1417.
52. Stratton IM, Adler AI, Neil HA, et al. Association of glycaemia with macrovascular and microvascular complications of type 2 diabetes (UKPDS 35): prospective observational study. BMJ 2000; 321:405–412.
53. Oizumi T, Daimon M, Jimbu Y, et al. Impaired glucose tolerance is a risk factor for stroke in a Japanese sample – the Funagata study. Metabolism 2008; 57:333–338.
54. Fuller JH, Shipley MJ, Rose G, Jarrett RJ, Keen H. Mortality from coronary heart disease and stroke in relation to degree of glycemia: the Whitehall study. BMJ 1983; 287:867–868.
55. Burchfiel CM, Curb D, Rodriguez BL, Abbott RD, Chiu D, Yano K. Glucose intolerance and 22-year stroke incidence. The Honolulu Heart Program. Stroke 1994; 25: 951–957.
56. Rastenyte D, Tuomilehto J, Domarkiene S, Cepaitis Z, Reklaitiene R. Risk factors for death from stroke in middle-aged Lithuanian men. Results from a 20-year prospective study. Stroke 1996; 27:672–676.
57. Qureshi AI, Giles WH, Croft JB. Impaired glucose tolerance and the likelihood of nonfatal stroke and myocardial infarction: the Third National Health and Nutrition Examination Survey. Stroke 1998; 29:1329–1332.
58. Manolio TA, Kronmal RA, Burke GL, O'Leary DH, Price TR, for the CHS Collaborative Research Group. Short-term predictors of incident stroke in older adults. The Cardiovascular Health Study. Stroke 1996; 27:1479–1486.
59. Cheung N, Rogers S, Couper DJ, Klein R, Sharrett AR, Wong TY. Is diabetic retinopathy an independent risk factor for ischemic stroke? Stroke 2007; 38:398–401.
60. Petitti DB, Bhatt H. Retinopathy as a risk factor for nonembolic stroke in diabetic subjects. Stroke 1995; 26:593–596.
61. Klein R, Sharrett AR, Klein BE, et al. The association of atherosclerosis, vascular risk factors, and retinopathy in adults with diabetes: the atherosclerosis risk in communities study. Ophthalmology 2002; 109:1225–1234.
62. Klein R, Klein BE, Moss SE, Cruickshanks KJ. Association of ocular disease and mortality in a diabetic population. Arch Ophtalmol 1999; 117:1487–1495.
63. Klein BE, Klein R, McBride PE, et al. Cardiovascular disease, mortality, and retinal microvascular characteristics in type 1 diabetes: Wisconsin epidemiologic study of diabetic retinopathy. Arch Intern Med 2004; 164:1917–1924.

64. Klein R, Klein BE, Moss SE, Wong TY. Retinal vessel caliber and microvascular and macrovascular disease in type 2 diabetes: XXI: the Wisconsin Epidemiologic Study of Diabetic Retinopathy. Ophthalmology 2007; 114:1884–1892.

65. Guerrero-Romero F, Rodriguez-Moran M. Proteinuria is an independent risk factor for ischemic stroke in non-insulin-dependent diabetes mellitus. Stroke 1999; 30:1787–1791.

66. Miettinen H, Haffner SM, Lehto S, Ronnemaa T, Pyorala K, Laakso M. Proteinuria predicts stroke and other atherosclerotic vascular disease events in nondiabetic and non-insulin-dependent diabetic subjects. Stroke 1996; 27:2033–2039.

67. Valmadrid CT, Klein R, Moss SE, Klein BE. The risk of cardiovascular disease mortality associated with microalbuminuria and gross proteinuria in persons with older-onset diabetes mellitus. Arch Intern Med 2000; 160:1093–1100.

68. Gall MA, Borch-Johnsen K, Hougaard P, Nielsen FS, Parving HH. Albuminuria and poor glycemic control predict mortality in NIDDM. Diabetes 1995; 44:1303–1309.

69. Spoelstra-De Man AM, Brouwer CB, Stehouwer CD, Smulders YM. Rapid progression of albumin excretion is an independent predictor of cardiovascular mortality in patients with type 2 diabetes and microalbuminuria. Diabetes Care 2001; 24:2097–2101.

70. Cohen JA, Estacio RO, Lundgren RA, Esler AL, Schrier RW. Diabetic autonomic neuropathy is associated with an increased incidence of strokes. Auton Neurosci 2003; 108:73–78.

71. Toyry JP, Niskanen LK, Lansimies EA, Partanen KP, Uusitupa MI. Autonomic neuropathy predicts the development of stroke in patients with non-insulin-dependent diabetes mellitus. Stroke 1996; 27:1316–1318.

72. Pinto A, Tuttolomondo A, Di Raimondo D, et al. Ischemic stroke in patients with diabetic foot. Int Angiol 2007; 26:266–269.

73. National Heart, Lung, and Blood Institute. National Cholesterol Education Program: Executive Summary of the Third report of the National Cholesterol Education Program (NCEP) Expert Panel on Detection, Evaluation and Treatment of High Blood Cholesterol in Adults (Adult Treatment Panel III). JAMA 2001; 285: 2486–2497.

74. World Health Organization Definition, diagnosis and classification of diabetes mellitus and its complications. Report of a WHO consultation. Part I: Diagnosis and classification of diabetes mellitus. Geneva: World Health Organization, 1999.

75. Alberti KG, Zimmet P, Shaw J. The metabolic syndrome – a new worldwide definition. Lancet 2005; 366:1059–1062.

76. Ninomiya JK, L'Italien G, Criqui MH, Whyte JL, Gamst A, Chen RS. Association of the metabolic syndrome with history of myocardial infarction and stroke in the Third National Health and Nutrition Examination Survey. Circulation 2004; 109:42–46.

77. Isomaa B, Almgren P, Tuomi T, et al. Cardiovascular morbidity and mortality associated with the metabolic syndrome. Diabetes Care 2001; 24:683–689.

78. Kurl S, Laukkanen JA, Niskanen L, et al. Metabolic syndrome and the risk of stroke in middle-aged men. Stroke 2006; 37:806–811.

79. Qiao Q, Laatikainen T, Zethelius B, et al. Comparison of definitions of metabolic syndrome in relation to the risk of developing stroke and coronary heart disease in Finnish and Swedish cohorts. Stroke 2009; 40:337–343.

80. Najarian RM, Sullivan LM, Kannel WB, Wilson PW, D'Agostino RB, Wolf PA. Metabolic syndrome compared with type 2 diabetes mellitus as a risk factor for stroke: the Framingham Offspring Study. Arch Intern Med 2006; 166:106–111.

81. Koren-Morag N, Goldbourt U, Tanne D. Relation between the metabolic syndrome and ischemic stroke or transient ischemic attack: a prospective cohort study in patients with atherosclerotic cardiovascular disease. Stroke 2005; 36:1366–1371.

82. Protopsaltis I, Korantzopoulos P, Milionis HJ, et al. Metabolic syndrome and its components as predictors of ischemic stroke in type 2 diabetic patients. Stroke 2008; 39: 1036–1038.

83. Bravata DM, Wells CK, Kernan WN, Concato J, Brass LM, Gulanski BI. Association between impaired insulin sensitivity and stroke. Neuroepidemiology 2005; 25: 69–74.

84. Adachi H, Hirai Y, Tsuruta M, Fujiura Y, Imaizumi T. Is insulin resistance or diabetes mellitus associated with stroke? An 18-year follow-up study. Diabetes Res Clin Pract 2001; 51:215–223.

85. Adler AI, Levy JC, Matthews DR, Stratton IM, Hines G, Holman RR. Insulin sensitivity at diagnosis of Type 2 diabetes is not associated with subsequent cardiovascular disease (UKPDS 67). Diabet Med 2005; 22:306–311.

86. Shinozaki K, Naritomi H, Shimizu T, et al. Role of insulin resistance associated with compensatory hyperinsulinemia in ischemic stroke. Stroke 1996; 27:37–43.

87. Zunker P, Schick A, Buschmann HC, et al. Hyperinsulinism and cerebral microangiopathy. Stroke 1996; 27:219–223.

88. Lindahl B, Dinesen B, Eliasson M, Roder M, Hallmans G, Stegmayr B. High proinsulin levels precede first-ever stroke in nondiabetic population. Stroke 2000; 31:2936–2941.

89. Burchfiel CM, Sharp DS, Curb JD, et al. Hyperinsulinemia and cardiovascular disease in elderly men: the Honolulu Heart Program. Arterioscler Thromb Vasc Biol 1998; 18: 450–457.

90. Pyorala M, Miettinen H, Laakso M, Pyorala K. Hyperinsulinemia and the risk of stroke in healthy middle-aged men: the 22-year follow-up results of the Helsinki Policemen Study. Stroke 1998; 29:1860–1866.

91. Pyorala M, Miettinen H, Laakso M, Pyorala K. Plasma insulin and all-cause, cardiovascular and noncardiovascular mortality. The 22-year follow-up results of the Helsinki Policemen Study. Diabetes Care 2000; 23:1097–1102.

92. Lakka HM, Lakka TA, Tuomilehto J, Sivenius J, Salonen JT. Hyperinsulinemia and the risk of cardiovascular death and acute coronary and cerebrovascular events in men: the Kuopio Ischaemic Heart Disease Risk Factor Study. Arch Intern Med 2000; 160:1160–1168.

93. Wiberg B, Sundström J, Zethelius B, Lind L. Insulin sensitivity measured by the euglycaemic insulin clamp and proinsulin levels as predictors of stroke in elderly men. Diabetologia 2009; 52:90–96.

94. Lithner F, Asplund K, Eriksson S, Hagg E, Strand T, Wester PO. Clinical characteristics in diabetic stroke patients. Diabete Metab 1988; 4:15–19.

95. Neaton JD, Wentworth DN, Cutler J, Stamler J, Kuller L. Risk factors for death from different types of stroke. Multiple Risk Factor Intervention Trial Research Group. Ann Epidemiol 1993; 3:493–499.

96. Janghorbani M, Hu FB, Willett WC, et al. Prospective study of type 1 and type 2 diabetes and risk of stroke subtypes: the Nurses' Health Study. Diabetes Care 2007; 30: 730–735.

97. Adams HP, Putman SF, Kassell NF, Torner JC. Prevalence of diabetes mellitus among patients with subarachnoid hemorrhage. Arch Neurol 1984; 41:1033–1035.

98. Bell ET. A post-mortem study of vascular disease in diabetes. Arch Pathol 1952; 53: 444–455.

99. Alex M, Baron EK, Goldenberg S, Blumenthal HT. An autopsy study of cerebrovascular accident in diabetes mellitus. Circulation 1962; 25:663–673.

100. Aronson SM. Intracranial vascular lesions in patients with diabetes mellitus. J Neuropathol Exp Neurol 1973; 32:183–196.

101. Njolstad I, Arnesen E, Lund-Larsen PG. Body height, cardiovascular risk factors, and risk of stroke in middle-aged men and women. A 14-year follow-up of the Finnmark Study. Circulation 1996; 94:2877–2882.

102. Jorgensen H, Nakayama H, Raaschou HO, Olsen TS. Stroke in patients with diabetes. The Copenhagen Stroke Study. Stroke 1994; 25:1977–1984.

103. Zia E, Pessah-Rasmussen H, Khan FA, et al. Risk factors for primary intracerebral hemorrhage: a population-based nested case-control study. Cerebrovasc Dis 2006; 21: 18–25.

104. Rodriguez BL, D'Agostino R, Abbott RD, et al. Risk of hospitalized stroke in men enrolled in the Honolulu Heart program and the Framingham Study: A comparison of incidence and risk factor effects. Stroke 2002; 33:230–236.

105. Gandolfo C, Caponnetto C, Del Sette M, Santoloci D, Loeb C. Risk factors in lacunar syndromes: a case-control study. Acta Neurol Scand 1988; 77:22–26.

106. Ghika A, Bogousslavsky J, Regli F. Infarcts in the territory of the deep perforators from the carotid system. Neurology 1989; 39:507–512.

107. Tuttolomondo A, Pinto A, Salemi G, et al. Diabetic and non-diabetic subjects with ischemic stroke: differences, subtype distribution and outcome. Nutr Metab Cardiovasc Dis 2008; 18:152–157.

108. Tuszynski MH, Petito CK, Levy DE. Risk factors and clinical manifestations of pathologically verified lacunar infarctions. Stroke 1989; 20:990–999.

109. Arboix A, Martii Vilalta JL, Garsia JH. Clinical study of 227 patients with lacunar infarcts. Stroke 1990; 21:842–847.

110. Horowitz DR, Tuhrim S, Weinberger JM, Rudolph SH. Mechanisms in lacunar infarction. Stroke 1992; 23:325–327.

111. Ohira T, Shahar E, Chambless LE, Rosamond WD, Mosley Jr. TH, Folsom AR. Risk factors for ischemic stroke subtypes: the Atherosclerosis Risk in Communities study. Stroke 2006; 37:2493–2498.

112. Kappelle LJ, van Gijn J. Lacunar infarcts. Clin Neurol Neurosurg 1986; 17:3–17.

113. Bejot Y, Catteau A, Caillier M, et al. Trends in incidence, risk factors, and survival in symptomatic lacunar stroke in Dijon, France, from 1989 to 2006. A population-based study. Stroke 2008; 39:1945–1951.

114. Jackson C, Sudlow C. Are lacunar strokes really different? A systematic review Stroke 2005; 36:891–901.

115. Chamorro A, Sacco RL, Mohr JP, et al. Clinical-computed tomographic correlations of lacunar infarction in the Stroke Data Bank. Stroke 1991; 22:175–181.

116. Petty GW, Brown RD, Whisnant JP, Sicks JRD, O'Fallon WM, Wiebers DO. Ischemic stroke subtypes: a population-based study of incidence and risk factors. Stroke 1999; 30: 2513–2516.

117. Lodder J, Bamford JM, Sandercock PAG, Jones LN, Warlow CP. Are hypertension or cardiac embolism likely causes of lacunar infarction? Stroke 1990; 21:375–381.

118. Tanne D, Yaari S, Goldbourt U. Risk profile and prediction of long-term ischemic stroke mortality. A 21-year follow-up in the Israeli Ischemic Heart Disease (IIHD) Project. Circulation 1998; 98:1365–1371.

119. Haheim LL, Holme I, Hjermann I, Leren P. Nonfasting serum glucose and the risk of fatal stroke in diabetic and nondiabetic subjects. 18-year follow-up of the Oslo Study. Stroke 1995; 26:774–777.

120. Pulsinelli WA, Levy DE, Sigsbee B, Scherer K, Plum F. Increased damage after ischemic stroke in patients with hyperglycemia with or without established diabetes mellitus. Am J Med 1983; 74:540–544.

121. Oppenheimer S, Halfbraid BI, Oswald GA, Yudkin JS. Diabetes mellitus and early mortality from stroke. BMJ 1985; 291:1014–1015.

122. Kushner M, Nencini P, Reivich M, et al. Relation of hyperglycemia early in ischemic brain infarction to cerebral anatomy, metabolism, and clinical outcome. Ann Neurol 1990; 28:129–135.

123. Kiers L, Davis SM, Larkins R, et al. Stroke topography and outcome in relation to hyperglycaemia and diabetes. J Neurol Neurosurg Psychiatry 1992; 55:263–270.

124. van Kooten F, Hoogerbrugge N, Naarding P, Koudstall PJ. Hyperglycemia in the acute phase of stroke is not caused by stress. Stroke 1993; 24:1129–1132.

125. Lai SM, Alter M, Friday G, Sobel E. Prognosis for survival after an initial stroke. Stroke 1995; 26:2011–2015.

126. Wong KS. Risk factors for early death in acute ischemic stroke and intracerebral hemorrhage: A prospective hospital-based study in Asia. Asian Stroke Advisory Panel. Stroke 1999; 30:2326–2330.

127. Oliveira TV, Gorz AM, Bittencourt PR. Diabetes mellitus as a prognostic factor in ischemic cerebrovascular disease. Arq Neuropsiquiatr 1988; 46:287–291.

128. Asplund K, Hagg E, Helmers C, Lithner F, Strand T, Wester PO. The natural history of stroke in diabetic patients. Acta Med Scand 1980; 297:417–424.
129. Hornig CR, Buttner T, Hoffmann O, Dorndorf W. Short-term prognosis of vertebrobasilar ischemic stroke. Cerebrovasc Dis 1992; 2:273–281.
130. Clavier I, Hommel M, Besson G, Noelle B, Perret JE. Long-term prognosis of symptomatic lacunar infarcts. A hospital-based study. Stroke 1994; 25:2005–2009.
131. Howard G, Toole JF, Frye-Pierson J, Hinshelwood LC. Factors influencing the survival of 451 transient ischemic attack patients. Stroke 1987; 18:552–557.
132. Simpson Jr. RK, Contant CF, Fischer DK, Cech DA, Robertson CS, Narayan RK. The influence of diabetes mellitus on outcome from subarachnoid hemorrhage. Diabetes Res 1991; 16:165–169.
133. Tuhrim S, Dambrosia JM, Price TR, et al. Intracerebral hemorrhage: external validation and extension of a model for prediction of 30-day survival. Ann Neurol 1991; 29:658–663.
134. Arboix A, Massons J, Garcia-Eroles L, Oliveres M, Targa C. Diabetes is an independent risk factor for in-hospital mortality from acute spontaneous intracerebral hemorrhage. Diabetes Care 2000; 23:1527–1532.
135. The Dutch TIA Trial Study Group. Predictors of major vascular events in patients with a transient ischemic attack or nondisabling stroke. Stroke 1993; 24:527–531.
136. Evans BA, Sicks JD, Whisnant JP. Factors affecting survival and occurrence of stroke in patients with transient ischemic attacks. Mayo Clin Proc 1994; 69:416–421.
137. Johnston SC, Gress DR, Browner WS, Sidney S. Short-term prognosis after emergency department diagnosis of TIA. JAMA 2000; 284:2901–2906.
138. Carlberg B, Asplund K, Hagg E. Factors influencing admission blood pressure levels in patients with acute stroke. Stroke 1991; 22:527–530.
139. Lefkovits J, Davis SM, Rossiter SC, et al. Acute stroke outcome: effects of stroke type and risk factors. Aust N Z J Med 1992; 22:30–35.
140. Sacco RL, Foulkes MA, Mohr JP, Wolf PA, Hier DB, Price TR. Determinants of early recurrence of cerebral infarction. The Stroke Data Bank. Stroke 1989; 20:983–989.
141. Hier DB, Foulkes MA, Swiontoniowski M, et al. Stroke recurrence within 2 years after ischemic infarction. Stroke 1991; 22:155–161.
142. Jorgensen HS, Nakayama H, Reith J, Raaschou HO, Olsen TS. Stroke recurrence: predictors, severity, and prognosis. The Copenhagen Stroke Study. Neurology 1997; 48:891–895.
143. Friday G, Alter M, Lai SM. Control of hypertension and risk of stroke recurrence. Stroke 2002; 33:2652–2657.
144. Censori B, Manara O, Agostinis C, et al. Dementia after first stroke. Stroke 1996; 27:1205–1210.
145. Luchsinger JA, Tang MX, Stern Y, Shea S, Mayeux R. Diabetes mellitus and risk of Alzheimer's disease and dementia with stroke in a multiethnic cohort. Am J Epidemiol 2001; 154:635–641.
146. Henon H, Durieu I, Guerouaou D, Lebert F, Pasquier F, Leys D. Poststroke dementia: Incidence and relationship to prestroke cognitive decline. Neurology 2001; 57:1216–1222.
147. Peres NS, Fane WC, Aronson SM. Central nervous system findings in a tenth decade autopsy population. Prog Brain Res 1973; 40:473–483.
148. Kameyama M, Fushimi H, Udaka F. Diabetes mellitus and cerebral vascular disease. Diab Res Clin Pract 1994; 24:S205–S208.
149. Iwase M, Yamamoto M, Yoshinari M, Ibayashi S, Fujishima M. Stroke topography in diabetic and nondiabetic patients by magnetic resonance imaging. Diabetes Res Clin Pract 1998; 42:109–116.
150. Cambon H, Derouesne C, Yelnik A, Duyckaerts C, Hauw JJ. Effect of diabetes mellitus and blood glucose on the size of cerebral infarction and causes of death. Neuropathological study of 77 cases of infarction in the sylvian artery area. Rev Neurol 1991; 147:727–734.
151. Mankovsky BN, Patrick JT, Metzger BE, Saver JL. The size of subcortical ischemic infarction in patients with and without diabetes mellitus. Clin Neurol Neurosurg 1996; 98:137–141.

152. Horowitz SH, Zito JL, Donnarumma R, Patel M, Alvir J. Clinical-radiographic correlations within the first five hours of cerebral infarctions. Acta Neurol Scand 1992; 86: 207–214.
153. Candelise I., Landi G, Orazio EN, Boccardi E. Prognostic significance of hyperglycemia in acute stroke. Arch Neurol 1985; 42:661–663.
154. Murros K, Fogelholm R, Kettunen S, Vuorela AL, Valve J. Blood glucose, glycosylated haemoglobin, and outcome of ischemic brain infarction. J Neurol Sci 1992; 111:59–64.
155. Toni D, De Michele M, Fiorelli M, et al. Influence of hyperglycemia on infarct size and clinical outcome of acute ischemic stroke in patients with intracranial arterial occlusion. J Neurol Sci 1994; 123:129–133.
156. Nathan DM, Cleary PA, Backlund JY, et al. Diabetes Control and Complications Trial/Epidemiology of Diabetes Interventions and Complications (DCCT/EDIC) Study Research Group. Intensive diabetes treatment and cardiovascular disease in patients with type 1 diabetes. N Engl J Med 2005; 353:2643–2653.
157. UK Prospective Diabetes Study (UKPDS) Group. Intensive blood-glucose control with sulphonylureas or insulin compared with conventional treatment and risk of complications in patients with type 2 diabetes (UKPDS 33). Lancet 1998; 352:837–853.
158. ADVANCE Collaborative Group, Patel A, MacMahon S, Chalmers J, et al. Intensive blood glucose control and vascular outcomes in patients with type 2 diabetes. N Engl J Med 2008; 358:2560–2572.
159. Action to Control Cardiovascular Risk in Diabetes Study Group, Gerstein HC, Miller ME, Byington RP, et al. Effects of intensive glucose lowering in type 2 diabetes. N Engl J Med 2008; 358:2545–2559.
160. Kuller LH, Velentgas P, Barzilay J, Beauchamp NJ, O'Leary DH, Savage PJ. Diabetes mellitus: subclinical cardiovascular disease and risk of incident cardiovascular disease and all-cause mortality. Arterioscler Thromb Vasc Biol 2000; 20:823–829.
161. UK Prospective Diabetes Study (UKPDS) Group. Effect of intensive blood-glucose control with metformin on complications in overweight patients with type 2 diabetes (UKPDS 34). Lancet 1998; 352:854–865.
162. Olsson J, Lindberg G, Gottsater M, et al. Increased mortality in Type II diabetic patients using sulfonylurea and metformin in combination: a population-based observational study. Diabetologia 2000; 43:558–560.
163. Wilcox R, Bousser MG, Betteridge DJ, et al. Effects of pioglitazone in patients with type 2 diabetes with or without previous stroke: results from PROactive (PROspective pioglitAzone Clinical Trial In macroVascular Events 04). Stroke 2007; 38:865–873.
164. Mazzone T, Meyer PM, Feinsten SB, et al. Effect of pioglitazone compared with glimepiride on carotid intima-media thickness in type 2 diabetes. A randomized trial. JAMA 2006; 296:E1–E10.
165. Weih M, Amberger N, Wegener S, Dirnagl U, Reuter T, Einhaupl K. Sulfonylurea drugs do not influence initial stroke severity and in-hospital outcome in stroke patients with diabetes. Stroke 2001; 32:2029–2032.
166. Kunte H, Schmidt S, Eliasziw M, et al. Sulfonylureas improve outcome in patients with type 2 diabetes and acute ischemic stroke. Stroke 2007; 38:2526–2530.
167. Asia Pacific Cohort Studies Collaboration, Kengne AP, Patel A, Barzi F, et al. Systolic blood pressure, diabetes and the risk of cardiovascular diseases in the Asia-Pacific region. J Hypertens 2007; 25:1205–1213.
168. Hu G, Sarti C, Jousilahti P, et al. The impact of history of hypertension and type 2 diabetes at baseline on the incidence of stroke and stroke mortality. Stroke 2005; 36:2538–2543.
169. UK Prospective Diabetes Study Group. Tight blood pressure control and risk of macrovascular and microvascular complications in type 2 diabetes: UKPDS 38. BMJ 1998; 317: 703–713.
170. Tuomilehto J, Rastenyte D, Birkenhager WH, et al. for the Systolic Hypertension in Europe Trial Investigators. Effects of calcium-channel blockade in older patients with diabetes and systolic hypertension. N Engl J Med 1999; 340:677–684.

171. Wang JG, Staessen JA, Gong L, Liu L, for the Systolic Hypertension in China (Syst-China) Collaborative Group. Chinese Trial on Isolated Systolic Hypertension in the Elderly. Arch Intern Med 2000; 160:211–220.

172. Curb JD, Pressel SL, Cutler JA, et al. Effect of diuretic-based antihypertensive treatment on cardiovascular disease risk in older diabetic patients with isolated systolic hypertension. Systolic Hypertension in the Elderly Program Cooperative Research Group. JAMA 1996; 276:1886–1892.

173. Hansson L, Zanchetti A, Carruthers SG, et al. for the HOT Study Group. Effects of intensive blood-pressure lowering and low-dose aspirin in patients with hypertension: principal results of the Hypertension Optimal Treatment (HOT) randomized trial. Lancet 1998; 351: 1755–1762.

174. Heart Outcomes Prevention Evaluation (HOPE) Study Investigators. Effects of ramipril on cardiovascular and microvascular outcomes in people with diabetes mellitus: results of the HOPE study and MICRO-HOPE substudy. Lancet 2000; 355:253–259.

175. Bosch J, Yusuf S, Pogue J, et al. for HOPE Investigators. Heart outcomes prevention evaluation. BMJ 2002; 324:699–702.

176. Patel A, MacMahon S, ADVANCE Collaborative Group. Effects of a fixed combination of perindopril and indapamide on macrovascular and microvascular outcomes in patients with type 2 diabetes mellitus (the ADVANCE trial): a randomized trial. Lancet 2007; 370: 829–840.

177. American Diabetes Association. Standards of medical care – 2008. Diabetes Care 2008; 31:S12–S54.

178. Rydén L, Standl E, Bartnik M, et al. Guidelines on diabetes, pre-diabetes, and cardiovascular diseases: executive summary. The Task Force on Diabetes and Cardiovascular Diseases of the European Society of Cardiology (ESC) and of the European Association for the Study of Diabetes (EASD). Eur Heart J 2007; 28:88–136.

179. Adler AI, Stratton IM, Neil HAW, et al. on behalf of the UK Prospective Study Group. Association of systolic blood pressure with macrovascular and microvascular complications of type 2 diabetes (UKPDS 36): prospective observational study. BMJ 2000; 321:412–419.

180. UK Prospective Diabetes Study Group. Efficacy of atenolol and captopril in reducing risk of macrovascular and microvascular complications in type 2 diabetes: UKPDS 39. BMJ 1998; 317:713–720.

181. Estacio RO, Jeffers BW, Hiatt WR, Biggerstaff SL, Gifford N, Schrier RW. The effect of nisoldipine as compared with enalapril on cardiovascular outcomes in patients with non-insulin-dependent diabetes and hypertension. N Engl J Med 1998; 338:645–652.

182. Tatti P, Pahr M, Byington RB, et al. Outcome results of the Fosinopril Versus Amlodipine Cardiovascular Events Randomized Trial (FACET) in patients with hypertension and NIDDM. Diabetes Care 1998; 21:597–603.

183. Hansson L, Lindholm LH, Niskanen L, et al. for the Captopril Prevention Project (CAPPP) study group. Effect of angiotensin-converting enzyme inhibition compared with conventional therapy on cardiovascular morbidity and mortality in hypertension: the Captopril Prevention Project (CAPP) randomized trial. Lancet 1999; 353:611–616.

184. Hansson L, Hedner T, Lund-Johansen P, et al. for the NORDIL Study Group. Randomised trial of effects of calcium antagonists compared with diuretics and b-blockers on cardiovascular morbidity and mortality in hypertension: the Nordic Diltiazem (NORDIL) study. Lancet 2000; 356:359–365.

185. Niskanen L, Hedner T, Hansson L, Lanke J, Niklason A, for the CAPPR study group. Reduced cardiovascular morbidity and mortality in hypertensive diabetic patients on first-line therapy with an ACE inhibitor compared with a diuretic/b-blocker-based treatment regimen: a subanalysis of the Captopril Prevention Project. Diabetes Care 2001; 24:2091–2096.

186. Hansson L, Lindholm LH, Ekbom T, et al. for the STOP-Hypertension-2 study group. Randomized trial of old and new antihypertensive drugs in elderly patients: cardiovascular mortality and morbidity the Swedish Trial in Old Patients with Hypertension-2 study. Lancet 1999; 354:1751–1756.

187. Lindholm L, Hansson L, Ekbom T, et al. for the STOP-Hypertension-2 Study Group. Comparison of antihypertensive treatment in preventing cardiovascular events in elderly diabetic patients: results from Swedish Trial in Old Patients with hypertension-2. J Hypertens 2002; 18:1671–1675.

188. Opie LH, Schall R. Evidence-based evaluation of calcium channel blockers for hypertension: equality of mortality and cardiovascular risk relative to conventional therapy. J Am Coll Cardiol 2002; 39:315–322.

189. Whelton PK, Barzilay J, Cushman WC, et al. for the ALLHAT Collaborative Research Group. Clinical outcomes in antihypertensive treatment of type 2 diabetes, impaired fasting glucose concentration, and normoglycemia: Antihypertensive and Lipid-Lowering Treatment to Prevent Heart Attack Trial (ALLHAT). Arch Intern Med 2005; 165:1401–1409.

190. Grossman E, Messerli FH. Are calcium antagonists beneficial in diabetic patients with hypertension? Am J Med 2004; 116:44–49.

191. Lindholm LH, Ibsen H, Dahlof B, et al. Cardiovascular morbidity and mortality in patients with diabetes in the Losartan Intervention For Endpoint reduction in hypertension study (LIFE): a randomised trial against atenolol. Lancet 2002; 359:1004–1010.

192. The ONTARGET Investigators. Telmasartan, ramipril, or both in patients at high risk for vascular events. N Engl J Med 2008; 358:1547–1559.

193. Ostergren J, Poulter NR, Sever PS, et al. for the ASCOT investigators. The Anglo-Scandinavian Cardiac Outcomes Trial: blood pressure-lowering limb: effects in patients with type II diabetes. J Hypertens 2008; 26:2103–2111.

194. Asia Pacific Cohort Studies Collaboration. Cholesterol, diabetes and major cardiovascular diseases in the Asia-Pacific region. Diabetologia 2007; 50:2289–2297.

195. Hitman GA, Colhoun H, Newman C, et al. for the CARDS Investigators. Stroke prediction and stroke prevention with atorvastatin in the Collaborative Atorvastatin Diabetes Study (CARDS). Diabet Med 2007; 24:1313–1321.

196. Sever PS, Poulter NR, Dahlöf B, et al. Reduction in cardiovascular events with atorvastatin in 2,532 patients with type 2 diabetes: Anglo-Scandinavian Cardiac Outcomes Trial–lipid-lowering arm (ASCOT-LLA). Diabetes Care 2005; 28:1151–1157.

197. Keech A, Colquhoun D, Best J, et al. for the LIPID Study Group. Secondary prevention of cardiovascular events with long-term pravastatin in patients with diabetes or impaired fasting glucose: results from the LIPID trial. Diabetes Care 2003; 26:2713–2721.

198. Goldberg RB, Mellies MJ, Sacks FM, et al. for the CARE Investigators. Cardiovascular events and their reduction with pravastatin in diabetic and glucose-intolerant myocardial infarction survivors with average cholesterol levels. Subgroup analyses in the Cholesterol And Recurrent Events (CARE) Trial. Circulation 1998; 98:2513–2519.

199. Pyorala K, Pedersen TR, Kjekshus J, Faergeman O, Olsson AG, Thorgeirsson G. Cholesterol lowering with simvastatin improves prognosis of diabetic patients with coronary heart disease. A subgroup analysis of the Scandinavian Simvastatin Survival Study (4S). Diabetes Care 1997; 20:614–620.

200. Collins R, Armitage J, Parish S, Sleight P, Peto R, and Heart Protection Study Collaborative Group. Effects of cholesterol-lowering with simvastatin on stroke and other major vascular events in 20536 people with cerebrovascular disease or other high-risk conditions. Lancet 2004; 363:757–767.

201. Shepherd J, Barter P, Carmena R, et al. Effect of lowering LDL cholesterol substantially below currently recommended levels in patients with coronary heart disease and diabetes: the Treating to New Targets (TNT) study. Diabetes Care 2006; 29:1220–1226.

202. Cholesterol Treatment Trialists' (CTT) Collaborators, Kearney PM, Blackwell L, Collins R, et al. Efficacy of cholesterol-lowering therapy in 18,686 people with diabetes in 14 randomised trials of statins: a meta-analysis. Lancet 2008; 371:117–125.

203. Keech A, Simes RJ, Barter P, et al. for the FIELD study investigators. Effects of long-term fenofibrate therapy on cardiovascular events in 9795 people with type 2 diabetes mellitus (the FIELD study): randomised controlled trial. Lancet 2005; 366:1849–1861.

204. Allemann S, Diem P, Egger M, Christ ER, Stettler C. Fibrates in the prevention of cardiovascular disease in patients with type 2 diabetes mellitus: meta-analysis of randomised controlled trials. Curr Med Res Opin 2006; 22:617–623.

205. Colwell JA. Aspirin therapy in diabetes (Technical review). Diabetes Care 1997; 20: 1767–1771.

206. He J, Whelton PK, Klag MJ. Aspirin and risk of hemorrhagic stroke: a meta-analysis of randomized controlled trials. JAMA 1998; 280:1930–1935.

207. Sacco RL, Adams R, Albers G, et al. American Heart Association; American Stroke Association Council on Stroke; Council on Cardiovascular Radiology and Intervention; American Academy of Neurology. Guidelines for prevention of stroke in patients with ischemic stroke or transient ischemic attack: a statement for healthcare professionals from the American Heart Association/American Stroke Association Council on Stroke: co-sponsored by the Council on Cardiovascular Radiology and Intervention: the American Academy of Neurology affirms the value of this guideline. Stroke 2006; 37:577–617.

208. Nicolucci A, De Berardis G, Sacco M, Tognoni G. AHA/ADA vs. ESC/EASD recommendations on aspirin as a primary prevention strategy in people with diabetes: how the same data generate divergent conclusions. Eur Heart J 2007; 28:1925–1927.

209. CAPRIE Steering Committee. A randomized, blinded, trial of clopidogrel versus aspirin in patients at risk of ischaemic events (CAPRIE). Lancet 1996; 348:1329–1339.

210. Diener HC, Bogousslavsky J, Brass LM, et al. for the MATCH investigators. Aspirin and clopidogrel compared with clopidogrel alone after recent ischaemic stroke or transient ischaemic attack in high-risk patients (MATCH): randomised, double-blind, placebo-controlled trial. Lancet 2004; 364:331–337.

211. Bhatt DL, Fox KA, Hacke W, et al. for the CHARISMA Investigators. Clopidogrel and aspirin versus aspirin alone for the prevention of atherothrombotic events. N Engl J Med 2006; 354:1706–1717.

212. Pfeffer MA, Jarcho JA. The charisma of subgroups and the subgroups of CHARISMA. N Engl J Med 2006; 354:1744–1746.

213. Sivenius J, Laakso M, Piekkinen Sr, Smets P, Lowenthal A. European stroke prevention study: effectiveness of antiplatelet therapy in diabetic patients in secondary prevention of stroke. Stroke 1992; 23:851–854.

214. ESPRIT Study Group, Halkes PH, van Gijn J, Kappelle LJ, Koudstaal PJ, Algra A. Aspirin plus dipyridamole versus aspirin alone after cerebral ischaemia of arterial origin (ESPRIT): randomised controlled trial. Lancet 2006; 367:1665–1673.

215. Halkes PH, Gray LJ, Bath PM, et al. Dipyridamole plus aspirin versus aspirin alone in secondary prevention after TIA or stroke: a meta-analysis by risk. Neurol Neurosurg Psychiatry 2008; 79:1218–1223.

216. Gaede P, Vedel P, Larsen N, Jensen GVH, Parving HH, Pedersen O. Multifactorial intervention and cardiovascular disease in patients with type 2 diabetes. N Engl J Med 2003; 348:383–393.

217. Gaede P, Lund-Andersen H, Parving HH, Pedersen O. Effect of a multifactorial intervention on mortality in type 2 diabetes. N Engl J Med 2008; 358:580–591.

218. Hu FB, Stampfer MJ, Solomon C, et al. Physical activity and risk for cardiovascular events in diabetic women. Ann Intern Med 2001; 134:96–105.

219. Rautio A, Eliasson M, Stegmayr B. Favorable Trends in the Incidence and Outcome in Stroke in Nondiabetic and Diabetic Subjects: Findings From the Northern Sweden MONICA Stroke Registry in 1985 to 2003. Stroke 2008; 39:3137–3144.

220. Goldstein LB, Adams R, Becker K, et al. Primary prevention of ischemic stroke. A statement for health care professionals from the stroke council of the American Heart Association. Stroke 2001; 32:280–293.

221. Ahari A, Bergqvist D, Troeng T, et al. Diabetes mellitus as a risk factor for early outcome after carotid endarterectomy – a population-based study. Eur J Vasc Endovasc Surg 1999; 18:122–126.

222. Pistolese GR, Appolloni A, Ronchey S, Martelli E. Carotid endarterectomy in diabetic patients. J Vasc Surg 2001; 33:148–154.
223. Cunningham EJ, Bond R, Mehta Z, Mayberg MR, Warlow CP, Rothwell PM. Long-term durability of carotid endarterectomy for symptomatic stenosis and risk factors for late post-operative stroke. Stroke 2002; 33:2658–2663.
224. Ballotta E, Da Giau G, Renon L. Is diabetes a risk factor for carotid endarterectomy? A prospective study. Surgery 2001; 129:146–152.
225. Rothwell PM, Eliasziw M, Gutnikov SA, Warlow CP, Barnett HJM, for the Carotid Endarterectomy Trialists Collaboration. Endarterectomy for symptomatic carotid stenosis in relation to clinical subgroups and timing of surgery. Lancet 2004; 363:915–924.

9   Hyperglycemia in Acute Stroke

Nyika D. Kruyt and Yvo W.B.M. Roos

CONTENTS

ABSTRACT

Hyperglycemia is frequently found (40–60%) after all kinds of stroke and it has been related to increased lesion size and poor clinical outcome. In this chapter, we will primarily focus on ischemic stroke; we will outline the incidence and natural course of post-stroke hyperglycemia and discuss the possible etiologies of post-stroke hyperglycemia. Subsequently, we will present an overview of various mechanisms that could explain how hyperglycemia is detrimental after ischemic stroke. Finally, we will address the question whether in-hospital hyperglycemia should be treated in stroke patients, and if so decided, the glucose levels that should be targeted and the difficulties that arise in achieving this.

From: *Contemporary Diabetes: Diabetes and the Brain*
Edited by: G. J. Biessels, J. A. Luchsinger (eds.), DOI 10.1007/978-1-60327-850-8_9
© Humana Press, a part of Springer Science+Business Media, LLC 2009

Key words: Acute stroke; Ischemic stroke; Hyperglycemia; Stress response; Diabetes mellitus; Insulin resistance; Reperfusion injury; Glycemic control.

BACKGROUND: STROKE

Stroke is a heterogeneous disorder and can be divided into ischemic stroke (80%), primary intracerebral hemorrhagic stroke (15%), and sub-arachnoid hemorrhage (5%).

Ischemic stroke can be further divided based on etiology into cardioem-bolic, artery-to-artery embolism, so-called large vessel, or in situ small-vessel (or lacunar) stroke.

Known major risk factors for ischemic stroke include hypertension, diabetes mellitus (DM), smoking, and atrial fibrillation. The major risk factor for primary intracerebral hemorrhage is hypertension (60–70% of patients). The remaining patients may have intracranial vascular malforma-tions (cavernous angiomas or arteriovenous malformations) or cerebral amy-loid angiopathy as the cause of the bleeding.

In the past 10–15 years, major advances have been made in the acute management of stroke. Most notably, the routine management of patients in stroke care units and specifically the use of thrombolytic therapy with recombinant tissue plasminogen activator (rtPA) within 3 h and the admin-istration of oral aspirin within 48 h of ischemic stroke have contributed to improved outcome. Despite this, stroke remains the second most common cause of death and the major cause of disability worldwide, and it is one of the major contributors to health-care costs in the industrialized countries (1).

Therefore, it remains of major importance to improve the treatment options for patients suffering from a stroke. Modifiable factors, associated with poor outcome after stroke, such as hyperglycemia, have the potential for being new treatment targets.

One of the drawbacks when reviewing the literature on hyperglycemia in acute stroke is that the distinction between stroke subtypes is not always clearly defined. Moreover, the definition of hyperglycemia varies substan-tially from study to study. In this chapter we will mainly focus on hyper-glycemia after ischemic stroke and just briefly discuss about other stroke subtypes. Concerning the definition of hyperglycemia, we adopted the defi-nition used in each separate study.

STROKE AND HYPERGLYCEMIA

Hyperglycemia is a frequent finding in various medical emergencies, and it has clearly been associated with poor outcome. Hyperglycemia is potentially modifiable, and in the past decade a number of trials have been published that investigated the potential beneficial effect of tight glycemic control on outcome in various acute diseases such as myocardial infarction or in patients admitted to an intensive care unit (ICU) *(2, 3)*. As a result, tight glycemic control has now worldwide become standard practice in the ICU. For several other patient groups treatment protocols have been adjusted to a more strict regulation of blood glucose levels.

Also after stroke, hyperglycemia is frequent and is independently associated with poor outcome. Although this is already known for a few decades, the 1994 guidelines for the treatment of ischemic stroke from the American Heart Association (AHA) did not make any recommendation for the treatment of hyperglycemia in these patients. More recent (2007) consensus papers recommended treating glucose levels more strictly, despite the lack of apparent evidence of a clinical benefit *(4–6)*.

In this chapter, focusing on ischemic stroke, we will first outline the incidence and the natural course of post-stroke hyperglycemia, next we will discuss the etiology of post-stroke hyperglycemia and the various mechanisms that could explain how acute hyperglycemia can be detrimental after ischemic stroke. Finally, we will address the question if in-hospital hyperglycemia should be treated, what such treatment should aim for, and the difficulties that arise when treating hyperglycemia in ischemic stroke patients.

HYPERGLYCEMIA AFTER STROKE

Incidence of Admission Hyperglycemia After Acute Stroke

In acute stroke, hyperglycemia on admission has been recognized for a long time, also in patients without pre-existing diabetes mellitus (DM) *(7)*. Despite considerable differences between studies concerning stroke subtypes, cut-off values used to define hyperglycemia (6–10 mmol/L), the condition under which glucose was assessed (random vs. fasting; capillary vs. plasma), and time between the ictus and glucose assessment, the rate of admission hyperglycemia is consistently high. In a systematic review the included studies reported that 8–63% of non-diabetic and 39–89% of diabetic stroke patients had hyperglycemia on admission *(8)*.

Only few studies investigated admission glucose levels in different stroke types. Studies that assessed glucose levels separately for ischemic or hemorrhagic stroke, however, report similar glucose levels, ranging between 7 and 8 mmol/L *(9–14)*. One study that specifically looked at clinical subtypes of ischemic stroke reports that hyperglycemia exists across all ischemic stroke subtypes, but is higher after cortical stroke *(15)*. This observation is supported by post hoc analyses of two large clinical trials including 1,375 patients within 6 h from stroke onset. In this report, glucose levels were also slightly higher in patients with cortical, compared to patients with subcortical infarctions (7.9 vs. 7.6 mmol/L) *(16)*.

Natural Course of Hyperglycemia Post-stroke

Although hyperglycemia on admission has been reported frequently, few studies have described the natural history of glucose levels during the clinical course of stroke. In a large clinical trial investigating the effect of tight glycemic control on outcome, glucose levels in the hyperglycemic control group declined spontaneously within the first 24 h *(17)*, and recently the post hoc analysis of another large clinical trial measuring blood glucose at 6 and 24 h post-ischemic stroke reports the same pattern *(18)*. Unfortunately neither of these trials report blood glucose levels beyond this time frame. In a prospective study that used a continuous glucose monitoring device, patients were monitored for 72 h after admission. It was also shown that both in non-diabetic as well as in diabetic stroke patients' glucose levels initially decrease, but after 24–88 h, glucose levels rose again *(19)*. This late (>24 h) hyperglycemic phase is probably the result of an underlying impairment of glucose metabolism once the patient resumes feeding after an initial fasting period *(20, 21)*.

In conclusion, admission hyperglycemia is a frequent finding after stroke, also in the absence of DM and it occurs irrespective of stroke (sub)type, although glucose levels seem to be somewhat higher in patients with cortical as compared to subcortical infarctions. Glucose levels decrease spontaneously during the first 24 h, but once patients resume feeding, glucose levels surge again, possibly indicating an underlying, previously subclinical, impairment of glucose metabolism.

ETIOLOGY OF HYPERGLYCEMIA IN ACUTE (ISCHEMIC) STROKE

Several mechanisms have been proposed to account for hyperglycemia after stroke. Most likely multiple mechanisms are interacting together at the same time. We will consider the most important mechanisms proposed (Fig. 1A).

Hyperglycemia Due to a Stress Response

Critical illnesses, including stroke, are accompanied by a generalized stress reaction with the activation of the hypothalamo–hypophyseal–adrenal axis (HPA axis). This activation leads to a subsequent increase in glucocorticoids (cortisol), and the activation of the sympathetic division of the autonomic nervous system, resulting in an increase in catecholamines *(22)*. Indeed, in the acute phase till the first week after stroke, increased levels of cortisol and catecholamines have been shown since the 1950s *(23, 24)*. Stress hormones are known to enhance both glycogenolysis and gluconeogenesis

Ischemic stroke

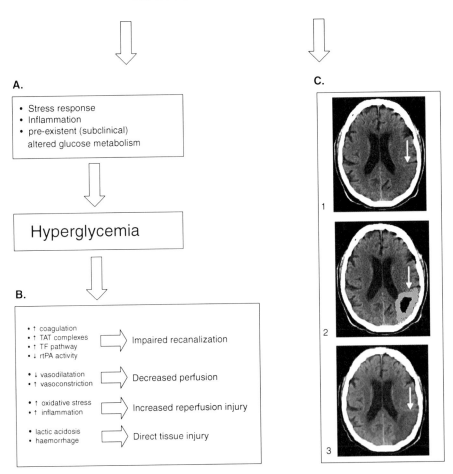

Fig. 1. The putative mechanisms involved in hyperglycemia and reduced penumbral salvage after ischemic stroke. (**A**) Mechanisms causing hyperglycemia after stroke. (**B**) Mechanisms that can explain how hyperglycemia causes the recruitment of penumbral tissue into the infarct. (**C**) Sequential CT scans of the brain in a patient with stroke. (1) Two hours after ischemic stroke: hypointense area in the left parieto-occipital lobe, indicating early edema and reduced perfusion (see *white arrow*). (2) Schematic representation of the ischemic penumbra, a rim of viable tissue (*grey*) at risk of infarction surrounding the infarct core (*black*). (3) Three days after ischemic stroke: attenuation of the hypointense area: penumbral tissue has been converted to infract tissue. : infarct core; – penumbral tissue. TAT: thrombin–antithrombin complexes; TF: tissue factor pathway; rt-PA: recombinant tissue plasminogen activator.

and also inhibit insulin-mediated glycogenesis, resulting in excessive glucose production and insulin resistance with hyperinsulinemia *(25–27)*. In experimental settings, infusion of these hormones in healthy volunteers caused a sustained increase in plasma glucose levels (60–80%) despite compensatory hyperinsulinemia *(28)*.

The hypothesis that stress causes hyperglycemia after stroke is supported by the observation that in many [but not all *(29)*] studies it is shown that a more severe stroke is accompanied by higher levels of stress hormones, with hyperglycemia *(30–33)*.

The exact mechanisms by which the HPA axis and the sympathetic nervous system are activated after stroke remain to be clarified, but probably originate at the supra-pituitary, cortical level. Interestingly, several studies have shown that stroke affecting the insular cortex, a brain area with many autonomic efferent projections, was associated with an increased rate of hyperglycemia *(34)* and an increased production of catecholamines, compared to non-insular stroke *(35)*. Other studies, however, could not confirm an association between insular infarction or insular hypoperfusion and hyperglycemia *(36, 37)*.

Finally, another interesting possibility is that the HPA axis is stimulated by cytokines in response to tissue damage due to stroke.

Hyperglycemia Due to Inflammation

Besides enhancement of the HPA axis, stroke is also accompanied by stimulation of the immune system with a subsequent release of cytokines *(38, 39)*. The immune system in turn has been linked to the activation of the HPA axis *(40)* and as such could facilitate the release of catecholamines with a subsequent rise in glucose levels as discussed in the previous paragraph.

Additionally, cytokines, in particular tumor necrosis factor-alpha (TNFα) which is known to increase after stroke *(38)*, have been linked directly to insulin resistance in both the liver and skeletal muscle, most likely through the modification of signaling properties of insulin receptor substrates *(41–43)*. There is also evidence, however, that an altered glucose metabolism in itself can stimulate the immune system, with the enhancement of cytokine release *(44)*. It remains therefore unclear as what is the cause and what is the effect.

Hyperglycemia as a Measure of Unrecognized Insulin Resistance

Various studies have shown that a substantial proportion of ischemic stroke patients without a previous history of DM appear to have insulin resistance or DM at follow-up. Three months after a stroke, 27–37% of non-diabetic stroke patients with hyperglycemia on admission appear to have an impaired glucose tolerance, and 21–38% of these patients appear to have DM *(45–47)*.

These observations have led to the hypothesis that hyperglycemia after ischemic stroke is in fact the resultant of an abnormal glucose metabolism already present, but not clinically manifest, prior to the stroke occurrence. This observation, however, does not fully explain the high rate of hyperglycemia and is unlikely to explain the high rate of hyperglycemia in patients with hemorrhagic stroke. Whereas, the incidence of ischemic stroke is consistently higher in patients with DM or insulin resistance, the rate of hemorrhagic stroke does not seem to be increased in patients with DM *(48)*. In the Honolulu Heart Study, for example, the incidence of ischemic stroke was more than twofold higher in diabetic patients compared to the general population (44.9 vs. 20.7 per 1,000), while the rate of hemorrhagic stroke was almost the same – 10.1 vs. 9.6 per 1,000 *(49)* (see also *Risk Factors for Stroke in Diabetic Subjects*, Chapter 8).

In conclusion, several mechanisms have been proposed to account for hyperglycemia after stroke. Possible mechanisms include a generalized stress reaction with an increase in catecholamines, the release of cytokines, or underlying subclinical and previously unrecognized DM or insulin resistance. Most probably the altered glucose metabolism and resulting hyperglycemia is multi-causal and differs for different stroke subtypes and from patient to patient.

ADMISSION HYPERGLYCEMIA AND CLINICAL OUTCOME AFTER STROKE

A retrospective study by Melamed *(7, 15)* showed in 1976 that hyperglycemia after stroke is frequent and relates to the severity of the stroke and in-hospital mortality. Since then many studies have reported similar associations and showed that this association is more pronounced if hyperglycemia persists during the first 24 h *(18)* or week *(50, 51)*.

Capes et al. performed a systematic review including a total of 33 studies and demonstrated that after stroke of either subtype (ischemic or hemorrhagic), the unadjusted relative risk of short-term mortality associated with admission glucose levels greater than 6–8 mmol/L was 3.1 [95% confidence interval (95%CI), 2.5–3.8] in non-diabetic patients and 1.3 (95%CI, 0.5–3.4) in diabetic patients *(8)*. For non-diabetic patients, glucose levels greater than 6.1–7.0 mmol/L were associated with a 3.3-fold higher risk of short-term mortality in patients with ischemic stroke – but not in non-diabetic patients with hemorrhagic stroke (2.4; 95%CI, 0.9–8.7) (Fig. 2). Recently, this observation was confirmed in a post hoc analysis of a large clinical stroke trial *(18)*. The review by Capes et al. showed also that after hemorrhagic stroke,

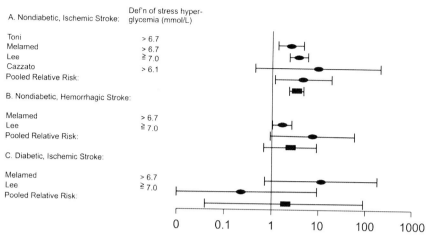

Fig. 2. Unadjusted relative risk (RR) of in-hospital or 30-day mortality after stroke in patients with stress hyperglycemia compared with those without stress hyperglycemia. In patients without known diabetes the pooled relative risk for ischemic stroke is 3.3 (95% confidence intervals (CI): 2.3–4.6) for hemorrhagic stroke: 2.4 (95%CI: 0.7–8.73). (From Capes et al. *(8).* Reprinted with permission from Lippincott Williams & Wilkins.)

admission hyperglycemia was not associated with higher short-term mortality in either diabetic or non-diabetic patients. Some of these data have to be interpreted with caution, however, because insufficient data could account for the lack of a significant correlation in the subgroup analyses. For example, more recent studies have convincingly demonstrated that admission hyperglycemia independently predicts poor outcome, also after hemorrhagic stroke *(10–12).*

The review by Capes et al. did not perform a subgroup analysis for patients with lacunar or non-lacunar stroke. Interestingly, in a small retrospective analysis that we performed *(52)* and in the post hoc analysis of three large clinical trials the association between hyperglycemia and poor outcome was confirmed, but only for patients with cortical stroke. In contrast, for patients with lacunar stroke hyperglycemia appears to be associated with improved, rather than poor outcome *(16, 53).* Many studies that related hyperglycemia to outcome have been performed before thrombolytic therapy with recombinant tissue plasminogen activator (rt-PA) became standard practice. Meanwhile, an increasing number of studies have demonstrated that hyperglycemia on admission also predicts poor outcome in patients treated with rt-PA. This association is even stronger than for non-rt-PA-treated patients *(12–14, 54, 55).* This has led to the suggestion that hyperglycemia may in part counterbalance the beneficial effect of rt-PA treatment *(54).*

In conclusion, admission hyperglycemia after stroke, either ischemic or hemorrhagic, is associated with poor outcome and this association is more pronounced (i) if hyperglycemia persists after the acute phase; (ii) in patients with cortical stroke; (iii) in patients without a history of DM, and (iv) in patients receiving rt-PA treatment. In contrast, after lacunar stroke high levels of blood glucose may predict improved outcome. These observations emphasize that stroke is a heterogeneous disorder and not a single entity and stress the need to study hyperglycemia after stroke for each stroke subtype separately.

GLUCOSE LEVELS AND LESION VOLUME

If hyperglycemia is indeed casually related to poor outcome after stroke, one would expect a relation between higher levels of blood glucose and an increased lesion volume. In hemorrhagic stroke, only little is known about the association between glucose levels and the size of the hemorrhage or its evolution during the clinical course. The evidence is limited to experimental settings where it has been shown that hyperglycemia exacerbates brain edema and peri-hematomal cell death after hemorrhagic stroke (56). In patients with ischemic stroke treated with rt-PA, hyperglycemia has been associated with an increased risk of hemorrhagic complications (57–59). In contrast to hemorrhagic stroke, research concerning hyperglycemia and lesion volume after ischemic stroke is much more extensive. Central in the pathophysiology of ischemic stroke is the concept of the ischemic penumbra (Fig. 1C). The penumbra is a rim of tissue surrounding the infarct core that consists of potentially salvageable hypoperfused tissue that is clinically not functional and at risk of infarction. For survival of the penumbra, restoration of the blood flow due to spontaneous or rt-PA-induced recanalization with adequate reperfusion is of paramount importance. In longitudinal imaging studies it has been shown that without reperfusion, the infarct core increases at the cost of penumbral tissue, a process that seems to be most important in the initial phase of stroke but has been shown to last up till 3–8 days post-ictus (60–62). In this context it is important to realize that it is not clear whether the concept of the penumbra applies to all types of stroke. For example, usually a penumbra does not exist after hemorrhagic stroke (63) and in most patients with subcortical or lacunar infarction there is no penumbra (64). As mentioned earlier, extensive research has been done on the association between hyperglycemia and (expansion of) infarct volume. Although there are inconsistencies (65–67), most studies did indeed report such an association (66, 68–72), and this association is more pronounced with persistent hyperglycemia (50).

In experimental studies an increased infarct volume associated with hyperglycemia is predominantly seen in animal models with medial cerebral artery occlusion, mimicking human cortical infarction. In contrast, in end-artery models, mimicking subcortical infarcts, this is not seen *(66, 67)*. Also, clinical studies that report such an association only included patients with cortical infarcts. These findings are therefore in line with the observation that in contrast to cortical infarction, hyperglycemia is not associated with worse clinical outcome after lacunar infarction. From a pathophysiological point of view, this may be explained by the presence or the absence of a penumbra in patients with cortical or subcortical stroke, respectively. The hypothesis that in cortical stroke hyperglycemia exerts its deleterious effects on the penumbra has been confirmed by a study which demonstrated that high levels of glucose were associated directly with decreased penumbral salvage and poor outcome *(71)* (Fig. 3).

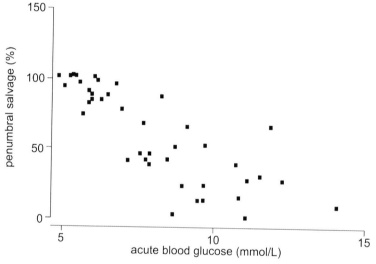

Fig. 3. Penumbral salvage vs. blood glucose. (From Parsons et al. *(71)*. Copyright 2002 American Neurological Association. Reprinted with permission of John Wiley & Sons, Inc.)

HOW DOES HYPERGLYCEMIA AFFECT THE ISCHEMIC BRAIN?

Although an accumulating number of studies have convincingly demonstrated an association between hyperglycemia and poor outcome after stroke, it remains controversial whether this association is causal, i.e., hyperglycemia is actually causing poor outcome.

Hyperglycemia could also be epiphenomenal to a more pronounced stress reaction with higher levels of blood glucose in more severe stroke. Indeed, higher levels of glucose have been associated with more severe stroke *(7, 73–75)*. On the other hand, most [but not all *(30, 76, 77)*] studies showed that the deleterious effect of hyperglycemia is independent of clinical severity *(7, 13, 53, 75, 76)*.

Several (mainly experimental) studies and observations from imaging studies have provided clues as to how impaired glucose metabolism resulting in hyperglycemia and insulin resistance could be detrimental to the ischemic brain. In this context, it is important to realize that the sequence of reactions that occur after arterial occlusion, leading to ischemia and ultimately to infarction, is complex and dynamic and will likely differ from patient to patient, depending among other factors on age, gender, and cardiovascular history. A dynamic interplay of multiple reactions will occur concomitantly over time and it is unlikely that any of these processes can be seen as the sole or dominant cause leading to infarction.

In the brain, glucose is transported via the glucose transporters (GLUT-1–3). These insulin independent transporters continuously transport glucose, leading to intracellular glucose accumulation when plasma glucose levels are high *(78)*. Hyperglycemia, both acute and chronic, can in turn induce a variety of biochemical changes and is believed to form the basis for many biochemical alterations involved in diabetic complications *(79)*.

In the following paragraphs we will outline the mechanisms thought to be responsible for acute hyperglycemia to be detrimental for the ischemic brain. These mechanisms involve impaired recanalization, impaired (re)perfusion, reperfusion injury, and direct detrimental effects of glucose (see also Fig. 1B).

Impaired Recanalization

As mentioned earlier, it was observed from clinical studies that hyperglycemia is capable of counterbalancing the beneficial effect of rt-PA treatment *(14, 54)*. This observation is supported by the results of a study that used Transcranial Doppler (TCD) imaging to assess rt-PA-induced recanalization in patients with middle cerebral artery occlusion. It was demonstrated that glucose levels exceeding 8.8 mmol/L were associated with a persistent occlusion [OR: 7.3 (95%CI) 1.3–42.3], suggesting that hyperglycemia hampers recanalization *(80)*. An explanation for this can be found in experimental studies that report a relation between an abnormal glucose metabolism and abnormal hemostasis. In these studies, hyperglycemia was shown to stimulate coagulation by increasing thrombin–antithrombin complexes and the tissue factor pathway *(81–84)*, and hyperinsulinemia was shown to decrease fibrinolytic activity by increasing plasminogen activator inhibitor (PAI) *(81, 85–87)*. Furthermore, both hyperglycemia and hyperinsulinemia have been shown to decrease the activity of rt-PA itself *(85)*. These observations support the hypothesis that an altered glucose metabolism impairs recanalization, probably due to increased coagulation and decreased fibrinolytic activity.

Interestingly, the detrimental effects of hyperglycemia were shown to be more pronounced in patients with early recanalization than in patients with delayed or no recanalization *(55)*. This suggests that hyperglycemia is also harmful more downstream of the occlusion and prevents the reperfusion of the penumbra.

Decreased Perfusion

Reperfusion of ischemic tissue is critical for penumbral salvage. In experimental stroke, hyperglycemia is associated with decreased reperfusion resulting in increased infarct volumes when compared to normoglycemic controls *(88–91)*. Cerebral blood flow (CBF) was reduced by 37% in hyperglycemic compared to normoglycemic rats *(89)*. After recanalization, penumbral blood flow was 60% of pre-ischemic values in hyperglycemic, vs. 89% in normoglycemic conditions *(92)*.

An important mechanism by which hyperglycemia appears to reduce CBF is by decreasing vasodilatation, which is necessary for optimal reperfusion. For example, glucose infusion for 6 h was shown to reduce endothelium-dependent vasodilatation in healthy humans *(93, 94)*.

Vasodilatation is predominantly mediated by endothelium-derived nitric oxide (NO) which is synthesized by endothelial NO synthetase (eNOS) *(95, 96)*. Reduction of eNOS gene expression has been reported in endothelial cells in a hyperglycemic environment *(97, 98)*, probably by reducing protein kinase C (PKC) *(99)*. Moreover, hyperglycemia can reduce the production of NO by increasing the activity of nicotinamide adenine dinucleotide phosphate (NADPH)-oxidase, also through the activation of PKC *(100)*. NADPH-oxidase in turn can reduce eNOS activity and, additionally, increases superoxide that neutralizes NO with the formation of peroxynitrite *(101, 102)*.

Besides reduced vasodilatation via the reduction of NO, hyperglycemia is also implicated in several signaling pathways involved in vascular function. Hyperglycemia stimulates the lipo-oxygenase and cyclo-oxygenase pathways, leading to enhanced formation of vasoconstrictive prostaglandins such as thromboxane A2 *(103, 104)*. Additionally, hyperglycemia can also alter the eicosanoid production affecting vascular tone resulting in vasoconstriction *(105)*.

Exacerbation of Reperfusion Injury

Although restoration of the blood flow to the ischemic tissue is essential for penumbral salvage, reperfusion itself can also induce injury. Hyperglycemia is associated with an exacerbation of this so-called reperfusion injury. The mechanisms by which reperfusion causes injury to the ischemic brain are complex and fall beyond the scope of this chapter. Here, we will only (briefly) consider the most important mechanisms where acute hyperglycemia appears to be involved. The more interested reader is referred to more specialized reviews on this topic *(79, 106, 107)*.

The hallmarks of reperfusion injury are oxidative stress and inflammation, and both these processes appear to be influenced by hyperglycemia. Oxidative stress is mainly caused by an imbalance between the production and neutralization of reactive oxygen species (ROS), such as superoxide and peroxides. These ROS have been shown to damage various components of the cell, including proteins, lipids, mitochondrial function, and DNA, which leads to an impaired blood–brain barrier (BBB) function, edema formation, and increased infarct volume *(106, 108–110)*.

Hyperglycemia increases the production of ROS through the activation of PKC, and through increased NADH production, and is as such associated with increased oxidative stress. In fact, increased oxidative stress by the formation of superoxide is considered one of the major pathways leading to hyperglycemic complications *(79)*.

Closely (inter)related to oxidative stress in the context of reperfusion injury is the inflammatory response *(106, 111)*. During ischemia the inflammatory response develops through the activation of pro-inflammatory cytokines (e.g., TNFα, interleukins, and cell adhesion molecules) and by the infiltration of inflammatory cells (e.g., leukocytes and macrophages). Inflammation can cause molecular and biochemical modifications resulting in tissue injury and increased infarction. Additionally, inflammation is a significant source of oxidative stress *(106, 107)*.

Hyperglycemia is shown to increase several pro-inflammatory transcription factors involved in inflammation, prominently nuclear factor κB(kappa beta), which plays a key role in the regulation of the inflammatory responses by enhancing pro-inflammatory cytokines and by promoting the adhesion of inflammatory cells *(106, 107, 111)*.

Other Mechanisms

Hyperglycemia has also been associated with several other mechanisms of tissue injury after infarction. Although controversial *(112)*, one of the most propagated ideas is that anaerobic glycolysis under hyperglycemic conditions is associated with the accumulation of lactic acid and a derangement in pH homeostasis which can in turn contribute to increased brain injury *(113–115)*. In humans, this hypothesis was supported by the previously mentioned observation that hyperglycemia correlates with greater lactate production and reduced penumbral salvage after infarction *(71)* (Fig. 3). Additionally, hyperglycemia may also directly affect mitochondrial function in the ischemic penumbra and cause significant intracellular acidosis *(115)*.

More recently, hyperglycemia has been associated with an increased rate of hemorrhagic complications after rt-PA treatment. In the National Institutes of Neurological Disorders and Stroke (NINDS) trial that investigated the effect of rt-PA treatment, a statistical trend was seen for severe hyperglycemia (>16.7 mmol/L) as a predictor of symptomatic hemorrhage *(116)*. In another study, hyperglycemia (>11.1 mmol/L) was associated with a 25% symptomatic hemorrhage rate and the odds ratio (OR) on symptomatic hemorrhage associated with each 5.5 mmol/L increment of admission glucose was 2.3 (95%CI: 1.1–4.8) *(57)*. These observations were later confirmed by two other studies *(57, 59)*. In all of these studies, however, DM was also associated with an increased rate of hemorrhage and hyperglycemia may therefore only be a marker of DM, which in turn has been associated with impairments of the blood–brain barrier and microvasculature that may result in an increased bleeding risk *(57, 117)*.

Taken together, hyperglycemia appears to be implicated on various levels in the dynamic reactions involved in cerebral infarction, ultimately leading to impaired penumbral salvage and increased infarct size. It is important, however, to realize that part of the evidence comes from experimental in vitro or animal studies which are an imperfect representation of human stroke. While stroke in humans is a very heterogeneous disease, with great variability in etiology, location, and severity, experimental models are usually performed in healthy young animals, comparable of equal age and gender and under standardized circumstances. Extrapolation to the situation in humans must therefore be done with great caution.

TREATMENT OF HYPERGLYCEMIA

Although the association between hyperglycemia and poor outcome is well established in stroke patients, it remains unclear if patients benefit from tight glycemic control. In experimental stroke reduction in blood, glucose with insulin to the lower physiological range (3–4 mmol/L) reduced infarction size *(118, 119)*. In human studies, treatment of hyperglycemia in patients with stroke remains the subject of debate.

Current guidelines from the American Heart Association (AHA) for the treatment of both ischemic *(6)* and hemorrhagic *(5)* stroke are cautious due to lack of evidence. Both guidelines state that "glucose concentrations (possibly >7.8–10.3 mmol/L) should probably trigger the administration of insulin." This recommendation is based on two observations: first, the increased risk of poor outcome associated with hyperglycemia; second, the accumulating evidence from trials in other medical emergencies than stroke which demonstrates that tight glycemic control improves outcome such as in patients admitted to the ICU (3, 120), patients with myocardial infarction (2, 121), or patients undergoing coronary artery bypass grafting (CABG) (122, 123). These results, however, cannot directly be extrapolated to patients with stroke and only a randomized clinical trial (RCT) can resolve this matter. Currently one RCT, the GIST-UK trial, has been published (17). The results of this very pragmatic trial did not favor tight glycemic control (OR for 90-day mortality: 1.1; 95%CI: 0.9–1.5). This trial, however, was affected by a premature discontinuation of patient recruitment (933 patients instead of the proposed sample size of 2,355 patients) and some other issues that will be outlined in the following paragraphs. In a retrospective study including 295 stroke patients, glycemic control was associated with a greater proportion of patients discharged home and a trend toward fewer in-hospital deaths (124).

The results of further trials that are currently still including patients or have recently been completed are eagerly awaited (125, 126). Although in these trials, clinical outcome is only a secondary outcome measure, the results can provide some indication of the effect of tight glycemic control on clinical outcome.

If one decides to treat hyperglycemia in patients with stroke, this poses several questions. It is not clear whether all type of stroke patients will benefit from glycemic control, which glucose levels should be targeted, and for how long this has to be maintained. Finally, although standard practice on the ICU, it is not clear how tight glycemic control can be practically implemented in stroke patients on a stroke care unit or regular ward.

We will address these questions in the following paragraphs, and we will attempt to give some directions for further research.

Who will Benefit from Glycemic Control?

The association between hyperglycemia and poor outcome varies for different stroke subtypes and is less clear in stroke patients with a history of DM compared to non-diabetic stroke patients (8, 16). These observations should warrant caution in selecting patients for treatment. In fact, the observation that hyperglycemia might even be beneficial in a subgroup of patients with lacunar infarction suggests that these patients should be abstained from intensive glycemic control maintaining glucose values in the lower physiological range. The GIST-UK trial included different types of stroke patients (including 21% lacunar infarction and 12% primary hemorrhagic stroke) irrespective of a previous history of DM (17% of included patients) *(17)*. This could have contributed to the lack of efficacy of glycemic control on clinical outcome. A more directed approach, by selecting patients with cortical ischemic stroke, such as is currently performed in the GRASP trial *(126)*, probably maximizes the probability to find a treatment effect associated with glycemic control. Such an approach does not suffer from a reduction in treatment effect due to the inclusion of patients where a minimal effect is anticipated and would therefore require fewer patients *(127)*.

What Glucose Levels should be Targeted?

Some lessons can be learned from trials in other patient populations regarding the target to aim for (Table 1). The DIGAMI I study *(2)*, a trial that investigated the clinical efficacy of glycemic control in patients with myocardial infarction, showed a significant 1-year mortality reduction of 29%. In a subsequent study, the DIGAMI II, these findings could not be reproduced *(128)*. The lack of efficacy in the DIGAMI II is probably explained by the observation that during the decade that separated these trials the routine treatment of hyperglycemia in patients admitted for myocardial infarction had been intensified. Due to this, in DIGAMI II the control patients had relatively low mean glucose levels (10.0 mmol/L) that are in fact comparable to the glucose levels of the treatment group in DIGAMI I (9.6 mmol/L). Tight glycemic control in DIGAMI II did not establish a contrast in the mean glucose levels between the treatment and control group which could explain the lack of treatment effect on clinical outcome.

Results from the GIST-UK trial in stroke patients (mean contrast in plasma glucose between the groups 0.57 mmol/L [*17*]) as well as the results from trials in other medical emergencies *(121, 129, 130)* also demonstrate that without a significant effect of tight glycemic control on the mean glucose level no benefit on clinical outcome was found. In contrast, most, but not all *(131, 132)*, trials that targeted glucose values in a lower physiological range (4.4–6.1. mmol/L), with intensive glucose control and/or that accomplished a contrast in the mean glucose levels between the treatment and control group, demonstrate a beneficial effect on clinical outcome when patients are treated for more than 2 days *(3, 120, 122, 123)*. We therefore suggest that for future clinical trials in stroke patients to be effective on clinical outcome, adequate glycemic control and targeting glucose levels in the lower physiological range are of paramount importance. Caution, however, is warranted as maintaining glucose values in the lower physiological range can result in an increase in (severe) hypoglycemic episodes with potential harmful effects *(132)*.

Table 1
Overview of glucose lowering trials

Author/Study name	Publication, Year	Target population (N)	Intervention (duration) and target glucose levels in treatment group (mmol/L)	Endpoint	Difference in mean glucose between treatment and controls	Treatment effect on clinical outcome
Malmberg/ DIGAMI 1 (2)	1995 and 1999	AMI (620)	IV insulin/24 h, followed by SC insulin ≥ 3 months Target: 7–11	Mortality at • 3 months • 1 year • 3.4 years	Yes	• 3 months: yes • 1 year: yes • 3.4 years: yes
Diaz/ ECLA study (121)	1998	AMI (407)	IV GIK/24 h Target: n.r.	Mortality • In-hospital	No	No
Ceremuzýnski (129)	1999	AMI (954)	IV GIK/24 h Target: n.r.	Mortality • In-hospital	No	No
vd Berghe (3) Ingels (134)	2001 and 2006	Surgical ICU (1,558)	IV insulin until discharge Target: 4.4–6.1	Mortality at • 1 year • 4 years	Yes	• 1 year: yes • 4 years. : yes
Furny (122)	2003	CABG (= 3,554)	IV insulin vs. SC insulin: peri- CABG until 3 days post CABG	Mortality • In-hospital	Yes	Yes

(continued)

Table 1
(continued)

Author/Study name	Publication, Year	Target population (N)	Intervention (duration) and target glucose levels in treatment group (mmol/L)	Endpoint	Difference in mean glucose between treatment and controls	Treatment effect on clinical outcome
			Target IV insulin: variable, starting at < 11.1, later < 9.7 Target SC insulin: target: <11.1			
Lazar (123)	2004	CABG (141)	IV GIK vs. SC insulin: peri-CABG till 12 h thereafter Target IV GIK: 7–11.1 Target SC insulin: <13.9	• Peri-CABG outcome • 2-year mortality	Yes	• Peri-CABG outcome: yes • 2-year mortality: yes
Malmberg/ DIGAMI II (128)	2005	AMI (1,253)	• IV insulin 24 h than SC insulin • IV insulin 24 h than standard control • Standard Target all three groups: 5–7	Mortality at • 2.1 years.	No	No

(continued)

Table 1
(continued)

Author/Study name	Publication, Year	Target population (N)	Intervention (duration) and target glucose levels in treatment group (mmol/L)	Endpoint	Difference in mean glucose between treatment and controls	Treatment effect on clinical outcome
Mehta/ CREATE-ECLA (130)	2005	AMI; (20,201)	IV GIK/24 h Target: n.r	Mortality • 1 month	No	No
Vd Berghe (120)	2006	Medical ICU (1,200)	IV insulin till discharge Target: 4.4–6.1	Mortality • in-hospital	Yes	All patients: no patients treated ≥ 3 days: yes
Gray GIST UK (17)	2007	Stroke (933)	IV GIK/24 h Target: 4–7	Mortality • 3 months	No	No
Gandhi (131)	2007	Cardiac surgery (371)	IV insulin intra-operative Target: 4.4–5.6	Composite endpoint • 30 days post surgery	Yes	No
Brunkhorst (132)	2008	Severe sepsis (537)	IV insulin Target: 4.4–6.1	Mortality • 28 days	Yes	No

AMI: acute myocardial infarction; ICU: intensive care unit; CABG: coronary artery bypass graft; IV: intravenous; SC: subcutaneous; GIK: glucose insulin potassium infusion; n.r.: not reported.

How long should treatment continue?

The same observations as for the target levels can be made concerning the duration glucose lowering treatment. Although from a pathophysiological point of view one could argue that glycemic control is not effective after disappearance of the penumbra (usually within 24 h), results from the ICU studies indicate that treatment should be continued after the acute phase as the beneficial effect on clinical outcome was much more pronounced in patients treated for more than 2 days (3, 120). Furthermore, trials with a shorter duration of glycemic control, for example, the (CREATE-) ECLA (24 h) and the GIST-UK trials (24 h), did not show a beneficial effect of glycemic control on outcome (17, 121, 130).

How can tight Glycemic Control be accomplished?

Finally, the question of *how* to accomplish and maintain glucose levels in the lower physiological range, also beyond the acute phase, appears to be difficult to answer in stroke patients. In contrast to an ICU, a stroke unit partially lacks the intensive treatment facilities available on the ICU. Patients will not generally have a direct venous or arterial access for frequent blood glucose monitoring and fewer personnel per patient will be available to execute the often laborious treatment algorithms.

Other factors may also hamper tight glycemic control in stroke patients. As outlined previously, in many stroke patients, glucose levels will be raised not only due to the ictus, but probably also as a result of previously unrecognized DM or insulin resistance. Moreover, the stress response that is associated with stroke can induce insulin resistance. This pre-existent or stroke-related insulin resistance may complicate glucose control. Furthermore, stroke patients generally resume feeding within 24 h from stroke. We (133) and others (20) have shown that especially post-prandial glucose surges appear to be a substantial contributor to recurrent hyperglycemia in stroke patients if the treatment paradigm consisted of a basal intravenous insulin scheme or predominantly meal-related subcutaneous insulin administration (Fig. 4). In order to avoid these post-prandial glucose surges, in a subsequent study we attempted to tackle this problem with continuous enteral feeding in addition to tight glycemic control with intravenous insulin. Although compared to hyperglycemic controls, the mean glucose values in the treatment group were low (5.8 vs. 8.0 mmol/L) and we managed to maintain glucose levels for a high percentage of time within a low physiological range during 5 consecutive days (55 vs. 14%); target: 4.4–6.1 mmol/L. The results were offset by a high incidence of hypoglycemic episodes (20% of patients were hypoglycemic, i.e., glucose <3.0 mmol/L), though glucose levels never fall below 2.4 mmol/L. Recently a pilot trial, including 46 diabetic

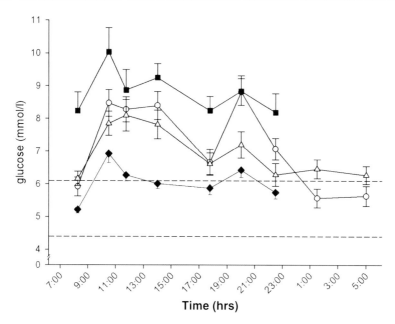

Fig. 4. Post-prandial hyperglycemia in a pilot study *(133)* investigating different algorithms to control post-stroke hyperglycemia. *Closed squares*: hyperglycemic controls (*N* = 10); *open triangles*: hyperglycemic patients treated with predominantly meal-related insulin (*N* = 10); *open circles*: hyperglycemic patients treated with predominantly basal insulin (*N* = 13); *closed diamonds*: normoglycemic controls (*N* = 16).

hyperglycemic ischemic stroke patients admitted to an ICU or an intermediate care unit, has showed promising results. Although the mean glucose levels remained relatively high, patients treated with intensive insulin for 3 consecutive days had lower mean glucose values than their controls (7.4 vs. 10.5 mmol/L) with 35% of patients suffering from a hypoglycemic episode (i.e., glucose <3.3 mmol/L) *(21)*.

In summary, we have to wait for the result of further randomized controlled trials (RCTs) in stroke patients that investigate the effect of tight glycemic control on clinical outcome. Results from experimental studies and clinical trials in other medical emergencies, however, seem promising. Hyperglycemic patients without a history of DM, with ischemic rather than hemorrhagic, and with cortical rather than lacunar stroke are expected to benefit most from tight glycemic control.

For tight glycemic control to improve clinical outcome, it seems to be important that such treatment maintains glucose levels within the lower physiological range, also after the acute phase of stroke. To accomplish this on a stroke unit, however, is difficult. Especially when patients resume feeding, post-prandial glucose surges contribute to recurrent hyperglycemia.

Moreover, tight glycemic control carries a substantial risk of hypoglycemic episodes that can potentially harm the patient.

CONCLUSIONS

- Admission hyperglycemia after stroke is a frequent finding (20–60%) in all types of stroke, irrespective of a previous history of DM.
- After an initial and spontaneous decline during the first 24 h, glucose levels rise again, probably as a result of post-prandial glucose surges when patients resume feeding.
- Hyperglycemia on admission and especially if persistent throughout the clinical course is an independent predictor of infarct volume and poor outcome. This association, however, is not as clear for patients with DM or for patients with lacunar-, rather than cortical infarction.
- Hyperglycemia after stroke could be the result of several mechanisms. Most important seem to be the increased stress and inflammatory response due to the stroke and the uncovering of previously unrecognized insulin resistance.
- Several, interrelated mechanisms could account for hyperglycemia to be detrimental after stroke. Most important seem to be an impaired recanalization, decreased perfusion, and an exacerbation of reperfusion injury.
- Currently, there is no sufficient evidence to support the implementation of tight glycemic control in stroke patients. This has to be investigated with an RCT.
- Before the initiation of an RCT, paradigms to obtain tight glycemic control should be optimized, aiming to maintain glucose values in the lower physiological range (probably 4.4–6.1 mmol/L), also after the acute phase (>2 days).
- To accomplish and maintain tight glycemic control in stroke patients is difficult and laborious, especially due to recurrent hyperglycemia, when patients resume feeding.
- Hyperglycemic patients with cortical ischemic stroke, and without DM, are likely to benefit most from tight glycemic control. Selecting these patients for an RCT will probably maximize the change to find a treatment effect on clinical outcome due to tight glycemic control.

RECOMMENDATIONS

- Blood glucose levels in stroke patients tend to rise after an initial decrease (24 h). We therefore recommend monitoring blood glucose levels also beyond the acute phase (i.e., >2 days).
- In the absence of evidence supporting tight glycemic control in stroke patients and because of the increased risk of hypoglycemia, we do not recommend the routine use of insulin infusion regimes in patients with moderate hyperglycemia (<10.0 mmol/L). We advise to follow the recommendations as published by the American Heart Association (AHA) (5,6) or the European Stroke Organization (ESO) (4), both stating that glucose concentrations exceeding 10.0 mmol/L should trigger insulin administration.

- Admission hyperglycemia after ischemic stroke could indicate underlying, previously unrecognized DM. We therefore recommend screening of ischemic stroke patients with admission hyperglycemia (glucose >7–8 mmol/L) for DM after the acute phase of the stroke.

REFERENCES

1. Donnan GA, Fisher M, Macleod M, Davis SM. Stroke. Lancet 2008; 371:1612–1623.
2. Malmberg K, Ryden L, Efendic S, et al. Randomized trial of insulin-glucose infusion followed by subcutaneous insulin treatment in diabetic patients with acute myocardial infarction (DIGAMI study): effects on mortality at 1 year. J Am Coll Cardiol 1995; 26: 57–65.
3. van den BergheG, Wouters P, Weekers F, et al. Intensive insulin therapy in the critically ill patients. N Engl J Med 2001; 345:1359–1367.
4. Guidelines for management of ischaemic stroke and transient ischaemic attack 2008. Cerebrovasc Dis 2008; 25:457–507.
5. Broderick J, Connolly S, Feldmann E, et al. Guidelines for the management of spontaneous intracerebral hemorrhage in adults: 2007 update: a guideline from the American Heart Association/American Stroke Association Stroke Council, High Blood Pressure Research Council, and the Quality of Care and Outcomes in Research Interdisciplinary Working Group. Circulation 2007; 116:e391–e413.
6. Adams HP Jr., del ZG, Alberts MJ, et al. Guidelines for the early management of adults with ischemic stroke: a guideline from the American Heart Association/American Stroke Association Stroke Council, Clinical Cardiology Council, Cardiovascular Radiology and Intervention Council, and the Atherosclerotic Peripheral Vascular Disease and Quality of Care Outcomes in Research Interdisciplinary Working Groups: The American Academy of Neurology affirms the value of this guideline as an educational tool for neurologists. Circulation 2007; 115:e478–e534.
7. Melamed E. Reactive hyperglycaemia in patients with acute stroke. J Neurol Sci 1976; 29:267–275.
8. Capes SE, Hunt D, Malmberg K, Pathak P, Gerstein HC. Stress hyperglycemia and prognosis of stroke in nondiabetic and diabetic patients: a systematic overview. Stroke 2001; 32: 2426–2432.
9. Passero S, Ciacci G, Ulivelli M. The influence of diabetes and hyperglycemia on clinical course after intracerebral hemorrhage. Neurology 2003; 61:1351–1356.
10. Fogelholm R, Murros K, Rissanen A, Avikainen S. Admission blood glucose and short term survival in primary intracerebral haemorrhage: a population based study. J Neurol Neurosurg Psychiatry 2005; 76:349–353.
11. Kimura K, Iguchi Y, Inoue T, et al. Hyperglycemia independently increases the risk of early death in acute spontaneous intracerebral hemorrhage. J Neurol Sci 2007; 255:90–94.
12. Saposnik G, Young B, Silver B, et al. Lack of improvement in patients with acute stroke after treatment with thrombolytic therapy: predictors and association with outcome. JAMA 2004; 292:1839–1844.
13. Bruno A, Levine SR, Frankel MR, et al. Admission glucose level and clinical outcomes in the NINDS rt-PA Stroke Trial. Neurology 2002; 59:669–674.
14. Leigh R, Zaidat OO, Suri MF, et al. Predictors of hyperacute clinical worsening in ischemic stroke patients receiving thrombolytic therapy. Stroke 2004; 35:1903–1907.
15. Scott JF, Robinson GM, French JM, O'Connell JE, Alberti KG, Gray CS. Prevalence of admission hyperglycaemia across clinical subtypes of acute stroke. Lancet 1999; 353: 376–377.
16. Uyttenboogaart M, Koch MW, Stewart RE, Vroomen PC, Luijckx GJ, De KJ. Moderate hyperglycaemia is associated with favourable outcome in acute lacunar stroke. Brain 2007; 130:1626–1630.

17. Gray CS, Hildreth AJ, Sandercock PA, et al. Glucose-potassium-insulin infusions in the management of post-stroke hyperglycaemia: the UK Glucose Insulin in Stroke Trial (GIST-UK). Lancet Neurol 2007; 6:397–406.

18. Yong M, Kaste M. Dynamic of Hyperglycemia as a Predictor of Stroke Outcome in the ECASS-II Trial. Stroke-Dallas 2008; 39:2749–2755.

19. Allport L, Baird T, Butcher K, et al. Frequency and temporal profile of poststroke hyperglycemia using continuous glucose monitoring. Diabetes Care 2006; 29:1839–1844.

20. Bruno A, Saha C, Williams LS, Shankar R. IV insulin during acute cerebral infarction in diabetic patients. Neurology 2004; 62:1441–1442.

21. Bruno A, Kent TA, Coull BM, et al. (2007) Treatment of Hyperglycemia In Ischemic Stroke (THIS). A Randomized Pilot Trial. Stroke-Dallas 2008; 39(2):384–389.

22. van den Berghe G. (2000) Novel insights into the neuroendocrinology of critical illness. Eur J Endocrinol 2000; 143:1–13.

23. Feibel JH, Hardy PM, Campbell RG, Goldstein MN, Joynt RJ. Prognostic value of the stress response following stroke. JAMA 1977; 238:1374–1376.

24. Oka M. Effect of cerebral vascular accident on the level of 17-hydroxycorticosteroids in plasma. Acta Med Scand 1956; 156:221–226.

25. Barth E, Albuszies G, Baumgart K, et al. Glucose metabolism and catecholamines. Crit Care Med 2007; 35:S508–S518.

26. Seematter G, Binnert C, Martin JL, Tappy L. Relationship between stress, inflammation and metabolism. Curr Opin Clin Nutr Metab Care 2004; 7:169–173.

27. Grimble RF. Inflammatory status and insulin resistance. Curr Opin Clin Nutr Metab Care 2002; 5:551–559.

28. Gelfand RA, Matthews DE, Bier DM, Sherwin RS. Role of counterregulatory hormones in the catabolic response to stress. J Clin Invest 1984; 74:2238–2248.

29. van Kooten F, Hoogerbrugge N, Naarding P, Koudstaal PJ. Hyperglycemia in the acute phase of stroke is not caused by stress. Stroke 1993; 24:1129–1132.

30. Tracey F, Crawford VL, Lawson JT, Buchanan KD, Stout RW. Hyperglycaemia and mortality from acute stroke. Q J Med 1993; 86:439–446.

31. Feibel JH, Hardy PM, Campbell RG, Goldstein MN, Joynt RJ. Prognostic value of the stress response following stroke. JAMA 1977; 238:1374–1376.

32. O'Neill PA, Davies I, Fullerton KJ, Bennett D. Stress hormone and blood glucose response following acute stroke in the elderly. Stroke 1991; 22:842–847.

33. Christensen H, Boysen G, Johannesen HH. Serum-cortisol reflects severity and mortality in acute stroke. J Neurol Sci 2004; 217:175–180.

34. Allport LE, Butcher KS, Baird TA, et al. Insular cortical ischemia is independently associated with acute stress hyperglycemia. Stroke 2004; 35:1886–1891.

35. Meyer S, Strittmatter M, Fischer C, Georg T, Schmitz B. Lateralization in autonomic dysfunction in ischemic stroke involving the insular cortex. Neuroreport 2004; 15:357–361.

36. Pettersen JA, Pexman JH, Barber PA, Demchuk AM, Buchan AM, Hill MD. Insular cortical ischaemia does not independently predict acute hypertension or hyperglycaemia within 3 h of onset. J Neurol Neurosurg Psychiatry 2006; 77:885–887.

37. Moreton FC, McCormick M, Muir KW. Insular cortex hypoperfusion and acute phase blood glucose after stroke: a CT perfusion study. Stroke 2007; 38:407–410.

38. Vila N, Castillo J, Davalos A, Chamorro A. Proinflammatory cytokines and early neurological worsening in ischemic stroke. Stroke 2000; 31:2325–2329.

39. Tarkowski E, Rosengren L, Blomstrand C, et al. Early intrathecal production of interleukin-6 predicts the size of brain lesion in stroke. Stroke 1995; 26:1393–1398.

40. Dunn AJ. Effects of cytokines and infections on brain neurochemistry. Clin Neurosci Res 2006; 6:52–68.

41. Plomgaard P, Bouzakri K, Krogh-Madsen R, Mittendorfer B, Zierath JR, Pedersen BK. Tumor necrosis factor-alpha induces skeletal muscle insulin resistance in healthy human subjects via inhibition of Akt substrate 160 phosphorylation. Diabetes 2005; 54: 2939–2945.

42. Rask-Madsen C, Dominguez H, Ihlemann N, Hermann T, Kober L, Torp-Pedersen C. Tumor necrosis factor-alpha inhibits insulin's stimulating effect on glucose uptake and endothelium-dependent vasodilation in humans. Circulation 2003; 108:1815–1821.

43. Hotamisligil GS, Spiegelman BM. Tumor necrosis factor alpha: a key component of the obesity-diabetes link. Diabetes 1994; 43:1271–1278.

44. Esposito K, Nappo F, Marfella R, et al. Inflammatory cytokine concentrations are acutely increased by hyperglycemia in humans: role of oxidative stress. Circulation 2002; 106: 2067–2072.

45. Gray CS, Scott JF, French JM, Alberti KG, O'Connell JE. Prevalence and prediction of unrecognised diabetes mellitus and impaired glucose tolerance following acute stroke. Age Ageing 2004; 33:71–77.

46. Kernan WN, Viscoli CM, Inzucchi SE, et al. Prevalence of abnormal glucose tolerance following a transient ischemic attack or ischemic stroke. Arch Intern Med 2005; 165:227–233.

47. Vancheri F, Curcio M, Burgio A, et al. Impaired glucose metabolism in patients with acute stroke and no previous diagnosis of diabetes mellitus. QJM 2005; 98:871–878.

48. Mankovsky BN, Ziegler D. Stroke in patients with diabetes mellitus. Diabetes Metab Res Rev 2004; 20:268–287.

49. Abbott RD, Donahue RP, MacMahon SW, Reed DM, Yano K. Diabetes and the risk of stroke. The Honolulu Heart Program. JAMA 1987; 257:949–952.

50. Baird TA, Parsons MW, Phanh T, et al. Persistent post-stroke hyperglycemia is independently associated with infarct expansion and worse clinical outcome. Stroke 2003; 34: 2208–2214.

51. Dora B, Mihci E, Eser A, et al. Prolonged hyperglycemia in the early subacute period after cerebral infarction: effects on short term prognosis. Acta Neurol Belg 2004; 104:64–67.

52. Kruyt ND, Nys GM, van der Worp HB, van Zandvoort MJ, Kappelle LJ, Biessels GJ. (2008) Hyperglycemia and cognitive outcome after ischemic stroke. J Neurol Sci 2008; 270: 141–147.

53. Bruno A, Biller J, Adams HP Jr., et al. Acute blood glucose level and outcome from ischemic stroke. Trial of ORG 10172 in Acute Stroke Treatment (TOAST) Investigators. Neurology 1999; 52:280–284.

54. Alvarez-Sabin J, Molina CA, Montaner J, et al. Effects of admission hyperglycemia on stroke outcome in reperfused tissue plasminogen activator–treated patients. Stroke 2003; 34:1235–1241.

55. Alvarez-Sabin J, Molina CA, Ribo M, et al. (2004) Impact of Admission Hyperglycemia on Stroke Outcome After Thrombolysis. Risk Stratification in Relation to Time to Reperfusion. Stroke-Dallas 2004;35(11):2493–2497.

56 Song EC, Chu K, Jeong SW, et al. Hyperglycemia exacerbates brain edema and perihematomal cell death after intracerebral hemorrhage. Stroke 2003; 34:2215–2220.

57. Demchuk AM, Morgenstern LB, Krieger DW, et al. Serum glucose level and diabetes predict tissue plasminogen activator-related intracerebral hemorrhage in acute ischemic stroke. Stroke 1999; 30:34–39.

58. Lansberg MG, Albers GW, Wijman CA. Symptomatic intracerebral hemorrhage following thrombolytic therapy for acute ischemic stroke: a review of the risk factors. Cerebrovasc Dis 2007; 24:1–10.

59. Tanne D, Kasner SE, Demchuk AM, et al. Markers of increased risk of intracerebral hemorrhage after intravenous recombinant tissue plasminogen activator therapy for acute ischemic stroke in clinical practice: the Multicenter rt-PA Stroke Survey. Circulation 2002; 105: 1679–1685.

60. Lansberg MG, O'Brien MW, Tong DC, Moseley ME, Albers GW. Evolution of cerebral infarct volume assessed by diffusion-weighted magnetic resonance imaging. Arch Neurol 2001; 58:613–617.

61. Beaulieu C, de Crespigny A, Tong DC, Moseley ME, Albers GW, Marks MP. Longitudinal magnetic resonance imaging study of perfusion and diffusion in stroke: evolution of lesion volume and correlation with clinical outcome. Ann Neurol 1999; 46:568–578.

62. Ritzl A, Meisel S, Wittsack HJ, et al. Development of brain infarct volume as assessed by magnetic resonance imaging (MRI): follow-up of diffusion-weighted MRI lesions. J Magn Reson Imaging 2004; 20:201–207.

63. Gass A. Is there a penumbra surrounding intracerebral hemorrhage? Cerebrovasc Dis 2007; 23:4–5.

64. Labelle M, Khiat A, Durocher A, Boulanger Y. Comparison of metabolite levels and water diffusion between cortical and subcortical strokes as monitored by MRI and MRS. Invest Radiol 2001; 36:155–163.

65. Toni D, De MM, Fiorelli M, et al. Influence of hyperglycaemia on infarct size and clinical outcome of acute ischemic stroke patients with intracranial arterial occlusion. J Neurol Sci 1994; 123:129–133.

66. Prado R, Ginsberg MD, Dietrich WD, Watson BD, Busto R. Hyperglycemia increases infarct size in collaterally perfused but not end-arterial vascular territories. J Cereb Blood Flow Metab 1988; 8:186–192.

67. Ginsberg MD, Prado R, Dietrich WD, Busto R, Watson BD. Hyperglycemia reduces the extent of cerebral infarction in rats. Stroke 1987; 18:570–574.

68. Murros K, Fogelholm R, Kettunen S, Vuorela AL, Valve J. Blood glucose, glycosylated haemoglobin, and outcome of ischemic brain infarction. J Neurol Sci 1992; 111: 59–64.

69. Berger L, Hakim AM. The association of hyperglycemia with cerebral edema in stroke. Stroke 1986; 17:865–871.

70. Els T, Klisch J, Orszagh M, et al. Hyperglycemia in patients with focal cerebral ischemia after intravenous thrombolysis: influence on clinical outcome and infarct size. Cerebrovasc Dis 2002; 13:89–94.

71. Parsons MW, Barber PA, Desmond PM, et al. Acute hyperglycemia adversely affects stroke outcome: a magnetic resonance imaging and spectroscopy study. Ann Neurol 2002; 52: 20–28.

72. Wagner KR, Kleinholz M, de Court, Myers RE. Hyperglycemic versus normoglycemic stroke: topography of brain metabolites, intracellular pH, and infarct size. J Cereb Blood Flow Metab 1992; 12:213–222.

73. Candelise L, Landi G, Orazio EN, Boccardi E. Prognostic significance of hyperglycemia in acute stroke. Arch Neurol 1985; 42:661–663.

74. Kagansky N, Levy S, Knobler H. The role of hyperglycemia in acute stroke. Arch Neurol 2001; 58:1209–1212.

75. Weir CJ, Murray GD, Dyker AG, Lees KR. Is hyperglycaemia an independent predictor of poor outcome after acute stroke? Results of a long term follow up study. BMJ 1997; 314:1303.

76. Woo E, Chan YW, Yu YL, Huang CY. Admission glucose level in relation to mortality and morbidity outcome in 252 stroke patients. Stroke 1988; 19:185–191.

77. Woo J, Lam CW, Kay R, Wong AH, Teoh R, Nicholls MG. The influence of hyperglycemia and diabetes mellitus on immediate and 3-month morbidity and mortality after acute stroke. Arch Neurol 1990; 47:1174–1177.

78. McEwen BS, Reagan LP. Glucose transporter expression in the central nervous system: relationship to synaptic function. Eur J Pharmacol 2004; 490:13–24.

79. Brownlee M. Biochemistry and molecular cell biology of diabetic complications. Nature 2001; 414:813–820.

80. Ribo M, Molina C, Montaner J, et al. Acute hyperglycemia state is associated with lower tPA-induced recanalization rates in stroke patients. Stroke 2005; 36:1705–1709.

81. Stegenga ME, van der Crabben SN, Levi M, et al. Hyperglycemia stimulates coagulation, whereas hyperinsulinemia impairs fibrinolysis in healthy humans. Diabetes 2006; 55: 1807–1812.

82. Rao AK, Chouhan V, Chen X, Sun L, Boden G. Activation of the tissue factor pathway of blood coagulation during prolonged hyperglycemia in young healthy men. Diabetes 1999; 48:1156–1161.

83. Gentile NT, Vaidyula VR, Kanamalla U, DeAngelis M, Gaughan J, Rao AK. Factor VIIa and tissue factor procoagulant activity in diabetes mellitus after acute ischemic stroke: impact of hyperglycemia. Thromb Haemost 2007; 98:1007–1013.
84. Vaidyula VR, Rao AK, Mozzoli M, Homko C, Cheung P, Boden G. Effects of hyperglycemia and hyperinsulinemia on circulating tissue factor procoagulant activity and platelet CD40 ligand. Diabetes 2006; 55:202–208.
85. Pandolfi A, Giaccari A, Cilli C, et al. Acute hyperglycemia and acute hyperinsulinemia decrease plasma fibrinolytic activity and increase plasminogen activator inhibitor type 1 in the rat. Acta Diabetol 2001; 38:71–76.
86. Festa A, D'Agostino R Jr., Mykkanen L, et al. Relative contribution of insulin and its precursors to fibrinogen and PAI-1 in a large population with different states of glucose tolerance. The Insulin Resistance Atherosclerosis Study (IRAS). Arterioscler Thromb Vasc Biol 1999; 19:562–568.
87. Meigs JB, Mittleman MA, Nathan DM, et al. Hyperinsulinemia, hyperglycemia, and impaired hemostasis: the Framingham Offspring Study. JAMA 2000; 283:221–228.
88. Yip PK, He YY, Hsu CY, Garg N, Marangos P, Hogan EL. Effect of plasma glucose on infarct size in focal cerebral ischemia-reperfusion. Neurology 1991; 41:899–905.
89. Quast MJ, Wei J, Huang NC, et al. Perfusion deficit parallels exacerbation of cerebral ischemia/reperfusion injury in hyperglycemic rats. J Cereb Blood Flow Metab 1997; 17:553–559.
90. Duckrow RB, Beard DC, Brennan RW. Regional cerebral blood flow decreases during hyperglycemia. Ann Neurol 1985; 17:267–272.
91. Kawai N, Keep RF, Betz AL, Nagao S. Hyperglycemia induces progressive changes in the cerebral microvasculature and blood-brain barrier transport during focal cerebral ischemia. Acta Neurochir Suppl 1998; 71:219–221.
92. Venables GS, Miller SA, Gibson G, Hardy JA, Strong AJ. The effects of hyperglycaemia on changes during reperfusion following focal cerebral ischaemia in the cat. J Neurol Neurosurg Psychiatry 1985; 48:663–669.
93. Beckman JA, Goldfine AB, Gordon MB, Garrett LA, Creager MA. Inhibition of protein kinase Cbeta prevents impaired endothelium-dependent vasodilation caused by hyperglycemia in humans. Circ Res 2002; 90:107–111.
94. Williams SB, Goldfine AB, Timimi FK, et al. Acute hyperglycemia attenuates endothelium-dependent vasodilation in humans in vivo. Circulation 1998; 97:1695–1701.
95. Vallance P, Collier J, Moncada S. Effects of endothelium-derived nitric oxide on peripheral arteriolar tone in man. Lancet 1989; 2:997–1000.
96. Fleming I, Busse R. Molecular mechanisms involved in the regulation of the endothelial nitric oxide synthase. Am J Physiol Regul Integr Comp Physiol 2003; 284:R1–R12.
97. Ding Y, Vaziri ND, Coulson R, Kamanna VS, Roh DD. Effects of simulated hyperglycemia, insulin, and glucagon on endothelial nitric oxide synthase expression. Am J Physiol Endocrinol Metab 2000; 279:E11–E17.
98. Du XL, Edelstein D, Dimmeler S, Ju Q, Sui C, Brownlee M. Hyperglycemia inhibits endothelial nitric oxide synthase activity by posttranslational modification at the Akt site. J Clin Invest 2001; 108:1341–1348.
99. Tesfamariam B, Brown ML, Cohen RA. Elevated glucose impairs endothelium-dependent relaxation by activating protein kinase C. J Clin Invest 1991; 87:1643–1648.
100. Inoguchi T, Li P, Umeda F, et al. High glucose level and free fatty acid stimulate reactive oxygen species production through protein kinase C-dependent activation of NAD(P)H oxidase in cultured vascular cells. Diabetes 2000; 49:1939–1945.
101. Cosentino F, Hishikawa K, Katusic ZS, Luscher TF. High glucose increases nitric oxide synthase expression and superoxide anion generation in human aortic endothelial cells. Circulation 1997; 96:25–28.
102. Bohlen HG, Nase GP. Arteriolar nitric oxide concentration is decreased during hyperglycemia-induced betaII PKC activation. Am J Physiol Heart Circ Physiol 2001; 280:H621–H627.

103. Natarajan R, Gu JL, Rossi J, et al. Elevated glucose and angiotensin II increase 12-lipoxygenase activity and expression in porcine aortic smooth muscle cells. Proc Natl Acad Sci USA 1993; 90:4947–4951.

104. Jawerbaum A, Franchi AM, Gonzalez ET, Novaro V, de Gimeno MA. Hyperglycemia promotes elevated generation of TXA2 in isolated rat uteri. Prostaglandins 1995; 50:47–56.

105. el-Kashef H. Hyperglycemia increased the responsiveness of isolated rabbit's pulmonary arterial rings to serotonin. Pharmacology 1996; 53:151–159.

106. Bemeur C, Ste-Marie L, Montgomery J. Increased oxidative stress during hyperglycemic cerebral ischemia. Neurochem Int 2007; 50:890–904.

107. Martini SR, Kent TA. Hyperglycemia in acute ischemic stroke: a vascular perspective. J Cereb Blood Flow Metab 2007; 27:435–451.

108. Bemeur C, Ste-Marie L, Desjardins P, et al. Dehydroascorbic acid normalizes several markers of oxidative stress and inflammation in acute hyperglycemic focal cerebral ischemia in the rat. Neurochem Int 2005; 46:399–407.

109. Li S, Zheng J, Carmichael ST. Increased oxidative protein and DNA damage but decreased stress response in the aged brain following experimental stroke. Neurobiol Dis 2005; 18:432–440.

110. Muralikrishna AR, Hatcher JF. Phospholipase A2, reactive oxygen species, and lipid peroxidation in cerebral ischemia. Free Radic Biol Med 2006; 40:376–387.

111. Garg R, Chaudhuri A, Munschauer F, Dandona P. Hyperglycemia, insulin, and acute ischemic stroke: a mechanistic justification for a trial of insulin infusion therapy. Stroke 2006; 37:267–273.

112. Schurr A. Lactate: the ultimate cerebral oxidative energy substrate? J Cereb Blood Flow Metab 2006; 26:142–152.

113. Siesjo BK. Acidosis and ischemic brain damage. Neurochem Pathol 1988; 9:31–88.

114. Katsura K, Asplund B, Ekholm A, Siesjo BK. Extra- and Intracellular pH in the Brain During Ischaemia, Related to Tissue Lactate Content in Normo- and Hypercapnic rats. Eur J Neurosci 1992; 4:166–176.

115. Anderson RE, Tan WK, Martin HS, Meyer FB. Effects of glucose and PaO2 modulation on cortical intracellular acidosis, NADH redox state, and infarction in the ischemic penumbra. Stroke 1999; 30:160–170.

116. Intracerebral hemorrhage after intravenous t-PA therapy for ischemic stroke. The NINDS t-PA Stroke Study Group. Stroke 1997; 28:2109–2118.

117. Hawkins BT, Lundeen TF, Norwood KM, Brooks HL, Egleton RD. Increased blood-brain barrier permeability and altered tight junctions in experimental diabetes in the rat: contribution of hyperglycaemia and matrix metalloproteinases. Diabetologia 2007; 50: 202–211.

118. Hamilton MG, Tranmer BI, Auer RN. Insulin reduction of cerebral infarction due to transient focal ischemia. J Neurosurg 1995; 82:262–268.

119. Zhu CZ, Auer RN. Optimal blood glucose levels while using insulin to minimize the size of infarction in focal cerebral ischemia. J Neurosurg 2004; 101:664–668.

120. van den BergheG, Wilmer A, Hermans G, et al. Intensive insulin therapy in the medical ICU. N Engl J Med 2006; 354:449–461.

121. Diaz R, Paolasso EA, Piegas LS, et al. Metabolic modulation of acute myocardial infarction. The ECLA (Estudios Cardiologicos Latinoamerica) Collaborative Group. Circulation 1998; 98:2227–2234.

122. Furnary AP, Gao G, Grunkemeier GL, et al. Continuous insulin infusion reduces mortality in patients with diabetes undergoing coronary artery bypass grafting. J Thorac Cardiovasc Surg 2003; 125:1007–1021.

123. Lazar HL, Chipkin SR, Fitzgerald CA, Bao Y, Cabral H, Apstein CS. Tight glycemic control in diabetic coronary artery bypass graft patients improves perioperative outcomes and decreases recurrent ischemic events. Circulation 2004; 109:1497–1502.

124. Gentile NT, Seftchick MW, Huynh T, Kruus LK, Gaughan J. Decreased mortality by normalizing blood glucose after acute ischemic stroke. Acad Emerg Med 2006; 13:174–180.

125. Samson Y. Efficacy and Safety of Continuous Intravenous Versus Usual Subcutaneous Insulin in Acute Ischemic Stroke (INSULINFARCT). 2008: (ClinicalTrials.gov Identifier: NCT00472381).
126. Johnston KC, Hall CE. Glucose Regulation in Acute Stroke Patients Trial (GRASP) Trial. 2008: (Clinical Trials.gov Identifier: NCT00282867).
127. Muir KW, Grosset DG. Neuroprotection for acute stroke: making clinical trials work. Stroke 1999; 30:180–182.
128. Malmberg K, Ryden L, Wedel H, et al. Intense metabolic control by means of insulin in patients with diabetes mellitus and acute myocardial infarction (DIGAMI 2): effects on mortality and morbidity. Eur Heart J 2005; 26:650–661.
129. Ceremuzynski L, Budaj A, Czepiel A. et al. Low-dose glucose-insulin-potassium is ineffective in acute myocardial infarction: results of a randomized multicenter Pol-GIK trial. Cardiovasc Drugs Ther 1999; 13:191–200.
130. Mehta SR, Yusuf S, Diaz R, et al. Effect of glucose-insulin-potassium infusion on mortality in patients with acute ST-segment elevation myocardial infarction: the CREATE-ECLA randomized controlled trial. JAMA 2005; 293:437–446.
131. Gandhi GY, Nuttall GA, Abel MD, et al. Intensive intraoperative insulin therapy versus conventional glucose management during cardiac surgery: a randomized trial. Ann Intern Med 2007; 146:233–243.
132. Brunkhorst FM, Engel C, Bloos F, et al. Intensive insulin therapy and pentastarch resuscitation in severe sepsis. N Engl J Med 2008; 358:125–139.
133. Vriesendorp TM, Roos YW, Kruyt ND, et al. Efficacy and safety of two 5-day insulin dosing regimens to achieve strict glycemic control in patients with acute ischemic stroke. J Neurol Neurosurg Psychiatry; in press.
134. Ingels C, Debaveye Y, Milants I, et al. Strict blood glucose control with insulin during intensive care after cardiac surgery: impact on 4-years survival, dependency on medical care, and quality-of-life. Eur Heart J 2006; 27:2716–2724.

IV   LONG-TERM CEREBRAL COMPLICATIONS IN DIABETES

10 Cognition in Children and Adolescents with Type 1 Diabetes

Christopher M. Ryan, PhD

CONTENTS

ABSTRACT

Diabetes has a marked effect on brain function and structure in children and adolescents. As a group, diabetic children are more likely to perform more poorly than their nondiabetic peers in the classroom and earn lower scores on measures of academic achievement and verbal intelligence. Specialized neuropsychological testing reveals evidence of dysfunction in a variety of cognitive domains, including sustained attention, visuoperceptual skills, and psychomotor speed. Children diagnosed early in life – before 7 years of age – appear to be most vulnerable, showing impairments on virtually all types of cognitive tests, with learning and memory skills being particularly affected. Results from neurophysiological, cerebrovascular, and neuroimaging studies also show evidence of CNS anomalies. Earlier research attributed diabetes-associated brain dysfunction to episodes of recurrent hypoglycemia, but more recent studies have

From: *Contemporary Diabetes: Diabetes and the Brain*
Edited by: G. J. Biessels, J. A. Luchsinger (eds.), DOI 10.1007/978-1-60327-850-8_10
© Humana Press, a part of Springer Science+Business Media, LLC 2009

generally failed to find strong support for that view. While there is growing evidence to suggest that elevated blood glucose levels may play an important role in the development of cognitive dysfunction in diabetic adults, there remains little compelling data for that possibility from pediatric studies, in part because of the many methodological shortcomings inherent in much of this research. In a systematic, critical review of the extant pediatric literature, this chapter addresses a variety of issues: Is it possible to identify one or more well-defined neurocognitive phenotypes characteristic of diabetes in childhood? Why – from developmental, biomedical, and psychosocial perspectives – are some diabetic children more likely to develop neurocognitive deficits? What is the pathophysiological basis for these brain anomalies?

Key words: Adolescents; Animal models of diabetes; Cerebral blood flow (CBF); Children; Chronic hyperglycemia; Cognitive dysfunction; Diabetic ketoacidosis (DKA); Electroencephalography (EEG); Hypoglycemia; Magnetic resonance imaging (MRI); Microvascular complications; Neuropsychological assessment.

INTRODUCTION

Children with diabetes have a greatly increased risk of manifesting mild neurocognitive dysfunction. This is an incontrovertible fact that has emerged from a large body of research conducted over the past 60 years [for reviews see *(1–4)*]. There is, however, less agreement about the details. How are these deficits manifested behaviorally? Who is at greatest risk? When are these most likely to occur? What pathophysiological mechanisms underlie their emergence? This chapter addresses each of those issues, highlighting what we currently know and identifying the sometimes enormous gaps in our knowledge.

Because the classroom may be where diabetes-associated cognitive dysfunction first becomes evident to adults, I begin with a discussion of how diabetic children differ from their nondiabetic peers in school. That is followed by an analysis of neuropsychological processes – attention, learning, memory, problem-solving, visuoperceptual skills, and psychomotor speed – that could be affected in the child with diabetes and could contribute to poorer classroom performance. To determine whether diabetes in childhood can be characterized by a unique "neurocognitive phenotype," other measures of brain function are also discussed, including results from electrophysiological, cerebrovascular, and neuroimaging studies. In an effort to identify possible pathophysiological mechanisms, I next review the relationship between neurocognitive outcomes and the three major classes of biomedical risk factors – episodes of recurrent hypoglycemia, ketoacidosis, and chronic hyperglycemia, as well as some possible psychosocial variables. This chapter closes with some thoughts about new research directions.

METHODOLOGICAL CONSIDERATIONS

Before embarking on this review of the pediatric literature, it may be especially instructive to identify some of the limitations and weaknesses inherent in much of the research conducted to date. Two broad problem areas are especially prevalent across studies: the failure to accurately and comprehensively ascertain the nature, severity, and course of the disease and its impact on both the child and the family, and the absence of large-scale studies from multiple research centers that consistently use a core battery of child-appropriate, valid, and reliable neurocognitive assessment measures.

When studying children with any type of chronic disorder, it is critically important to be able to identify and document, for each child, the nature and extent of their disease process from both a biomedical and a psychosocial perspective. For the diabetic child, we ought to – but hardly ever – have medical, metabolic, and psychosocial data from diagnosis onward. Did the child experience ketoacidosis and/or cerebral edema around the time of diagnosis or anytime thereafter? Since diagnosis, how often and for what duration did the child experience excessively low – and excessively high – glucose values, and how were these episodes of hypoglycemia and hyperglycemia operationalized? When did the child begin to show evidence of microvascular complications and other comorbid conditions like blood pressure elevations, and how did these progress over time? How did the child cope psychologically with the diagnosis of diabetes and with diabetes-related events, like the occurrence of a hypoglycemic seizure or coma? Each of these biomedical and psychosocial variables may influence the phenomenology, measurement, and/or etiology of neurocognitive outcomes, but they are rarely captured by researchers or incorporated into analyses.

It is also critically important for researchers to be able to delineate, in a meaningful and reliable fashion, the neurocognitive characteristics of each child and any acute state – depression, anxiety, low blood glucose values – that might influence cognitive performance at the time of that assessment. Ordinarily, this is accomplished by administering a battery of psychometrically sound neuropsychological tests, assessing mood state, and measuring blood glucose periodically during the assessment session. Unfortunately, there are no universally agreed upon standards for selecting such tests, particularly when assessing children (or adults!) with diabetes, despite pleas for the establishment of a "core" battery (5), as has happened in research with other neurocognitive disorders like dementia (6, 7). Lack of consistency in neuropsychological assessment across research groups challenges our ability to rationally aggregate results from many smaller cross-sectional studies.

This problem has been compounded further by researchers who have either failed to assess neuropsychological function in a comprehensive fashion or have used tests with questionable, or unknown, psychometric properties for a pediatric population. As an example, a number of seminal studies either ignored the assessment of learning and memory skills completely *(8)*, used tests that had been developed for adults but not children *(9)*, or relied on mnestic tests from the research laboratory with questionable or unproven psychometric properties *(10, 11)*. This would, at least in part, explain why there exists no consensus about the impact of diabetes on a cognitive process which is a key determinant to classroom success: effective learning and memory abilities *(11–14)*.

Longitudinal studies in which subjects are evaluated repeatedly over an extended period of time present an additional set of problems *(15, 16)*. Not only may practice or familiarity effects from repeated exposure to the same materials reduce the sensitivity of the test to subtle declines in cognition *(17)*, but the use of different cognitive tests (which can have very different psychometric properties) at different ages to account for qualitative and quantitative variations in the normal course of cognitive development may further complicate the researcher's ability to detect meaningful changes over time *(18)*.

Those methodological issues notwithstanding, extant research on diabetic children's brain function has identified a number of themes that emerge in this review. All other things being equal, children diagnosed with type 1 diabetes early in life – within the first 5–7 years of age – have the greatest risk of manifesting neurocognitive dysfunction, the magnitude of which is greater than that seen in children with a later onset of diabetes. The development of brain dysfunction seems to occur within a relatively brief period of time, often appearing within the first 2–3 years following diagnosis. It is not limited to performance on neuropsychological tests, but is manifested on a wide range of electrophysiological measures as marked neural slowing. Somewhat surprisingly, the magnitude of these effects does not seem to worsen appreciably with increasing duration of diabetes – at least through early adulthood.

SCHOOL PERFORMANCE

As a group, diabetic children earn somewhat lower grades in school as compared to their nondiabetic classmates, are more likely to fail or repeat a grade, perform more poorly on formal tests of academic achievement, and have lower IQ scores, particularly on tests of verbal intelligence. The most compelling evidence for a link between diabetes and poorer school outcomes has been provided by a Swedish population-based register study involving

5,159 children who developed diabetes between July 1997 and July 2000 and 1,330,968 nondiabetic children *(19)*. Those who developed diabetes very early in life (diagnosis before 2 years of age) had a significantly increased risk of not completing school as compared to either diabetic patients diagnosed after that age or to the reference population. Small, albeit statistically reliable between-group differences were noted in school marks, with diabetic children, regardless of age at diagnosis, consistently earning somewhat lower grades. Of note is their finding that the diabetic sample had a significantly lower likelihood of getting a high mark (passed with distinction or excellence) in two subjects and was less likely to take more advanced courses. The authors conclude that despite universal access to active diabetes care, diabetic children – particularly those with a very early disease onset – had a greatly increased risk of somewhat lower educational achievement.

Similar results have been reported by a number of smaller studies [for reviews see *(20, 21)*]. In a 10-year follow-up of diabetic and nondiabetic children participating in the prospective Melbourne Royal Children's Hospital (RCH) cohort study *(22)*, Northam and her associates reported that only 68% of her diabetic sample completed 12 years of school, as compared to 85% of the nondiabetic comparison group *(23)*. Although age at onset was not examined in that analysis, other reports on this cohort have indicated that those children with an earlier onset of diabetes had an elevated risk of cognitive dysfunction *(13, 24)*. Children with diabetes, especially those with an earlier onset, have also been found to require more remedial educational services and to be more likely to repeat a grade *(25–28)*, to earn lower school grades over time *(29)*, to experience somewhat greater school absenteeism *(28, 30–32)*, to have a two to threefold increase in rates of depression *(33–35)*, and to manifest more externalizing behavior problems *(25)*. On standardized tests of academic achievement, diabetic children generally perform somewhat worse than their healthy peers; this effect was most notable on measures of reading *(26, 31, 36–38)* and has been associated with poorer metabolic control *(39)*.

Performance on measures of verbal intelligence – particularly those that assess vocabulary knowledge and general information about the world – is frequently compromised in diabetic children *(9, 14, 26, 40)* and in adults *(41)* with a childhood onset of diabetes. The few studies that have followed subjects over time have noted that verbal IQ scores tend to decline as the duration of diabetes increases *(13, 15, 29)*. These effects appear to be more pronounced in boys and in those children with an earlier onset of diabetes. Whether this phenomenon is a marker of cognitive decline or whether it reflects a delay in cognitive development cannot yet be determined because sufficiently large numbers of diabetic and nondiabetic children have not been followed serially from childhood into early adulthood.

Since optimal performance in school and on formal tests of vocabulary and reading is largely dependent on exposure to a specific body of knowledge that is normally presented in a classroom setting, it is possible, but remains unproven, that psychosocial processes (e.g., school absence, depression, distress, externalizing problems) *(42)*, and/or multiple and prolonged periods of classroom inattention and reduced motivation secondary to acute and prolonged episodes of hypoglycemia *(43–45)* may be contributing to the poor academic outcomes characteristic of children with diabetes. Although it may seem more reasonable to attribute poorer school performance and lower IQ scores to diabetes-associated disruption of specific neurocognitive processes (e.g., attention, learning, memory) secondary to brain dysfunction, there is little compelling evidence to support that possibility at the present time. Remarkably, no efforts have been made to predict scholastic achievement from neurocognitive variables in diabetic children.

IDENTIFYING NEUROCOGNITIVE PHENOTYPES

Drawing on results from cognitive, electrophysiological, cerebrovascular, and neuroimaging evaluations, researchers have attempted to delineate one or more distinct neurocognitive phenotypes characteristic of patients with diabetes *(46)*. At the present time this effort may best be considered as a "work in progress" because the accuracy of any phenotype is completely dependent on the comprehensiveness of the assessment. This has been especially problematic in the pediatric research arena where until very recently, most studies of brain function were relatively small in scope and restricted to the administration of a limited number of cognitive tests or the measurement of brain waves. Nevertheless, as the remainder of this section indicates, a pattern of results is beginning to appear in diabetic children which is remarkably similar to that seen in adults with type 1 or type 2 diabetes.

Cognitive Manifestations

Children and adults who develop diabetes within the first 5–7 years of life may show moderate cognitive dysfunction that can affect all cognitive domains, although the specific pattern varies, depending both on the cognitive domain assessed and on the child's age at assessment. Data from a recent meta-analysis of 19 pediatric studies have indicated that effect sizes tend to range between ~ 0.4 and 0.5 for measures of learning, memory, and attention, but are lower for other cognitive domains *(47)*. For the younger child with an early onset of diabetes, decrements are particularly pronounced on visuospatial tasks that require copying complex designs, solving jigsaw puzzles, or using multi-colored blocks to reproduce designs, with girls more likely to earn lower scores than boys *(8)*. By adolescence and early adult-hood, gender differences are less apparent and deficits occur on measures of attention, mental efficiency, learning, memory, eye–hand coordination, and "executive functioning" *(13, 26, 40, 48–50)*. Not only do children with an early onset of diabetes often – but not invariably – score lower than healthy comparison subjects, but a subset earn scores that fall into the "clinically impaired" range defined as scores that are more than 2 standard deviations beyond the mean value for nondiabetic comparison subjects *(49)*. According to one estimate, the prevalence of clinically significant impairment is approximately four times higher in those diagnosed within the first 6 years of life as compared to either those diagnosed after that age or to nondiabetic peers (25 vs. 6%) *(49)*. Nevertheless, it is important to keep in mind that not all early onset diabetic children show cognitive dysfunction, and not all tests within a particular cognitive domain differentiate diabetic from nondiabetic subjects. Why certain tests are more sensitive to diabetes-related variables than others remains unknown and unexamined.

The interpretation of the early onset literature is complicated by the fact that in a number of studies, investigators have stratified their diabetic samples in terms of presence or absence of severe hypoglycemic events rather than earlier or later age at onset *(14, 51)*. As a consequence, cognitive dysfunction has been attributed to severe hypoglycemia, but that may be in error insofar as severe hypoglycemia and onset age tend to be interrelated. Data from both epidemiologic *(52)* and cross-sectional studies *(53)* show that children with an early onset of diabetes have a greatly increased risk of severe hypoglycemia when compared to those with a later onset (45 vs. 13%). The use of more intensive therapeutic regimens further increases the risk of severe hypoglycemia *(54)*, particularly in those with an earlier onset of diabetes *(55)*, perhaps because of a heightened sensitivity to insulin in young patients *(56)*.

Children and adolescents with a later onset of diabetes also manifest cognitive dysfunction, particularly on tests requiring sustained attention, visuoperceptual skills, and psychomotor speed *(2, 9, 11, 13, 14, 37)*. The magnitude of these effects tends to be relatively modest, with estimates generally approximating ~ 0.2 or less *(47)*, although there is much variation across different studies. Whether learning and memory skills are also compromised – as they clearly are in children with an earlier onset of diabetes – remains controversial *(12)*. Some studies have reported no evidence of mnestic deficits *(9)* while others sometimes *(11, 37, 57)* but not invariably *(14)* find deficits on certain types of memory tests, particularly those having a visuospatial component. The extent to which "higher order" cognitive processes are compromised cannot be determined at the present time because of limited ascertainment. With very few exceptions *(13)*, problem-solving and executive functions have not been evaluated in children with diabetes.

Regardless of age at onset, cognitive abnormalities may appear relatively early in the course of diabetes. This is best demonstrated in the Melbourne RCH study, which remains the largest, longest prospective study of children conducted to date. At study entry, there were no differences on any cognitive measure between a representative sample of 90 newly diagnosed diabetic children and 84 healthy children drawn from the community *(22)*. Two years later, those children diagnosed early in life (defined as <4 years) manifested a marked developmental delay insofar as their scores on Vocabulary and Block Design tests improved less over time, as compared to either children with a later onset of diabetes or healthy controls *(58)*. At the 6-year follow-up visit, diabetic children performed worse than nondiabetic subjects on a broad array tests measuring attention, processing speed, long-term memory, and executive skills. These effects were seen in both the early onset and the later onset subgroups, but their magnitude was greater in those diagnosed before 4 years of age *(13)*. No other study of children or adults has yet measured cognition comprehensively since the time of diagnosis and compared the results with a matched group of nondiabetic subjects assessed serially at the same time periods.

Electrophysiological Changes

Slowed neural activity, measured at rest by electroencephalogram (EEG) and in response to sensory stimuli, is common in children with diabetes. On tests of auditory- or visual-evoked potentials (AEP; VEP), children and adolescents with more than a 2-year history of diabetes show significant slowing, as indexed by the increased latencies *(59)*. Not only were these effect sizes large (Cohen's d: 1.0–1.2), but 37% of the sample had latencies considered to be abnormal. In contrast, those children with a briefer duration of diabetes had normal latencies. EEG recordings have also demonstrated abnormalities in diabetic adolescents in very good metabolic control. Compared to age-matched healthy control subjects, the diabetic patients showed significant increases in delta and theta (slow wave) activity, significant declines in alpha peak frequency – greatest in frontal brain areas, and declines in alpha, beta, and gamma fast wave activity that are most pronounced in posterior temporal regions *(60)*. Changes in central slow wave activity were also correlated with reductions in peripheral nerve conduction velocities. Poor metabolic control and severe hypoglycemia were correlated with one another and were associated with the increase in slow wave activity and the reduction in alpha peak frequency. Similar results have been reported in other studies of diabetic children *(61)* and adults *(62, 63)*.

EEG abnormalities have also been associated with childhood diabetes. One large study noted that 26% of their diabetic subjects had abnormal EEG recordings, as compared to 7% of healthy controls *(64)*. Both earlier age at onset and episodes of severe hypoglycemia were strong predictors of pathology in that study and in several other earlier studies *(65–67)*. Although most commentators have assumed that it was the severe hypoglycemic event that caused those EEG abnormalities, there is now some evidence to suggest the obverse: diabetic children with EEG abnormalities recorded at diagnosis may be more likely to experience a seizure or coma (i.e., a severe hypoglycemic event) when blood glucose levels subsequently fall *(68)*. The assumption made by those authors is that the EEG abnormality reflects brain damage that has a genetic or perinatal origin rather than some metabolic perturbation secondary to the onset of diabetes *(69)*. This intriguing possibility – that seizures occur in some diabetic children during hypoglycemia because of the presence of pre-existing brain dysfunction – requires further study.

Cerebral Blood Flow

Little is known about changes in cerebral blood flow (CBF) in children with diabetes. The single study that used single-photon emission tomography (SPECT) found that children with diabetes had lower levels of cerebral perfusion bilaterally as compared to healthy comparison subjects. Basal ganglia and frontal regions showed the greatest reduction in perfusion, followed by parietal and temporal regions *(70)*. This pattern is very similar to that reported in adults with type 1 diabetes *(71)*. No associations were found between CBF measures and neuropsychological test results, duration of diabetes, and HbA1c values, but the sample was small. Despite the recent success of MRI technologies like continuous arterial spin labeling (CASL) *(72)* in identifying regional differences in cerebral blood flow, this noninvasive, nonradioactive technique has not yet been utilized in studies of children and adolescents.

Brain Structure Anomalies

A very large neuroimaging literature indicates that adults with either type 1 or type 2 diabetes manifest structural changes in a number of brain regions [for comprehensive critical reviews see *(73, 74)*], but until very recently, there had been little pediatric research on this topic. In what may be the largest study to date, MRI scans were acquired from 108 diabetic and 51 age-matched nondiabetic children, 7–17 years of age, and voxel-based morphometry techniques were used to quantify between-group differences in gray- and white-matter volumes, and to correlate those values with measures of recurrent severe hypoglycemia and chronic hyperglycemia *(75)*.

Although brain volumes were found to be comparable in the two groups, analyses restricted to the diabetic sample showed statistically reliable relationships between metabolic variables and specific brain regions. Compared to those children with no past history of severe hypoglycemia, those who experienced 1 or more episodes of severe hypoglycemia had smaller gray-matter volumes in the left (but not right) temporal–occipital region. This left-sided lateralization is consistent with findings from a study of young adults with type 1 diabetes *(76)* as well as with several case reports of adults experiencing very severe hypoglycemic episodes *(77–79)*. Chronic hyperglycemia – estimated since diagnosis from serial HbA1c values – was also found to be associated with less cortical volume in right posterior regions (particularly the right cuneus and precuneus). Those regions have also been identified in adults as being sensitive to higher lifetime HbA1c values *(76)*. Less white matter was also associated with chronic hyperglycemia in these diabetic children. Parietal regions were particularly affected, with these relationships stronger in the right, as compared to the left, hemisphere.

One needs to be cautious about over-interpreting these data, primarily because there was no evidence that as a group, diabetic children have significantly less brain volume than their carefully matched nondiabetic peers. Nevertheless, the fact that within-group analyses revealed limited, but statistically reliable, relationships between certain brain regions and metabolic variables in these children which are analogous to what has been reported in diabetic adults who were studied with a similar neuroimaging paradigm *(76)* supports the view that the brain is compromised by diabetes. Moreover, measurable structural changes seem to occur relatively early in the course of the disease since these diabetic children had diabetes for 6.7 years, on average. Whether these modest structural anomalies impact cognitive function remains unknown: no relationships between neuroimaging data and neuropsychological test performance have yet been reported in children with diabetes.

A second study, restricted to 62 younger children who developed diabetes early in life (before 6 years of age), noted a very high rate (29%) of clinically significant structural changes in the central nervous system *(80)* which were evident relatively soon after diagnosis (mean diabetes duration $\sim$ 7 years). The most common anomaly was mesial temporal sclerosis, a condition that ordinarily occurs in less than 1% of the normal pediatric population *(81)* and is usually associated with temporal lobe epilepsy. Not only was the prevalence of this abnormality greatly elevated, occurring in 16% of the early onset sample, but it was unrelated to a past history of severe hypoglycemia. On the other hand, gray-matter volumes were smaller in the subgroup of children who experienced severe hypoglycemia (seizure or coma) as compared to those with no such history (724 vs. 764 cm^3; $d = 0.5$), regardless of whether hypoglycemia occurred before or after 6 years of age. Reductions in white-matter volume were also reported in this study, but that was dependent on the timing of the hypoglycemic event: children who experienced their first hypoglycemic seizure before 6 years of age had less white matter than those who experienced severe hypoglycemia after that age (490 vs. 531 cm^3; $d =$ 0.6); the latter group did not differ from those with no events. Because of marked differences in methodology, these volumetric data are not entirely comparable to those reported by either Perantie et al. in children *(75)* or by Musen et al. in adults *(76)*. Nevertheless, they provide additional support for the view that the child's brain is sensitive to chronically elevated blood glucose levels – as evidenced by the appearance of mesial temporal sclerosis – and to severe hypoglycemic events.

Brain Metabolites

Indirect evidence of neural damage has also come from studies using MRI spectroscopy to measure brain metabolites. Diabetic children in very poor control (mean HbA1c = 11.9%) showed marked reductions in *N*-acetyl-aspartate (NAA) – a marker of neuronal death and dysfunction – in two brain areas: pons and posterior parietal white matter *(82)*. Reductions in choline-containing compounds were also evident in the pons, consistent with the view that the integrity of phospholipid cell membranes, including myelin, may be compromised significantly because of diabetes. Similar reductions in NAA have also been noted in diabetic adults in poor metabolic control *(83)*, in hyperglycemic rats *(84)*, and in diabetic children following an episode of moderately severe hypoglycemia *(85)*. In that latter study, NAA was reduced in frontal and temporal brain regions, as well as in the basal ganglia shortly after the hypoglycemic event. However, those effects were transient; when the children were subsequently re-evaluated 6 months later, the NAA values began to approach normality. Thus, the possibility exists – although remains untested – that the changes in brain metabolites found in poorly controlled diabetic children may not actually reflect permanent neuronal damage but may merely be a consequence of acute hyperglycemia and be reversible following improved metabolic control.

Neurocognitive Phenotypes for the Child with Diabetes: The Search Continues

Despite an increasing interest in brain function in children with diabetes, the research described in this chapter provides, at best, an incomplete picture of neurocognitive status. We do know that children with diabetes earn somewhat lower scores in school, have lower IQ scores, perform more poorly on visuoperceptual and attentional tasks, and are somewhat slower on a variety of mental efficiency tests as compared to their nondiabetic peers. The magnitude of these effects is quite small, unless the child developed diabetes early in life; then, a subset of those children may show moderately severe impairment. Other cognitive domains (e.g., learning, memory, problem-solving, language skills) are also compromised to some extent in children with an earlier age at onset, but there is less consensus as to whether they are affected in children with a later onset of diabetes.

Consistent with the mental slowing is the neural slowing noted on a variety of electrophysiological measures obtained either while the child is quietly resting or in response to sensory stimuli. One would assume that a robust relationship would exist between these cognitive and electrophysiological measures but remarkably this has not been studied in children. Other measures of brain function and structure also reveal some extremely modest effects in a very limited number of brain regions. Those findings are sufficient for a "proof-of-concept" demonstration – that is, that the brain is indeed affected to some extent in children with diabetes. At the present time, however, this body of research is insufficient to provide an accurate, comprehensive, and integrated delineation of those neurocognitive characteristics.

BIOMEDICAL RISK FACTORS

Three types of diabetes-related biomedical variables have been linked to the appearance of neurocognitive anomalies in children with diabetes: moderately severe episodes of hypoglycemia, ketoacidosis, and chronic hyperglycemia. Our understanding of these associations remains imperfect, unfortunately, because so few studies have adequately ascertained those biomedical variables in pediatric samples. Rather than capturing most, or even a representative number, of those events over the course of the diabetic child's disease, the best investigators have been able to do is to estimate metabolic control from one or a handful of glycosylated hemoglobin values, count severe hypoglycemic episodes retrospectively (missing virtually all episodes of nocturnal hypoglycemia), and rely on often incomplete medical records or parents' delayed recall to quantify the number, duration, and severity of episodes of ketoacidosis.

Severe Hypoglycemia

Animal research *(86)* and a series of dramatic case reports *(77, 87–92)* have provided compelling support for the argument that under certain circumstances, hypoglycemia is capable of producing irreversible structural and functional damage to the CNS, although the exact pathophysiological processes remain incompletely understood *(93)*. Yet in virtually all of those instances, the degree of hypoglycemia was "profound," i.e., blood glucose levels typically fell below 1.5 mmol/l (27 mg/dl), persisted for an extended period of time, and were accompanied by coma or seizure, or an essentially flat (isoelectric) EEG. Moreover, most of the diabetic patients described in these case reports were older adults who may have also had some other conditions that could affect brain integrity (e.g., history of chronic alcohol abuse) or who may have manifested wildly fluctuating blood glucose levels (e.g., history of "brittle" diabetes). Although this form of profound hypoglycemia can lead to extraordinary brain morbidity, it seems to be atypical, occurring remarkably infrequently in diabetic patients as a group, with even fewer published reports of such events occurring in children and adolescents.

On the other hand, "severe" hypoglycemic events, defined as a blood glucose value below 3.8 mmol/l (70 mg/dl) *with* loss of consciousness or seizure, and "moderately severe" hypoglycemic events, defined as a blood glucose value below 3.0 mmol/l (55 mg/dl) *without* loss of consciousness or seizure *(43)*, are far more common in diabetic patients of any age (see Chapter 6). Rates of severe hypoglycemia in children and adolescents are approximately 20 per 100 patient years, although the exact value varies somewhat, depending on type of diabetes management regimen and level of glycemic control *(54)*.

Poorer neurocognitive outcomes have been associated with recurrent episodes of severe hypoglycemia in several small, cross-sectional pediatric studies *(51, 64, 70, 94, 95)*, but as noted above, these effects were often moderated by age at onset. That is, children with an earlier age of diabetes onset and a history of severe hypoglycemia were most likely to perform poorly on a limited number of cognitive tests or show more EEG abnormalities, whereas those with a later age at onset were less likely to show deficits, regardless of the presence or absence of severe hypoglycemia. Other studies of children, adolescents, and young adults have either found no robust relationship between severe hypoglycemic events and multiple measures of brain function *(14, 96–99)* or have been unable to accurately attribute neurocognitive dysfunction to severe hypoglycemia in subjects who may have had elevated (or highly variable) blood glucose values over an extended time period *(13, 40, 60)*.

Null results from a subgroup analysis of the Diabetes Control and Complication Trial (DCCT) study cohort provide the most compelling evidence to date that severe hypoglycemia does *not* lead to readily detectable cognitive dysfunction in adolescents or young adults *(16)*. Subjects who enrolled in the DCCT as adolescents (13–19 years of age) were followed over a period of approximately 18 years and were reassessed repeatedly with a comprehensive battery of neuropsychological tests as well as with multiple detailed biomedical measures, including careful prospective ascertainment of severe hypoglycemia (defined as seizure or coma). Of the 249 adolescents who entered the DCCT, 175 (76% of surviving eligible subjects) completed the follow-up cognitive test battery, with half the subjects ($N = 88$) never having an episode of severe hypoglycemia while the remainder experiencing one or more events. Despite a high incidence of severe hypoglycemia ($N = 249$ episodes), there was no relationship between cumulative number of hypoglycemic events and change in cognitive functioning over time within any of the eight cognitive domains assessed. The major limitation of this study is its focus on adolescence – a period when most brain development has already occurred *(100)*. Whether the brain of the younger diabetic child would be more vulnerable to the effects of severe hypoglycemia is an issue that has not yet been settled, although similar null results have been reported from two smaller clinical studies that carefully ascertained hypoglycemic events and measured cognitive function in diabetic children who were 6–15 years of age *(98, 99)*.

Ketoacidosis

Diabetic ketoacidosis (DKA) results from an absolute or relative deficiency in circulating insulin, combined with increased levels of counter-regulatory hormones. The resulting acceleration in catabolism is accompanied by increased glucose production in the kidney and liver and reduced peripheral glucose utilization which leads to hyperglycemia, hyperosmolarity, ketogenesis, and metabolic acidosis *(101)* (see Chapter 7). DKA occurs frequently during the onset of diabetes, with rates ranging from 37 (for those diagnosed before 4 years of age) to 15% in older adolescents *(102)*. For a very small proportion of children (<1%), DKA eventuates into clinically significant cerebral edema, although perhaps as many as half of the non-symptomatic children may manifest evidence of subclinical brain swelling, characterized by a narrowing of the lateral ventricles *(103)*.

The effects of DKA on neurocognitive function have been studied only infrequently, with the focus generally being on acute changes in brain electrical activity, as indexed by EEG recording *(69)*, and brain tissue integrity, as measured by diffusion-weighted MRI *(104)*. Most of the studies previously described in this chapter have either not collected information on DKA or have not incorporated that information into their analyses *(13–15, 37, 49)*. The few reports linking cognitive dysfunction to DKA have tended to be secondary findings; to the best of our knowledge, no neurocognitive study has been explicitly designed to explicitly compare outcomes in individuals with and without a clearly documented history of DKA. Nevertheless, several casual observations suggest possible links between DKA and changes in the CNS measured several years after the event. For example,

26 of the adolescents participating in the DCCT experienced one or more episodes of DKA and subsequently showed declines over the 18-year follow-up period on measures of learning; in contrast, those with no history of DKA showed improvements over time *(16)*. Smaller studies have also reported that children with DKA were more likely to manifest reductions in cerebral blood flow *(70)* and earn somewhat lower scores on certain cognitive tests, with the magnitude and pattern of results varying depending on the age when DKA occurred *(18)*. Those latter observations led the authors to speculate that DKA-associated cognitive dysfunction may require an extended period of time to develop, with specific manifestations being dependent on the stage of brain maturation and the sensitivity of different brain substrates to metabolic insults. These very thoughtful speculations clearly require additional study.

Chronic Hyperglycemia

A very large body of research on *adults* with diabetes now demonstrates that the risk of developing a wide range of neurocognitive changes – poorer cognitive function, slower neural functioning, abnormalities in cerebral blood flow and brain metabolites, and reductions or alterations in gray- and white-brain matter – is associated with chronically elevated blood glucose values and the occurrence of clinically significant microvascular and macrovascular diabetic complications [for reviews see *(105, 106)* and Chapter 11]. In contrast, no pediatric neurocognitive studies have yet evaluated the impact of comorbid medical conditions like elevated blood pressure or early microvascular changes like background retinopathy or subclinical peripheral neuropathy, despite the fact that these are evident in children within 5 years of diagnosis *(107)* and have been found to predict cognitive dysfunction in adults with and without diabetes *(108–110)*. On the other hand, multiple small studies have examined the relationship between HbA1c values and neurocognitive measures in children. In some instances chronic hyperglycemia has been operationalized by averaging several HbA1c values collected over an extended period of time *(60)*; in other studies, composite estimates of chronic hyperglycemia have been generated by calculating the percentage of time from diagnosis that the child exceeded a "poor control" threshold [HbA1c > 9.5%] *(13)* or by adding the *z*-score of median lifetime HbA1c values to the *z*-score of diabetes duration *(14)*. This approach has often [but not invariably – see *(37, 95)*] revealed statistically reliable relationships between exposure to hyperglycemia and neural slowing *(59, 60)*, structural changes in brain gray and white matter *(75)*, and poorer performance on at least a subset of neuropsychological tests *(13–15, 111)*, although the magnitude of these effects may be moderated by age at onset, i.e., the relationships are strongest in those with an early onset of diabetes *(15)*.

Animal research also supports the position that chronic hyperglycemia, as induced by streptozotocin (STZ), can adversely affect the integrity of the CNS (see Chapters 16 and 17). Compared to healthy controls, young adult diabetic rats showed slowed neural processing (longer latencies of auditory- and visual-evoked potentials) after 3–4 months of diabetes. As duration increased further, there was a corresponding increase in evoked potential latencies which was subsequently reversed following the initiation of insulin therapy *(112)*. Spatial learning skills, assessed in a water maze, were also impaired, with the magnitude of those learning deficits linked to reductions in hippocampal plasticity *(113)*.

Very young rats that experienced STZ-induced hyperglycemia between 4 and 8 weeks of age showed especially notable structural CNS abnormalities. Within the cortex of the hyperglycemic rats, neurons were more closely packed together, were smaller than normal, and had less myelin, as indicated by reductions in the amount of protein, fatty acids, and cholesterol. Similar results were seen in the hippocampus, where the density of both astrocytes and neurons was greater, with many more smaller neurons. In contrast, recurrent bouts of moderately severe hypoglycemia had minimal effects on brain structure *(114)*. More recently, this group has identified changes in the neuronal structure that were characterized by reductions in dendritic branching and spine density *(115)*. These structural abnormalities were accompanied by increased levels of sorbitol (indicative of alterations in the activity of the cerebral polyol pathway) and decreases in taurine (thought to serve as a trophic factor for normal neuronal development). While the hyperglycemic rats showed normal learning performance on a water maze task, their delayed recall on that task was significantly impaired. Again, these changes were limited to animals made diabetic with STZ at 4 weeks of age; recurrent bouts of hypoglycemia had no impact on CNS structure or function.

Taken together, the limited animal research on this topic complements the extant pediatric work and provides quite compelling support for the view that even relatively brief bouts of chronically elevated blood glucose values can induce structural and functional changes to the brain. Rodent models have been used previously to study the impact of diabetes on the CNS in adults *(116)*. The very elegant work by Malone and his associates *(114, 115)* is some of the first to explore the effects of diabetes and glucose fluctuations in the developing organism and demonstrates the value of animal models in searching for the pathophysiological basis for brain dysfunction in children with diabetes.

Psychological Stress and Mood Disorder

In addition to the biomedical risk factors described above, one needs to entertain the possibility that some of the neurocognitive problems noted in children may be exacerbated (or obscured) by the occurrence of anxiety and mood disorders – most typically depression and anxiety – that are often *(33, 35, 117)* although not invariably *(118)* seen in children and adolescents with diabetes. A growing literature on nondiabetic children has demonstrated that depression is associated with reductions in whole brain volumes, with changes particularly apparent in the frontal lobes *(119)*, the amygdala *(120)*, and the basal ganglia *(121)*; whether the hippocampus is affected remains unresolved *(120, 122)*. Generalized anxiety disorders are also associated with structural changes, with one study reporting increases in white- and gray-matter volumes in the superior temporal gyrus *(123)*. It is noteworthy that young adults with a childhood onset of diabetes manifest changes in this same brain region, although they are more likely to show decreases in gray-matter density, rather than increases *(76)*. Why this region appears to be sensitive to anxiety and diabetes remains unknown. Magnetic resonance spectroscopy studies have identified changes in brain metabolites *(124)*, particularly brain choline levels, suggestive of diminished cell growth or myelination in the left dorsolateral frontal cortex *(125)*, although there is no complete agreement in this regard *(126)*. Although research has begun on the possible synergistic effects of depression and diabetes on CNS integrity in adults with type 2 diabetes *(127)*, similar studies have not yet been initiated in diabetic children.

PATHOPHYSIOLOGICAL MODELS: ARE WE THERE YET?

Based on this critical review of the pediatric literature, it should be obvious that we are not yet in a position to make strong statements about the etiology of neurocognitive dysfunction in the child with diabetes. Indeed, only one attempt has been made to address some of those findings, with the "diathesis" or vulnerability model *(50)* offering an explanation for why it is that children with an early onset of diabetes seem to be especially likely to manifest significant brain abnormalities. According to this model, in the very young child diagnosed with diabetes, chronically elevated blood glucose levels interfere with normal brain maturation at a time when those neurodevelopmental processes are particularly labile, as they are during the first 5–7 years of life *(128–131)*. The resulting alterations in brain organization that occur during this "sensitive period" will not only lead to delayed cognitive development and lasting cognitive dysfunction, but may also induce a predisposition or diathesis that increases the individual's sensitivity to subsequent insults to the brain, as could be initiated by the prolonged neuroglycopenia that occurs during an episode of hypoglycemia.

Data from most, but not all, research are consistent with that view. In general, children with an early onset of diabetes are more likely to manifest mild-to-moderately severe cognitive impairment on a variety of cognitive and neurophysiological measures. Furthermore, those who experienced an episode of severe hypoglycemia either during, or after, the end of this sensitive period were more likely [but not inevitably – see *(98)*] to show marked cognitive dysfunction as compared to either those with a later onset of diabetes (and severe hypoglycemia) or those with an early onset of diabetes but without seizures *(13, 40, 51)*. Because *some* neurodevelopmental processes continue through adolescence and early adulthood *(132, 133)*, chronically elevated blood glucose levels may also adversely affect brain structure and function in individuals with a later onset of diabetes, but to a far lesser degree. Again that prediction is consistent with findings from many of the neuropsychological studies discussed previously. Compared to their nondiabetic peers, many children and adolescents diagnosed after 6 or 7 years of age show relatively circumscribed cognitive dysfunction that is quite small in magnitude and more often than not, unrelated to the presence or absence of severe hypoglycemia.

Research is only now beginning to focus on plausible pathophysiological mechanisms. We know from animal studies that a relatively brief exposure to chronically elevated blood glucose values can lead to a series of changes in neuronal structure and in brain chemistry *(114, 115)*. Normally, brain glucose levels are tightly regulated at the blood–brain barrier (BBB) by active glucose transporters (e.g., GLUT 1) that up- or down-regulate based on glucose values in the peripheral circulation *(134)*. Recent research has suggested that the development of diabetes per se may lead to at least transient increases in the permeability of the BBB to glucose (and other molecules) *(135)*. Thus it is certainly plausible that around the time of diagnosis, excessive amounts of glucose rapidly flood into the brain and by disrupting normal metabolic and neurotropic processes, trigger structural and functional damage to the CNS in the diabetic child. Validation of this possibility will require additional research that uses animal models to specifically examine the neural and metabolic changes occurring in the brain shortly after the initiation of diabetes.

FUTURE DIRECTIONS

Are the cognitive deficits seen in children with diabetes preventable or reversible? To date, there has been absolutely no research on this topic. In contrast, studies of older adults with type 2 diabetes have demonstrated some modest improvements on a very limited subset of cognitive tasks following interventions that led to better metabolic control *(136–139)*. To what extent are the cognitive deficits seen in children initiated or exacerbated by the development of subclinical (or clinical) microvascular complications of diabetes? Again, there is essentially no literature on this. Psychosocial stressors – do they contribute appreciably to some of the classroom problems or neurocognitive abnormalities seen in diabetic children? Are the deficits seen in children merely developmental delays that disappear as the child grows into adulthood or do they reflect permanent and irreversible brain dysfunction? These and many other questions have not yet been addressed and will remain unanswered until prospective studies are initiated that follow large numbers of newly diagnosed children over an extended period of time. Moreover, underlying pathophysiological mechanisms cannot be disentangled until appropriate animal research has been done; it is unfortunate that to date, few basic scientists have focused on what happens at the time of diabetes onset and shortly thereafter and even fewer have examined the extent to which those findings are moderated by maturation. For all of us, there is much exciting research ahead!

REFERENCES

1. Ryan C. Neuropsychological consequences and correlates of diabetes in childhood. In: Holmes CS, ed. Neuropsychological and Behavioral Aspects of Diabetes. New York, NY: Springer-Verlag, 1989; 58–84.
2. Desrocher M, Rovet J. Neurocognitive correlates of type 1 diabetes in childhood. Child Neuropsychol 2004; 10:36–52.
3. Rovet JF. Diabetes. In: Yeates KW, Ris MD, Taylor HG, eds. Pediatric Neuropsychology: Research, Theory, and Practice. New York, NY: Guilford Press, 2000; 336–365.
4. Northam EA, Rankins D, Cameron FJ. Therapy Insight: The impact of type 1 diabetes on brain development and function. Nature Clinical Practice: Neurology 2006; 2:78–86.
5. Strachan MWJ, Frier BM, Deary IJ. Cognitive assessment in diabetes: The need for consensus. Diabet Med 1997; 14:421–422.
6. Waldemar G, Dubois B, Emre M, et al. Recommendations for the diagnosis and management of Alzheimer's disease and other disorders associated with dementia: EFNS guideline. Eur J Neurol 2007; 14:e1–e26.
7. Hachinski V, Iadecola C, Petersen RC, et al. National Institute of Neurological Disorders and Stroke – Canadian Stroke Network vascular cognitive impairment harmonization standards. Stroke 2006; 37:2220–2241.
8. Rovet JF, Ehrlich RM, Hoppe MG. Intellectual deficits associated with the early onset of insulin-dependent diabetes mellitus in children. Diabetes Care 1987; 10:510–515.
9. Ryan C, Vega A, Longstreet C, Drash L. Neuropsychological changes in adolescents with insulin-dependent diabetes mellitus. J Consult Clin Psychol 1984; 52:335–342.
10. Wolters CA, Yu SL, Hagen JW, Kail, R. Short-term memory and strategy use in children with insulin-dependent diabetes mellitus. J Consult Clin Psychol 1996; 64:1397–1405.
11. Hershey T, Bhargava N, Sadler M, White NH, Craft S. Conventional vs. intensive diabetes therapy in children with type 1 diabetes: Effects on memory and motor speed. Diabetes Care 1999; 22:1318–1324.
12. Ryan CM. Memory and metabolic control in children. Diabetes Care 1999; 22:1242–1244.
13. Northam EA, Anderson PJ, Jacobs R, Hughes M, Warne GL, Werther GA. Neuropsychological profiles of children with type 1 diabetes 6 years after disease onset. Diabetes Care 2001; 24:1541–1546.

14. Perantie DC, Lim A, Wu J, et al. Effects of prior hypoglycemia and hyperglycemia on cognition in children with type 1 diabetes mellitus. Pediatric Diabetes 2008; 9:87–95.
15. Schoenle EJ, Schoenle D, Molinari L, Largo RH. Impaired intellectual development in children with Type 1 diabetes: Association with HbA1c, age at diagnosis, and sex. Diabetologia 2002; 45:108–114.
16. Musen G, Jacobson AM, Ryan CM, et al. Impact of diabetes and its treatment on cognitive function among adolescents who participated in the Diabetes Control and Complications Trial. Diabetes Care 2008; 31:1933–1938.
17. McCaffrey RJ, Westervelt HJ. Issues associated with repeated neuropsychological assessments. Neuropsychol Rev 1995; 5:203–221.
18. Rovet JF, Ehrlich RM, Czuchta D. Intellectual characteristics of diabetic children at diagnosis and one year later. J Pediatr Psychol 1990; 15:775–788.
19. Dahlquist G, Källén B, Swedish Childhood Diabetes Study Group. School performance in children with type 1 diabetes: A population-based register study. Diabetologia 2007; 50:957–964.
20. Taras H, Potts-Datema W. Chronic health conditions and student performance at school. J Sch Health 2005; 75:255–266.
21. Rovet JF, Ehrlich RM, Czuchta D, Akler M. Psychoeducational characteristics of children and adolescents with insulin-dependent diabetes mellitus. J Learn Disabil 1993; 26:7–22.
22. Northam E, Anderson P, Wether G, Adler R, Andrewes D. Neuropsychological complications of insulin dependent diabetes in children. Child Neuropsychol 1995; 1:74–87.
23. Northam E. Screening for psychosocial problems in type 1 diabetes Pediatric Diabetes 2008; 9:5.
24. Lin A, Northam E, Rankins D, Humphreys L, Werther G, Cameron F. Neuropsychological profiles of young people with type 1 diabetes 12–15 years after disease onset. Pediatric Diabetes 2008; 9:17.
25. Rovet J, Ehrlich R, Hoppe M. Behaviour problems in children with diabetes as a function of sex and age of onset of disease. J Child Psychol Psychiatry 1987; 28:477–491.
26. Hagen JW, Barclay CR, Anderson BJ, et al. Intellective functioning and strategy use in children with insulin-dependent diabetes mellitus. Child Dev 1990; 61:1714–1727.
27. Rovet JF, Ehrlich RM, Hoppe M. Specific intellectual deficits in children with early onset diabetes mellitus. Child Dev 1988; 59:226–234.
28. Holmes CS, Dunlap WP, Chen RS, Cornwell JM. Gender differences in the learning status of diabetic children. J Consult Clin Psychol 1992; 60:698–704.
29. Kovacs M, Goldston D, Iyengar S. Intellectual development and academic performance of children with insulin-dependent diabetes mellitus: A longitudinal study. Dev Psychol 1992; 28:676–684.
30. McCarthy AM, Lindgren S, Mengeling MA, Tsalikian E, Engvall, JC. Effects of diabetes on learning in children. Pediatrics 2002; 109:1–10.
31. Ryan C, Longstreet C, Morrow LA. The effects of diabetes mellitus on the school attendance and school achievement of adolescents. Child Care, Health, Dev 1985; 11:229–240.
32. Glaab L, Brown R, Daneman D. School attendance in children with type 1 diabetes. Diabet Med 2005; 22:421–426.
33. Grey M, Whittemore R, Tamborlane WV. Depression in Type 1 diabetes in children: Natural history and correlates. J Psychosom Res 2002; 53:907–911.
34. Northam EA, Matthews LK, Anderson PJ, Cameron FJ, Werther GA. Psychiatric morbidity and health outcome in Type 1 diabetes: Perspectives from a prospective longitudinal study. Diabet Med 2004; 22:152–157.
35. Kovacs M, Goldston D, Obrosky DS, Bonar LK. Psychiatric disorders in youths with IDDM: Rates and risk factors. Diabetes Care 1997; 20:36–44.
36. Gath A, Alison M, TBaum JD. Emotional, behavioural, and educational disorders in diabetic children. Arch Dis Child 1980; 55:371–375.
37. Kaufman FR, Epport K, Engilman R, Halvorson M. Neurocognitive functioning in children diagnosed with diabetes before age 10 years. J Diabetes Complications 1999; 13:31–38.

38. Holmes CS, Richman L. Cognitive profiles of children with insulin-dependent diabetes. J Dev Behav Pediatr 1985; 6:323–326.
39. McCarthy AM, Lindgren S, Mengeling MA, Tsalikian E, Engvall JC. Factors associated with academic achievement in children with Type 1 diabetes. Diabetes Care 2003; 26:112–117.
40. Rovet J, Alverez M. Attentional functioning in children and adolescents with IDDM. Diabetes Care 1997; 20:803–810.
41. Brands AMA, Biessels GJ, De Haan EHF, Kappelle LJ, Kessels RPC. The effects of type 1 diabetes on cognitive performance: A meta-analysis. Diabetes Care 2005; 28:726–735.
42. Aronen ET, Vuontela V, Steenari MR, Salmi J, Carlson S. Working memory, psychiatric symptoms, and academic performance at school. Neurobiol Learn Mem 2005; 83: 33–42.
43. Ryan C, Gurtunca N, Becker D. Hypoglycemia: A complication of diabetes therapy in children. Pediatr Clin North Am 2005; 52:1705–1733.
44. McAulay V, Deary IJ, Sommerfield AJ, Frier BM. Attentional functioning is impaired during acute hypoglycaemia in people with Type 1 diabetes. Diabet Med 2006; 23:26–31.
45. McAulay V, Deary IJ, Sommerfield AJ, Matthews G, Frier BM. Effects of acute hypoglycemia on motivation and cognitive interference in people with type 1 diabetes. J Clin Pharmacol 2006; 26:143–151.
46. Ryan CM. Diabetes mellitus and neurocognitive function. In: Pfaff D, Arnold A, Et-gen A, Fahrbach S, Rubin R, eds. Hormones, Brain and Behavior. San Diego, CA: Harcourt Brace, 2008.
47. Gaudieri PA, Chen R, Greer TF, Holmes CS. Cognitive function in children with type 1 diabetes: A meta-analysis. Diabetes Care 2008; 31:1892–1897.
48. Ferguson SC, Blane A, Wardlaw JM, et al. Influence of an early-onset age of type 1 diabetes on cerebral structure and cognitive function. Diabetes Care 2005; 28:1431–1437.
49. Ryan C, Vega A, Drash A. Cognitive deficits in adolescents who developed diabetes early in life. Pediatrics 1985; 75:921–927.
50. Ryan CM. Why is cognitive dysfunction associated with the development of diabetes early in life? The diathesis hypothesis. Pediatric Diabetes 2006; 7:289–297.
51. Bjørgaas M, Gimse R, Vik T, Sand T. Cognitive function in Type 1 diabetic children with and without episodes of hypoglycaemia. Acta Paediatr 1997; 86:148–153.
52. Barkai L, Vámosi I, Lukács K. Prospective assessment of severe hypoglycaemia in diabetic children and adolescents with impaired and normal awareness of hypoglycaemia. Diabetologia 1998; 41:898–903.
53. Lteif AN, Schwenk WF. Type 1 diabetes mellitus in early childhood: Glycemic control and associated risk of hypoglycemic reactions. Mayo Clin Proc 1999; 74:211–216.
54. Jones TW, Davis EA. Hypoglycemia in children with type 1 diabetes: Current issues and controversies. Pediatric Diabetes 2003; 4:143–150.
55. Wagner VM, Grabert M, Holl RW. Severe hypoglycaemia, metabolic control and diabetes management in children with type 1 diabetes in the decade after the Diabetes Control and Complications Trial – a large scale multicentre study. Eur J Pediatr 2005; 164:73–79.
56. Ternand C, Go VLW, Gerich JE, Haymond MW. Endocrine pancreatic response of children with onset of insulin-requiring diabetes before age 3 and after age 5. J Pediatr 1982; 101:36–39.
57. Hershey T, Lillie R, Sadler M, White NH. Severe hypoglycemia and long-term spatial memory in children with type 1 diabetes mellitus: A retrospective study. J Intern Neuropsychol Soc 2003; 9:740–750.
58. Northam EA, Anderson PJ, Werther GA, Warne GL, Adler RG, Andrewes D. Neuropsychological complications of IDDM in children 2 years after disease onset. Diabetes Care 1998; 21:379–384.
59. Seidl R, Birnbacher R, Hauser E, Gernert G, Freilinger M, Schober E. Brainstem auditory evoked potentials and visually evoked potentials in young patients with IDDM. Diabetes Care 1996; 19:1220–1224.

60. Hyllienmark L, Maltez J, Dandenell A, Ludviggson J, Brismar T. EEG abnormalities with and without relation to severe hypoglycaemia in adolescents with type 1 diabetes. Diabetologia 2005; 48:412–419.
61. Bjørgaas M, Sand T, Gimse R. Quantitative EEG in Type 1 diabetic children with and without episodes of severe hypoglycemia: a controlled, blind study. Acta Neurol Scand 1996; 93:398–402.
62. Howorka K, Pumprla J, Saletu B, Anderer P, Krieger M, Schabmann A. Decrease of vigilance assessed by EEG-mapping in Type 1 diabetic patients with history of recurrent severe hypoglycaemia. Psychoneuroendocrinology 2000; 25:85–105.
63. Brismar T, Hyllienmark L, Ekberg K, Johansson BL. Loss of temporal lobe beta power in young adults with type 1 diabetes mellitus. Neuroreport 2002; 13:2469–2473.
64. Soltész G, Acsádi G. Association between diabetes, severe hypoglycemia, and electroencephalographic abnormalities. Arch Dis Child 1989; 64:992–996.
65. Eeg-Olofsson O. Hypoglycemia and neurological disturbances in children with diabetes mellitus. Acta Paediatr Scand 1997; 91–95.
66. Haumont D, Dorchy H, Pelc S. EEG abnormalities in diabetic children: Influence of hypoglycemia and vascular complications. Clin Pediatr 1979; 18:750–753.
67. Gilhaus KH, Daweke H, Lülsdorf HG, Sachsse R, Sachsse B. EEG-Veränderungen bei diabetischen Kindern. Dtsch Med Wochenschr 1973; 98:1449–1454.
68. Tupola S, Saar P, Rajantie J. Abnormal electroencephalogram at diagnosis of insulin-dependent diabetes mellitus may predict severe symptoms of hypoglycemia in children. J Pediatr 1998; 133:792–794.
69. Tsalikian E, Becker DJ, Crumrine PK, Daneman D, Drash AL. Electroencephalographic changes in diabetic ketosis in children with newly and previously diagnosed insulin-dependent diabetes mellitus. J Pediatr 1981; 98:355–359.
70. Salem MAK, Matta LF, Tantawy AAG, Hussein M, Gad GI. Single photon emission tomography (SPECT) study of regional cerebral blood flow in normoalbuminuric children and adolescents with type 1 diabetes. Pediatric Diabetes 2002; 3:155–162.
71. Quirce R, Carril JM, Jiménez-Bonilla JF, et al. Semi-quantitative assessment of cerebral blood flow with 99mTc-HMPAO SPET in type 1 diabetic patients with no clinical history of cerebrovascular disease. Eur J Nucl Med 1997; 24:1507–1513.
72. Last D, Alsop DC, Abduljalil AM, et al. Global and regional effects of Type 2 diabetes on brain tissue volumes and cerebral vasoreactivity. Diabetes Care 2007; 30: 1193–1199.
73. Jongen C, Biessels GJ. Structural brain imaging in diabetes: A methodological perspective. Eur J Pharmacol 2008; 585:208–218.
74. van Harten B, De Leeuw FE, Weinstein HC, Scheltens P, Biessels GJ. Brain imaging in patients with diabetes: A systematic review. Diabetes Care 2006; 29:2539–2548.
75. Perantie DC, Wu J, Koller JM, et al. Regional brain volume differences associated with hyperglycemia and severe hypoglycemia in youth with type 1 diabetes. Diabetes Care 2007; 30:2331–2337.
76. Musen G, Lyoo IK, Sparks CR, et al. Effects of Type 1 diabetes on gray matter density as measured by voxel-based morphometry. Diabetes 2006; 55:326–333.
77. Auer RN, Hugh J, Cosgrove E, Curry B. Neuropathologic findings in three cases of profound hypoglycemia. Clin Neuropathol 1989; 8:63–68.
78. Chalmers J, Risk MTA, Kean DM, Grant R, Ashworth B, Campbell IW. Severe amnesia after hypoglycemia. Diabetes Care 1991; 14:922–925.
79. Foster JW, Hart RG. Hypoglycemic hemiplegia: two cases and a clinical review. Stroke 1987; 18:944–946.
80. Ho MS, Weller NJ, Ives FJ, et al. High prevalence of structural CNS abnormalities in early onset type 1 diabetes. J Pediatr 2008; 153:385–390.
81. Ng YT, McGregor AL, Duane DC, Jahnke HK, Bird CR, Wheless JW. Childhood mesial temporal sclerosis. J Child Neurol 2006; 21:512–517.
82. Sarac K, Akinci A, Alkan A, Baysal T, Özcan C. Brain metabolite changes on proton magnetic resonance spectroscopy in children with poorly controlled type 1 diabetes. Neuroradiology 2005; 47:562–565.

83. Kreis R, Ross BD. Cerebral metabolic disturbances in patients with subacute and chronic diabetes mellitus: Detection with proton MR spectroscopy. Radiology 1992; 184:123–130.

84. Biessels GJ, Braun KPJ, de Graaf RA, van Eijsden P, Gispen WH, Nicolay K. Cerebral metabolism in streptozotocin-diabetic rats: an in vivo magnetic resonance spectroscopy study. Diabetologia 2001; 44:346–353.

85. Rankins D, Wellard RM, Cameron F, McDonnell C, Northam E. The impact of acute hypo-glycemia on neuropsychological and neurometabolite profiles in children with type 1 dia-betes. Diabetes Care 2005; 28:2771–2773.

86. Auer RN. Hypoglycemic brain damage. Metab Brain Dis 2004; 19:169–175.

87. Gold AE, Deary IJ, Jones RW, O'Hare JP, Reckless JPD, Frier BM. Severe deterioration in cognitive function and personality in five patients with long-standing diabetes: a complica-tion of diabetes or a consequence of treatment? Diabet Med 1994; 11:499–505.

88. Fujioka M, Okuchi K, Hiramatsu K, Sakaki T, Sakaguchi S, Ishii Y. Specific changes in human brain after hypoglycemic injury. Stroke 1997; 28:584–587.

89. Boeve BF, Bell DG, Noseworthy JH. Bilateral temporal lobe MRI changes in uncomplicated hypoglycemic coma. Can J Neurol Sci 1995; 22:56–58.

90. Jung SL, Kim BS, Lee KS, Yoon KH, Byun JY. Magnetic resonance imaging and diffusion-weighted imaging changes after hypoglycemic coma. J Neuroimaging 2005; 15:193–196.

91. Mori F, Nishie M, Houszen H, Yamaguchi J, Wakabayashi K. Hypoglycemic encephalopathy with extensive lesions in the cerebral white matter. Neuropathology 2006; 26:147–152.

92. Strachan MWJ, Abraha HD, Sherwood RA, et al. Evaluation of serum markers of neuronal damage following severe hypoglycaemia in adults with insulin-treated diabetes mellitus. Diabetes Metab Res Rev 1999; 15:5–12.

93. Suh SW, Hamby AM, Swanson RA. Hypoglycemia, brain energetics, and hypoglycemic neuronal death. Glia 2007; 55:1280–1286.

94. Rovet JF, Ehrlich RM. The effect of hypoglycemic seizures on cognitive function in children with diabetes: A 7-year prospective study. J Pediatr 1999; 134:503–506.

95. Hershey T, Perantie DC, Warren SL, Zimmerman EC, Sadler M, White NH. Frequency and timing of severe hypoglycemia affects spatial memory in children with type 1 diabetes mellitus. Diabetes Care 2005; 28:2372–2377.

96. Weinger K, Jacobson AM, Musen G, et al. The effects of type 1 diabetes on cerebral white matter. Diabetologia 2008; 51:417–425.

97. Ferguson SC, Blane A, Perros P, et al. Cognitive ability and brain structure in type 1 dia-betes: Relation to microangiopathy and preceding severe hypoglycemia. Diabetes 2003; 52:149–156.

98. Strudwick SK, Carne C, Gardiner J, Foster JK, Davis EA, Jones TW. Cognitive function-ing in children with early onset type 1 diabetes and severe hypoglycemia. J Pediatr 2005; 147:680–685.

99. Wysocki T, Harris MA, Mauras N, et al. Absence of adverse effects of severe hypoglycemia on cognitive function in school-aged children with diabetes over 18 months. Diabetes Care 2003; 26:1100–1105.

100. Shaw P, Greenstein D, Lerch J, et al. Intellectual ability and cortical development in children and adolescents. Nature 2006; 440:676–679.

101. Wolfsdorf JI, Craig ME, Daneman D, et al. Diabetic ketoacidosis. Pediatric Diabetes 2007; 8:28–43.

102. Rewers A, Klingensmith GJ, Davis C, et al. Presence of diabetic ketoacidosis at diagnosis of diabetes mellitus in youth: The Search for Diabetes in Youth Study. Pediatrics 2008; 121:e1258–e66.

103. Glaser NS, Wootton-Gorges SL, Buonocore MH, et al. Frequency of sub-clinical cerebral edema in children with diabetic ketoacidosis. Pediatric Diabetes 2006; 7:75–80.

104. Glaser NS, Marcin JP, Wootton-Gorges SL, et al. Correlation of clinical and biochemical findings with diabetic ketoacidosis-related cerebral edema in children using magnetic reso-nance diffusion-weighted imaging. J Pediatr 2008; 153:541–546.

105. Ryan CM. Diabetes and brain damage: More (or less) than meets the eye? Diabetologia 2006; 49:2229–2233.

106. Wessels AM, Scheltens P, Barkhof F, Heine RJ. Hyperglycaemia as a determinant of cognitive decline in patients with type 1 diabetes. Eur J Pharmacol 2008; 585:88–96.

107. Derosa G, Avanzini MA, Geroldi D, et al. Matrix metalloproteinase 2 may be a marker of microangiopathy in children and adolescents with type 1 diabetes mellitus. Diabetes Res Clin Pract 2005; 70:119–125.

108. Wong TY, Mosley TH, Klein R, et al. Retinal microvascular changes and MRI signs of cerebral atrophy in healthy, middle-aged people. Neurology 2002; 61:806–811.

109. Cooper LS, Wong TY, Klein R, et al. Retinal microvascular abnormalities and MRI-defined subclinical cerebral infarction: The Atherosclerosis Risk in Communities Study. Stroke 2006; 37:82–86.

110. Reitz C, Tang MX, Manly J, Mayeux R, Luchsinger JA. Hypertension and the risk of mild cognitive impairment. Arch Neurol 2007; 64:1734–1740.

111. Rovet J, Ehrlich R, Hoppe M. Specific intellectual deficits associated with the early onset of insulin-dependent diabetes mellitus in children. Child Dev 1988; 59:226–234.

112. Biessels GJ, Cristino NA, Rutten GJ, Hamers FPT, Erkenlens DW, Gispen WH. Neurophysiological changes in the central and peripheral nervous system of streptozotocin-diabetic rats: Course of development and effects of insulin treatment. Brain 1999; 122:757–768.

113. Biessels GJ, Kamel A, Ramakers GM, et al. Place learning and hippocampal synaptic plasticity in streptozotocin-induced diabetic rats. Diabetes 1996; 45:1259–1266.

114. Malone JI, Hanna SK, Saporta S. Hyperglycemic brain injury in the rat. Brain Res 2006; 1076:9–15.

115. Malone JI, Hanna S, Saporta S, et al. Hyperglycemia NOT hypoglycemia alters neuronal dendrites and impairs spatial memory. Pediatric Diabetes 2008; 9:531–539.

116. Biessels GJ, Gispen WH. The impact of diabetes on cognition: What can be learned from rodent models? Neurobiol Aging 2005; 26S: S36–S41.

117. Blanz BJ, Rensch-Riemann BS, Fritz-Sigmund DI, Schmidt MH. IDDM is a risk factor for adolescent psychiatric disorders. Diabetes Care 1993; 16:1579–1587.

118. Jacobson AM, Hauser ST, Willett JB, et al. Psychological adjustment to IDDM: 10-year follow-up of an onset cohort of child and adolescent patients. Diabetes Care 1997; 20:811–818.

119. Steingard RJ, Renshaw PF, Hennen J, et al. Smaller frontal lobe white matter volumes in depressed adolescents. Biol Psychiatry 2002; 52:413–417.

120. Rosso IM, Cintron CM, Steingard RJ, Renshaw PF, Young AD, Yurgelun-Todd DA. Amygdala and hippocampus volumes in pediatric major depression. Biol Psychiatry 2005; 57:21–26.

121. Matsuo K, Rosenberg DR, Easter PC, et al. Striatal volume abnormalities in treatment-naïve patients diagnosed with pediatric major depressive disorder. J Child Adolesc Psychopharmacol 2008; 18:121–131.

122. MacMaster FP, Kusumakar V. Hippocampal volume in early onset depression. BMC Medicine 2004; 2:1–6.

123. De Bellis M, Keshavan MS, Shifflett H, et al. Superior temporal gyrus volumes in pediatric generalized anxiety disorder. Biol Psychiatry 2002; 51:553–562.

124. Unal SS, Port JD, Mrazek DA. Magnetic resonance spectroscopic studies of pediatric mood disorders: A selective review. Curr Opin Pediatr 2005; 17:619–625.

125. Caetano SC, Fonseca M, Olvera RL, et al. Proton spectroscopy study of the left dorsolateral prefrontal cortex in pediatric depressed patients. Neurosci Lett 2005; 384: 321–326.

126. Farchione TR, Moore GJ, Rosenberg DR. Proton magnetic resonance spectroscopic imaging in pediatric major depression. Biol Psychiatry 2002; 52:86–92.

127. Ajilore O, Haroon E, Kumaran S, et al. Measurement of brain metabolites in patients with type 2 diabetes and major depression using proton magnetic resonance spectroscopy. Neuropsychopharmacology 2007; 32:1224–1231.

128. Caviness VS, Kennedy DN, Bates JF, Makris N. The developing human brain: a morphometric profile. In: Thatcher RW, Lyon GR, Rumsey J, Krasnegor N, eds. Developmental

Neuroimaging: Mapping the Development of Brain and Behavior. San Diego, CA: Academic Press, 1997; 3–14.

129. Chugani HT. A critical period of brain development: Studies of cerebral glucose utilization with PET. Prev Med 1998; 27: 184–188.

130. Huttenlocher PR, Dabholkar AS. Regional differences in synaptogenesis in human cerebral cortex. J Comp Neurol 1997; 387:167–178.

131. Rapoport JL, Gogtay N. Brain neuroplasticity in healthy, hyperactive, and psychotic children: Insights from neuroimaging. Neuropsychopharmacology 2008; 33:181–197.

132. Lebel C, Walker L, Leemans A, Phillips L, Beaulieu C. Microstructural maturation of the human brain from childhood to adulthood. Neuroimage 2008; 40:1044–1055.

133. Giorgio A, Watkins KE, Douaud G, et al. Changes in white matter microstructure during adolescence. Neuroimage 2008; 39:52–61.

134. McEwen BS, Reagan LP. Glucose transporter expression in the central nervous system: Relationship to synaptic function. Eur J Pharmacol 2004; 490:13–24.

135. Hawkins BT, Lundeen TF, Norwood KM, Brooks HL, Egleton RD. Increased blood-brain barrier permeability and altered tight junctions in experimental diabetes in the rat: Contribution of hyperglycaemia and matrix metalloproteinases. Diabetologia 2007; 50:202–211.

136. Ryan CM, Freed MI, Rood JA, Cobitz AR, Waterhouse BR, Strachan MWJ. Improving metabolic control leads to better working memory in adults with Type 2 diabetes. Diabetes Care 2006; 29:345–351.

137. Gradman TJ, Laws A, Thompson LW, Reaven GM. Verbal learning and/or memory improves with glycemic control in older subjects with non-insulin-dependent diabetes mellitus. J Am Geriatr Soc 1993; 41:1305–1312.

138. Naor M, Steingruber HJ, Westhoff K, Schottenfeld-Naor Y, Gries AF. Cognitive function in elderly non-insulin-dependent diabetic patients before and after inpatient treatment for metabolic control. J Diabetes Complications 1997; 11:40–46.

139. Areosa Sastre A, Grimley Evans J. Effect of the treatment of Type II diabetes mellitus on the development of cognitive impairment and dementia. The Cochrane Database of Systematic Reviews 2004:4.

Cognition in Adults with Type 1 Diabetes

Augustina M.A. Brands, Roy P.C. Kessels, and Christopher M. Ryan

CONTENTS

ABSTRACT

In this chapter, the literature on the neuropsychology of type 1 diabetes is reviewed. First, the pattern and magnitude of cognitive impairments in adults with type 1 diabetes are discussed. Cognitive decrements are limited to only some cognitive domains and can best be characterised as a slowing of mental

From: *Contemporary Diabetes: Diabetes and the Brain*
Edited by: G. J. Biessels, J. A. Luchsinger (eds.), DOI 10.1007/978-1-60327-850-8_11
© Humana Press, a part of Springer Science+Business Media, LLC 2009

speed and a diminished mental flexibility, whereas learning and memory are generally spared. Also, the cognitive decrements are mild in magnitude (i.e. within 0.5 SD of the mean of the control group) and seem neither to be progressive over time, nor to be substantially worse in older adults. Next, we focus on the results of neuroimaging studies. These studies suggest that type 1 diabetic patients have relatively subtle reductions in brain volume but these structural changes may be more pronounced in patients with an early disease onset. Furthermore, we will highlight several possible risk factors and confounding variables, including psychiatric comorbidity, recurrent hypoglycaemia, and chronic hyperglycaemia, and we will address the apparent paradox between evidence of end-organ damage in the brain as a result of diabetes versus evidence of cognitive resilience. Finally, we will discuss the implications of these findings for understanding their effects on daily life.

Key words: Neuropsychological assessment; Mental speed; Mental flexibility; Neuroimaging; Cognitive resilience

INTRODUCTION

Neuropsychology, the study of brain–behaviour relationships, has traditionally examined cognitive dysfunction secondary to neurological diseases or psychiatric disorders. With the rise of the subspecialty area 'medical neuropsychology', however, it has become apparent that many medical conditions may also affect the structure and function of the central nervous system (CNS). Diabetes mellitus has received much attention in that regard, and there is now an extensive literature demonstrating that adults with type 1 diabetes have an elevated risk of CNS anomalies. This literature is no longer limited to small cross-sectional studies in relatively selected populations of young adults with type 1 diabetes, but now includes studies that investigated the pattern and magnitude of neuropsychological decrements and the associated neuroradiological changes in much more detail, with more sensitive measurements, in both younger and older patients. This chapter sets out to review this literature and discuss the implications of these findings. First, the pattern and magnitude of cognitive impairments in adults with type 1 diabetes are discussed. Furthermore, we will highlight several possible risk factors and confounding variables including psychiatric comorbidity, recurrent hypoglycaemia, and chronic hyperglycaemia. We will address the apparent paradox between evidence of end-organ damage in the brain as a result of diabetes versus evidence of cognitive resilience. Finally, we will discuss the implications of these findings for understanding their effects on daily life.

COGNITION IN YOUNG TO MIDDLE-AGED ADULT PATIENTS WITH TYPE 1 DIABETES

Individuals with type 1 diabetes have repeatedly been reported to show modest performance deficits in a wide range of neuropsychological tests compared with non-diabetic controls. In the last decades numerous studies were published on cognition and diabetes in adults. However, the results of these studies are relatively heterogeneous with respect to the severity and nature of the affected cognitive domains, which is probably due to the wide variation with respect to patient characteristics and psychometric tests used in these studies. Recently, a meta-analysis has been performed to resolve this heterogeneity. The advantage of the meta-analytic technique is that it in effect combines all the research on one topic into one large study with many participants, thereby increasing the power. The meta-analysis clearly showed that cognitive function is mildly impaired in patients with type 1 diabetes relative to healthy controls (Fig. 1) *(1)*. In this meta-analysis, 33 studies were identified (including a total number of 660 patients) that had

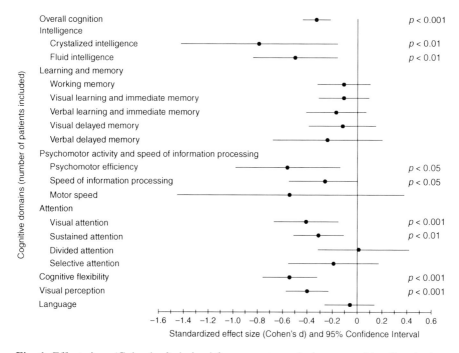

Fig. 1. Effect sizes (Cohen's *d*) derived from a meta-analysis on cognitive functioning in type 1 diabetes. (From Brands et al. *(1)*. Copyright © 2005 *American Diabetes Association*, Diabetes Care®, Vol. 28, 2005; 726–735. Reprinted with permission from *The American Diabetes Association*.)

included healthy matched control groups and used reliable neuropsychological tests at normal blood glucose values. Of note, as is also pointed out by Kodl and Seaquist *(2)*, the methodological strength of the included studies varies. Possible confounding variables that may affect neurocognitive performance include age, education level, sex, history of other chronic illnesses, psychiatric comorbidity, neurological disorders, substance abuse, absence from school, socio-economic status, and hypoglycaemia or hyperglycaemia during testing. The studies in this meta-analysis controlled for at least some of these factors, but only few controlled for all of them.

Meta-analyses on case–control studies report findings in terms of effect sizes (Cohen's *d*), that is, the standardised difference between the experimental group and the compared group *(3)*. This effect size provides information about how large a difference is evident across all studies. Compared to non-diabetic controls, the type 1 diabetic group demonstrated a significant overall lowered performance, as well as impairment in the cognitive domains intelligence, implicit memory, speed of information processing, psychomotor efficiency, visual and sustained attention, cognitive flexibility, and visual perception. There was no difference in explicit memory, motor speed, selective attention, or language function. See Chapter 4 for more detailed information on the different cognitive domains.

These results strongly support the hypothesis that there is a relationship between cognitive dysfunction and type 1 diabetes. Clearly, there is a modest, but statistically significant, lowered cognitive performance in patients with type 1 diabetes compared to non-diabetic controls. The pattern of cognitive findings does not suggest decline in all cognitive domains, but is characterised by a slowing of mental speed and a diminished mental flexibility. Patients with type 1 diabetes seem to be less able to flexibly apply acquired knowledge in a new situation. These findings suggest that patients with diabetes have difficulty with cognitively demanding or effortful tasks *(4)*. Cognitive tasks are 'effortful' when they are completely novel to the person and rely on new information-processing strategies or when they require rapid responding. Indeed, the cognitive decrements in diabetic patients can be described in terms of mental-effort problems *(4)*. Central to the mental-effort hypothesis is a limited attentional capacity. Attentional effort reflects the allocation of cognitive and behavioural resources. Patients have to invest more effort to reach the same level of performance as controls.

Similar ideas have been formulated to describe the pattern of cognitive decrements seen in normal ageing processes *(5, 6)*. For example, beginning in the twenties, a continuous, regular decline occurs for processing-intensive tasks (including speed of information processing, working memory, and delayed recall measures), whereas verbal knowledge of the world (as measured by vocabulary tests) increases across the life span *(5, 6)*. A large body of literature on cognitive functioning in ageing persons indicates that older people display deficits in cognitive domains such as memory, processing speed, attention, and executive function *(7, 8)*. This suggests that tasks requiring substantial mental effort, because they rely heavily on processing speed or involve novel and complex stimuli, are more susceptible to decline than tasks in which performance depends on automatic processing, i.e. over-learned skills, knowledge, and expertise. The common element of tasks tapping mental effort is that they require a substantial amount of cognitive control. More precisely, successful performance of such tasks critically depends on the internal representation, maintenance, and updating of context information in the service of exerting control over thoughts and behaviour *(7)*. Additionally, the resource view asserts that energy or resources that are needed during task performance are limited in their availability *(9)*. Especially controlled processes, in contrast to automatic processes, require more resources *(9)*. It could be hypothesised that patients with diabetes may be depleted of resources earlier in life than control subjects, but it is not clear how this depletion works. In all, the cognitive problems we see in type 1 diabetes mimics the patterns of cognitive ageing.

Although the magnitude of these cognitive decrements is relatively modest (within one half standard deviation of the control group, i.e. an equivalent effect size of less than 0.5), moderate forms of cognitive dysfunction can potentially hamper everyday activities and may result in problems in more demanding situations such as academic achievement or vocational situations. Consequently, they can have a negative impact on the quality of life of patients. An alternative view is that although the patient group as a whole may show only modest cognitive dysfunction, a subset of patients within this group with greater cognitive deterioration may exist. However, so far no studies have identified such a subgroup. One of the problems with much of this research is that it is conducted in patients who are seen in specialised medical centres where care is very good. Other aspects of population selection may also have affected the results. Persons who participate in research projects that include a detailed work-up at a hospital tend to be less affected than persons who refuse participation. Possibly, specific studies that recruit type 1 adults from the community, with individuals being in poorer health, would result in greater cognitive deficits, affecting daily life, in that subset of patients. Another shortcoming of the earlier studies on cognition is the fact that cognitive measures were usually restricted to those seeking clinical (rather than subclinical) deficits, while subjects tended to be relatively healthy, cooperative diabetic adults.

COGNITIVE PERFORMANCE IN OLDER PEOPLE WITH TYPE 1 DIABETES

Studies addressing cognition in type 1 diabetes predominantly examined cognition in children or young to middle-aged adults. However, it could be hypothesised that the cognitive effects of type 1 diabetes might be more pronounced in older individuals. A recent study compared the cognitive performance in 40 patients with type 1 diabetes with a mean age of 60 years with 40 age- and education-matched controls. Also, cognitive performance was related to measures of psychological well-being and cerebral magnetic resonance imaging (MRI) findings, i.e. cortical and subcortical atrophies and periventricular and deep white-matter abnormalities *(10)*. The diabetes group performed significantly worse than controls on speed of information processing (Cohen's d <0.4). No significant between-group differences were found on any of the MRI rating scales and cognitive performance was unrelated to MRI findings. Although the type 1 diabetic patients reported significantly more depressive and cognitive complaints, depressive symptoms were not correlated with cognition in this group.

Both the pattern and the severity of cognitive dysfunction in this study of older individuals are comparable with the results of the previous meta-analysis, which included only studies using adults under the age of 50. These results suggest that there may be only limited progression of cognitive deterioration over time in type 1 diabetic patients. This is in line with the very limited progression of cognitive deterioration reported in the few longitudinal studies that exist on cognitive functioning in type 1 diabetic patients who are available *(11–14)*. In order to draw firm conclusions, future longitudinal studies should examine the course of cognitive impairment in older people with type 1 diabetes in more detail.

MRI FINDINGS IN TYPE 1 DIABETES

As discussed in the previous sections, neurocognitive research suggests that type 1 diabetes is primarily associated with psychomotor slowing and reductions in mental efficiency. This pattern is more consistent with damage to the brain's white matter than with grey-matter abnormalities. Unfortunately, the relation between cognitive impairments and structural changes in the brain is a topic that has not yet been investigated in sufficient detail in patients with type 1 diabetes. The combined results of the papers discussed below indicate that MRI changes in the brain of patients with type 1 diabetes are relatively subtle. In terms of effect sizes, these are at best large enough to distinguish the patient group from the control group, but not large enough to classify an individual subject as being patient or control. Figure 2a and b

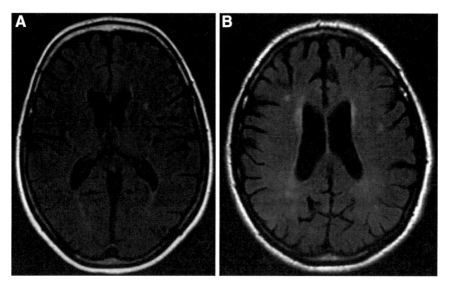

Fig. 2. Example of mild age-related white-matter lesions and atrophy in a person of 60 (**a**) and 71 (**b**) years of age.

gives an illustration of age-related white-matter lesions and atrophy that can be found in type 1 diabetes, but it is important to note that brain alterations in type 1 diabetes are not profoundly different from the age-related changes on brain MRI seen in control subjects of the same age.

The first neuropathological report on structural changes in the brain was performed in the 1960s *(15)*. That study showed that patients with severe diabetic complications showed signs of cerebral atrophy. The few studies on structural changes in the brain in patients with type 1 diabetes that have been published in the 1990s *(16, 17)* reported findings that were comparable to MRI findings in non-diabetic groups, in that similar rates of (silent) infarcts and white-matter lesion (WML) severity have been reported in random samples from the general population of the same age group *(18–20)*. It should be noted, however, that these early studies used small sample sizes, included relatively young patient groups, and used rather insensitive rating scales.

More recent studies used voxel-based morphometry (VBM) analysis of the MRI data. VBM is a sensitive method to detect subtle brain alterations in grey or white matter and thus is appropriate for use in evaluating brain-structural changes in diabetic patients. Still, these detailed studies on structural brain changes come up with contradictory reports. For example, one small study in 13 type 1 diabetic patients reported a 3% decrease in total cerebral volume, whereas hippocampal volume did not differ between type 1 diabetic patients and control subjects *(21)*. Recently, an interesting paper on the effects of type 1 diabetes on grey-matter densities (GMD) as measured by VBM was published *(22)*. This study investigated whether lower GMD in patients with type 1 diabetes were present, and if so, whether they were associated with glycaemic control and/or a history of severe hypoglycaemic events. It was found that, compared with healthy controls, patients with type 1 diabetes showed lower GMD in several brain areas. Especially the posterior, temporal, and cerebellar regions of the brain were affected. They concluded that the data suggest that areas of the brain such as the hippocampus and parahippocampal gyrus that contribute to memory and the superior temporal gyrus and angular gyrus that are important in language processing show GMD loss. This density loss was associated with both hyperglycaemia and hypoglycaemia.

Another study using VBM *(23)* investigated GMD loss in two groups of type 1 diabetic patients (with and without proliferative diabetic retinopathy) in comparison with an age- and education-matched control group of healthy participants. It showed that the patients with retinopathy, compared to the patients without retinopathy, showed reduced GMD in four brain areas: the right inferior frontal gyrus, right occipital lobe, left cerebellum, and left middle frontal gyrus. Two of these regions, the right inferior frontal gyrus and the right occipital lobe, also showed reduced GMD in comparison with the healthy participants. The patient group without retinopathy did not show reduced GMD compared with healthy participants.

Another recent study by Weinger and colleagues *(24)* examined white-matter (WM) integrity in a larger sample of young adults with type 1 diabetes of long duration and in a group of demographically similar non-diabetic adults. This study reported a similar prevalence of grade 1 and grade 2 WM hyperintensities in young adults with or without diabetes mellitus. These WM hyperintensities were not associated with depressive history or with clinical characteristics of diabetes including retinopathy, history of severe hypoglycaemia or lifetime glycaemic control. Moreover, these were not robustly associated with the cognitive test scores of either people with diabetes or in age-matched controls. These findings are consistent with those of another study *(10)* that obtained MRI and cognitive measures from 40 older diabetic participants and 40 age-matched non-diabetic comparison participants, although it has to be mentioned that this study used rather insensitive rating scales.

On the other hand, a study by Wessels and colleagues *(25)* showed that patients with a microvascular complication had a significantly smaller white-matter volume than non-diabetic controls ($p = 0.04$), and smaller white-matter volume was associated with worse performance on the domains of speed of information processing and attention and executive function. Also a co-occurrence of retinopathy (as a marker of microvascular damage) and brain abnormalities evidence was reported in another study *(26)*. That study showed that background retinopathy was associated with small punctate WM lesions corresponding to enlarged perivascular spaces.

The neuroradiological reports discussed here all used a cross-sectional design. Cross-sectional designs do not permit a distinction between acquired volume loss as a possible consequence of diabetes duration and a diminished development of brain tissue as a consequence of early diabetes onset. In theory, longitudinal studies could provide more details on the course of structural brain abnormalities and thus provide more insight into the underlying processes.

Furthermore, future studies using more sensitive neuroimaging paradigms, such as fMRI, might be more informative with respect to the apparent subtle changes in brain functioning. One example of such a study *(27)* reported a different pattern of brain activation in a group of patients with type 1 diabetes during a cognitively demanding working-memory task. Patients with diabetic retinopathy showed significantly less de-activation in the anterior cingulate and the right orbital frontal gyrus than those without retinopathy. Since the actual performance on this task was similar in the two groups, this different pattern of brain activation may reflect a compensatory mechanism *(27)*.

PSYCHIATRIC COMORBIDITY IN DIABETES MELLITUS: IS THERE A RELATIONSHIP WITH COGNITIVE IMPAIRMENT?

The prevalence of psychiatric disorders, in particular depression and anxiety disorders which are known to have a negative effect on cognition *(28, 29)*, is increased in type 1 diabetes. In a recent meta-analysis, odds ratios and prevalence of depression were estimated for both type 1 and type 2 diabetes, from 42 studies having a combined sample size of 21,351 subjects *(30)*. The main conclusion is that diabetes doubles the odds ratio. A difference in the prevalence of depression in type 1 compared to type 2 diabetes could not be established.

This increased prevalence of depression might result from an inability to cope with the stress associated with diabetes and its complicated treatment that requires strict compliance, but neurophysiological alterations in serotonin and dopamininergic activity in diabetic patients could also be involved *(31, 32)*. Disturbances in glucocorticoid metabolism may play an additional role, since several authors have suggested a relation between type 1 diabetes and a dysregulation of the hypothalamic–pituitary–adrenal axis activity *(33, 34)*.

Other biomedical factors may also play a role, since it has been reported that depressive symptoms are related to white-matter abnormalities *(35)* and severity of diabetic complications *(36)*. The association between white-matter abnormalities and depressive symptoms in older people has been labelled 'vascular depression' *(37)*. Others refer to the co-occurrence of cognitive impairments, depressed mood, and vascular dysfunction as 'vascular dementia' *(38)* or 'pseudo dementia', i.e. geriatric depression with reversible cognitive deficits *(37)*. The question of how psychological well-being is related to cognition or MRI abnormalities in type 1 diabetes has not been intensively examined yet. There are a few reports on a potential interrelationship between subclinical depressive symptoms, cognitive dysfunction, and MRI findings *(10, 24)*. These studies failed to find a clear association between these variables in their participants.

Although it is assumed that even mild-to-moderately severe levels of psychological distress have a negative impact on neuropsychological performance, the empirical evidence in diabetes suggests otherwise. The finding that psychological distress, cognitive functioning, and MRI abnormalities do not correlate *(10)* is in agreement with recent studies in healthy persons *(39)*, as well as with clinical studies of patients with chronic diseases such as multiple sclerosis *(40)* or psychiatric patients *(41)*. Together these studies imply that, unless depression or anxiety levels cross a 'clinical threshold', they do not have a serious impact on cognitive functioning. The relation between depression and diabetes is discussed in more detail in Chapter 14.

RISK FACTORS FOR COGNITIVE DYSFUNCTION

Clearly, the above-mentioned results indicate that the subtle cognitive decrements in speed of information processing and mental flexibility found in diabetic patients are not merely caused by acute metabolic derangements or psychological factors, but point to end-organ damage in the central nervous system. Although some uncertainty remains about the exact pathogenesis, several mechanisms through which diabetes may affect the brain have now been identified more clearly.

Hypoglycaemia

Until recently, most research on the pathophysiological basis of diabetic encephalopathy in type 1 diabetes was aimed at the hypothesis that hypoglycaemic events are the primary cause of neurocognitive dysfunction in type 1 diabetes. The issue whether or not repeated episodes of severe hypoglycaemia result in permanent mild cognitive impairment has been debated extensively in the literature. Several studies reported deleterious effects of repeated episodes of severe hypoglycaemia on cognition *(42–44)*. One study even reported severe deterioration in cognitive function and personality in five patients with diabetes *(45)*. The meta-analysis on the effect of type 1 diabetes on cognition *(1)* does not support the idea that there are important negative effects from recurrent episodes of severe hypoglycaemia on cognitive functioning, and large prospective studies did not confirm the earlier observations as well *(12, 46)*. Neither frequency of severe hypoglycaemia nor previous treatment-group assignment was associated with decline in any cognitive domain *(11, 12)*. Thus, there is no evidence for a linear relationship between recurrent episodes of hypoglycaemia and permanent brain dysfunction in adults. The reason for this may be that, despite the acute energy failure in the brain associated with hypoglycaemia, there might be a period in which the central nervous system is resistant to hypoglycaemia-induced damage *(47)*. This 'brain-damage free period' contrasts with immediate brain damage caused by other acute effects in the brain, such as hypoxia or ischaemia *(48)*. It has been argued that the brain actively attempts to cope with or compensate for pathology, which could be based on more efficient utilisation of brain networks or on enhanced ability to recruit alternate brain networks as needed *(49)*.

Hyperglycaemia

Toxic effects of high glucose levels are mediated by an enhanced flux of glucose along the so-called polyol and hexosamine pathways, disturbances of intracellular second messenger pathways, an imbalance in the generation and scavenging of reactive oxygen species, and by advanced glycation of important functional and structural proteins *(50)*. These mechanisms directly affect brain tissue and may lead to microvascular changes in the brain *(51)*. It could be hypothesised that these toxic effects of high glucose levels result in the initial damage to the brain. Indeed, there is evidence that cognitive changes can be detected in type 1 diabetic patients without significant vascular damage. For example, some studies using electrophysiological responses of specific CNS structures to visual, auditory, or somatosensory stimuli (evoked potentials) showed abnormalities that could be assessed before other complications *(52–56)*.

Still, microvascular complications that develop in the course of diabetes as a result of chronic hyperglycaemia, such as retinopathy and neuropathy, do appear to be associated with impaired cognition. A recent review by Kodl and Seaquist *(2)* also points out that metabolic control appears to play a role in cognitive dysfunction in type 1 diabetic patients. Functions, such as psychomotor efficiency, motor speed, attention, and memory *(12, 57)*, are improved with better glycaemic control. Furthermore, the 18-year follow-up of the Diabetes Control and Complications Trial showed that patients with higher HbA1c levels declined relatively more on motor speed and psychomotor efficiency than patients with lower HbA1c levels, but it is important to note that no other cognitive domain was related to HbA1c levels in a similar way *(12)*.

Evidence for the involvement of microvascular abnormalities in the pathogenesis of diabetic encephalopathy comes from several studies. For example, in a study in which adults with type 1 diabetes were followed for over a 7-year period, only patients with significant proliferative retinopathy showed a decline in measures of psychomotor efficiency *(58)*. Also, a higher degree of structural brain damage has been reported in diabetic patients with clinically significant retinopathy *(26)*. In line with this, a recent study suggested a link between reduced cortical grey matter and increased severity of retinopathy in diabetic patients *(22)*. Importantly, microvascular abnormalities in the retina (i.e. microaneurysms) are associated with similar patterns of cognitive deficits (namely, psychomotor slowing) in middle-aged adults without diabetes *(59)*. This is in agreement with experimental models of diabetes, demonstrating 'toxic' effects of hyperglycaemia on the brain as is discussed extensively in Chapter 17.

Cerebral microvascular pathology in diabetes may result in a decrease of regional cerebral blood flow and an alteration in cerebral metabolism, which could partly explain the occurrence of cognitive impairments. It could be hypothesised that vascular pathology disrupts white-matter integrity in a way that is akin to what one sees in peripheral neuropathy and as such could perhaps affect the integrity of neurotransmitter systems and as a consequence limits cognitive efficiency. These effects are likely to occur diffusely across the brain. Indeed, this is in line with MRI findings and other reports. If an individual is performing a cognitive task that reflects the operation of structures in multiple brain regions, and requires the integration of that neural information rapidly, then anyone who has even mild diffuse brain damage will show the types of impairments that can be found in diabetic patients (e.g. on effortful tasks that require rapid responding). This could be analogous to what is seen in individuals who have suffered mild-to-moderate closed head injuries, where the damage is primarily to white-matter integrity.

Interactive Effects

Another important issue is the interaction between different disease variables. In particular, patients with diabetes onset before the age of 5 *(60)* (see also Chapter 10) and patients with advanced microangiopathy might be more sensitive to the effects of hypoglycaemic episodes or elevated HbA1c levels. In this respect it is also important to note that in the large longitudinal study that addressed the effects of hypoglycaemia on cognition, patients with advanced microvascular complications were not included at baseline (11). Indeed, some studies (57, 61) that addressed the effect of hypoglycaemic episodes in patients with microvascular complications do report adverse effects of recurrent hypoglycaemia in this subpopulation.

The pattern and severity of cognitive changes in study populations of adult diabetic patients with an average age at diabetes onset below 15 were comparable to those with an average age at onset above this age (1). It should be noted, however, that studies that assessed cognition in children with diabetes observed that a very early age at onset (before the age of 5) appears to be associated with more severe impairments of cognitive performance (60, 62). Also, decrements in cognitive function have been observed as early as 2 years after the diagnosis (63). It is important to consider the possibility that the developing brain is more vulnerable to the effect of diabetes (see also Chapter 10). Ryan and colleagues (64) found that 24% of adolescents with diabetes that was diagnosed before the age of 5 show neuropsychological decrements compared with 6% of those diagnosed later and 6% of controls. Of course, one must take into consideration that multiple school and classroom absences, family disruptions, and other psychosocial problems associated with chronic illness may interfere with learning and with accurate cognitive assessment (64–66).

THE PARADOX: DIABETIC ENCEPHALOPATHY VERSUS COGNITIVE RESILIENCE

Although the combined results of the studies discussed in this chapter provide compelling evidence for the adverse effects of type 1 diabetes on the brain, several observations are incongruent with the concept of slowly progressing end-organ damage. First, the results from the study in older patients with type 1 diabetes (10) suggest that although patients suffer from significant peripheral complications, there is only a limited effect on the brain. In this context it is important to note that Ryan (6, 7) recently pointed out that the majority of cross-sectional studies on type 1 diabetic patients, including patients with childhood onset, typically have found quite modest cognitive decrements that hardly meet the criteria for 'clinical relevance'. These observations suggest that diabetic patients have a remarkable level of what might be best conceptualised as neurocognitive resilience (67). This line of reasoning counters the concept of 'diabetic encephalopathy', which predicts a gradual, but apparently relentless, decline over time (68, 69). If there is no inexorable neurocognitive deterioration in the vast majority of diabetic patients, the question arises as to what protects the brain from diabetes-related vascular and metabolic damage (67). The concept of 'cognitive reserve' could be of interest here *(70)*. The notion of reserve against brain damage stems from the repeated observation in clinical research that there is no direct relationship between the degree of brain pathology or brain damage and the clinical manifestation of that damage *(70)*.

IMPLICATIONS FOR CLINICAL PRACTICE

The concept of diabetic encephalopathy is probably not a useful one to describe the neurocognitive complications of type 1 diabetes in individual patients, given the relative subtlety of impairments in most cases. Indeed, cognitive disturbances relative to age-matched controls appear to be more pronounced in patients with type 2 diabetes than in patients with type 1 diabetes (see also Chapter 12). These differential effects of type 1 and type 2 diabetes on the brain are likely to be explained by differences in the pathophysiology, treatment, and comorbid conditions.

Figure 1 clearly indicates that the combined effects of type 1 diabetes and its associated conditions lead to cognitive impairment of a magnitude in the order of an effect size of 0.5 (overall cognition). Although such an effect size is relevant when comparing *different* groups, one has to acknowledge that in relation to the total variation *within* a group of individuals this effect size is rather modest. The relevance of such a difference in cognitive performance for differential diagnosis in clinical practice is fairly limited *(71)*. Nevertheless, the large variation in cognitive performance indicates that individual patients may present with cognitive impairments that are clinically relevant and hamper everyday functioning. Neuropsychological assessment may help to unravel the underlying decrements that may or may not be related to the diabetic complications or brain alterations. In general, sensitive neuropsychological tests relying on mental effort should be used to detect the subtle cognitive changes that can be expected in patients with diabetes. Furthermore, a clinician should also give attention to other risk factors of cognitive problems, such as depression.

REFERENCES

1. Brands AMA, Biessels GJ, De Haan EHF, Kappelle LJ, Kessels RPC. The effects of type 1 diabetes on cognitive performance: A meta-analysis. Diabetes Care 2005; 28:726–735.
2. Kodl CT, Seaquist ER. Cognitive dysfunction and diabetes mellitus. Endocr Rev 2008; 29:494–511.
3. Cohen, J. Statistical power analysis for the behavioral sciences. 2nd ed. Hillsdale, NJ: Erlbaum, 1988.
4. Kahneman D. Attention and effort. Englewood Cliffs, NJ: Prentice Hall Inc., 1973.
5. Park DC, Lautenschlager G, Hedden T, Davidson NS, Smith AD, Smith PK. Models of visuospatial and verbal memory across the adult life span. Psychol Aging 2002; 17:299–320.

6. Salthouse TA. What and when of cognitive aging. Curr Dir Psychol Sci 2004; 13: 140–144.

7. Braver TS, Barch DM. A theory of cognitive control, aging cognition, and neuromodulation. Neurosci Biobehav Rev 2002; 26:809–817.

8. Tisserand DJ, Jolles J. On the involvement of prefrontal networks in cognitive ageing. Cortex 2003; 39:1107–1128.

9. Wickens CD. Processing resources in attention. In: Parasuraman R, ed. Varieties of attention. Orlando, FL: Academic Press, 1984.

10. Brands AMA, Kessels RPC, Hoogma RPLM, et al. Cognitive performance, psychological well-being and brain MRI in older patients with type 1 diabetes. Diabetes 2006; 55(6):1800.

11. DCCT Research Group Effects of intensive diabetes therapy on neuropsychological function in adults in the Diabetes Control and Complications Trial. Ann Int Med 1996; 124:379–388.

12. Diabetes Control and Complications Trial/Epidemiology of Diabetes Interventions and Complications Study Research Group, Jacobson AM, Musen G, Ryan CM, et al. Long-term effect of diabetes and its treatment on cognitive function. N Engl J Med 2007; 356:1842–1852.

13. Ryan CM, Williams TM. Effects of insulin-dependent diabetes on learning and memory efficiency in adults. J Clin Exp Neuropsychol 1993; 15:685–700.

14. Reichard P, Pihl M, Rosenqvist U, Sule J. Complications in IDDM are caused by elevated blood glucose level: The Stockholm Diabetes Intervention Study (SDIS) at 10-year follow up. Diabetologia 1996; 39:1483–1488.

15. Reske-Nielsen E, Lundbaek K, Rafaelsen OJ. Pathological changes in the central and peripheral nervous system of young long-term diabetics. Diabetologia 1965; 1: 233–241.

16. Dejgaard A, Gade A, Larsson H, Balle V, Parving A, Parving HH. Evidence for diabetic encephalopathy. Diabet Med 1991; 8:162–167.

17. Lunetta M, Damanti AR, Fabbri G, Lombardo M, Di Mauro M, Mughini L. Evidence by magnetic resonance imaging of cerebral alterations of atrophy type in young insulin-dependent diabetic patients. J Endocrinol Invest 1994; 17:241–245.

18. de Leeuw F, de Groot J, Achten E, et al. Prevalence of cerebral white-matter lesions in elderly people: a population based magnetic resonance imaging study. The Rotterdam Scan Study. J Neurol Neurosurg Psychiatry 2001; 70:9–14.

19. Vermeer SE, den Heijer T, Koudstaal PJ, Oudkerk M, Hofman A, Breteler MMB. Incidence and Risk Factors of Silent Brain Infarcts in the Population-Based Rotterdam Scan Study. Stroke 2003; 34:392–396.

20. Ylikoski A, Erkinjuntti T, Raininko R, Sarna S, Sulkava R, Tilvis R. White-matter hyperintensities on MRI in the neurologically nondiseased elderly. Analysis of cohorts of consecutive subjects aged 55 to 85 years living at home. Stroke 1995; 26:1171–1177.

21. Lobnig BM, Krömeke O, Optenhostert-Porst C, Wolf OT. Hippocampal volume and cognitive performance in longstanding Type 1 diabetic patients without macrovascular complications. Diabet Med 2006; 23:32–39.

22. Musen G, Lyoo IK, Sparks CR, et al. Effects of type 1 diabetes on gray matter density as measured by voxel-based morphometry. Diabetes 2006; 55:326–332.

23. Wessels AM, Simsek S, Remeijnse PL, et al. Voxel-based morphometry demonstrates reduced grey matter density on brain MRI in patients with diabetic retinopathy. Diabetologia 2006; 49:2474–2480.

24. Weinger K, Jacobson AM, Musen G, et al. The effects of type 1 diabetes on cerebral white matter. Diabetologia 2008; 51:417–425.

25. Wessels AM, Rombouts SA, Remeijnse PL, et al. Cognitive performance in type 1 diabetes patients is associated with cerebral white matter volume. Diabetologia 2007; 50:1763–1769.

26. Ferguson SC, Blane A, Perros P, et al. Cognitive ability and brain structure in type 1 diabetes: relation to microangiopathy and preceding severe hypoglycemia. Diabetes 2003; 52: 149–156.

27. Wessels AM, Rombouts SA, Simsek S, et al. Microvascular disease in type 1 diabetes alters brain activation: a functional magnetic resonance imaging study. Diabetes 2006; 55: 334–340.

28. Elderkin-Thompson V, Kumar A, Bilker WB, et al. Neuropsychological deficits among patients with late-onset minor and major depression. Arch Clin Neuropsychol 2003; 18: 529–549.
29. Lockwood KA, Alexopoulos GS, van Gorp WG. Executive dysfunction in geriatric depression. Am J Psychiatry 2002; 159:1119–1126.
30. Anderson RJ, Freedland KE, Clouse RE, Lustman PJ. The prevalence of comorbid depression in adults with diabetes: a meta-analysis. Diabetes Care 2001; 24:1069–1078.
31. Broderick PA, Jacoby JH. Serotonergic function in diabetic rats: psychotherapeutic implications. Biol Psychiatry 1988; 24:234–239.
32. Lackovic Z, Salkovic M, Kuci Z, Relja M. Effect of long-lasting diabetes mellitus on rat and human brain monoamines. J Neurochem 1990; 54:143–147.
33. Prestele S, Aldenhoff J, Reiff J. The HPA-axis as a possible link between depression, diabetes mellitus and cognitive dysfunction. Fortschritte der Neurologie-Psychiatrie 2003; 71: 24–36.
34. Roy M, Collier B, Roy A. Dysregulation of the hypothalamo-pituitary-adrenal axis and duration of diabetes. J Diabet Complications 1991; 5:218–220.
35. Jorm AF, Anstey KJ, Christensen H, de Plater G, Kumar R, Wen W, Sachdev P. MRI hyperintensities and depressive symptoms in a community sample of individuals 60–64 years old. Am J Psychiatry 2005; 162:699–704.
36. Leedom L, Meehan WP, Procci W, Zeidler A. Symptoms of depression in patients with type II diabetes mellitus. Psychosomatics 1991; 32:280–286.
37. Alexopoulos GS, Meyers BS, Young RC, Campbell S, Silbersweig D, Charlson M. 'Vascular depression' hypothesis. Arch Gen Psychiatry 1997; 54:915–922.
38. Baldwin RC, Gallagley A, Gourlay M, Jackson A, Burns A. Prognosis of late life depression: a three-year cohort study of outcome and potential predictors. Int J Geriatr Psychiatry 2006; 21:57–63.
39. Waldstein SR, Ryan CM, Jennings JR, Muldoon MF, Manuck SB. Self-reported levels of anxiety do not predict neuropsychological performance in healthy men. Arch Clin Psychol 1997; 122:567–574.
40. Lovera J, Bagert B, Smoot KH, et al. Correlations of perceived deficits questionnaire of multiple sclerosis quality of life inventory with Beck depression inventory and neuropsychological tests. J Rehab Res Devel 2006; 43:73–82.
41. O'Jile JR, Schrimsher GW, O'Bryant SE. The relation of self-report of mood and anxiety to CVLT-C, CVLT, and CVLT-2 in a psychiatric sample. Arch Clin Neuropsychol 2005; 20: 547–553.
42. Bale RN. Brain damage in diabetes mellitus. Br J Psychiatry 1973; 122:337–341.
43. Sachon C, Grimaldi A, Digy JP, Pillon B, Dubois B, Thervet F. Cognitive function, insulin-dependent diabetes and hypoglycemia. J Int Med 1992; 231:471–475.
44. Wredling R, Levander S, Adamson U, Lins PE. Permanent neuropsychological impairment after recurrent episodes of severe hypoglycemia in man. Diabetologia 1990; 33:152–157.
45. Gold AE, Deary IJ, Jones RW, O'Hare JP, Reckless JP, Frier BM. Severe deterioration in cognitive function and personality in five patients with long-standing diabetes: a complication of diabetes or a consequence of treatment? Diabet Med 1994; 11:499–505.
46. Reichard P, Berglund A, Britz A, Levander S, Rosenqvist U. Hypoglycaemic episodes during intensified insulin treatment: increased frequency but no effect on cognitive function. J Int Med 1991; 229:9–16.
47. Chabriat H, Sachon C, Levasseur M, et al. Brain metabolism after recurrent insulin induced hypoglycemic episodes: a PET study. J Neurol Neurosurg Psychiatry 1994; 57:1360–1365.
48. Fehm HL, Kern W, Peters A. The selfish brain: competition for energy resources. Prog Brain Res 2006; 153:129–140.
49. Stern Y. What is cognitive reserve? Theory and research application of the reserve concept. J Int Neuropsychol Soc 2002; 8:448–460.
50. Brownlee M. Biochemistry and molecular cell biology of diabetic complications. Nature 2001; 414:813–820.

51. Biessels GJ, van der Heide LP, Kamal A, Bleys RLAW, Gispen WH. Ageing and diabetes: implications for brain function. Eur J Pharmacol 2002; 441:1–14.
52. Seidl R, Birnbacher R, Hauser E, Bernert G, Freilinger M, Schober E. Brainstem auditory evoked potentials and visually evoked potentials in young patients with IDDM. Diabetes Care 1996; 19:1220–1224.
53. Pozzessere G, Rizzo P, Valle E, et al. A longitudinal study of multimodal evoked potentials in diabetes mellitus. Diabet Res 1989; 10:17–20.
54. Pozzessere G, Valle E, de Crignis S, et al. Abnormalities of cognitive functions in IDDM revealed by P300 event-related potential analysis. Comparison with short-latency evoked potentials and psychometric tests. Diabetes 1991; 40:952–958.
55. Pietravalle P, Morano S, Cristina G, et al. Early complications in type 1 diabetes: central nervous system alterations preceded kidney abnormalities. Diabet Res Clin Prac 1993; 21: 143–154.
56. Donald MW, Erdahl DL, Surridge DH, Monga TN, Lawson JS, Bird CE, Letemendia FJ. Functional correlates of reduced central conduction velocity in diabetic subjects. Diabetes 1984; 33:627–633.
57. Ryan CM, Williams TM, Finegold DN, Orchard TJ. Cognitive dysfunction in adults with type 1 (insulin-dependent) diabetes mellitus of long duration: effects of recurrent hypoglycemia and other chronic complications. Diabetologia 1993; 36:329–334.
58. Ryan CM, Geckle MO, Orchard TJ. Cognitive efficiency declines over time in adults with type 1 diabetes: effects of micro- and macrovascular complications. Diabetologia 2003; 46: 940–948.
59. Wong TY, Klein R, Sharrett AR, et al. Cerebral white matter lesions, retinopathy, and incident clinical stroke. JAMA 2002; 288:67–74.
60. Ryan CM. Memory and metabolic control in children. Diabetes Care 1999; 22:1239–1241.
61. Reichard P, Britz A, Rosenqvist U. Intensified conventional insulin treatment and neuropsychological impairment. Br Med J 1991; 303:1439–1442.
62. Schoenle EJ, Schoenle D, Molinari L, Largo RH. Impaired intellectual development in children with type1 diabetes: association with HbA1c, age at diagnosis and sex. Diabetologia 2002; 45:108–114.
63. Northam EA, Anderson PJ, Werther GA, Warne GL, Andrewes D. Predictors of change in the neuropsychological profiles of children with type 1 diabetes 2 years after disease onset. Diabetes Care 1999; 22:1438–1444.
64. Ryan CM, Longstreet C, Morrow L. The effects of diabetes mellitus on the school attendance and school achievement of adolescents. Child Care Health Devel 1985; 11:229–240.
65. Ryan CM. Why is cognitive dysfunction associated with the development of diabetes early in life? The diathesis hypothesis. Pediatr Diabet 2006; 7:289–297.
66. Ho MS, Weller NJ, Ives FJ, et al. Prevalence of structural central nervous system abnormalities in early-onset type 1 diabetes mellitus. J Pediatr 2008; 153:385–390.
67. Ryan CM. Diabetes and brain damage: more (or less) than meets the eye? Diabetologia 2006; 49:2229–2233.
68. DeJong RN. The nervous system complications in diabetes mellitus with special reference to cerebrovascular changes. J Nerv Ment Dis 1950; 111:181–206.
69. Reske-Nielsen E, Lundbaek K, Rafaelsen OJ. Pathological changes in the central and peripheral nervous system of young long-term diabetics. Diabetologia 1965; 1:233–241.
70. Satz, P. Brain reserve capacity on symptom onset after brain injury: a formulation and review of evidence for threshold theory. Neuropsychology 1993; 7:273–295.
71. Zakzanis K, Leach L, Kaplan E. Neuropsychological differential diagnosis. Lisse: Swets and Zeitlinger, 1999.

12 Cognition in Type 2 Diabetes or Pre-diabetic Stages

Esther van den Berg, Yael D. Reijmer, and Geert Jan Biessels

CONTENTS

ABSTRACT

This chapter addresses the effects of type 2 diabetes mellitus on cognitive functioning. It covers the nature and severity of cognitive decrements in relation to diabetes and "pre-diabetic stages." Possible risk factors and pathophysiological mechanisms, such as vascular risk factors, hypoglycemia and hyperglycemia, microvascular and macrovascular complications, depression, genetic factors, and lifestyle, will be examined. Moreover, the chapter provides a description of structural changes in the brain, such as infarcts, white-matter hyperintensities, and brain atrophy in relation to diabetes and cognitive

From: *Contemporary Diabetes: Diabetes and the Brain*
Edited by: G. J. Biessels, J. A. Luchsinger (eds.), DOI 10.1007/978-1-60327-850-8_12
© Humana Press, a part of Springer Science+Business Media, LLC 2009

functioning. In the final sections of the chapter the implications for clinical practice and directions for future research will be discussed.

Key words: Cognitive functioning; Pre-diabetic stages; Metabolic syndrome; Brain imaging; Treatment; Clinical care.

INTRODUCTION

A 68-year-old patient with type 2 diabetes visits your clinic because of memory difficulties. He complains that "things are not going as they used to" and that he keeps forgetting things, like where he put his car keys or what he has to buy in the grocery store. He has to rely more and more on his calendar to remember appointments.

How would you evaluate these complaints? What is the relation to diabetes? Would you offer treatment? What would you tell him?

This chapter addresses the effects of type 2 diabetes mellitus on cognitive functioning and may help you to answer these questions. The chapter covers the nature and severity of cognitive decrements in relation to diabetes and "pre-diabetic stages," possible risk factors, pathophysiological mechanisms, structural changes in the brain, and implications for clinical practice.

COGNITIVE FUNCTIONING IN TYPE 2 DIABETES

Screening Tests and Neuropsychological Examination

In 1922, Miles and Root were the first to describe a possible relation between diabetes and cognitive dysfunction. They observed worse performance of patients with diabetes on measures of memory, arithmetic, and psychomotor speed compared to non-diabetic persons *(1)*. Since then, numerous studies have examined the relation between type 2 diabetes and cognitive functioning *(2–4)*. Study designs varied, from case–control to population-based sampling and from cross-sectional to longitudinal, as did the cognitive outcome measures, which varied from a full neuropsychological assessment to screening tests or a clinical diagnosis of dementia. The next section of this chapter offers a brief overview of these studies.

Thus far, the most commonly used screening test is the Mini-Mental State Examination [MMSE *(5)*]. MMSE scores range from 0 to 30 and although different cut-off scores are used, a score of 23 or below is considered an indication of cognitive impairment and 18 or below an indication of severe cognitive impairment *(6)*. The advantages and limitations of the MMSE for cognitive assessment in relation to diabetes are discussed in Chapter 4. Cross-sectional population-based studies in older individuals generally showed a 1- to 2-point lower score for patients with diabetes compared to control participants, while the scores of both groups were generally in the normal range of 24–27 (7–9). Other studies showed a 25–50% increased risk of an "impaired" score, i.e., a score below a certain threshold (7, 10). Longitudinal studies tend to show an increased decline in MMSE score of time for patients with diabetes compared to non-diabetic persons (11–14). This additional decline is relatively modest in size, for example, an extra 0.5 MMSE point decline over a 2-year interval (12).

Cognitive functioning is comprised of multiple cognitive domains, such as memory, information-processing speed, language, visuoconstruction, perception, attention, and executive functions, which can be impaired selectively [Chapter 4, (15)]. A neuropsychological examination is well-suited to examine these domains in detail and to detect relatively modest impairments in individual persons. A substantial number of studies have assessed the effect of type 2 diabetes on cognitive functioning with psychometric tests. The majority of these studies reported subtle decrements in individuals with type 2 diabetes relative to non-diabetic controls (2, 4). The cognitive domains that were assessed vary markedly between studies. Memory has been assessed most commonly, usually through tests that require a patient to repeat a short paragraph or recall a list of unrelated words that is presented to them repeatedly, for example, the Wechsler Memory Scale-Logical Memory (16) or the Rey Auditory Verbal Learning Test (17). Many studies also included a measure of information-processing speed. This involves tests in which the ability to process information within a limited amount of time is essential, such as the Digit Symbol Test of the Wechsler Adults Intelligence Scale, third edition (WAIS-III (18)), where patients are asked to copy as many symbols according to a code key in 2 min. These tests are known to be sensitive to cognitive decline and are thus used in many studies. The cognitive domains of attention and, closely related, mental flexibility have received increasing attention in recent years. Tests that are used to measure these functions include Digit Span (WAIS-III) for basic attentional processes or the Stroop Color Word Test (19) for more complex, selective attention. Mental flexibility involves the planning and monitoring of behavior and is assessed by tests such as the Trail Making Test (Part B) (20), where patients are asked to alternately connect letters and digits, and Verbal Fluency (21), where patients are asked to reproduce as many words as possible that begin with a specified letter of the alphabet over 1 min.

Cross-sectional case–control studies (mostly with sample sizes < 50) generally showed worse performance for patients with diabetes compared to age-, sex-, and education-matched control participants on measures of attention, memory, processing speed, and cognitive flexibility (22–24). Cross-sectional population-based studies in larger cohorts such as the Atherosclerosis Risk in Communities (ARIC) study and the Framingham study reported a similar pattern of cognitive decrements *(25, 26)*. The domains of perception, visuoconstruction, and language have been examined in only a minority of studies and reliable conclusions on the effect of diabetes on these domains can therefore not be drawn at this point.

The magnitude of cognitive decrements is often expressed in so-called effect sizes (see Chapter 4). Effect sizes below 0.2 are considered small, between 0.2 and 0.8 medium, and above 0.8 large *(27)*. The effect sizes of the decrements reported in non-demented persons with type 2 diabetes are mild to moderate and range from 0.2 to 0.8 relative to non-diabetic controls, with a median effect size around ~0.4 *(28)*.

Several studies have examined the impact of diabetes on cognitive functioning longitudinally *(11, 12, 29–33)*. These studies showed a 1.5- to 2-fold increased risk for patients with diabetes to perform in the "impaired" range at follow-up *(11, 29, 31)*. Other longitudinal studies showed a 1.5- to 2-fold greater decline over time on measures of processing speed, mental flexibility, and memory *(11, 12, 30, 32, 34)*. The aforementioned studies generally matched or adjusted their analysis for the confounding effects of age, sex, and educational level. Since depression is known to hamper cognitive functioning, many studies also adjusted their results for depressive symptoms.

In summary, the majority of studies in patients with type 2 diabetes reported moderate reductions in neuropsychological test performance, mainly in memory, information-processing speed, and mental flexibility, a pattern that is also observed in aging-related cognitive decline. There was some variation in the pattern of affected domains between studies, which may not only reflect differences in methods and population characteristics, but may also be due to the fact that the observed cognitive decrements are relatively subtle and rather non-specific.

PRE-DIABETES AND COGNITION

Pre-diabetic Stages

The progression from normal glucose tolerance to type 2 diabetes is a gradual process which generally proceeds unnoticed. In most cases, the very first changes in insulin and glucose metabolism already occur years before type 2 diabetes is actually diagnosed. Essential to type 2 diabetes is the reduction of insulin sensitivity in the tissue, referred to as insulin resistance *(35)* (see Chapter 2). Insulin resistance results in a compensatory increase in insulin secretion of the pancreas and abnormal plasma insulin levels, referred to as hyperinsulinemia. Eventually, the pancreas may fail to secrete enough insulin to overcome the insulin resistance and as a consequence insulin-dependent glucose uptake will drop and blood glucose concentrations rise. Depending on the glucose levels at this stage, this is referred to as impaired glucose tolerance or diabetes. Impaired glucose tolerance is defined as fasting blood glucose concentration above normal (6.1 mmol/l) and below the diabetic value (7.0 mmol/l) as well as a 2-h post-load glucose concentrations between 7.8 and 11.1 mmol/l. Higher fasting blood glucose or 2-h post-load concentrations with diabetes symptoms, such as increased urine output or unusual thirst is classified as diabetes (36). Because insulin resistance, hyperinsulinemia, and impaired glucose tolerance predispose to the development of diabetes in non-diabetic individuals these metabolic abnormalities are often referred to as pre-diabetes. However, not all individuals with insulin resistance or hyperinsulinemia will develop glucose intolerance and diabetes and each condition may occur in isolation.

Insulin resistance and disturbances in glucose metabolism often co-occur with other vascular risk factors such as hypertension, dyslipidemia, and obesity. The co-occurrence of these risk factors is usually referred to as the "the metabolic syndrome." Reaven postulated in 1988 (37) that insulin resistance should be regarded as the central driving force in this syndrome and that traditional vascular risk factors such as hypertension, diabetes, dyslipidemia and, later on, also abdominal obesity are all part of it. Since then, multiple definitions of the syndrome have been postulated, including or excluding different risk factors. The ATP-III criteria are currently the most widely applied (Table 1) (38). The metabolic syndrome predisposes to both atherosclerotic cardiovascular disease and type 2 diabetes and may also be considered a pre-diabetic condition (37, 38).

In the context of this book, which deals with cerebral complications of diabetes, it is important to address the potential impact of these pre-diabetic conditions on the brain. Indeed, several factors that are associated with insulin resistance, glucose intolerance, and the metabolic syndrome

Table 1
Criteria for the metabolic syndrome

ATP-III criteria (38)	
Impaired glucose metabolism	Fasting blood glucose ≥ 6.1 mmol/l or use of insulin/oral glucose-lowering medication
Hypertension	Blood pressure ≥ 130/85 mmHg or use of antihypertensive medication
Elevated triglycerides	Triglycerides ≥ 1.7 mmol/l
Low HDL cholesterol	HDL cholesterol < 1.3 mmol/l for women and <1.0 mmol/l for men
Abdominal obesity	Waist circumference > 88 cm for women and >102 cm for men

HDL, high-density cholesterol.

are known to be associated with an increased risk of cognitive decline and dementia. In the next section the potential impact of these factors on cognition will be addressed.

Hyperinsulinemia, Glucose Intolerance, and Cognition

Acute rises of peripheral blood glucose and insulin, after, for example, glucose ingestion, may directly influence cognitive performance (see Chapter 18). Indeed, acute improvement of cognitive performance has been reported after ingestion of glucose *(39)*. However, these changes are temporary. The consequences of long-term exposure to elevated blood glucose or insulin levels, which are considered in this chapter, may be quite different.

Population-based studies showed that persons with hyperinsulinemia, but no diabetes, have an increased risk for cognitive decrements compared to persons with normal blood insulin levels *(40–43)*. The cognitive domains mostly affected were memory, attention, and mental flexibility. One study found evidence for greater cognitive decline over a 6-year period for persons with hyperinsulinemia compared to those without *(43)*. The observed effects were at least partially independent of cardiovascular disease, hypertension, and other risk factors associated with the insulin resistance syndrome.

Similar changes are observed in persons with poor glucoregulation. In the studies mentioned here, participants were classified as having impaired glucose tolerance according to the formal definition *(36)* or an abnormal glucose recovery index after a glucose tolerance test *(44)*. In these studies poor glucoregulation was associated with reduced performance on a variety of cognitive tests, mainly measuring verbal memory (word list and story recall) *(41, 44–47)*. The observed changes in cognitive functioning were relatively small, with effect sizes ranging from 0.1 to 0.2 and thus appear to be somewhat less pronounced than in type 2 diabetes. Not all case–control studies found a relationship between glucose regulation and cognitive performance *(48, 49)*. Only two out of six longitudinal studies found an increased risk for cognitive decline for persons with impaired glucose tolerance at baseline *(29, 31, 32, 50–52)*. However, one of these two studies was the only study that measured glucose tolerance at baseline and during follow-up *(50)*. Cognitive changes in persons with poor glucoregulation are primarily observed in older individuals, although this association is demonstrated in younger adults as well *(45, 46)*.

The Metabolic Syndrome and Cognition

A number of studies have examined cognitive functioning in persons with the metabolic syndrome *(53–58)*. A cross-sectional study showed worse cognitive performance for person with the metabolic syndrome compared to those without on the MMSE and measures of memory, information-processing speed, and fluid intelligence (effect size ∼–0.3) *(53)*. Three longitudinal studies that examined the association between the metabolic syndrome and cognitive functioning also showed a 1.2- to 4-fold increased risk of cognitive decline over time *(54–56)*. In contrast, one longitudinal study in a population-based sample of very old persons (>85 years) showed that the metabolic syndrome was actually associated with a *decelerated* cognitive decline *(57)*, but the implications of this observation are still unclear. Three of the aforementioned studies also reported an interaction with inflammation *(54–56)*, where individuals with the metabolic syndrome and high levels of inflammation were at greatest risk of cognitive impairment.

While the number of studies that assessed cognitive functioning in persons with the metabolic syndrome is still limited, the relation between individual components of the metabolic syndrome, in particular hypertension, and cognitive functioning has been examined more extensively. Cross-sectional studies generally showed a decreased performance for hypertensive persons compared to normotensive individuals in memory, processing speed, and cognitive flexibility *(25, 59)* with effect sizes that are comparable to those found in studies on cognitive functioning in diabetes. Longitudinal studies tended to show increased risk of cognitive decline *(60, 61)*, although not invariably *(62)*. Interestingly, in these studies an interaction with age is observed where hypertension in midlife was associated with an increased risk of late-life cognitive impairment and dementia, while the link between hypertension at a more advanced age and cognitive functioning was less clear. In fact, some studies showed inverse effects where in old age low blood pressure was actually associated with decreased cognitive performance *(63)*.

Some studies on cognitive functioning in relation to obesity showed worse cognitive performance in persons with a BMI over 25 or 30 kg/m^2 *(61, 64)* compared to normal-weight individuals, but others failed to show such associations *(54)*. Studies that assessed obesity at midlife generally showed a more consistent relation with worse cognitive performance than studies that assessed obesity at late-life. Similar to obesity, the findings of studies on the relation between dyslipidemia and cognition are not always consistent. Some studies reported an increased risk of cognitive impairment associated with high levels of total cholesterol or triglycerides *(56, 65)*, whereas other studies showed inverse associations where high cholesterol was associated with better cognition or low cholesterol with worse cognition *(66, 67)*. For a more detailed overview on the relative impact of each of these vascular risk factors on cognition we refer to two recent reviews from our group *(28, 68)*.

All in all, disturbances in glucose and insulin metabolism and associated vascular risk factors are associated with modest reductions in cognitive performance in "pre-diabetic stages." Consequently, it may well be that the cognitive decrements that can be observed in patients with type 2 diabetes also start to develop before the actual onset of the diabetes. In this regard it is important to note that the size and profile of the cognitive decrements associated with insulin resistance, hyperinsulinemia, impaired glucose tolerance, the metabolic syndrome and its components are similar to each other and to the cognitive decrements found in type 2 diabetes. Because the different vascular and metabolic risk factors that are clustered in the metabolic syndrome are strongly interrelated, the contribution of each of the individual factor will be difficult to assess. Rather than teasing out the individual contributions of risk factors it could be more rewarding to assess shared etiology or consequences, such as atherosclerosis or insulin resistance, and develop treatment strategies directed at these common components.

BRAIN IMAGING IN TYPE 2 DIABETES

Structural Changes in Normal Aging

Aging-related changes on brain imaging include vascular lesions and focal and global atrophy. Vascular lesions include (silent) brain infarcts and white-matter hyperintensities (WMHs). WMHs are common in the general population and their prevalence increases with age, approaching 100% by the age of 85 *(69)*. The prevalence of lacunar infarcts also increases with age, up to 5% for symptomatic infarcts and 30% for silent infarcts by the age of 80 *(70)*. In normal aging, the brain gradually reduces in size, which becomes particularly evident after the age of 70 *(71)*. This loss of brain volume is global, including enlargement of the ventricles (subcortical atrophy) and cortical sulci (cortical atrophy). Figure 1 shows examples of these aging-related changes in the brain, which can be detected on computed tomography (CT) or magnetic resonance imaging (MRI).

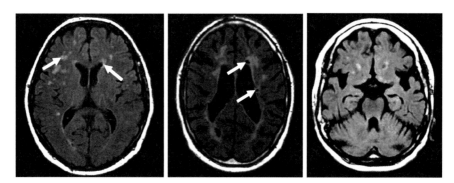

Fig. 1. White-matter hyperintensities, infarctions, and atrophy of the brain. These MRI images (FLAIR-sequence) show typical age-related changes of the brain that are often relatively more pronounced in older patients with type 2 diabetic. The picture on the left shows punctuate deep (*left arrow*) and periventricular (*right arrow*) white-matter hyperintensities. The middle picture shows subcortical lacunar infarctions and enlarged ventricles. The picture on the right shows global cortical atrophy.

Brain Imaging in Patients with Type 2 Diabetes and Pre-diabetic Stages

Population-based studies reported an increased prevalence and incidence of lacunar infarcts in patients with type 2 diabetes *(70, 72–74)*. A recent systematic review showed that patients with diabetes have a 2-fold increased risk of (silent) infarcts compared to non-diabetic persons *(75)*. The relationship between type 2 diabetes and WMHs is subject to debate. Several large population-based studies did not observe a significant association between diabetes and WMHs *(75–77)*. The use of relatively crude, insensitive WMH rating scales may explain some of the inconsistencies. Recent case–control studies that applied a more refined WMH rating scale and volumetric measurements reported a modest increase in WMH severity in patients with type 2 diabetes *(78–81)*, and there are now clear indications that diabetes is a risk factor for WMH progression *(82)*.

Brain atrophy can be assessed with relatively simple measures such as ordinal rating scales or one-dimensional ventricle-to-brain ratios or more sophisticated techniques such as fully automated volumetry. Modest degrees of global atrophy have been demonstrated in patients with type 2 diabetes with each of these techniques *(75, 83, 84)*. Given the association between type 2 diabetes and Alzheimer's disease (see also Chapter 13) atrophy in specific brain regions such as the medial temporal lobe is of particular interest. Some population-based studies have indeed shown that type 2 diabetes was associated with reduced hippocampal and/or amygdalar volumes on MRI *(77, 85)* and a 3-fold increased risk of severe medial temporal lobe atrophy *(74)*. Although abnormalities in hippocampal volume may be an early manifestation of brain atrophy in type 2 diabetes *(86)*, it is not yet clear whether temporal lobe structures are particularly vulnerable to diabetes-related atrophy.

To date, the number of studies that specifically addressed the relation between brain abnormalities and cognitive functioning in patients with type 2 diabetes is limited. Some studies showed that, within a group of patients with type 2 diabetes, cognitive functioning was related to white-matter hyperintensities, atrophy, and the presence of infarcts *(78, 87)*. Another study observed an independent association between periventricular white-matter lesion and motor speed, but no association between other MRI measures and cognitive performance *(9)*.

Some evidence exists that the aforementioned brain imaging abnormalities start to develop in the pre-diabetic stage. One study found that reduced peripheral glucose regulation was not only associated with smaller hippocampal volume, but also with decreased general cognitive performance and memory performance in healthy elderly *(47)*. Moreover, hyperinsulinemia, impaired glucose tolerance, insulin resistance, and the metabolic syndrome are previously reported as risk factors for lacunar infarcts, atrophy, and white-matter hyperintensities *(77, 88–91)*. WMHs and infarcts have also been associated with diabetes-related complications such as retinal microvascular disease *(92)* and microalbuminuria *(91)*. However, there are inconsistencies between studies, possibly partially due to confounding effects of other associated risk factors.

Vascular risk factors that are closely related to diabetes, such as hypertension, dyslipidemia, and obesity, have been examined in more detail in relation to abnormalities on brain MRI. Hypertension is one of the most important risk factors for stroke in the general population *(70)* and is also strongly associated with WMHs *(93)*. Dyslipidemia is also strongly associated with stroke, but associations with lacunar infarcts, WMHs, or atrophy are less clear *(89, 94, 95)*. Obesity appears to be associated with reduced global brain volume and hippocampal volume *(96, 97)*. Some studies showed an independent relationship between obesity and lacunar infarcts *(88)* and WMHs *(98)*, but others failed to show such associations *(72, 90)*.

DETERMINANTS AND MECHANISMS

Possible risk factors for changes in cognitive functioning and brain structure in patients with type 2 diabetes include diabetes-specific factors (e.g., hyperglycemia, glucose-lowering therapy, microvascular complications), factors that are linked to diabetes but are not specific to the disease (e.g., hypertension, stroke, depression), genetic factors and demographic, socio-economic, and lifestyle factors (Fig. 2). All of these risk factors may affect cognitive functioning at different times during life span, but there are still relatively few studies that have specifically addressed these risk factors in relation to cognition in patients with type 2 diabetes.

Genetic Factors

Genetic predisposition possibly plays a role in the association between type 2 diabetes, cognitive impairment, and dementia, but thus far only the role of the apolipoprotein (APOE) genotype and the Pro12Ala polymorphism of peroxisome proliferator-activated receptor-gamma (PPARG) genotype has been examined. The presence of the APOE ε4 allele is a risk factor for the development of Alzheimer's disease *(99)*. Patients with type 2 diabetes who carry the APOE ε4 allele appeared to have a 2-fold increased risk of dementia compared to persons with either of these risk factors in isolation *(100, 101)*. Data on the risk of cognitive impairment in non-demented persons are limited. Some studies reported an interaction with APOE where APOE ε4 allele carriers who had diabetes had the highest risk of cognitive decline *(14, 102, 103)*. Results of the Rancho Bernardo Study *(32)*,

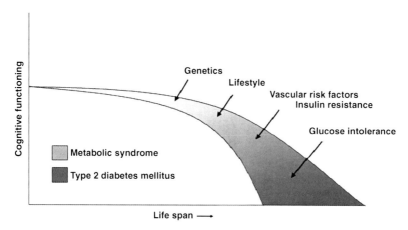

Fig. 2. Relation between type 2 diabetes, related risk factors and cognitive decline. It shows a putative course of development for cognitive dysfunction in type 2 diabetes. In our view, impaired cognitive functioning in patients with type 2 diabetes develops against a background of genetic predisposition and socio-economic and lifestyle factors. In midlife, the presence of vascular risk factors such as hypertension and obesity starts to play an important role, together with insulin resistance, both by increasing the risk of developing diabetes and atherosclerotic vascular disease and by independent associations with cognitive decline and dementia later in life. The development of hyperglycemia, glucose intolerance, and microvascular and macrovascular complications that are associated with type 2 diabetes then further accelerates diabetes-associated brain dysfunction.

however, failed to show such interaction. A recent study on the role of PPARG Pro12Ala further suggested that risk of cognitive decline is greater in Pro12Ala carriers who develop diabetes *(104)*.

Demographics and Lifestyle

Several demographic factors, such as socio-economic status, age, and sex, are associated with both type 2 diabetes and cognitive dysfunction. For example, women with a lower socio-economic status or a lower educational level have 20–60% increased odds of having type 2 diabetes *(105)*. In addition, the risk of cognitive decline and dementia is increased for persons with lower socio-economic status or educational level *(106, 107)*. Factors such as gender and ethnic background also affect the incidence of vascular disease and vascular risk factors *(108–110)*. These demographic factors may therefore play a role in the association between type 2 diabetes and cognitive decline. The majority of studies that were reviewed in earlier sections of this chapter take the possible confounding effects of sex, ethnicity, and level of education into account, but systematic examination of the potential role of these demographic factors in the association between diabetes and cognitive functioning is lacking. Examination of the results of studies that specifically assessed cognitive functioning in women (111), or men (112), with type 2 diabetes shows essentially the same cognitive impairments across both sexes. The impact of ethnicity is unclear, but the results of studies that adjusted their analyses for ethnic background (25, 49) were similar to those of studies who did not explicitly adjust for this variable. Moreover, the risk of dementia in relation to diabetes was quite consistent across populations from different continents (113).

The effects of age deserve special attention, as type 2 diabetes is particularly common among older individuals. Also, age is an important risk factor for both cognitive decline and type 2 diabetes. As was mentioned in an earlier section of this chapter, the pattern of neuropsychological deficits in younger patients with diabetes, with mild impairments across the cognitive domains, and the largest effects in the domains, verbal memory, information-processing speed, and executive functioning, resembles the pattern of cognitive decline seen in older persons without diabetes (114, 115). The effects of age and type 2 diabetes on cognitive functioning may thus interact, which is supported by both studies in patients with type 2 diabetes and in experimentally diabetic rodents (116). Such interaction would also be plausible from a mechanistic point of view as several of the mechanisms that are assumed to mediate the toxic effects of hyperglycemia on the brain, such as oxidative stress, the accumulation of advanced glycation end-products, and microangiopathy are also implicated in brain aging (117).

Lifestyle factors, such as smoking and diet, are associated with both type 2 diabetes (118, 119) and with cognitive decline and dementia (120, 121). Similar to demographic factors, such as sex and socio-economic status, these factors are potentially confounding factors in the association between type 2 diabetes and cognitive decline. More importantly, these factors are potentially modifiable, which may reduce the risk of both type 2 diabetes and cognitive impairment.

(Midlife) Vascular Risk Factors

As was described in the previous paragraphs, hypertension, obesity, and dyslipidemia are associated with cognitive decline and may thus be involved in the association between type 2 diabetes and cognitive decline. Thus far, studies on the role of vascular risk factors in the association between diabetes and impaired cognition have focused on hypertension. Several studies have shown cumulative or interactive effects of hypertension and type 2 diabetes (26, 122). Other studies, however, do not confirm these results (11, 31, 32, 74). Studies that failed to show interaction or additive associations tend to involve study populations of relatively high age (>70). A recent review on vascular risk factors for dementia has shown that for many vascular risk factors the risk of late-life dementia is generally largest in studies that measured the risk factor in midlife (compared to late-life) and had a long follow-up time *(68)*. These results suggest that midlife hypertension, even in pre-diabetic stages, may indeed be additive to the effects of type 2 diabetes on cognitive functioning later in life.

Data on the effect of (midlife) lipid levels and obesity on cognitive functioning in patients with type 2 diabetes are limited. A recent longitudinal study on predictors of cognitive impairment and dementia in older ($\geq$70) patients with diabetes showed that higher baseline total cholesterol level was associated with a 30% decreased risk of cognitive impairment after 7 years *(123)*. Higher baseline waist-to-hip ratio was associated with a 50% decreased risk of cognitive impairment in this study. In addition, a cross-sectional study showed a modest association between the use of lipid-lowering drugs and better cognitive performance *(124)*.

Hyperglycemia and Hypoglycemia

Studies in patients with type 1 diabetes suggest that chronic exposure to hyperglycemia may have a negative impact on cognitive function *(125)*. Several studies in patients with type 2 diabetes reported similar findings. Longer duration of type 2 diabetes was associated with a greater risk of cognitive impairment *(9, 11, 26)* and elevated HbA1c levels, which reflect chronic hyperglycemia, are found to be associated with impaired cognition in type 2 diabetes *(9, 32, 78, 126–128)*, although not invariably *(129, 130)*. Figure 3 shows a dose–response relation between quartiles of HbA1c and cognitive performance [adapted from *(131)*]. A study on acute effects of hyperglycemia further added to these findings that hyperglycemia may be associated with short-term fluctuations in cognitive functioning *(132)*. For these acute fluctuations the relationship with glucose levels is non-linear, and there may be a threshold of glucose levels around 15 mmol/l when cognitive functioning starts to get affected *(132)*.

Hypoglycemia is a well-known complication of glucose-lowering therapy. Although severe hypoglycemic episodes are much less common in type 2 than in type 1 diabetes, such episodes may have detrimental effects on the brain. Data on the impact of hypoglycemic episodes on cognition in type 2 diabetes are limited. A cross-sectional study did not find an association between the prevalence of hypoglycemic episodes and cognition *(78)*. A recent longitudinal study observed an association between the prevalence of severe hypoglycemia and the prevalence of cognitive impairment and dementia at follow-up, but showed no difference in the baseline prevalence

HbA1c quartiles

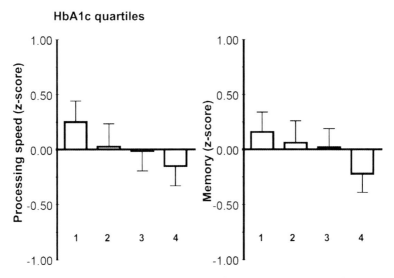

Fig. 3. Relation between HbA1c level and performance on two cognitive domains. (Adapted from Tiehuis et al. *(131)* with permission from Future Medicine Ltd.)

of hypoglycemic episodes in persons who developed cognitive impairment after 7 years follow-up and those who did not *(123)*. In type 1 diabetes a meta-analysis *(125)* and results from the Diabetes Control and Complications Trial (DCCT) *(133)* provided no evidence for an association between the occurrence of hypoglycemic episodes and impaired cognition, despite the fact that small case series suggested that such an association might exist *(134)*.

Microvascular and Macrovascular Complications

In general, longer duration of diabetes and worse glycemic control are associated with an increased prevalence, progression, and severity of microvascular end-organ complications both in type 1 as well as in type 2 diabetes *(135, 136)*. In adults with type 1 diabetes the occurrence of microvascular complications is associated with reduced cognitive performance *(137)* and accelerated cognitive decline *(138)*. Moreover, type 1 diabetes is associated with decreased white-matter volume of the brain and diminished cognitive performance in particular in patients with retinopathy *(139)*. Microvascular complications are also thought to play a role in the development of cognitive decline in patients with type 2 diabetes, but studies that have specifically examined this association are scarce.

Macrovascular disease, including previous vascular events, presence of plaques in the carotid arteries, and presence of peripheral arterial atherosclerotic disease, is associated with age-related cognitive impairment *(140)* in the general population. Type 2 diabetes is associated with an increased risk of macrovascular complications. In a recent study in patients with type 2 diabetes macrovascular atherosclerotic disease appeared to be the most consistent determinant of impaired cognition and brain MRI abnormalities *(78)*. In addition, peripheral artery disease was associated with a 2- to 5-fold increased risk of developing cognitive impairment or dementia in a population of older patients with type 2 diabetes *(123)* and a history of cerebrovascular disease was associated with a 3-fold increased risk of a low MMSE score *(141)*.

Depression

A recent meta-analysis reported that patients with type 2 diabetes have a 2-fold increased risk of depression compared to non-diabetic persons *(142)*. The prevalence of major depressive disorder in patients with type 2 diabetes was estimated at 11% and depressive symptoms were observed in 31% of the patients. A recent study in 907 elderly patients with type 2 diabetes showed that higher depression scores were associated with a 10% increased risk of cognitive impairment, measured with MMSE *(141)*. However, the exact nature of the relation between type 2 diabetes and depression is incompletely understood. Depression may result from coping with chronic disease or from metabolic consequences of type 2 diabetes, even at the level of cerebral neurotransmitters. Conversely, depression may even predispose the development of type 2 diabetes *(143)*. Although depressive symptoms probably play a role in the etiology of diabetes-associated cognitive decrements, only a proportion of the patients with diabetes develop clinically relevant depressive symptoms. It is therefore unlikely that depression explains the whole association between diabetes and cognition. Moreover, the majority of studies that assessed cognition in relation to diabetes controlled for the potential confounding effects of depression. Chapter 14 offers a more detailed overview of relation between diabetes and depression.

TREATMENT OPPORTUNITIES

Currently there are no established specific treatment measures to prevent or ameliorate cognitive impairments in patients with diabetes. However, some of the factors that are discussed in the previous sections of this chapter, in particular blood glucose levels and vascular risk factors, are potential targets for intervention and are increasingly being examined in treatment studies that include cognition as an outcome measure.

There are indications that cognitive dysfunction in patients with type 2 diabetes is partially reversible with improvement of glycemic control

(144–148), though not invariably *(149)*. These observations will need to be confirmed in properly designed randomized clinical trials on the effects of intensified glucose-lowering therapy versus standard treatment *(150)*. A recent randomized trial comparing the effects of rosiglitazone to glyburide therapy found similar and statistically significant cognitive improvement in both treatment groups on measures of working memory, but not on learning and cognitive speed *(144)*. The magnitude of the improvement was correlated with the degree to which fasting plasma glucose improved (correlation coefficient $r = 0.30$). The DCCT trial, however, showed no differences in cognitive functioning after 6.5 years between type 1 diabetes patients who received conventional treatment versus those who received intensive treatment *(151)*. Cognitive performance also remained similar in the two groups after 18 years of follow-up *(133)*.

Regarding the effects of improved glycemic control on cognition, it is difficult to disentangle the interplay between (1) patient factors, which demand a particular therapy, (2) potential direct effects of treatment on the brain, and (3) indirect effects of treatment on the brain, through modulation of glucose levels. This complex interplay, which prohibits inferences on causality, is clearly reflected in observations from the Rotterdam study, where patients receiving insulin treatment had the highest risk of developing dementia [OR 4.3 (95% CI 1.7–10.5)], oral glucose-lowering medication was associated with an intermediate risk [OR 2.4 (95% CI 1.4–4.1)] and the lowest risk was found in patients who received no drug treatment [OR 1.3 (95% CI 0.7–2.3)] (152).

It is yet uncertain whether reductions in the level of vascular risk factors will prevent cognitive decline in patients with type 2 diabetes. Studies in the general population thus far do not consistently demonstrate that modifications of vascular risk factors can delay cognitive decline or dementia *(153–155)*, despite the fact that such treatment effectively prevents macrovascular events such as stroke or myocardial infarction. Limitations of the available studies, including timing and duration of the interventions, may be a source of this uncertainty and vascular risk factors remain a promising target for therapy. Results from further studies on this topic are therefore eagerly awaited. A study in a small cohort of hyperlipidemic patients with type 2 diabetes who were treated with atorvastatin showed that verbal memory improvement was associated with improvement of the diabetic dyslipidemia profile, regardless of high- or low-dose atorvastatin *(156)*.

Other approaches include physical activity, lowering of glucocorticoid levels, and reducing oxidative stress. Certain types of physical activity, including light and moderate exercise, appear to be beneficial to cognitive functioning in patients with type 2 diabetes *(157)*. In a small randomized, placebo-controlled study administration of the 11β-hydroxysteroid dehydrogenase inhibitor carbenoxolone improved verbal memory after 6 weeks in 12 patients with type 2 diabetes *(158)*. Moreover, reduction of oxidative stress by taking high-dose antioxidant supplements after a high-fat meal prevented an acute post-prandial decline in delayed verbal memory in 16 patients with type 2 diabetes *(159)*.

IMPLICATIONS FOR CLINICAL CARE

In the previous sections of this review we have summarized the results from studies on cognition and brain imaging in groups of patients with diabetes. How should these results be translated to the level of an individual patient who attends your clinic (Table 2)? Obviously, not all patients with type 2 diabetes will experience changes in cognitive functioning and cognitive impairments in a patient with type 2 diabetes are not always due to diabetes. Moreover, while subtle cognitive decrements may be an early manifestation of dementia in the years to come, not all patients with cognitive impairments progress to frank dementia.

Nevertheless, in our view the cognitive decrements as discussed in this chapter should have implications for clinical care for individual patients with type 2 diabetes. Clinicians should be aware of the fact that cognitive decrements are relatively more common among patients with diabetes. We hope that this book will contribute to this awareness, which should lead to an increased degree of suspicion and alertness with regard to possible cognitive deterioration. In this respect it is important to note that cognitive complaints as spontaneously expressed by the patient are often a poor indicator of the severity of cognitive decrements. People with moderate disturbances may express marked complaints, while people with marked disturbances of cognition often do not complain at all. If one suspects that cognition may be affected in an individual patient it is of particular importance to get an impression of the impact of the "cognitive disturbances" on day-to-day functioning. Ask about the impact on professional, household, leisure, and social activities. It is also essential to supplement the history given by the patient with one given by a partner, relative, or close friend. Table 3 offers some questions that can be used for screening purposes. If this initial screening step provides indications for cognitive decrements it is important to get insight into the course of development, nature, and extent of the cognitive problems. Changes in behavior, mood, and personality should also be addressed. For a brief and simple cognitive screening the MMSE is widely used. When a structured interview and the MMSE indeed point to a decline in cognitive functioning further examination is indicated. Depending on the nature and severity of the complaints and the expertise of the clinician, patients can be referred to a specialist in the field of cognitive

Table 2
A typical case – continued

The 68-year-old patient whom we introduced in the beginning of this chapter was first diagnosed with type 2 diabetes 10 years ago. He is currently treated with oral glucose-lowering drugs. His A1c levels generally varied between 6 and 7%. There are no known microvascular complications. He is slightly overweight and has elevated blood pressure. When he visits his general practitioner together with his wife, his complaints are rather vague. He noticed "things were not going as they used to" and he kept "forgetting things.". His wife mentions that her husband used to be a good cook, but nowadays he is not able to organize a proper meal without forgetting an ingredient or he lets something burn. When he comes back from the grocery store, there is always something missing. The first changes were noticed by his wife and children about a year ago. Since then the mistakes occurred more frequent. After the structured interview the general practitioner has no evidence for depression or stressful life events. The patient seems emotionally stable but worried about the whole situation. He is afraid of becoming demented. The cognitive problems he reports are primarily related to memory and attention functions.

The practitioner decides to refer the patient for neuropsychological assessment to obtain more detailed information about the cognitive profile. The assessment reveals no focal impairments, but shows a profile of mental slowing and some difficulty in processing unstructured material, with test scores falling in the 20th to 30th percentile compared to an age- and education-matched norm group. Based on this information the practitioner sees no need for further examination. He ensures them that the patient is not demented, but that the diabetes may cause the process of normal cognitive aging to go somewhat faster. The patient decides to improve his diet and starts exercising in order to further improve his glycemic control. His blood pressure will be treated by medication. From that moment on, extra attention is given to the cognitive status and control of potential risk factors.

deterioration, such as a neurologist or geriatrician to undergo more extensive physical and (neuro)psychological examination (Table 4). A neuropsychological assessment can help to quantify the exact cognitive profile and severity of the problems. Diabetes is generally associated with relatively mild impairments, mainly in attention, memory, information-processing speed, and executive function. Rapid cognitive decline or severe cognitive impairment, especially in persons under the age of 60 is indicative of other underlying pathology. Potentially treatable causes of cognitive decline such as depression should be excluded. People who are depressed often present with complaints of concentration or memory. Other potentially influencing factors such as hypothyroidism, alcohol dependence syndrome, and drug use (e.g., use of benzodiazepines, opioids, anticholinergics, and tricyclic

Table 3
Relevant issues in the examination of a patient with type 2 diabetes with complaints in cognitive functioning

Changes in cognitive functioning?
- Memory: forgetting recent activities and news items, losing things
- Attention, mental flexibility, and planning: concentration and distractibility (reading, watching TV), doing two simultaneous tasks, forgetting appointments
- Course of development: slow decrease in functioning or clear decline in the previous year?
- Cognitive screening measure: Mini-Mental State Examination (MMSE)

Changes in daily functioning?
- Instrumental activities: using telephone, managing money, cooking, managing medication
- Does spouse/family member take over these activities?
- Questionnaires: Instrumental Activities of Daily Living (IADL) *(160)*

Changes in mood and behavior?
- Agitation and aggression: not cooperative, not allowing someone to help, impatience, easily irritated
- Depression, sadness
- Anxiety: nervous, unable to relax
- Apathy: decreased interest in normal activities of self and others, indifference
- Questionnaires: Beck Depression Inventory (BDI) *(161)*, Neuropsychiatric Inventory (NPI) *(162)*

antidepressants) should also be considered. Hence, the diagnostic work-up in patients with diabetes with cognitive dysfunction is in essence identical to that of people without diabetes.

Based on the outcome of the diagnostic assessment an etiologic diagnosis may be formed (see also Chapter 5). When diabetes is identified as the sole risk factor for the cognitive complaints in an individual patient and the nature and severity of the cognitive decrements are compatible with what one would expect in relation with diabetes, this can be conveyed to the patient and partner/family. It is important to provide a balanced view on the risk of further cognitive decline and the potential relation with diabetes-related risk factors. The course of development of the complaints should be monitored by the clinician, patient, and his family. There is as yet no evidence-based treatment for diabetes-related cognitive decline. A pragmatic approach is to monitor and treat vascular and metabolic risk factors. Although the evidence for this approach is limited to the reduction of the risk and progression of macrovascular events and microvascular complications, it might also

Table 4
Recommendations for further examination concerning patients with suspected cognitive decline[1]

Laboratory assessment[2]
– A1c and glucose level
– Hb, Ht, MCV, BSE, TSH, creatinine
– Consider vitamin B_1, B_6, B_{12}, foliumzuur, Na, K

Neuropsychological assessment
Consider in order to
– Quantify cognitive impairments
– Determine which cognitive domains are affected (attention, memory, language, visual perception, orientation, executive functions)
– Assess the role of mood disorders
– Assess personality changes

Brain imaging[2]
– MRI or CT is recommended in case of frank cognitive impairments
– Additional arguments to perform brain imaging: rapid cognitive decline, focal neurological deficits, early onset of cognitive impairments (<65 years)

[1]The diagnostic work-up for persons with suspected cognitive decline is essentially identical for person with or without type 2 diabetes.
[2]Consult local guidelines, see also Chapter 5 and, for example *(163, 164)*.

minimize the detrimental effects of diabetes on the brain. If an etiologic diagnosis other than diabetes alone is made, such as (early) Alzheimer's disease or vascular dementia the management of the patient should be performed according to guidelines for these conditions (see also Chapter 5). Finally, in patients in whom no specific therapy can be offered, the physician can offer guidance of the patient and his or hers next of kin, especially when loss of function and behavioral changes set in.

CONCLUSIONS AND DIRECTIONS FOR FURTHER RESEARCH

The development of cognitive impairments in patients with type 2 diabetes appears to represent a continuum, with an onset in the pre-clinical stages of diabetes and a gradual progression thereafter. Although the data on cognitive decrements are difficult to translate to the individual patient, there is a substantial impact at the population level. Currently 6–8% of all cases of late-life dementia may be attributed to type 2 diabetes *(68)*. Owing to the western lifestyle and aging of the population, the prevalence of type 2 diabetes is likely to increase and so is the incidence of cognitive decline and dementia attributable to type 2 diabetes.

Because of the lack of specific therapy, there is a need for further mechanistic studies. Gaining more insight into the causal relationship and interaction of different risk factors is crucial to develop effective treatment strategies. Besides improvement of therapy, interventions should aim to prevent the development of diabetes and associated risk factors. Changes in diet and lifestyle are in this regard modifiable risk factors and the effectiveness of these strategies during different diabetic stages should be investigated.

REFERENCES

1. Miles WR, Root HF. Psychologic tests applied in diabetic patients. Arch Intern Med 1922; 30:767–777.
2. Stewart R, Liolitsa D. Type 2 diabetes mellitus, cognitive impairment and dementia. Diabet Med 1999; 16:93–112.
3. Strachan MWJ, Deary IJ, Ewing FME, Frier BM. Is type II diabetes associated with an increased risk of cognitive dysfunction? A critical review of published studies. Diabetes Care 1997; 20:438–445.
4. Awad N, Gagnon M, Messier C. The relationship between impaired glucose tolerance, type 2 diabetes, and cognitive function. J Clin Exp Neuropsychol 2004; 26:1044–1080.
5. Folstein MF, Folstein SE, McHugh PR. "Mini-mental state". A practical method for grading the cognitive state of patients for the clinician. J Psychiatr Res 1975; 12:189–198.
6. Tombaugh TN, McIntyre NJ. The Mini-Mental State Examination: a comprehensive review. J Am Geriatr Soc 1992; 40:922–935.
7. Hiltunen LA, Keinanen-Kiukaanniemi SM, Laara EM. Glucose tolerance and cognitive impairment in an elderly population. Public Health 2001; 115:197–200.
8. Vanhanen M, Koivisto K, Karjalainen L, et al. Risk for non-insulin-dependent diabetes in the normoglycaemic elderly is associated with impaired cognitive function. NeuroReport 1997; 8:1527–1530.
9. van Harten B, Oosterman J, Muslimovic D, van Loon BJ, Scheltens P, Weinstein HC. Cognitive impairment and MRI correlates in the elderly patients with type 2 diabetes mellitus. Age Ageing 2007; 36164–36170.
10. Nguyen HT, Black SA, Ray LA, Espino DV, Markides KS. Predictors of decline in MMSE scores among older Mexican Americans. J Gerontol A Biol Sci Med Sci 2002; 57:M181-M185.
11. Gregg EW, Yaffe K, Cauley JA, et al. Is diabetes associated with cognitive impairment and cognitive decline among older women? Study of Osteoporotic Fractures Research Group. Arch Intern Med 2000; 160:174–180.
12. Hassing LB, Grant MD, Hofer SM, et al. Type 2 diabetes mellitus contributes to cognitive decline in old age: a longitudinal population-based study. J Int Neuropsychol Soc 2004; 10:599–607.
13. Wu JH, Haan MN, Liang J, Ghosh D, Gonzalez HM, Herman WH. Impact of diabetes on cognitive function among older Latinos: a population-based cohort study. J Clin Epidemiol 2003; 56:686–693.
14. Haan MN, Shemanski L, Jagust WJ, Manolio TA, Kuller L. The role of APOE epsilon4 in modulating effects of other risk factors for cognitive decline in elderly persons. JAMA 1999; 282:40–46.
15. Lezak MD, Howieson DB, Loring DW. Neuropsychological Assessment. 4th ed. New York, NY: Oxford Press; 2004.

16. Wechsler D. Wechsler Memory Scale – III. San Antonio, TX: Psychological Corporation; 1997.

17. van der Elst W, van Boxtel MP, van Breukelen GJ, Jolles J. Rey's verbal learning test: normative data for 1855 healthy participants aged 24–81 years and the influence of age, sex, education, and mode of presentation. J Int Neuropsychol Soc 2005; 11:290–302.

18. Wechsler D. Wechsler Adult Intelligence Scale – III. San Antonio, TX: Psychological Corporation; 1997.

19. Stroop JR. Studies of interference in serial verbal reactions. J Exp Psychol 1935; 18: 643–662.

20. Corrigan JD, Hinkeldey NS. Relationships between parts A and B of the Trail Making Test. J Clin Psychol 1987; 43:402–409.

21. Deelman BG, Koning-Haanstra M, Liebrand WBG. SAN test, een afasietest voor auditief en mondeling taalgebruik. Lisse: Swets & Zeitlinger; 1981.

22. Dey J, Misra A, Desai NG, Mahapatra AK, Padma MV. Cognitive function in younger type II diabetes. Diabetes Care 1997; 20:32–35.

23. Ryan CM, Geckle MO. Circumscribed cognitive dysfunction in middle-aged adults with type 2 diabetes. Diabetes Care 2000; 23:1486–1493.

24. Reaven GM, Thompson LW, Nahum D, Haskins E. Relationship between hyperglycemia and cognitive function in older NIDDM patients. Diabetes Care 1990; 13:16–21.

25. Cerhan JR, Folsom AR, Mortimer JA, et al. Correlates of cognitive function in middle-aged adults. Atherosclerosis Risk in Communities (ARIC) Study Investigators. Gerontology 1998; 44:95–105.

26. Elias PK, Elias MF, D'Agostino RB., et al. NIDDM and blood pressure as risk factors for poor cognitive performance. The Framingham Study. Diabetes Care 1997; 20:1388–1395.

27. Cohen J. Statistical Power Analysis for the Behavioral Sciences. 2nd ed. Hillsdale, NJ: Laurence Erlbaum; 1988.

28. van den Berg E, Kloppenborg RP, Kessels RPC, Kappelle LJ, Biessels GJ. Type 2 diabetes mellitus, hypertension, dyslipidemia and obesity: a systematic comparison of their impact on cognition. Biochimica et biophysica acta 2009; 1792:470–481.

29. Kumari M, Marmot M. Diabetes and cognitive function in a middle-aged cohort: findings from the Whitehall II study. Neurology 2005; 65:1597–1603.

30. Knopman D, Boland LL, Mosley T, et al. Cardiovascular risk factors and cognitive decline in middle-aged adults. Neurology 2001; 56:42–48.

31. Fontbonne A, Berr C, Ducimetiere P, Alperovitch A. Changes in cognitive abilities over a 4-year period are unfavorably affected in elderly diabetic subjects: results of the Epidemiology of Vascular Aging Study. Diabetes Care 2001; 24:366–370.

32. Kanaya AM, Barrett-Connor E, Gildengorin G, Yaffe K. Change in cognitive function by glucose tolerance status in older adults: a 4-year prospective study of the Rancho Bernardo study cohort. Arch Intern Med 2004; 164:1327–1333.

33. van den Berg E, de Craen AJ, Biessels GJ, Gussekloo J, Westendorp RG. The impact of diabetes mellitus on cognitive decline in the oldest of the old: a prospective population-based study. Diabetologia 2006; 49:2015–2023.

34. Cukierman T, Gerstein HC, Williamson JD. Cognitive decline and dementia in diabetes – systematic overview of prospective observational studies. Diabetologia 2005; 48: 2460–2469.

35. Nijpels G. Determinants for the progression from impaired glucose tolerance to non-insulin-dependent diabetes mellitus. Eur J Clin Invest 1998; 28(Suppl 2):8–13.

36. American Diabetes Association. Standards of medical care for patients with diabetes mellitus. Diabetes Care 2002; 25:213–229.

37. Reaven GM. Banting lecture 1988. Role of insulin resistance in human disease. Diabetes 1988; 37:1595–1607.

38. Adult Treatment Panel III. Executive summary of the third report of the National Cholesterol Education Program (NCEP) Expert Panel on Detection, Evaluation, And Treatment

of High Blood Cholesterol In Adults (Adult Treatment Panel III). JAMA 2001; 285: 2486–2497.

39. Manning CA, Stone WS, Korol DL, Gold PE. Glucose enhancement of 24-h memory retrieval in healthy elderly humans. Behav Brain Res 1998; 93:71–76.

40. Kuusisto J, Koivisto K, Mykkänen L, et al. Essential hypertension and cognitive function: the role of hyperinsulinemia. Hypertension 1993; 22:771–779.

41. Kalmijn S, Feskens EJM, Launer LJ, Stijnen T, Kromhout D. Glucose intolerance, hyper-insulinaemia and cognitive function in a general population of elderly men. Diabetologia 1995; 38:1096–1102.

42. Abbatecola AM, Paolisso G, Lamponi M, et al. Insulin resistance and executive dysfunction in older persons. J Am Geriatr Soc 2004; 52:1713–1718.

43. Young SE, Mainous III AG, Carnemolla M. Hyperinsulinemia and cognitive decline in a middle-aged cohort. Diabetes Care 2006; 29:2688–2693.

44. Messier C, Tsiakas M, Gagnon M, Desrochers A, Awad N. Effect of age and glucoregulation on cognitive performance. Neurobiol Aging 2003; 24:985–1003.

45. Messier C, Desrochers A, Gagnon M. Effect of glucose, glucose regulation, and word imagery value on human memory. Behav Neurosci 1999; 113:431–438.

46. Awad N, Gagnon M, Desrochers A, Tsiakas M, Messier C. Impact of peripheral glucoregu-lation on memory. Behav Neurosci 2002; 116:691–702.

47. Convit A, Wolf OT, Tarshish C, de Leon MJ. Reduced glucose tolerance is associated with poor memory performance and hippocampal atrophy among normal elderly. Proc Natl Acad Sci USA 2003; 100:2019–2022.

48. Fuh JL, Wang SJ, Hwu CM, Lu SR. Glucose tolerance status and cognitive impairment in early middle-aged women. Diabet Med 2007; 24:788–791.

49. Lindeman RD, Romero LJ, LaRue A, et al. A biethnic community survey of cognition in participants with type 2 diabetes, impaired glucose tolerance, and normal glucose tolerance: the New Mexico Elder Health Survey. Diabetes Care 2001; 24:567–572.

50. Vanhanen M, Koivisto K, Kuusisto J, et al. Cognitive function in an elderly population with persistent impaired glucose tolerance. Diabetes Care 1998; 21:398–402.

51. Yaffe K, Blackwell T, Kanaya AM, Davidowitz N, Barrett-Connor E, Krueger K. Diabetes, impaired fasting glucose, and development of cognitive impairment in older women. Neu-rology 2004; 63:658–663.

52. Scott RD, Kritz-Silverstein D, Barrett-Connor E, Wiederholt WC. The association of non-insulin-dependent diabetes mellitus and cognitive function in an older cohort. J Am Geriatr Soc 1998; 46:1217–1222.

53. Dik MG, Jonker C, Comijs HC, et al. Contribution of metabolic syndrome components to cognition in older individuals. Diabetes Care 2007; 30:2655–2660.

54. Yaffe K, Kanaya A, Lindquist K, et al. The metabolic syndrome, inflammation, and risk of cognitive decline. JAMA 2004; 292:2237–2242.

55. Yaffe K, Haan M, Blackwell T, Cherkasova E, Whitmer RA, West N. Metabolic syndrome and cognitive decline in elderly Latinos: findings from the Sacramento Area Latino Study of Aging study. J Am Geriatr Soc 2007; 55:758–762.

56. Komulainen P, Lakka TA, Kivipelto M, et al. Metabolic syndrome and cognitive function: a population-based follow-up study in elderly women. Dement Geriatr Cogn Disord 2007; 23:29–34.

57. van den Berg E, Biessels GJ, de Craen AJ, Gussekloo J, Westendorp RG. The metabolic syndrome is associated with decelerated cognitive decline in the oldest old. Neurology 2007; 69:979–985.

58. Gatto NM, Henderson VW, St John JA, McCleary C, Hodis HN, Mack WJ. Metabolic syn-drome and cognitive function in healthy middle-aged and older adults without diabetes. Neu-ropsychol Dev Cogn B Aging Neuropsychol Cogn 2008:1–15.

59. Harrington F, Saxby BK, McKeith IG, Wesnes K, Ford GA. Cognitive performance in hyper-tensive and normotensive older subjects. Hypertension 2000; 36:1079–1082.

60. Reinprecht F, Elmstahl S, Janzon L, ndre-Petersson L. Hypertension and changes of cognitive function in 81-year-old men: a 13-year follow-up of the population study "Men born in 1914", Sweden. J Hypertens 2003; 21:57–66.

61. Wolf PA, Beiser A, Elias MF, Au R, Vasan RS, Seshadri S. Relation of obesity to cognitive function: importance of central obesity and synergistic influence of concomitant hypertension. The Framingham Heart Study. Curr Alzheimer Res 2007; 4:11–16.

62. Hebert LE, Scherr PA, Bennett DA, et al. Blood pressure and late-life cognitive function change: a biracial longitudinal population study. Neurology 2004; 62:2021–2024.

63. Paran E, Anson O, Reuveni H. Blood pressure and cognitive functioning among independent elderly. Am J Hypertens 2003; 16:818–826.

64. Gunstad J, Paul RH, Cohen RA, Tate DF, Spitznagel MB, Gordon E. Elevated body mass index is associated with executive dysfunction in otherwise healthy adults. Compr Psychiatry 2007; 48:57–61.

65. de Frias CM, Bunce D, Wahlin A, et al. Cholesterol and triglycerides moderate the effect of apolipoprotein E on memory functioning in older adults. J Gerontol B Psychol Sci Soc Sci 2007; 62:112–118.

66. Zhang J, Muldoon MF, McKeown RE. Serum cholesterol concentrations are associated with visuomotor speed in men: findings from the third National Health and Nutrition Examination Survey, 1988–1994. Am J Clin Nutr 2004; 80:291–298.

67. Henderson VW, Guthrie JR, Dennerstein L. Serum lipids and memory in a population based cohort of middle age women. J Neurol Neurosurg Psychiatry 2003; 74:1530–1535.

68. Kloppenborg RP, van den Berg E, Kappelle LJ, Biessels GJ. Diabetes and other vascular risk factors for dementia: Which factor matters most? A systematic review. Eur J Pharmacol 2008; 585:97–108.

69. de Leeuw FE, de Groot JC, Achten E, et al. Prevalence of cerebral white matter lesions in elderly people: a population based magnetic resonance imaging study. The Rotterdam Scan Study. J Neurol Neurosurg Psychiatry 2001; 70:9–14.

70. Vermeer SE, Koudstaal PJ, Oudkerk M, Hofman A, Breteler MM. Prevalence and risk factors of silent brain infarcts in the population- based Rotterdam Scan Study. Stroke 2002; 33: 21–25.

71. Scahill RI, Frost C, Jenkins R, Whitwell JL, Rossor MN, Fox NC. A longitudinal study of brain volume changes in normal aging using serial registered magnetic resonance imaging. Arch Neurol 2003; 60:989–994.

72. Vermeer SE, Hollander M, van Dijk EJ, Hofman A, Koudstaal PJ, Breteler MM. Silent brain infarcts and white matter lesions increase stroke risk in the general population: the Rotterdam Scan Study. Stroke 2003; 34:1126–1129.

73. Longstreth Jr.WT, Bernick C, Manolio TA, Bryan N, Jungreis CA, Price TR. Lacunar infarcts defined by magnetic resonance imaging of 3660 elderly people: the Cardiovascular Health Study. Arch Neurol 1998; 55:1217–1225.

74. Korf ES, van Straaten EC, de Leeuw FE, et al. Diabetes mellitus, hypertension and medial temporal lobe atrophy: the LADIS study. Diabet Med 2007; 24:166–171.

75. van Harten B, de Leeuw FE, Weinstein HC, Scheltens P, Biessels GJ. Brain imaging in patients with diabetes: a systematic review. Diabetes Care 2006; 29:2539–2548.

76. Schmidt R, Launer LJ, Nilsson LG, et al. Magnetic resonance imaging of the brain in diabetes: the Cardiovascular Determinants of Dementia (CASCADE) Study. Diabetes 2004; 53:687–692.

77. den Heijer T, Vermeer SE, van Dijk EJ, et al. Type 2 diabetes and atrophy of medial temporal lobe structures on brain MRI. Diabetologia 2003; 46:1604–1610.

78. Manschot SM, Brands AM, van der Grond J, et al. Brain magnetic resonance imaging correlates of impaired cognition in patients with type 2 diabetes. Diabetes 2006; 55: 1106–1113.

79. Jongen C, van der Grond J, Kappelle LJ, Biessels GJ, Viergever MA, Pluim JP. Automated measurement of brain and white matter lesion volume in type 2 diabetes mellitus. Diabetologia 2007; 50:1509–1516.

80. van Harten B, Oosterman JM, Potter van Loon BJ, Scheltens P, Weinstein HC. Brain lesions on MRI in elderly patients with type 2 diabetes mellitus. Eur Neurol 2007; 57: 70–74.
81. Last D, Alsop DC, Abduljalil AM, et al. Global and regional effects of type 2 diabetes on brain tissue volumes and cerebral vasoreactivity. Diabetes Care 2007; 30:1193–1199.
82. Gouw AA, van der Flier WM, Fazekas F, et al. Progression of white matter hyperintensities and incidence of new lacunes over a 3-year period: the Leukoaraiosis and Disability study. Stroke 2008; 39:1414–1420.
83. Last D, Alsop DC, Abduljalil AM, et al. Global and regional effects of type 2 diabetes on brain tissue volumes and cerebral vasoreactivity. Diabetes Care 2007; 30:1193–1199.
84. Jongen C, Biessels GJ. Structural brain imaging in diabetes: a methodological perspective. Eur J Pharmacol 2008; 585:208–218.
85. Korf ES, White LR, Scheltens P, Launer LJ. Brain aging in very old men with type 2 diabetes: the Honolulu-Asia Aging Study. Diabetes Care 2006; 29:2268–2274.
86. Gold SM, Dziobek I, Sweat V, et al. Hippocampal damage and memory impairments as possible early brain complications of type 2 diabetes. Diabetologia 2007; 50:711–719.
87. Akisaki T, Sakurai T, Takata T, et al. Cognitive dysfunction associates with white matter hyperintensities and subcortical atrophy on magnetic resonance imaging of the elderly diabetes mellitus Japanese elderly diabetes intervention trial (J-EDIT). Diabetes Metab Res Rev. 2006; 22:376–384.
88. Tanizaki Y, Kiyohara Y, Kato I, et al. Incidence and risk factors for subtypes of cerebral infarction in a general population: the Hisayama study. Stroke 2000; 31:2616–2622.
89. Knopman DS, Mosley TH, Catellier DJ, Sharrett AR. Cardiovascular risk factors and cerebral atrophy in a middle-aged cohort. Neurology 2005; 65:876–881.
90. Murray AD, Staff RT, Shenkin SD, Deary IJ, Starr JM, Whalley LJ. Brain white matter hyperintensities: relative importance of vascular risk factors in nondemented elderly people. Radiology 2005; 237:251–257.
91. Anan F, Masaki T, Iwao T, et al. The role of microalbuminuria and insulin resistance as significant risk factors for white matter lesions in Japanese type 2 diabetic patients. Curr Med Res Opin 2008; 24:1561–1567.
92. Longstreth Jr.W, Larsen EK, Klein R, et al. Associations between findings on cranial magnetic resonance imaging and retinal photography in the elderly: the Cardiovascular Health Study. Am J Epidemiol 2007; 165:78–84.
93. de Leeuw FE, de Groot JC, Oudkerk M, et al. Hypertension and cerebral white matter lesions in a prospective cohort study. Brain 2002; 125:765–772.
94. Vermeer SE, den Heijer T, Koudstaal PJ, Oudkerk M, Hofman A, Breteler MM. Incidence and risk factors of silent brain infarcts in the population-based Rotterdam Scan Study. Stroke 2003; 34:392–396.
95. Longstreth Jr. WT, Manolio TA, Arnold A, et al. Clinical correlates of white matter findings on cranial magnetic resonance imaging of 3301 elderly people. The Cardiovascular Health Study. Stroke 1996; 27:1274–1282.
96. Jagust W, Harvey D, Mungas D, Haan M. Central obesity and the aging brain. Arch Neurol 2005; 62:1545–1548.
97. Ward MA, Carlsson CM, Trivedi MA, Sager MA, Johnson SC. The effect of body mass index on global brain volume in middle-aged adults: a cross sectional study. BMC Neurol 2005; 5:23.
98. Gustafson D, Lissner L, Bengtsson C, Bjorkelund C, Skoog I. A 24-year follow-up of body mass index and cerebral atrophy. Neurology 2004; 63:1876–1881.
99. Slooter AJ, Tang MX, van Duijn CM, et al. Apolipoprotein E epsilon4 and the risk of dementia with stroke. A population-based investigation. JAMA 1997; 277:818–821.
100. Xu WL, Qiu CX, Wahlin A, Winblad B, Fratiglioni L. Diabetes mellitus and risk of dementia in the Kungsholmen project: a 6-year follow-up study. Neurology 2004; 63:1181–1186.
101. Peila R, Rodriguez BL, Launer LJ. Type 2 diabetes, APOE gene, and the risk for dementia and related pathologies: The Honolulu-Asia Aging Study. Diabetes 2002; 51:1256–1262.

102. Blair CK, Folsom AR, Knopman DS, Bray MS, Mosley TH. Boerwinkle E. APOE genotype and cognitive decline in a middle-aged cohort. Neurology 2005; 64:268–276.
103. Craft S, Asthana S, Schellenberg G, et al. Insulin metabolism in Alzheimer's disease differs according to apolipoprotein E genotype and gender. Neuroendocrinology 1999; 70:146–152.
104. Johnson W, Harris SE, Starr JM, Whalley LJ, Deary IJ. PPARG Pro12Ala genotype and risk of cognitive decline in elders? Maybe with diabetes. Neurosci Lett 2008; 434:50–55.
105. Robbins JM, Vaccarino V, Zhang H, Kasl SV. Socioeconomic status and type 2 diabetes in African American and non-Hispanic white women and men: evidence from the Third National Health and Nutrition Examination Survey. Am J Public Health 2001; 91:76–83.
106. Evans DA, Beckett LA, Albert MS, et al. Level of education and change in cognitive function in a community population of older persons. Ann Epidemiol 1993; 3:71–77.
107. Stern Y, Gurland B, Tatemichi TK, Tang MX, Wilder D, Mayeux R. Influence of education and occupation on the incidence of Alzheimer's disease. JAMA 1994; 271:1004–1010.
108. Yusuf S, Hawken S, Ounpuu S, et al. Effect of potentially modifiable risk factors associated with myocardial infarction in 52 countries (the INTERHEART study): case-control study. Lancet 2004; 364:937–952.
109. Harris MI, Flegal KM, Cowie CC, et al. Prevalence of diabetes, impaired fasting glucose, and impaired glucose tolerance in U.S. adults. The Third National Health and Nutrition Examination Survey, 1988–1994. Diabetes Care 1998; 21:518–524.
110. Froehlich TE, Bogardus Jr. ST, Inouye SK. Dementia and race: are there differences between African Americans and Caucasians? J Am Geriatr Soc 2001; 49:477–484.
111. Soininen H, Puranen M, Helkala EL, Laakso M, Riekkinen PJ. Diabetes mellitus and brain atrophy: a computed tomography study in an elderly population. Neurobiol Aging 1992; 13:717–721.
112. Mooradian AD. Diabetic complications of the central nervous system. Endocr Rev 1988; 9:346–356.
113. Biessels GJ, Staekenborg S, Brunner E, Brayne C, Scheltens P. Risk of dementia in diabetes mellitus: a systematic review. Lancet Neurol 2006; 5:64–74.
114. Tisserand DJ, Jolles J. On the involvement of prefrontal networks in cognitive ageing. Cortex 2003; 39:1107–1128.
115. Ryan CM, Geckle M. Why is learning and memory dysfunction in Type 2 diabetes limited to older adults? Diabetes Metab Res Rev 2000; 16:308–315.
116. Kamal A, Biessels GJ, Duis SEJ, Gispen WH. Learning and hippocampal synaptic plasticity in streptozotocin-diabetic rats: interaction of diabetes and ageing. Diabetologia 2000; 43:500–506.
117. Biessels GJ, van der Heide LP, Kamal A, Bleys RL, Gispen WH. Ageing and diabetes: implications for brain function. Eur J Pharmacol 2002; 441:1–14.
118. Egede LE, Zheng D. Modifiable cardiovascular risk factors in adults with diabetes: prevalence and missed opportunities for physician counseling. Arch Intern Med 2002; 162: 427–433.
119. Berry EM. Dietary fatty acids in the management of diabetes mellitus. Am J Clin Nutr 1997; 66:991S-7S.
120. Launer LJ, Andersen K, Dewey ME, et al. Rates and risk factors for dementia and Alzheimer's disease: results from EURODEM pooled analyses. EURODEM Incidence Research Group and Work Groups. European Studies of Dementia. Neurology 1999; 52: 78–84.
121. Petot GJ, Friedland RP. Lipids, diet and Alzheimer disease: an extended summary. J Neurol Sci 2004; 226:31–33.
122. Hassing LB, Hofer SM, Nilsson SE, et al.. Comorbid type 2 diabetes mellitus and hypertension exacerbates cognitive decline: evidence from a longitudinal study. Age Ageing 2004.
123. Bruce DG, Davis WA, Casey GP, et al. Predictors of cognitive impairment and dementia in older people with diabetes. Diabetologia 2008; 51:241–248.
124. Manschot SM, Biessels GJ, de Valk H, et al. Metabolic and vascular determinants of impaired cognitive performance and abnormalities on brain magnetic resonance imaging in patients with type 2 diabetes. Diabetologia 2007; 50:2388–2397.

125. Brands AM, Biessels GJ, De Haan EH, Kappelle LJ, Kessels RP. The effects of type 1 diabetes on cognitive performance: a meta-analysis. Diabetes Care 2005; 28:726–735.
126. Perlmuter LC, Hakami MK, Hodgson-Harrington C, et al. Decreased cognitive function in aging non-insulin-dependent diabetic patients. Am J Med 1984; 77:1043–1048.
127. Jagusch W, v Cramon Renner R, Hepp KD. Cognitive function and metabolic state in elderly diabetic patients. Diab Nutr Metab 1992; 5:265–274.
128. Munshi M, Grande L, Hayes M, et al. Cognitive dysfunction is associated with poor diabetes control in older adults. Diabetes Care 2006; 29:1794–1799.
129. Worrall GJ, Chaulk PC, Moulton N. Cognitive function and glycosylated hemoglobin in older patients with type II diabetes. J Diabetes Complic 1996; 10:320–324.
130. Lowe LP, Tranel D, Wallace RB, Welty TK. Type II diabetes and cognitive function. A population-based study of Native Americans. Diabetes Care 1994; 17:891–896.
131. Tiehuis AM, van den Berg E, Kappelle LJ, Biessels GJ. Cognition and dementia in Type 2 diabetes: brain imaging correlates and metabolic and vascular risk factors. Aging Health 2007; 3:361–373.
132. Cox DJ, Kovatchev BP, Gonder-Frederick LA, et al. Relationships between hyperglycemia and cognitive performance among adults with type 1 and type 2 diabetes. Diabetes Care 2005; 28:71–77.
133. Jacobson AM, Musen G, Ryan CM, et al. Long-term effect of diabetes and its treatment on cognitive function. N Engl J Med 2007; 356:1842–1852.
134. Gold AE, Deary IJ, Jones RW, O'Hare JP, Reckless JP, Frier BM. Severe deterioration in cognitive function and personality in five patients with long-standing diabetes: a complication of diabetes or a consequence of treatment? Diabet Med 1994; 11:499–505.
135. Wong TY, Klein R, Islam FM, et al. Diabetic retinopathy in a multi-ethnic cohort in the United States. Am J Ophthalmol 2006; 141:446–555.
136. Epidemiology of Diabetes Interventions and Complications (EDIC) Research Group. Effect of intensive diabetes treatment on carotid artery wall thickness in the epidemiology of diabetes interventions and complications. Diabetes 1999; 48:383–390.
137. Ferguson SC, Blane A, Perros P, et al. Cognitive ability and brain structure in type 1 diabetes: relation to microangiopathy and preceding severe hypoglycemia. Diabetes 2003; 52: 149–156.
138. Ryan CM, Geckle MO, Orchard TJ. Cognitive efficiency declines over time in adults with Type 1 diabetes: effects of micro- and macrovascular complications. Diabetologia 2003; 46:940–948.
139. Wessels AM, Rombouts SA, Remijnse PL, et al. Cognitive performance in type 1 diabetes patients is associated with cerebral white matter volume. Diabetologia 2007; 50: 1763–1769.
140. Breteler MM, Claus JJ, Grobbee DE, Hofman A. Cardiovascular disease and distribution of cognitive function in elderly people: the Rotterdam Study. BMJ 1994; 308:1604–1608.
141. Umegaki H, Iimuro S, Kaneko T, Araki A, et al. Factors associated with lower Mini Mental State Examination scores in elderly Japanese diabetes mellitus patients. Neurobiol Aging 2008; 29:1022–1026.
142. Anderson RJ, Freedland KE, Clouse RE, Lustman PJ. The prevalence of comorbid depression in adults with diabetes: a meta-analysis. Diabetes Care 2001; 24:1069–1078.
143. Knol MJ, Twisk JW, Beekman AT, Heine RJ, Snoek FJ, Pouwer F. Depression as a risk factor for the onset of type 2 diabetes mellitus. A meta-analysis. Diabetologia 2006; 49:837–845.
144. Ryan CM, Freed MI, Rood JA, Cobitz AR, Waterhouse BR, Strachan MW. Improving metabolic control leads to better working memory in adults with type 2 diabetes. Diabetes Care 2006; 29:345–351.
145. Gradman TJ, Laws A, Thompson LW, Reaven GM. Verbal learning and/or memory improves with glycemic control in older subjects with non-insulin-dependent diabetes mellitus. J Am Geriat Soc 1993; 41:1305–1312.
146. Meneilly GS, Cheung E, Tessier D, Yakura C, Tuokko H. The effect of improved glycemic control on cognitive functions in the elderly patient with diabetes. J Gerontol 1993; 48:M117-M121.

147. Naor M, Steingruber HJ, Westhoff K, Schottenfeld-Naor Y, Gries AF. Cognitive function in elderly non-insulin-dependent diabetic patients before and after inpatient treatment for metabolic control. J Diabetes Complications 1997; 11:40–46.

148. Abbatecola AM, Rizzo MR, Barbieri M, et al. Postprandial plasma glucose excursions and cognitive functioning in aged type 2 diabetics. Neurology 2006; 67:235–240.

149. Mussell M, Hewer W, Kulzer B, Bergis K, Rist F. Effects of improved glycaemic control maintained for 3 months on cognitive function in patients with Type 2 diabetes. Diabet Med 2004; 21:1253–1256.

150. Areosa Sastre A, Grimley Evans V. Effect of the treatment of Type II diabetes mellitus on the development of cognitive impairment and dementia. Cochrane Database Syst Rev, 2002:CD003804.

151. Austin EJ, Deary IJ. Effects of repeated hypoglycemia on cognitive function: a psychometrically validated reanalysis of the Diabetes Control and Complications Trial data. Diabetes Care 1999; 22:1273–1277.

152. Ott A, Stolk RP, Van Harskamp F, Pols HA, Hofman A, Breteler MM. Diabetes mellitus and the risk of dementia: The Rotterdam Study. Neurology 1999; 53:1937–1942.

153. McGuinness B, Todd S, Passmore P, Bullock R. The effects of blood pressure lowering on development of cognitive impairment and dementia in patients without apparent prior cerebrovascular disease. Cochrane Database Syst Rev 2006:CD004034.

154. Feigin V, Ratnasabapathy Y, Anderson C. Does blood pressure lowering treatment prevents dementia or cognitive decline in patients with cardiovascular and cerebrovascular disease? J Neurol Sci 2005; 229–230:151–155.

155. Li G, Higdon R, Kukull WA, et al. Statin therapy and risk of dementia in the elderly: a community-based prospective cohort study. Neurology 2004; 63:1624–1628.

156. Berk-Planken I, de KI, Stolk R, Jansen H, Hoogerbrugge N. Atorvastatin, diabetic dyslipidemia, and cognitive functioning. Diabetes Care 2002; 25:1250–1251.

157. Colberg SR, Somma CT, Sechrist SR. Physical activity participation may offset some of the negative impact of diabetes on cognitive function. J Am Med Dir Assoc 2008; 9: 434–438.

158. Sandeep TC, Yau JL, MacLullich AM, Noble J, Deary IJ, Walker BR, Seckl JR. 11Beta-hydroxysteroid dehydrogenase inhibition improves cognitive function in healthy elderly men and type 2 diabetics. Proc Natl Acad Sci USA 2004; 101:6734–6739.

159. Herman Chui M, Greenwood CE. Antioxidant vitamins reduce acute meal-induced memory deficits in adults with type 2 diabetes. Nutrition Research 2008; 28:423–429.

160. Lawton MP, Brody EM. Assessment of older people: self-maintaining and instrumental activities of daily living. Gerontologist 1969; 9:179–186.

161. Beck AT, Steer AR, Brown GK. Beck Depression Inventory – Second Edition: Manual. San Antonio, TX: Psychological Corporation; 1996.

162. Cummings JL, Mega M, Gray K, Rosenberg-Thompson S, Carusi DA, Gornbein J. The Neuropsychiatric Inventory: comprehensive assessment of psychopathology in dementia. Neurology 1994; 44:2308–2314.

163. Knopman DS, DeKosky ST, Cummings JL, et al. Practice parameter: diagnosis of dementia (an evidence-based review). Report of the Quality Standards Subcommittee of the American Academy of Neurology. Neurology 2001; 56:1143–1153.

164. Scheltens P, Fox N, Barkhof F, De CC. Structural magnetic resonance imaging in the practical assessment of dementia: beyond exclusion. Lancet Neurol 2002; 1:13–21.

13

Type 2 Diabetes, Related Conditions, and Dementia

José Alejandro Luchsinger

CONTENTS

ABSTRACT

The objective of this chapter is to provide a comprehensive review of the evidence linking type 2 diabetes and its related conditions, adiposity and

From: *Contemporary Diabetes: Diabetes and the Brain*
Edited by: G. J. Biessels, J. A. Luchsinger (eds.), DOI 10.1007/978-1-60327-850-8_13
© Humana Press, a part of Springer Science+Business Media, LLC 2009

hyperinsulinemia, with dementia. The mechanisms for these associations remain to be elucidated, but may include cerebrovascular and non-vascular mechanisms. Elevated adiposity in middle age is related to a higher risk of dementia. The evidence relating adiposity in old age to dementia is conflicting. Several studies have shown that hyperinsulinemia, a consequence of higher adiposity and insulin resistance is also related to a higher risk of dementia. Hyperinsulinemia is a risk factor for diabetes, and numerous studies have shown a relation of type 2 diabetes with higher dementia risk. In general, these associations are stronger for vascular dementia than for Alzheimer's disease. The implication of these associations is that a large proportion of the world population may be at increased risk of Alzheimer's disease given the trends for increasing prevalence of overweight, obesity, hyperinsulinemia, and diabetes. However, if proven causal, these associations also present a unique opportunity for prevention and treatment of dementia.

Key words: Adiposity; Overweight; Obesity; Hyperinsulinemia; Diabetes; Alzheimer's disease; Vascular dementia; Dementia; Mild cognitive impairment.

INTRODUCTION

This chapter covers the evidence relating type 2 diabetes (T2D) and its related conditions to the diagnostic forms of cognitive impairment identified in clinical practice and research, dementia and mild cognitive impairment (MCI). The chapter by Van den Berg covers the association between T2D and cognitive impairment assessed as a continuous measure, not as a diagnostic entity. The chapter by Van de Pol et al. has a comprehensive review of cognitive diagnostic categories. This chapter will cover Alzheimer's disease (AD), the most frequent form of dementia, and vascular dementia (VD), the second most frequent form. It will also cover MCI and its two main forms, amnestic MCI, thought to be a transitional stage to AD, and non-amnestic MCI, thought to be in the continuum of vascular forms of cognitive impairment. These forms of cognitive impairment are relevant to this chapter not only because T2D is a cerebrovascular risk factor, potentially affecting VD, but also because there is evidence linking it to AD.

The main emphasis of this book is on diabetes. However, T2D is a proxy for prior exposure to elevated adiposity and insulin resistance, and persons with T2D suffer not only the effects of impaired glycemia but also of exposure to years or decades of the effects of elevated adiposity and insulin resistance. Thus, this chapter will cover the evidence linking adiposity, insulin resistance (and hyperinsulinemia), and T2D to the diagnostic forms of cognitive impairment.

TYPE 2 DIABETES AND ITS RELATED CONDITIONS

There is a concerning epidemic of obesity, insulin resistance, and T2D in the world *(1)*. With the aging of the population and greater longevity, the long-term consequences of these conditions are serious and burdensome. Adiposity refers to the amount of adipose (fat) tissue in the body *(2)*. Some refer to adiposity as "fatness" or obesity. Adiposity is a continuum, and the normal or ideal threshold of adiposity is not clear. However, as adiposity increases it is associated with higher risk of insulin resistance, diabetes, hypertension, dyslipidemia, cardiovascular disease, degenerative joint disease, cancer, and respiratory diseases *(3, 4)*. Definitions of a high level of adiposity have been devised using existing measures and according to their relationship with adverse outcomes *(5)*. Adiposity is usually measured indirectly with anthropological measures *(6)* such as the body mass index (BMI), defined as weight in kilograms divided by height in meters squared (kg/m^2). BMI is strongly correlated with total body fat tissue and is a good indirect measure of adiposity *(4)*, although this correlation decreases in older age *(7)*. Another commonly used measure of adiposity is waist circumference. Waist circumference is meant to measure the accumulation of adipose tissue in the abdomen, the largest depot of adipose tissue, and thus, perhaps it is a more direct measure of adiposity compared to BMI *(6, 8)*. Elevated waist circumference is also related to a higher risk of T2D, hypertension, dyslipidemia, and heart disease, and some studies have shown that it is a better predictor of adverse cardiovascular outcomes compared to BMI *(9)*, and some have advocated its use as the best measure of adiposity *(6)*. A commonly used cutoff to define elevated waist circumference is 102 cm for men and 88 cm for women *(9)*. Other less frequently used anthropologic measures of adiposity include skinfolds and waist-to-hip ratio *(6)*. Overweight (BMI $\geq$25 and <30 kg/m^2) and obesity (BMI $\geq$30 kg/m^2) *(10)* and elevated waist circumference *(11)* are increasing in adults in the United States. More concerning, these trends are also observed in children and adolescents *(12)*. Two-thirds of the United States population are overweight or obese *(12)*; 30% are obese, and the prevalence of obesity is higher in women than men.

Insulin sensitivity is the ability of insulin to dispose of a glucose load. Insulin resistance refers to the resistance of tissues that dispose of glucose to the actions of insulin. Insulin resistance results in an increase in insulin secretion in the pancreas in order to overcome that insulin resistance. Fasting insulin levels are used in epidemiological studies as indicators of the risk of T2D *(13–16)*. Fasting insulin is accepted as a measure of insulin resistance that is highly correlated with more complicated measures of insulin resistance such as the euglycemic clamp *(17)* and the homeostasis model assessment *(18)*.

Glucose intolerance and diabetes are abnormal elevations of blood glucose that put people at risk for microvascular (nephropathy, neuropathy, and retinopathy) and macrovascular diseases (coronary artery disease, cerebrovascular disease, and peripheral vascular disease) *(19)*. The American Diabetes Association currently defines diabetes as a fasting glucose elevation >126 mg/dl and glucose intolerance as an elevation of glucose between 110 and 126 mg/dl *(20)*. It is difficult to establish an absolute threshold for the definition of glucose intolerance and diabetes. Previously, the definition of diabetes was a fasting glucose >140 mg/dl, and people currently defined as having diabetes were then considered non-diabetic *(21)*. It is likely that the diabetes definition will change again and persons currently considered to have glucose intolerance will be considered to be diabetic. This underlines the caveats of using cutoffs to define conditions that have continuous (linear or non-linear) associations with disease: depending on the cutoff use, persons at risk may be classified as normal or abnormal (and vice versa). This is true for measures of adiposity, insulin resistance, and measures of glucose tolerance.

Adiposity, hyperinsulinemia, glucose intolerance, and diabetes are often treated as separate constructs and have been separately related to the risk of dementia *(22)*. However, they are related sequentially and often occur simultaneously, and understanding this relationship is fundamental in the study of the role of adiposity, insulin resistance, and T2D with dementia. Keeping glucose in normal levels is achieved by the balance between the ability of peripheral tissues (muscle, adipose tissue, liver) to take glucose into cells and the pancreas' ability to secrete insulin, the hormone in charge of glucose tissue uptake *(19)*. Thus, abnormal glucose levels are caused by a resistance of tissues to the action of insulin (insulin resistance) and by the pancreas' inability to secrete enough insulin at normal levels or higher than normal insulin levels (hyperinsulinemia) to overcome insulin resistance in tissues *(23)*. Insulin resistance increases with age, and the organism maintains normal glucose levels as long as it can produce enough insulin (hyperinsulinemia). Some individuals are less capable than others to mount sustained hyperinsulinemia and will develop glucose intolerance and T2D *(23)*. Other individuals with insulin resistance will maintain normal glucose levels at the expense of hyperinsulinemia but their pancreas will eventually "burn out," will not be able to sustain hyperinsulinemia, and will develop glucose intolerance and diabetes *(23)*. Others will continue having insulin resistance, may have or not have glucose intolerance, will not develop diabetes, but will have hyperinsulinemia and suffer its consequences. The most frequent modifiable determinant of insulin resistance and hyperinsulinemia is adiposity *(2, 24)*, although adipose tissue is not the only factor. Insulin resistance can reside in other tissues, including muscle, liver, and the pancreas itself *(25)*. The

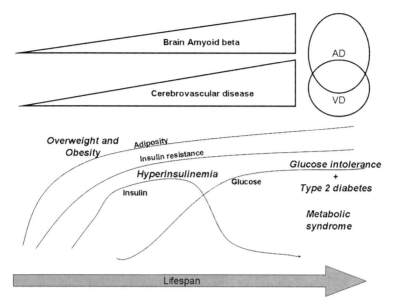

Fig. 1. Natural history of the continuum of adiposity, insulin resistance, hyperinsuline-mia, glucose intolerance, and type 2 diabetes. Increased adiposity causes insulin resis-tance and hyperinsulinemia. Insulin levels may decrease over time due to pancreatic fail-ure, resulting in glucose intolerance and type 2 diabetes. Adiposity, hyperinsulinemia, glucose intolerance, and type 2 diabetes could increase brain amyloid beta deposition and cerebrovascular disease. Cerebrovascular disease leads to vascular dementia (VD). The joint effects of amyloid beta deposition and cerebrovascular disease could lead to Alzheimer's disease (AD).

natural history linking adiposity to insulin resistance to hyperinsulinemia to glucose intolerance and diabetes for most persons could be summarized in the following way (Fig. 1).

Elevations of adiposity result in insulin resistance, causing the pancreas to increase insulin to abnormal levels to sustain normal glucose, and if and when the pancreas can no longer sustain hyperinsulinemia, glucose intoler-ance and diabetes will ensue. However, the overlap between these processes is not complete *(26)*. Not all persons with higher adiposity will develop insulin resistance and hyperinsulinemia, but most will. Not all persons with insulin resistance and hyperinsulinemia will develop glucose intolerance and diabetes, and this depends on genetic and other susceptibility factors that are not completely understood *(25, 26)*. Some adults develop diabetes without going through insulin resistance and hyperinsulinemia, but it is thought that most will.

The susceptibility to adiposity, that is, the risk of developing the above-described sequence in response to adiposity, varies by gender *(4)* and particularly by ethnicity. For example, Chinese and Southeast Asians are more susceptible than Europeans to developing insulin resistance with comparable increases of adiposity (2). The distribution of factors related to insulin resistance and the metabolic syndrome, including adiposity, is different in whites and blacks (27). Thus, conventional ways to classify adiposity may not capture its relation with adverse outcomes and this should be taken into account. High adiposity and hyperinsulinemia are both accompanied by dyslipidemia, hypertension, and inflammation (24), and these should also be taken into account.

One implication of this continuum from a research standpoint is that if we examine diabetes as an exposure, we classify persons without diabetes who may have increased adiposity, hyperinsulinemia, and even glucose intolerance as not exposed. This kind of misclassification would result in an underestimation of the true relation between T2D and dementia if it is random (not conditional on exposure and disease).

Another implication of the continuum described above is that when an epidemiologic study finds a relation between the components of this continuum and dementia we cannot be certain if we are looking at a surrogate marker of one of the other components (e.g., T2D is a marker of past adiposity or hyperinsulinemia, obesity is a marker of hyperinsulinemia) or if the important exposure is the one we are examining. The answer could be that there is an aggregate effect of all the components of the continuum. The metabolic syndrome, an increasingly popular term in clinical practice and research and reported to be associated with a higher risk of cognitive decline (28), is a constellation of adiposity, hypertension, glucose intolerance, and dyslipidemia that is associated mainly with insulin resistance and hyperinsulinemia (29, 30). However, the definition of the metabolic syndrome is somewhat arbitrary, intended to capture the clustering of cardiovascular risk factors particularly in middle-aged populations, and its validity in elderly populations at risk for dementia is not clear (30). The difficulty of arriving at precise metabolic syndrome criteria is reflected by the fact that, over the years, at least six different definitions have been developed that share several characteristics (29).

RISK FACTORS FOR DEMENTIA AND THEIR RELATION TO ADIPOSITY, HYPERINSULINEMIA, AND TYPE 2 DIABETES

Among demographic characteristics, old age (31), low education (32, 33), and being Caribbean Hispanic or African American (34) have been related to a higher risk of AD in New York City. Weight decreases with old age and frailty (35), and BMI in older age may not reflect that of middle age. In the United States, higher adiposity has been related to lower education and socioeconomic position *(21)*. Being overweight or obese is an indication of high adiposity and is more prevalent in blacks and Hispanics compared to whites *(10)*, who have been reported to have a higher risk of AD *(36)*. Thus, it is possible that the association between adiposity and AD is partially explained by older age, lower socioeconomic and educational status, and ethnicity.

Among environmental risk factors, diet *(37)*, physical activity *(32)*, and vascular risk factors *(22)* have attracted increasing interest. The evidence for various dietary factors is conflicting *(37)* and no solid conclusions can be drawn at this time. Higher caloric and fat intake may be related to a higher risk of dementia *(38)*, and higher caloric and fat intake are related to increased adiposity *(3, 4)*, hyperinsulinemia, and T2D. Several studies have found that increased physical activity is inversely related to dementia *(39)*. High physical activity is typically accompanied by low adiposity *(4)*, lower hyperinsulinemia, and lower T2D risk which may be the explanation for the beneficial effects.

In terms of vascular risk factors, hypertension, dyslipidemia, diabetes, hyperinsulinemia, the metabolic syndrome, homocysteine, smoking, and heart disease are potential risk factors for Alzheimer's disease and vascular dementia *(22)*. High adiposity, hyperinsulinemia, and diabetes are clearly related to the metabolic syndrome *(29)*, dyslipidemia *(40)*, and hypertension *(41)*, and these can be reversed or prevented by weight loss, by the reduction of insulin resistance, and by the prevention of T2D *(3, 42, 43)*. Smoking, another potential risk factor for AD *(22)*, is related to weight loss and low weight and thus may produce the appearance of a relation between low BMI and AD through confounding. This type of confounding may partially explain the U-shaped associations found between BMI and other outcomes such as mortality *(44)*.

In summary, many of the putative risk factors for AD and VD are related to the continuum of high adiposity, hyperinsulinemia, and T2D.

MECHANISMS LINKING TYPE 2 DIABETES AND RELATED CONDITIONS TO MILD COGNITIVE IMPAIRMENT AND DEMENTIA

Detailed descriptions of the mechanisms linking T2D to cognitive impairment can be found in other chapters. This summary of mechanisms intends to put into perspective the epidemiologic evidence reviewed later in this chapter. We will classify the mechanisms linking adiposity, hyperinsulinemia, and T2D to dementia as cerebrovascular and non-cerebrovascular. It seems fair to say that it is clearly established that adiposity, hyperinsulinemia, and T2D are vascular risk factors, are accompanied by other vascular risk factors such as hypertension and dyslipidemia, and are risk factors for cerebrovascular disease. Thus, it is expected that these conditions increase the risk of VD, which is determined by the presence of cerebrovascular disease. The mechanisms linking adiposity, hyperinsulinemia, and T2D with AD are not as certain, and this summary emphasizes these mechanisms.

CEREBROVASCULAR DISEASE

Cerebrovascular disease and stroke are related to a higher risk of AD (45, 46). It is not clear whether cerebrovascular disease has a direct action on the amyloid cascade. It may cause brain damage aggregated to amyloid neurotoxicity that may decrease the threshold for the clinical manifestation of AD (47). An autopsy study showed that large vessel cerebrovascular disease, but not small vessel disease or infarcts, was related to a higher frequency of brain neuritic plaques (48), the pathologic hallmark of AD (31). Adiposity, hyperinsulinemia, and T2D (3), and related vascular risk factors such as hypertension and dyslipidemia are related to a higher risk of cerebrovascular disease (49). Thus, adiposity, hyperinsulinemia, and diabetes may affect AD risk indirectly through vascular risk factors and cerebrovascular disease.

NON-CEREBROVASCULAR MECHANISMS

Hyperinsulinemia

As described previously, one of the main consequences of adiposity is insulin resistance and hyperinsulinemia (2). The role of insulin in AD has attracted increasing attention (50) and is covered in more detail in Chapter 18. Insulin can cross the blood–brain barrier from the periphery to the central nervous system and compete with Aβ for insulin-degrading enzyme (IDE) in the brain, including the hippocampus (51). Insulin is also produced in the brain and may alternatively have a beneficial effect on amyloid clearance (52). Peripheral hyperinsulinemia may inhibit brain insulin production which in turn results in impaired amyloid clearance and a higher risk of AD (52). Thus, it is possible that decreasing peripheral hyperinsulinemia and increasing brain insulin levels have the same beneficial effect on AD. A study found that rosiglitazone, which decreases insulin resistance and decreases peripheral insulin levels, and is used in the treatment of T2D, may also be beneficial in Alzheimer's disease (53). Interestingly, intranasal insulin, delivered with direct access to the brain without accessing the periphery has a similar effect (52). Manipulation of insulin levels in humans has been demonstrated to affect cognition and levels of amyloid β in the cerebrospinal fluid (54, 55), supporting the potential direct role of insulin in Alzheimer's disease.

Advanced Products of Glycosylation

Advanced glycosylation products are direct products of glucose intolerance and diabetes and are responsible for their related end-organ damage *(56)*. Advanced glycosilation products can be identified immunohistochemically in senile plaques and neurofibrillary tangles, the pathologic hallmarks of AD *(31)*. Glycation of amyloid β enhances its aggregation in vitro. Furthermore, receptors for advanced glycosilation products have been found to be specific cell-surface receptors for amyloid β, thus potentially causing neuronal damage *(56)*.

Adipokines and Cytokines

Adipose tissue used to be conceived as a passive depot of energy in the form of fats. Recent evidence shows that adipose tissue is active and produces a series of substances that are important in metabolism (adipokines) and inflammation (cytokines). The adipokines include adiponectin *(57)*, leptin *(58)*, and resistin *(58)*, and the inflammatory cytokines include tumor necrosis factor-α and interleukin-6 *(58)*, all correlated with insulin resistance and hyperinsulinemia. It is unclear at this point whether adipokines and cytokines produced by adipose tissue are directly related to AD or whether they are only markers of insulin resistance and hyperinsulinemia. This distinction may be important in the exploration of therapeutic targets.

EPIDEMIOLOGIC EVIDENCE OF THE RELATION BETWEEN TYPE 2 DIABETES AND RELATED CONDITIONS TO MILD COGNITIVE IMPAIRMENT AND DEMENTIA

Adiposity

Few studies have explored the association between adiposity and AD, and several reveal conflicting findings. Elevated BMI in middle age may be associated with higher dementia risk *(59, 60)*. A recent study showed that central adiposity in middle age was related to a higher risk of dementia in older age *(61)*. Higher BMI at ages 70, 75, and 79 years may also predict higher dementia risk *(62)*. However, there have been reports of no association at mid-life *(63)* and of lower BMI related to higher AD risk *(64, 65)* at older ages. There are several explanations for this apparent paradox. First, age of the adiposity measure in relation to clinical dementia onset varies across studies. Throughout life, there may exist critical periods in which risk or protective factors may have more or less impact. Second, several studies have reported weight loss preceding dementia onset *(63, 66)* that may precede diagnosis by decades *(67)*. Understanding the reverse causality observed for

adiposity parameters in relation to dementia onset *(68)* is critical for interpretation of study findings. Third, anthropometric characteristics of populations vary around the world. If baseline BMI, whether measured at mid-life
or late-life, is within a healthy range (e.g., <25 kg/m^2), with low prevalence
of overweight and obesity, the risky effects of high adiposity may be less
likely observed. Finally, another potential explanation is ethnicity. One study
in Japanese Americans showed no association of high adiposity with AD
(63). A study in Northern New York City *(69)* found that in younger elderly
(65–76 years of age), the association between BMI quartiles and AD resembles a U-shaped curve, while in the oldest old (>76 years) higher BMI is
related to a lower AD risk. This U-shaped association has been reported for
the relation between adiposity and cardiovascular mortality *(70)* and underscores the difficulty in studying the effects of adiposity in older age *(71)*.
This study also found that higher waist circumference is related to higher
AD risk in the younger elderly, but not in the oldest. In late life, low BMI
may also be a sign of frailty due to sarcopenia *(35, 72)* or the consequence
of hyperinsulinemia *(73)*, one of the putative mechanisms linking adiposity
and AD.

Recent publications from 2007 to 2008 encapsulate the paradoxes mentioned above, but also seem to explain them. One study in California found
that central adiposity in middle age is a predictor of dementia *(61)*. A study
in New York City found that higher waist circumference was related to a
higher risk of VD, but the findings for AD were similar for persons of age
65–75 years, but not for persons of age 76 years and older *(69)*. The study
in New York City also found that BMI in persons of age 65–75 years had a
U-shaped association with dementia, while there was an inverse association
in persons of age 76 years and older. Similarly, a study in Sweden found
an inverse association between BMI and dementia in persons 75 years and
older. Finally, these findings could be explained by a recent study in Min-
nesota, which found that weight loss may precede dementia by more than 10
years.

Hyperinsulinemia

Several cross-sectional studies show an association between hyperinsulinemia and an increased risk of AD *(74–76)*. Two longitudinal studies, one
in elderly Japanese Americans in Hawaii *(77)*, and another in elderly Black,
Caribbean Hispanic, and non-Hispanic whites in New York City *(78)* found
that the risk of incident AD was higher in persons with hyperinsulinemia.
These studies also found that the risk of AD related to hyperinsulinemia was
higher among persons with the APOE-ε4. There is a paucity of prospective

epidemiologic studies exploring the relation between markers of hyperinsulinemia and AD and more are needed.

Type 2 Diabetes

Diabetes has been related to a twofold higher risk of developing MCI among postmenopausal women *(79)*. A multiethnic study in elderly from New York City found that diabetes was related to a doubling of the risk of cognitive impairment-no dementia (similar to MCI) with stroke, although the effect on cognitive impairment-no dementia without stroke was weaker after adjusting for demographic variables and the presence of Apo E-ε(epsilon)4 allele *(80)*. An Italian study showed a non-statistically significant increase of MCI with diabetes in an elderly population *(81)*, while a Canadian study found that diabetes was related only to vascular cognitive impairment-no dementia *(82)*. A study in New York City found that diabetes was related to a higher risk of both amnestic and non-amnestic MCI, underlining the importance of T2D for both AD-related and vascular cognitive impairment *(83)*. A recent study from Olmstead County, MN, found that T2D itself was not related to MCI, but longer T2D duration and the presence of complications were related to a higher risk of MCI *(84)*.

Diabetes has been found to be consistently related to VD, but its relation to AD is less clear. A study on Japanese subjects aged 65 years and older found that diabetes was related to a doubling of the risk of Alzheimer's disease and a tripling of the risk of VD *(85)*. A longitudinal study from the Netherlands in over 5,000 subjects aged 55 years and older without dementia at baseline found a doubling of the risk of AD *(86)*. This association was stronger in subjects with diabetes who reported insulin treatment. Another European study found that the risk of all cause-dementia was doubled by T2D, but this relation was weaker for AD *(87)*. A study from Rochester, MN, found a doubling of AD in relation to diabetes *(88)*, similar to the study from the Netherlands. A study on catholic nuns, priests, and brothers of age 55 years and older found that diabetes was associated with a 70% higher risk of AD *(89)*. The Honolulu Asia Aging study also found that diabetes in old age was related to an 80% higher risk of AD and AD pathology on autopsy, particularly in subjects with the APOE-ε4 allele *(90)*, the only known genetic risk factor for sporadic AD *(91)*. One study from Canada found that diabetes had a weak non-statistically significant relation to AD, but was related to a doubling of VD risk. A Swedish study found a similar non-significant relation to AD and more than a doubling of the risk of VD *(92)*. A prospective study in over 1,000 subjects from New York City who were mostly African American and Caribbean Hispanic, with a mean age of 75 years, and without dementia at baseline found 40% increased risk of AD, which was not statistically significant after adjustment for other variables, but diabetes was significantly related to significantly higher risk of a composite outcome of AD and cognitive impairment-no dementia (80). The risk of AD was also increased in those treated with insulin, indicating a higher risk of AD in subjects with long-standing diabetes. This study also found a tripling of the risk of VD in relation to T2D. A recent reanalysis of these data with longer follow-up showed that the risk of AD associated with T2D was stronger than previously reported, independent of other vascular conditions (hypertension, heart disease, stroke) and not explained by misclassification of VD cases as AD (93). A study in Sweden found that T2D increased the risk of VD but not of AD (92) and that this risk was higher in the presence of hypertension and heart disease. The same study recently reported that borderline T2D was associated with a higher risk of AD in persons without the APOE-ε4 allele (94), and this association was stronger in the presence of hypertension. The Cardiovascular Health Study recently reported that the risks of AD and mixed dementia (mixed AD and VD) were four times higher in persons with type 2 diabetes and the APOE-ε4 allele compared to those with neither factor (95).

Few studies have examined if T2D in middle age leads to the development of dementia in older age. One study in the United States (96) and another in Israel (97) found that T2D at mid-life increased the risk of dementia in the elderly. However, a study in Japanese Americans found no association between diabetes in middle age and dementia (98).

The diagnosis of diabetes is somewhat arbitrary and many cases go undetected. Few studies have examined the relation between continuous measures of glycemia and dementia. One study in postmenopausal women found that the risk of MCI and dementia increased with each 1% elevation in glycosylated hemoglobin, a stable measure of glucose levels, even in women without diabetes (99). Glycosylated hemoglobin in persons without T2D correlates with both glucose intolerance and insulin resistance, and this study underscores the continuous nature of the relation between these constructs and higher dementia risk.

Metabolic Syndrome

There is limited evidence on the association between the metabolic syndrome and dementia in the elderly. One study in 2,632 Black and White elders found that the metabolic syndrome was associated with a higher risk of cognitive decline, particularly among those with high inflammatory markers (28). A cross-sectional study in Europeans found that AD prevalence was higher in persons with the metabolic syndrome (100). The discrepancy between these studies could be due to the fact that our study was conducted in an older population, ethnically diverse, and with a high prevalence of vascular risk factors *(93)*. In Japanese Americans the metabolic syndrome in middle age was associated with VD, but not AD *(101)*. In New York City the metabolic syndrome was not related to AD risk, while T2D and hyperinsulinemia, the very constructs that the metabolic syndrome attempts to capture, were *(102)*.

SUMMARY AND CAVEATS OF THE EVIDENCE

The study of the association between adiposity and dementia is full of inconsistencies and caveats. The evidence could be summarized as showing that elevated adiposity in middle age is related to higher dementia risk, while the evidence for adiposity in older age is mixed. The epidemiologic evidence linking insulin resistance to dementia is limited by the small number of studies. Numerous studies have related T2D with a higher risk of dementia. The evidence is stronger for VD than for AD, which is expected given the status of T2D as a cerebrovascular risk factor. There are less studies relating T2D with MCI than there are relating T2D with dementia. They seem to indicate that type 2 diabetes is related both to amnestic MCI, thought to precede AD, and to non-amnestic MCI, thought to be more strongly related to cerebrovascular disease.

Some studies show strong associations between T2D and AD despite taking vascular disease and stroke into account. However, the diagnosis of AD is usually done in the absence of brain imaging evidence of cerebrovascular disease, and most cerebrovascular disease may not present as a clinical stroke. Thus, not using brain imaging evidence of cerebrovascular disease for the diagnosis of dementia may result in underestimating the role of cerebrovascular disease in the relation between T2D and AD. This caveat also applies to adiposity and insulin resistance.

Measures of adiposity and risk factors that are part of the metabolic syndrome change with age in ways that may underestimate the effects of high adiposity, dyslipidemia, and blood pressure. In fact, high adiposity in the oldest old may be a marker of health and is related to decreased mortality *(71)*.

Since these risk factors increase morbidity and mortality, survival bias is an issue in cohorts of elderly persons. Persons with the worst adiposity, hyperinsulinemia, and diabetes may die before inclusion into a study, before having the opportunity to develop dementia, or are too frail to participate in studies.

This review describes adiposity, insulin resistance, and T2D as a continuum, but in reality they may be quite heterogeneous, particularly in the elderly, in whom they do not always overlap, and in whom more complicated sub-phenotypes with different pathological significance may exist *(26)*.

As explained before, the definition of normal for adiposity, hyperinsulinemia, and diabetes is somewhat arbitrary and may differ by gender and ethnic
background. This lends itself to misclassification of persons as having or not
having a condition, and this can bias the results of epidemiologic studies.

Lastly, we attempt a reductionist approach to separate the effects of glucose, insulin, components of the metabolic syndrome (hypertension, dyslipidemia), and possibly products of adipose tissue (adipokines, cytokines) on
the risk of cognitive impairment. We also try to separate the associations of
these conditions with AD and vascular cognitive impairment. There is such
overlap in these conditions that this reductionist approach is a very difficult
if not an impossible task. However, we should not be discouraged in isolat-
ing the mechanisms relating these conditions to AD and VD, in particular
because of the potential for interventions including specific drugs, but should
always take into account that the overlaps invariably exist.

IMPLICATIONS FOR THE PREVENTION
AND TREATMENT OF DEMENTIA

There is very strong evidence that adiposity, hyperinsulinemia, and T2D
are related to cognitive impairment syndromes, whether AD, VD, or MCI,
and whether the main mechanism is cerebrovascular disease or non-vascular
mechanisms. However, more evidence is needed to establish causation. If
the relation between these conditions and dementia were to be causal, the
public health implications are enormous. As explained before, two-thirds of
the adult population in the United States are overweight or obese, and the
short-term trend is for this to worsen. These trends are also being observed
worldwide. With increasing life expectancy we are likely to increasingly
see the cognitive consequences of increased adiposity, hyperinsulinemia,
and T2D in old age. We estimated that in New York City the presence
of diabetes or hyperinsulinemia in elderly people could account for 39%
of cases of AD *(78)*. However, the other implication is that a large proportion of cases of AD could be preventable or treatable. The Finnish
Diabetes Prevention Study (FDPS) *(103)* demonstrated that T2D can be
prevented with lifestyle interventions. The Diabetes Prevention Program
(DPP) in the United States demonstrated that T2D can be prevented through
lifestyle interventions or metformin *(43)*, and this effect was largely mediated by improvements in insulin sensitivity and reductions in insulin levels *(104)*. Cognition ancillary studies are planned for both the FDPS and
DPP. These cognition ancillary studies will be unique opportunities to
answer whether the prevention of diabetes through improvement in adiposity and insulin sensitivity is related to improvements in the risk of cognitive impairment. Rosiglitazone, an insulin sensitizer, used not only in the

treatment of T2D but also shown to be effective in prevention *(105)* has shown preliminary promise *(106)* in the treatment of AD, particularly in persons without the APOE-ε4 allele *(53)*. Phase III trials of rosiglitazone are under way although concerns about its safety may limit this drug's usefulness *(107, 108)*. Another important question is whether intense treatment can decrease the risk of cognitive impairment and Alzheimer's disease in persons with T2D. Moreover, it is important to answer whether treatment of T2D with drugs that increase insulin levels vs. insulin sensitizers affects cognitive impairment. Some of these questions will be answered by a cognition ancillary study in the Action to Control Cardiovascular Risk in Diabetes (ACCORD) clinical trial *(109)*. Elucidating the mechanisms linking adiposity, hyperinsulinemia, and T2D to dementia will help identify specific targets for treatment and more research is needed in this regard.

ACKNOWLEDGMENTS

Support for this work was provided by grants from the National Institutes of Health (AG026413, AG07232, MD00206), by the Alzheimer's Association (IIRG-05-15053), and by the Florence and Herbert Irving Clinical Research Scholar's Award.

REFERENCES

1. Hill JO, Bessesen D. What to do about the metabolic syndrome? Arch Intern Med 2003; 163(4):395–397.
2. Reaven GM, Laws A. Insulin resis2tance: the metabolic syndrome X. Totowa, NJ: Humana Press; 1999.
3. Poirier P, Giles TD, Bray GA, et al. Obesity and cardiovascular disease: Pathophysiology, evaluation, and effect of weight loss: an update of the 1997 American Heart Association Scientific Statement on Obesity and Heart Disease from the Obesity Committee of the Council on Nutrition, Physical Activity, and Metabolism. Circulation 2006; 113(6):898–918.
4. Pi-Sunyer FX. The obesity epidemic: Pathophysiology and consequences of obesity. Obes Res 2002; 10(90002):97S–104S.
5. Clinical Guidelines on the Identification, Evaluation, and Treatment of Overweight and Obesity in Adults–The Evidence Report. National Institutes of Health [published erratum appears in Obes Res 1998 Nov; 6(6):464]. Obes Res 1998; 6(90002):51S–209S.
6. Mueller WH, Wear ML, Hanis CL, et al. Which measure of body fat distribution is best for epidemiologic research? Am J Epidemiol 1991; 133(9):858–869.
7. Baumgartner RN, Heymsfield SB, Roche AF. Human body composition and the epidemiology of chronic disease. Obes Res 1995; 3(1):73–95.
8. Wahrenberg H, Hertel K, Leijonhufvud B-M, Persson L-G, Toft E, Arner P. Use of waist circumference to predict insulin resistance: retrospective study. BMJ 2005; 330(7504): 1363–1364.
9. Janssen I, Katzmarzyk PT, Ross R. Waist circumference and not body mass index explains obesity-related health risk. Am J Clin Nutr 2004; 79(3):379–384.
10. Flegal KM, Carroll MD, Ogdan CL, Johnson CL. Prevalence and trends in obesity among US adults, 1999–2000. JAMA 2002; 288(14):1723–1727.

11. Ford ES, Mokdad AH, Giles WH. Trends in waist circumference among U.S. adults. Obes Res 2003; 11(10):1223–1231.

12. Hedley AA, Ogden CL, Johnson CL, Carroll MD, Curtin LR, Flegal KM. Prevalence of overweight and obesity among US children, adolescents, and adults, 1999–2002. JAMA 2004; 291(23):2847–2850.

13. Lillioja S, Mott DM, Spraul M, et al. Insulin resistance and insulin secretory dysfunction as precursors of non-insulin-dependent diabetes mellitus. Prospective studies of Pima Indians. N Engl J Med 1993; 329(27):1988–1992.

14. Haffner SM, Stern MP, Mitchell BD, Hazuda HP, Patterson JK. Incidence of type II diabetes in Mexican Americans predicted by fasting insulin and glucose levels, obesity, and body-fat distribution. Diabetes. 1990; 39(3):283–288.

15. Lundgren H, Bengtsson C, Blohme G, Lapidus L, Waldenstrom J. Fasting serum insulin concentration and early insulin response as risk determinants for developing diabetes. Diabet Med 1990; 7(5):407–413.

16. Charles MA, Fontbonne A, Thibult N, Warnet JM, Rosselin GE, Eschwege E. Risk factors for NIDDM in white population. Paris prospective study. Diabetes 1991; 40(7): 796–799.

17. Laakso M. How good a marker is insulin level for insulin resistance? Am J Epidemiol 1993; 137(9):959–965.

18. Haffner SM, Miettinen H, Stern MP. The homeostasis model in the San Antonio Heart Study. Diabetes Care 1997; 20(7):1087–1092.

19. DeFronzo RA. Pharmacologic therapy for type 2 diabetes mellitus. Ann Intern Med 2000; 133(1):73–74.

20. ClarkJr. MJ, Sterrett JJ, Carson DS. Diabetes Guidelines: a summary and comparison of the recommendations of the American Diabetes Association, Veterans Health Administration, and American Association of Clinical Endocrinologists. Clin Ther 2000; 22(8): 899–910.

21. Luchsinger JA. Diabetes. In: Aguirre-Molina M, Molina CW, Zambrana RE, eds. Health issues in the Latino community. San Francisco, CA: Jossey-Bass; 2001:277–300.

22. Luchsinger J, Mayeux R. Cardiovascular risk factors and Alzheimer's disease. Curr Atheroscler Rep 2004; 6(4):261–266.

23. Festa A, Williams K, D' Agostino R, Jr., Wagenknecht LE, Haffner SM. The natural course of {beta}-cell function in nondiabetic and diabetic individuals: The Insulin Resistance Atherosclerosis Study. Diabetes 2006; 55(4):1114–1120.

24. Reaven G. Insulin resistance, type 2 diabetes mellitus, and cardiovascular disease: the end of the beginning. Circulation 2005; 112(20):3030–3032.

25. Accili D. Lilly Lecture 2003: The struggle for mastery in insulin action: from triumvirate to republic. Diabetes 2004; 53(7):1633–1642.

26. Ferrannini E, Balkau B. Insulin: in search of a syndrome. Diabet Med 2002; 19(9):724–729.

27. Kraja AT, Hunt SC, Pankow JS, et al. An evaluation of the metabolic syndrome in the Hyper-GEN study. Nutr Metab (Lond) 2005; 2(1):2.

28. Yaffe K, Kanaya A, Lindquist K, et al. The metabolic syndrome, inflammation, and risk of cognitive decline. JAMA 2004; 292(18):2237–2242.

29. Grundy SM, Cleeman JI, Daniels SR, et al. Diagnosis and management of the metabolic syndrome: An American Heart Association/National Heart, Lung, and Blood Institute Scientific Statement. Circulation 2005; 112(17):2735–2752.

30. Luchsinger JA. A work in progress: the metabolic syndrome. Sci Aging Knowledge Environ 2006(10):pe19.

31. Cummings JL. Alzheimer's disease. N Engl J Med 2004; 351(1):56–67.

32. Scarmeas N, Zarahn E, Anderson KE, et al. Association of life activities with cerebral blood flow in Alzheimer disease: implications for the cognitive reserve hypothesis. Arch Neurol 2003; 60(3):359–365.

33. Scarmeas N, Stern Y. Cognitive reserve and lifestyle. J ClinExp Neuropsychol 2003; 25(5):625–633.

34. Tang MX, Cross P, Andrews H, et al. Incidence of AD in African-Americans, Caribbean Hispanics, and Caucasians in northern Manhattan. Neurology 2001; 56(1):49–56.
35. Morley JE. Anorexia, sarcopenia, and aging. Nutrition 2001; 17(7–8):660–663.
36. Tang M-X, Maestre G, Tsai W-Y. Relative risk of Alzheimer's disease and age-at-onset base of APOE genotypes among elderly among elderly African Americans, Caucasians and Hispanics in New York City. Am J Hum Genet 1996; 58:554–574.
37. Luchsinger JA, Mayeux R. Dietary factors and Alzheimer's disease. Lancet Neurol 2004; 3(10):579–587.
38. Luchsinger JA, Tang MX, Shea S, Mayeux R. Caloric intake and the risk of Alzheimer disease. Arch Neurol 2002; 59(8):1258–1263.
39. Larson EB, Wang L, Bowen JD, et al. Exercise is associated with reduced risk for incident dementia among persons 65 years of age and older. Ann Intern Med 2006; 144(2):73–81.
40. Morgan JM, Capuzzi DM. Hypercholesterolemia. The NCEP Adult Treatment Panel III Guidelines. Geriatrics 2003; 58(8):33–38; quiz 41.
41. Chobanian AV, Bakris GL, Black HR, et al. The Seventh Report of the Joint National Committee on Prevention, Detection, Evaluation, and Treatment of High Blood Pressure: the JNC 7 report.[see comment][erratum appears in JAMA. 2003 Jul (9); 290(2):197]. JAMA 2003; 289(19):2560–2572.
42. Orchard TJ, Temprosa M, Goldberg R, et al. The effect of metformin and intensive lifestyle intervention on the metabolic syndrome: The Diabetes Prevention Program Randomized Trial. Ann Intern Med 2005; 142(8):611–619.
43. Diabetes Prevention Program Research Group. Reduction in the incidence of type 2 diabetes with lifestyle intervention or metformin. N Engl J Med 2002; 346(6):393–403.
44. Allison DB, Faith MS, Heo M, Kotler DP. Hypothesis concerning the U-shaped relation between body mass index and mortality. Am J Epidemiol 1997; 146(4):339–349.
45. Vermeer SE, Prins ND, den Heijer T, Hofman A, Koudstaal PJ, Breteler MM. Silent brain infarcts and the risk of dementia and cognitive decline. N Engl J Med 2003; 348(13): 1215–1222.
46. Honig LS, Tang MX, Albert S, et al. Stroke and the risk of Alzheimer disease. Arch Neurol 2003; 60(12):1707–1712.
47. Snowdon DA, Greiner LH, Mortimer JA, Riley KP, Greiner PA, Markesbery WR. Brain infarction and the clinical expression of Alzheimer disease. The Nun Study. JAMA 1997; 277(10):813–817.
48. Honig LS, Kukull W, Mayeux R. Atherosclerosis and AD: Analysis of data from the US National Alzheimer's Coordinating Center. Neurology 2005; 64(3):494–500.
49. Sacco RL, Benjamin EJ, Broderick JP, et al. American Heart Association Prevention Conference. IV. Prevention and rehabilitation of stroke. Risk factors.[see comment]. Stroke 1997; 28(7):1507–1517.
50. Strachan MWJ. Insulin and cognitive function. Lancet 2003; 362(9392):1253.
51. Farris W, Mansourian S, Chang Y, et al. Insulin-degrading enzyme regulates the levels of insulin, amyloid beta-protein, and the beta-amyloid precursor protein intracellular domain in vivo. Proc Natl Acad Sci USA 2003; 100(7):4162–4167.
52. Reger MA, Watson GS, Frey WH, 2nd, et al. Effects of intranasal insulin on cognition in memory-impaired older adults: modulation by APOE genotype. Neurobiol Aging 2006; 27(3):451–458.
53. Risner ME, Saunders AM, Altman JF, et al. Efficacy of rosiglitazone in a genetically defined population with mild-to-moderate Alzheimer's disease. Pharmacogenomics J 2006; 6(4):246–254.
54. Watson GS, Bernhardt T, Reger MA, et al. Insulin effects on CSF norepinephrine and cognition in Alzheimer's disease. Neurobiol Aging 2006; 27(1):38–41.
55. Watson GS, Craft S. Modulation of memory by insulin and glucose: neuropsychological observations in Alzheimer's disease. Eur J Pharmacol 2004; 490(1–3):97–113.
56. Yamagishi S, Nakamura K, Inoue H, Kikuchi S, Takeuchi M. Serum or cerebrospinal fluid levels of glyceraldehyde-derived advanced glycation end products (AGEs) may be a

promising biomarker for early detection of Alzheimer's disease. Med Hypotheses 2005; 64(6):1205–1207.

57. Trujillo ME, Scherer PE. Adiponectin – journey from an adipocyte secretory protein to biomarker of the metabolic syndrome. J Int Med 2005; 257(2):167–175.

58. Yu YH, Ginsberg HN. Adipocyte signaling and lipid homeostasis: sequelae of insulin-resistant adipose tissue. Circ Res 2005; 96(10):1042–1052.

59. Kivipelto M, Ngandu T, Fratiglioni L, et al. Obesity and vascular risk factors at midlife and the risk of dementia and Alzheimer disease. Arch Neurol 2005; 62(10):1556–1560.

60. Whitmer RA, Gunderson EP, Barrett-Connor E, Quesenberry CP, Jr, Yaffe K. Obesity in middle age and future risk of dementia: a 27 year longitudinal population based study. BMJ 2005:bmj.38446.466238.E466230.

61. Whitmer RA, Gustafson DR, Barrett-Connor E, Haan MN, Gunderson EP, Yaffe K. Central obesity and increased risk of dementia more than three decades later. Neurol Mar 26 2008.

62. Gustafson D, Rothenberg E, Blennow K, Steen B, Skoog I. An 18-year follow-up of overweight and risk of Alzheimer disease. Arch Intern Med 2003; 163(13):1524–1528.

63. Stewart R, Masaki K, Xue Q-L, et al. A 32-year prospective study of change in body weight and incident dementia: The Honolulu-Asia Aging Study. Arch Neurol 2005; 62(1):55–60.

64. Atti AR, Palmer K, Volpato S, Winblad B, De Ronchi D, Fratiglioni L. Late-life body mass index and dementia incidence: nine-year follow-up data from the Kungsholmen Project. J Am Geriatr Soc 2008; 56(1):111–116.

65. Nourhashemi F, Deschamps V, Larrieu S, et al. Body mass index and incidence of dementia: the PAQUID study. Neurology 2003; 60(1):117–119.

66. Buchman AS, Wilson RS, Bienias JL, Shah RC, Evans DA, Bennett DA. Change in body mass index and risk of incident Alzheimer disease. Neurology 2005; 65(6):892–897.

67. Knopman DS, Edland SD, Cha RH, Petersen RC, Rocca WA. Incident dementia in women is preceded by weight loss by at least a decade. Neurology 2007; 69(8):739–746.

68. White H, Pieper C, Schmader K, Fillenbaum G. Weight change in Alzheimer's disease. J Am Geriatr Soc 1996; 44(3):265–272.

69. Luchsinger JA, Patel B, Tang MX, Schupf N, Mayeux R. Measures of adiposity and dementia risk in elderly persons. Arch Neurol 2007; 64(3):392–398.

70. Stevens J, Cai J, Pamuk ER, Williamson DF, Thun MJ, Wood JL. The effect of age on the association between body-mass index and mortality. N Engl J Med 1998:1–7.

71. Stevens J. Impact of age on associations between weight and mortality. Nutr Rev 2000; 58:129–137.

72. Morley JE, Thomas DR, Wilson M-MG. Cachexia: pathophysiology and clinical relevance. Am J Clin Nutr 2006; 83(4):735–743.

73. Wedick NM, Mayer-Davis EJ, Wingard DL, Addy CL, Barrett-Connor E. Insulin resistance precedes weight loss in adults without diabetes: The Rancho Bernardo Study. Am J Epidemiol 2001; 153(12):1199–1205.

74. Razay G, Wilcock GK. Hyperinsulinaemia and Alzheimer's disease. Age Ageing 1994; 23:396–399.

75. Kuusisto J, Koivisto K, Mykkanen L, et al. Association between features of the insulin resistance syndrome and Alzheimer's disease independently of apolipoprotein E4 phenotype: cross sectional population based study. BMJ 1997; 315(7115):1045–1049.

76. Stolk RP, Breteler MM, Ott A, et al. Insulin and cognitive function in an elderly population. The Rotterdam Study. Diabetes Care 1997; 20:792–795.

77. Peila R, Rodriguez BL, White LR, Launer LJ. Fasting insulin and incident dementia in an elderly population of Japanese-American men. Neurology 2004; 63(2):228–233.

78. Luchsinger JA, Tang M-X, Shea S, Mayeux R. Hyperinsulinemia and risk of Alzheimer disease. Neurology 2004; 63(7):1187–1192.

79. Yaffe K, Blackwell T, Kanaya AM, Davidowitz N, Barrett-Connor E, Krueger K. Diabetes, impaired fasting glucose, and development of cognitive impairment in older women. Neurology 2004; 63(4):658–663.

80. Luchsinger JA, Tang MX, Stern Y, Shea S, Mayeux R. Diabetes mellitus and risk of Alzheimer's disease and dementia with stroke in a multiethnic cohort. Am J Epidemiol 2001; 154(7):635–641.
81. Solfrizzi V, Panza F, Colacicco AM, et al. Vascular risk factors, incidence of MCI, and rates of progression to dementia. Neurology 2004; 63(10):1882–1891.
82. MacKnight C, Rockwood K, Awalt E, McDowell I. Diabetes mellitus and the risk of dementia, Alzheimer's disease and vascular cognitive impairment in the Canadian Study of Health and Aging. Dement Geriatr Cogn Disord 2002; 14(2):77–83.
83. Luchsinger JA, Reitz C, Patel B, Tang M-X, Manly JJ, Mayeux R. Relation of diabetes to mild cognitive impairment. Arch Neurol 2007; 64(4):570–575.
84. Roberts RO, Geda YE, Knopman DS, et al. Association of duration and severity of diabetes mellitus with mild cognitive impairment. Arch Neurol 2008; 65(8):1066–1073.
85. Yoshitake T, Kiyohara Y, Kato I, et al. Incidence and risk factors of vascular dementia and Alzheimer's disease in a defined elderly Japanese population: the Hisayama Study. Neurology 1995; 45(6):1161–1168.
86. Ott A, Stolk RP, van Harskamp F, Pols HA, Hofman A, Breteler MM. Diabetes mellitus and the risk of dementia: The Rotterdam Study. Neurology 1999; 53(9):1937–1942.
87. Brayne C, Gill C, Huppert FA, et al. Vascular risks and incident dementia: results from a cohort study of the very old. Dement Geriatr Cogn Disord 1998; 9(3):175–180.
88. Leibson CL, Rocca WA, Hanson VA, et al. Risk of dementia among persons with diabetes mellitus: a population- based cohort study. Am J Epidemiol 1997; 145(4):301–308.
89. Arvanitakis Z, Wilson RS, Bienias JL, Evans DA, Bennett DA. Diabetes mellitus and risk of Alzheimer disease and decline in cognitive function. Arch Neurol 2004; 61(5):661–666.
90. Peila R, Rodriguez BL, Launer LJ, Honolulu-Asia Aging S. Type 2 diabetes, APOE gene, and the risk for dementia and related pathologies: The Honolulu-Asia Aging Study. Diabetes 2002; 51(4):1256–1262.
91. Ritchie K, Lovestone S. The dementias. Lancet 2002; 360(9347):1759–1766.
92. Xu WL, Qiu CX, Wahlin A, Winblad B, Fratiglioni L. Diabetes mellitus and risk of dementia in the Kungsholmen project: a 6-year follow-up study. Neurology 2004; 63(7): 1181–1186.
93. Luchsinger JA, Reitz C, Honig LS, Tang MX, Shea S, Mayeux R. Aggregation of vascular risk factors and risk of incident Alzheimer disease. Neurology 2005; 65(4):545–551.
94. Xu W, Qiu C, Winblad B, Fratiglioni L. The effect of borderline diabetes on the risk of dementia and Alzheimer's disease. Diabetes 2007; 56(1):211–216.
95. Irie F, Fitzpatrick AL, Lopez OL, et al. Enhanced risk for Alzheimer disease in persons with type 2 diabetes and APOE epsilon4: the Cardiovascular Health Study Cognition Study. Arch Neurol 2008; 65(1):89–93.
96. Whitmer RA, Sidney S, Selby J, Johnston SC, Yaffe K. Midlife cardiovascular risk factors and risk of dementia in late life. Neurology 2005; 64(2):277–281.
97. Schnaider Beeri M, Goldbourt U, Silverman JM, et al. Diabetes mellitus in midlife and the risk of dementia three decades later. Neurology 2004; 63(10):1902–1907.
98. Curb JD, Rodriguez BL, Abbott RD, et al. Longitudinal association of vascular and Alzheimer's dementias, diabetes, and glucose tolerance. Neurology 1999; 52(5):971–975.
99. Yaffe K, Blackwell T, Whitmer RA, Krueger K, Barrett Connor E. Glycosylated hemoglobin level and development of mild cognitive impairment or dementia in older women. J Nutr Health Aging 2006; 10(4):293–295.
100. Vanhanen M, Koivisto K, Moilanen L, et al. Association of metabolic syndrome with Alzheimer disease: A population-based study. Neurology 2006; 67(5):843–847.
101. Kalmijn S, Foley D, White L, et al. Metabolic cardiovascular syndrome and risk of dementia in Japanese- American elderly men. The Honolulu-Asia aging study. Arterioscler Thromb Vasc Biol 2000; 20(10):2255–2260.
102. Muller M, Tang MX, Schupf N, Manly JJ, Mayeux R, Luchsinger JA. Metabolic syndrome and dementia risk in a multiethnic elderly cohort. Dement Geriatr Cogn Disord 2007; 24(3):185–192.

103. Tuomilehto J, Lindstrom J, Eriksson JG, et al. Prevention of type 2 diabetes mellitus by changes in lifestyle among subjects with impaired glucose tolerance. N Engl J Med 2001; 344(18):1343–1350.
104. The Diabetes Prevention Program Research G. Role of Insulin Secretion and Sensitivity in the Evolution of Type 2 Diabetes in the Diabetes Prevention Program: Effects of lifestyle intervention and metformin. Diabetes 2005; 54(8):2404–2414.
105. DREAM investigators. Effect of rosiglitazone on the frequency of diabetes in patients with impaired glucose tolerance or impaired fasting glucose: A randomised controlled trial. Lancet 2006; 368(9541):1096–1105.
106. Watson GS, Cholerton BA, Reger MA, et al. Preserved cognition in patients with early Alzheimer disease and amnestic mild cognitive impairment during treatment with rosiglitazone: A preliminary study. Am J Geriatr Psychiatry 2005; 13(11):950–958.
107. Nathan DM, Berkwits M. Trials that matter: rosiglitazone, ramipril, and the prevention of type 2 diabetes. Ann Intern Med 2007; 146(6):461–463.
108. Nathan DM. Rosiglitazone and cardiotoxicity – weighing the evidence. N Engl J Med 2007:NEJMe078117.
109. Williamson JD, Miller ME, Bryan RN, et al. The action to control cardiovascular risk in diabetes memory in diabetes study (ACCORD-MIND): rationale, design, and methods. Am J Cardiol 2007; 99(12A):112i–122i.

14   Diabetes and Depression

Maria D. Llorente and
Julie E. Malphurs

ONTENTS

ABSTRACT

Diabetes mellitus affects about 20% of adults older than 65 years of age and its prevalence among Americans is reaching epidemic proportions. In cross-sectional studies, diabetes mellitus has been associated with various

From: _Contemporary Diabetes: Diabetes and the Brain_
Edited by: G. J. Biessels, J. A. Luchsinger (eds.), DOI 10.1007/978-1-60327-850-8_14
© Humana Press, a part of Springer Science+Business Media, LLC 2009

complications and comorbid conditions, especially psychiatric disorders. The relationship between diabetes and depression is particularly complex. Evidence demonstrates high co-occurrence of these disorders, with associated poorer medical outcomes. Studies have also shown an increased risk for Alzheimer's disease and more rapid cognitive decline for diabetic patients. The neuroanatomic changes that occur in depression, as well as the neurochemical, neuroendocrine, and resultant inflammatory effects that occur in patients with co-occurring depression and diabetes, are reviewed. The range of treatments for depression including pharmacologic and non-pharmacologic is discussed, with particular consideration of impact of these treatments on patients with diabetes and/or cognitive impairment.

Key words: Depressive disorder; Brain chemistry; Diabetes mellitus; Cognitive impairment; Antidepressant treatment; Neuroanatomy in depression.

BACKGROUND

Thomas Willis (1621–1675), a pioneer in the brain and nervous system and one of the founders of clinical neuroscience, speculated just prior to his death that diabetes was caused by "long sorrow, melancholy, and other depressions" *(1)*. Research findings to date have still failed to yield definitive support for his theory. Most studies have been cross-sectional in nature, limiting the conclusions that can be drawn regarding causality, and the relationship between diabetes and depression is complicated by factors that are associated with both conditions. As the number of persons impacted by both of diabetes and depression will continue to increase with the aging of the population, it is most important to be aware of the strong relationship between these two chronic and demanding illnesses.

EPIDEMIOLOGY OF DIABETES AND DEPRESSION

Approximately 16% of the population will suffer from depression at any time during their lifetime *(2)*. This lifetime prevalence will increase significantly with age, as well as with the existence of a co-occurring physical condition. The number of Americans with diagnosed diabetes is projected to increase 165% from 11 million in 2000 to 29 million in 2050, with the largest percent increase occurring among those persons aged 75 years and older (+271% in older women; +437% in older men) *(3)*.

Prevalence of Comorbidity of Depression and Diabetes

Psychiatric illnesses in general may be more common among persons with diabetes than in community-based samples, specifically affective and anxiety-related disorders *(4)*. Persons with diabetes are twice as likely to have depression as non-diabetic persons *(5)*. A review of 20 studies on the comorbidity of depression and diabetes found that the average prevalence was about 15%, and ranged from 8.5 to 40%, three times the rate of depressive disorders found in the general adult population of the United States (4–7). The rates of clinically significant depressive symptoms among persons with diabetes are even higher – ranging from 21.8 to 60.0% (8). Recent studies have indicated that persons with type II diabetes, accompanied by either major or minor depression, have significantly higher mortality rates than non-depressed persons with diabetes (9–10).

Clinical Outcomes Related to Co-occurring Diabetes and Depression

Diabetes, similar to depression, is a chronic illness that can impact multiple physical and physiological systems in the body. Physical symptoms are often assumed to be related to diabetes with little to no consideration given to the potential impact of co-occurring mood or other psychological conditions. Diabetes symptoms may, in fact, be unreliable indicators of poor glycemic control when symptoms of depression are present in an individual. A study of typical diabetes-related symptoms was conducted and found that depression, not diabetes (glycemic control), was the better predictor of most diabetes-related symptoms when both diabetes and depression are present (11).

Persons with diabetes and depressive symptoms have mortality rates nearly twice as high as persons with diabetes and no depressive symptomatology (9). Persons with co-occurring medical illness and depression also have higher health care utilization leading to higher direct and indirect health care costs (12–13) and it has been suggested that co-occurring medical illness and depression may be key barriers to achieving treatment goals (14).

A meta-analysis of the relationship between depression and diabetes (types I and II) indicated that an increase in the number of depressive symptoms is associated with an increase in the severity and number of diabetic complications, including retinopathy, neuropathy, and nephropathy (15–17). Compared to persons with either diabetes or depression alone, individuals with co-occurring diabetes and depression have shown poorer adherence to dietary and physical activity recommendations, decreased adherence to hypoglycemic medication regimens, higher health care costs, increases in HgbA1c levels, poorer glycemic control, higher rates of retinopathy, and macrovascular complications such as stroke and myocardial infarction, higher ambulatory care use, and use of prescriptions (14, 18–22).

Diabetes and depressive symptoms have been shown to have strong independent effects on physical functioning, and individuals experiencing either of these conditions will have worse functional outcomes than those with neither or only one condition (19–20). Nearly all of diabetes management is conducted by the patient and those with co-occurring depression may have poorer outcomes and increased risk of complications due to less adherence to glucose, diet, and medication regimens *(19, 21, 23)*. The lowest adherence to dietary and exercise recommendations is among older adults with the highest levels of depressive symptom severity *(21, 24)*. Increasing physical activity has been shown to improve both diabetic and depression outcomes *(24, 25)* and a program promoting walking is safe for most patients, including those with medical illness *(14, 25, 26)*. There is some evidence that treatment of depression with antidepressant and/or cognitive-behavioral therapies can improve glycemic control and glucose regulation without any change in the treatment for diabetes *(27, 28)* (see also: *Depression Treatment Considerations for Diabetic Patients*).

Challenges in the Identification of Depression in Non-mental Health Settings

Clinicians treating diabetic patients must have a high index of suspicion regarding the possible presence of depressive symptoms and/or major depressive disorder. All patients with diabetes, at a minimum, should be screened for depressive symptoms on an annual basis and administered appropriate treatments. A simple two-question patient self-administered screen is clinically effective in easily identifying many of these patients (Table 1) *(29)*. Providing this service to patients not only alleviates depressive symptoms, but also has a significant impact on improving mental and physical functioning, adherence with disease self-management and medication regimens, and diabetes outcomes, including HgbA1c levels.

Table 1
Two-question screen for depression

1. During the past month have you often been bothered by feeling down, depressed, or hopeless?
2. During the past month have you often been bothered by little interest or pleasure in doing things?

From: PRIME-MD Patient Health Questionnaire (Primary Care Evaluation of Mental Disorders). Spitzer RL, Kroenke K, Williams JBW. Validation and utility of a self-report version of the PRIME-MD. *JAMA* 1999; 282:1737–1744. Copyright © 2002–2007 Pfizer Inc.

PATHOPHYSIOLOGIC RELATIONSHIP BETWEEN DIABETES AND DEPRESSION

Depression has important clinical relevance to diabetes due to its potential association with poor glycemic control and decreased adherence to treatment regimens. However, it is still unclear what etiology is behind the strong association between these two illnesses. There are several possible mechanisms to explain the relationship between depressive symptoms and DM, and none have been absolutely supported by an evidence-base to date. A very recent study *(30)* examined the bidirectional relationship between diabetes and depressive symptoms using a multi-ethnic, longitudinal cohort of men and women with atherosclerosis and determined that persons with depressive symptoms are at a significantly increased risk of developing diabetes even after controlling for demographic, metabolic, and inflammatory factors. What is clear is that there exists clinical and neurological evidence that diabetes and depression are linked, primarily through dysregulation of the hypothalamo-pituitary-adrenal (HPA) axis (see *Neuroendocrine Findings Associated with Depression*), but the direction of the causality remains under debate *(30, 31)*.

Diabetes as a Risk Factor for Depression

One view is that depressive symptoms are triggered by the existence of diabetes. Depressive symptoms are associated with biochemical changes related to the diabetes (i.e., hyperglycemia, inflammation, activation of the hypothalamic–pituitary–adrenal axis, stress) and may be important factors in disrupting overall metabolic control *(7, 32, 33)*. Further, the presence of depression and depressive symptoms may present as a result of lifestyle choices (i.e., poor diet, no physical activity) and psychological stress associated with managing the illness that are frequently associated with the presence of diabetes. Treated type II diabetes has been associated with a significantly higher chance of developing depressive symptoms, even after controlling for BMI and co-morbidities *(30)*, and well-functioning older adults with diabetes are at nearly twice the risk of developing depressive symptoms than those without diabetes *(34)*.

Depression as a Risk Factor for Diabetes

An alternative explanation for the relationship between depression and diabetes views the development of diabetes as the result of pre-existing depression. This view suggests that (1) neurohormonal changes induced by depression, such as hypercortisolism, can lead to insulin resistance and to the development of diabetes, and (2) behavioral factors associated with depression, including lack of physical activity and poor diet, increase the risk for the development of diabetes *(24, 32, 35–38)*.

The presence of depression may adversely impact the function of a number of neurotransmitters, including serotonin, norepinephrine, dopamine, acetylcholine, and GABA *(7)*. Depressive symptoms are also associated with increased inflammation *(39)* and inflammatory markers are established risk factors for type II diabetes *(40)*. Further, depressive symptoms and major depression can cause abnormalities in the hypothalamic–pituitary–adrenal (HPA) axis and other hormonal irregularities *(41)*. Meta-analyses have identified an association between depression and hyperglycemia, but the mechanism and directionality of the association have not been determined *(7, 23)*.

The increase in glycosylated hemoglobin (HgbA1c) levels attributed to depression alone has ranged from 1.8 to 3.3% *(23, 42)*. A meta-analysis of depression and studies of glycemic control confirmed the association of depression with hyperglycemia, but was unable to reveal the mechanism or the direction of the association *(23)*. The association between depression and glycemic control has recently been observed in ethnic minority groups with diabetes as well *(43)*. In addition, treatment and subsequent improvement in depression has been significantly associated with improvement in glycemic control (see also: *Treatment Considerations*).

Diabetes and Depression as Clinical Outcomes of a Common Pathophysiologic Pathway

It is extremely difficult to establish an evidence-base for either of these explanations due to the lack of control populations and standardized measurements. The role of stress in the development of depression as well as in glucose regulation has been well established, and the impact of stress can be nearly impossible to disentangle in studies of diabetes and depression. While the relationship between diabetes and depression clearly exists, the causative nature of this relationship may always be difficult to determine due to the circular directionality of these two illnesses. Depression may be a cause or a result of diabetes and both the direction and the mechanism of this relationship may vary over time. There is a growing research base that confirms the bidirectional association between diabetes and depression *(30, 44)*. Regardless of the etiology of these illnesses in a patient, the outcomes for both illnesses worsen when they co-occur, than with either illness alone. Providers should be aware of the strong relationship between diabetes and depression and provide appropriate treatment and management of both illnesses.

NEUROANATOMICAL FINDINGS ASSOCIATED WITH DEPRESSION

A number of studies have used magnetic resonance imaging to examine volumetric differences in the brains of adults with major depressive disorder (MDD). Overall brain size is not affected, but certain brain regions have received attention. In particular, in looking at the symptom complex during a depressive episode, one could postulate that the following brain regions are likely involved: (1) frontal lobe areas which are involved in executive functioning, cognitions (hopelessness, guilt) and motivation; (2) hypothalamus which mediate neurovegetative symptoms including appetite, sleep, energy metabolism, and autonomic functioning; (3) hippocampus and amygdala, involved in the formation and storage of memories. These areas have indeed received attention. Discrepant study findings have occurred and may be attributed to several factors, including variations in study populations (medicated vs. untreated, unipolar vs. bipolar samples, younger vs. older subjects), scan parameters (such as scan thickness), and inclusion of anatomic areas that are difficult to delineate (such as the amygdala). Nevertheless, several consistent findings have been reported.

In two recent meta-analyses of MRI studies measuring hippocampal and amygdalar volumes, MDD patients had lower bilateral hippocampal volumes relative to controls *(45)*, averaging an 8% reduction on the left, and a 10% reduction on the right *(46)*. Several studies have found a positive relationship between smaller hippocampal volume and longer duration of illness, larger total number of depressed episodes, and poor response to antidepressants *(47–49)*. Inclusion of the amygdala in combined measurements is a confounder, however, and no differences were observed in amygdalar volumes alone or combined with the hippocampus.

Similarly, neuroanatomic changes in the frontal lobes have been implicated in depressive disorders. Lesions of the orbitofrontal cortex increase the risk for developing depression, and metabolic activity is more reduced in this brain region in depressed vs. non-depressed Parkinson's patients. Lower cortical volume in the subgenual prefrontal cortex and orbitofrontal cortex occurs more often in depressed subjects compared to non-depressed controls *(50, 51)*. Further, decreased glial cell counts, density, as well as smaller neuronal size have been reported in the prefrontal, anterior cingulate, and orbitofrontal cortices of patients with MDD *(52, 53)*. Reduction in the gray matter of the anterior subgenual cingulate cortex persists across illness episodes, correlates with illness severity, appears early in the course of illness, and has been found prior to illness onset in patients with significant family history of MDD.

Regional volumetric losses have also been reported in diabetic patients. For example, type II diabetic patients had smaller hippocampal volumes even after controlling for vascular disease *(54)*, and associated decrements in memory *(55)*. Type I diabetic patients were found to be more likely to have superior temporal gyrus gray matter density loss compared to controls *(56)*. Diabetes and depressive states have both been found to be associated with chronic stress and hypercortisolemia. Elevated levels of glucocorticoids have been found to be neurotoxic to gray matter cells of the frontal lobe as well as hippocampal neurons and may in part explain the similar findings.

NEUROENDOCRINE FINDINGS ASSOCIATED
WITH DEPRESSION

The hypothalamic–pituitary–adrenal (HPA) axis mediates the ability of an organism to respond to threats, including stress. Interestingly, the determining characteristics of stressors which provoke depression in humans (namely entrapment, humiliation, and loss) provoke animal models of depression. Following exposure to a stressor, the hypothalamus releases corticotrophin-releasing hormone (CRH) which in turn stimulates the release of adrenocorticotrophic hormone (ACTH) by the anterior pituitary gland. This causes the adrenal glands to release glucocorticoids, including cortisol. Glucocorticoids interact with receptors in most body tissues, particularly in the regulation of energy metabolism. Glucocorticoids eventually bind corticosteroid receptors in the hippocampus which then act to inhibit further production of CRH and ACTH, shutting down the loop. This "fast feedback" operates over the course of minutes. This system allows the "flight or fight" response, in which pulse and blood pressure increase, gastrointestinal and immunologic responses are suppressed, and glucose is mobilized to the muscles. In times of chronic stress, however, the HPA axis remains activated. This occurs through up-regulation of the hypothalamus and down-regulation of the corticosteroid receptors which mediate the negative feedback regulation, especially those in the hippocampus.

Pathological elevations of glucocorticoids occur and are associated with depression, with as many as 50% of Cushing's disease patients having significant depressive symptoms (57). Studies have consistently found that approximately half of depressed patients have hypothalamic–pituitary–adrenal (HPA)-axis hyperactivity. There is also a direct correlation between peripheral cortisol levels and depression symptom severity. While the key neuroregulator of the HPA axis is CRH, whose effects are mediated by neuropeptides and catecholamines (serotonin, dopamine, norepinephrine), impaired negative feedback control by glucocorticoid and mineralocorticoid receptors (GR and MR, respectively) in the hippocampus has also been implicated (so-called glucocorticoid resistance). Additional evidence for HPA hyperactivity is the finding of enlarged pituitary and adrenal glands in depressed patients. Impairments in HPA axis and elevated serum cortisol levels are similarly implicated in complications of types I and II diabetes. Poor glycemic control is associated with increased plasma levels of cortisol and greater sensitivity to both acute and chronic stress, contributing to the frequent co-occurrence of diabetes and depression.

Many animal studies have demonstrated that glucocorticoids are toxic to the hippocampus and decrease the proliferation of oligodendrocyte precursors (58). In addition, these cells are also sensitive to excitotoxic effects of excess glutamate, which is known to occur in depressive states. In chronic stress states, high cortisol levels can overstimulate the hippocampus, leading to cell death and further diminishing the inhibitory regulation of the HPA axis (59, 60).

THE INFLAMMATORY RESPONSE AND DEPRESSION

Excess inflammation may also play a role in the development of depression and contribute to poor response to antidepressants. A recent study found that an increased inflammatory state at baseline predicted incident onset of depression in elderly individuals without a prior history of depression, suggesting that excess inflammation precedes depression (61). Inflammatory mediators can lead to glutamate-receptor agonism and increase glutamate release. Recently, glutamate has been implicated in depression. During both acute and remitted phases of illness, depressed patients have elevated levels of glutamate in some brain regions. Activation of NMDA receptors by glutamate can then activate microglia and cause further release of inflammatory mediators, and more glutamate release, as well as inhibition of amino acid removal by astroglia. Inflammatory mediators can activate both neurotoxic and neurotrophic microglia. It has been hypothesized that imbalance between T-helper cell type 1 (Th1) mediator (which induces neurotoxic microglia) and the T-helper cell type 2 (Th2) mediator (which induces neuroprotective microglia) may play a role in depression. A Th1 response activates macrophages which secrete pro-inflammatory mediators. A Th2 response is characterized by antibody production and anti-inflammatory mediators, which inhibit the Th1 response. This balance prevents excess inflammation. A subgroup of depressed patients consistently have elevated plasma levels of pro-inflammatory mediators (62, 63), which decrease with antidepressant treatment (64, 65), suggesting that a possible mechanism of action for antidepressants is reduction of inflammation. In depressive states, this inappropriate balance can also shift the microglial phenotype toward a neurotoxic one, impairing neuroplasticity and causing loss of neurons.

NEUROCHEMICAL FINDINGS ASSOCIATED WITH DEPRESSION AND DIABETES

The role of some catecholamines (most notably, dopamine and serotonin) in depression has received much attention. For example, the mesolimbic dopamine pathway allows an organism to analyze the environment and its cues and to express appropriate approach or avoidance behaviors. One animal model for depression, which exposes mice to daily bouts of social defeat, followed by protected sensory contact with the aggressor characterizes the actions of this pathway *(66)*. Mice are exposed to a different aggressor each day for 10 days, screened for social behavior, and then exposed to an unfamiliar mouse enclosed in a wire mesh cage. Social approach toward the unfamiliar mouse is then measured. Control mice spend most of the time interacting socially. The defeated mice displayed intensive aversive responses. This response persisted for up to 4 weeks following the stressor. Social interactions in these defeated mice improved with chronic administration of fluoxetine or imipramine, but not chlordiazepoxide, suggesting that depression and not anxiety was primarily mediating the response. The social defeat exposure increased brain-derived neurotrophic factor (BDNF), a key regulator of the mesolimbic dopamine pathway, in the nucleus accumbens. The source of BDNF is thought to be the ventral tegmental area since BDNF mRNA is expressed in high levels there, but is barely detectable in the nucleus accumbens neurons. Deletion of the BDNF gene led to an antidepressant-like effect in defeated mice. To demonstrate the complexities of these circuits and to illustrate that neuropeptides serve different functions in different brain regions, increased BDNF in the hippocampus exerts an antidepressant effect. During depressive episodes, hippocampal serotonin 5-HT2A receptors are up-regulated. This serves to decrease BDNF *(67)*. On the other hand, BDNF in the hippocampus exerts an antidepressant effect, thus illustrating that neuropeptides have differing effects in varied neuronal circuits. Mesolimbic dopamine abnormalities are also associated with obesity and diabetes. Specifically, people with a single copy of the Taq1A1 allele (a gene that codes for fewer dopamine receptors) were more likely to overeat and be obese.

Serotonin abnormalities have also been described in depressed subjects. Lower brainstem levels of both serotonin (5-HT) and its metabolite 5-hydroxyindoleacetic acid (5-HIAA), as well as fewer serotonin transporter (SERT) binding sites and more post-synaptic 5-HT1A receptors in the prefrontal cortex all suggest reduced serotonin brain function which also correlated with suicidality *(68)*. A recent study found significantly fewer receptors in various brain regions of depressed individuals, especially in the hippocampus *(67)*. It is possible that this could be due to volume loss and hippocampal damage or may resemble the pathophysiology of diabetes in which people still make insulin, but the receptors are unresponsive.

RELATIONSHIP BETWEEN DEPRESSION AND VASCULAR DISEASE

A frequently replicated neuroimaging finding in depression is an increase in hyperintensities in the white matter and deep gray matter of the basal ganglia. In a large study of more than 3,000 elderly, severity of hyperintensity lesions was significantly associated with depression severity. These signal intensities are due to cerebrovascular disease more commonly in depression.

Further, several studies have consistently found that depression is a risk factor for cardiovascular disease and has a direct impact on cardiovascular mortality following a heart attack (69). Depression is as strong a predictor of poor outcome following an MI as the best-established risk factor, left ventricular dysfunction. Similarly, there is equally compelling evidence that coronary artery disease, stroke, and peripheral vascular disease are all associated with high rates of depression. There is little relationship between hypertension or cholesterol and depression.

Chronic pro-inflammatory cytokine activation is also associated with coronary artery syndromes and thought to mediate the relationship between depression and cardiovascular disease, as well as that between cardiovascular disease and diabetes (70, 71). Specifically, interleukin-6 (IL-6) and tumor necrosis factor-α (TNF-α) increase hyperglycemia and interfere with lipid metabolism. They are important in the pathogenesis of atherosclerosis. As symptoms of stress increase, so does systemic inflammation, increasing cardiovascular risk (72).

RELATIONSHIP BETWEEN DEPRESSION AND COGNITIVE IMPAIRMENT

Certain symptoms of cognitive impairment (psychomotor retardation, loss of affect, concentration, and memory difficulties) are frequent among persons with depression and other mood disorders, and prevalence of both cognitive impairment and depression increases significantly with age (73). People with depression have been shown to perform worse on tests of cognitive performance and neuropsychological measures than non-depressed persons (73).

Similar to the relationship between diabetes and depression, dementia and depression have been closely linked and the directionality of this relationship remains uncertain (31, 73). Depression is highly prevalent among persons with dementia, and several studies have suggested that a history of depression may increase dementia risk.

Volumetric changes of the hippocampus offer one possible explanation of recent findings that depression is a risk factor for dementia. Many patients with MDD report cognitive impairment, even in euthymic states. For example, when compared with controls, euthymic women with recurrent depression showed smaller bilateral hippocampal volumes and lower verbal memory scores, a neuropsychological measure of hippocampal function (74). Further, the severity of deficits correlates with total number of depressive episodes *(75)*, and a smaller hippocampus, especially on the left, is predictive of incident dementia at 5-year follow-up in older depressed persons *(76)*.

DEPRESSION TREATMENT CONSIDERATIONS FOR DIABETIC PATIENTS

Despite the lack of a definitive cause–effect model to explain the significant relationship between depression and diabetes, reports on the effects of treatment for depression have shown promise on outcomes for both diseases. Treatment for depression in patients with diabetes has demonstrated benefits on glycemic control as well as mood and even insulin sensitivity *(32, 77)*. There is evidence that both antidepressant medication and psychotherapeutic treatments can improve both depressive and diabetic outcomes in patients with both illnesses. Recently, collaborative care models in primary care using case management interventions for the treatment of depression have shown promise in improving outcomes in patients with diabetes *(78, 79)*.

Antidepressant Medications

Antidepressants, as a group, are equally effective in the treatment of depression. For a given individual, however, one medication will be more effective and/or tolerable than another. In current practice, the choice of medication is primarily based on side effects one wants to avoid (such as urinary retention or confusion secondary to anticholinergic effects in patients with benign prostatic hypertrophy or cognitive symptoms) or side effects that are desirable (such as sedation in patients with significant reports of insomnia). Additional considerations in diabetic patients include avoiding antidepressant medications which can increase weight gain, or which dysregulate glucose metabolism, and whether one wants to additionally target diabetic neuropathic pain. This has been recently reviewed *(80)*. Most current evidence supports the use of serotonin-reuptake inhibitors to treat depression *(81)*.

A limited open-label study of sertraline indicated that patients with diabetes (HgbA1c > 8) and depressive symptoms showed decreases in depressive symptoms and a statistically significant decrease in HgbA1c from an average 9.2 to 8.8 *(82)*. Several studies of fluoxetine in patients with diabetes and depression have indicated reductions in weight and in HbA1c to near-normal levels (<7) *(83)*, and significant reductions in depressive symptoms in diabetic patients have occurred in addition to improvement in glycemic control *(23, 84)*. A double-blind placebo-controlled study of nortriptyline showed considerable effect on depressive symptomatology while at the same time indicating significant improvement in glucose control in patients with diabetes and depression *(85)*. In a recent open-label treatment trial, depressed, diabetic patients treated with bupropion had significantly reduced depressive symptomatology as well as improved glycemic control which was unrelated to improvements in self-care or weight loss *(27)*.

Rubin and colleagues (2008) *(1)* recently reported that among participants in a diabetes prevention program, use of antidepressants significantly increased the risk of subsequently developing diabetes. The authors postulate that use of antidepressants could be a marker for the actual cause of increased diabetes risk, namely, severe, chronic depression *(1)*. A meta-analysis conducted in Canada indicated that persons with depression and treated with antidepressants (both tricyclics and SSRIs) had an increased risk of developing type II diabetes, but persons treated with SSRIs only had a significantly reduced risk of developing diabetes *(28)*.

More double-blind, controlled studies of antidepressant treatments need to be conducted on larger populations of patients with diabetes and depression in order to obtain an evidence-base with which to establish treatment guidelines for use. Currently, the evidence suggests that treatment of depression improves both depressive symptoms as well as diabetes symptoms at clinically, if not statistically, significant levels.

Mechanism of Action

These agents act by increasing serotonergic functioning, which in turn increases insulin sensitivity and reduces plasma glucose. Most studies have investigated fluoxetine (doses up to 60 mg/day) and sertraline. Patients' depressive symptoms responded, and they experienced weight loss, decreased fasting plasma glucose, and lowered HgbA1c levels. Catecholamines, on the other hand, are associated with insulin resistance and hyperglycemia. Depressed diabetic patients who were administered nortriptyline, a norepinephrine-reuptake inhibitor, had poorer glycemic control. Other tricyclic antidepressants can increase food cravings, increase weight, and raise serum glucose levels. Because both catecholamines and serotonin have been implicated in diabetic neuropathy, dual-action antidepressants may be the preferred agents, particularly in non-depressed subjects.

One important finding is that treatment of depression seems to be able to halt atrophy of the hippocampus and may even lead to stimulation of neurogenesis of hippocampal cells *(86)*. Similarly, antidepressants directly increase the expression and function of corticosteroid receptors in the brain, enhancing the negative feedback loop and reducing pathological HPA-axis hyperactivity.

Future Directions for Antidepressant Treatments

The notion of targeting the HPA axis directly to treat depression in diabetes is intriguing. Three major pathways are currently under investigation and include administration of (1) CRH antagonists; (2) glucocorticoid receptor (GR) antagonists; (3) steroid-synthesis inhibitors.

CRH antagonists: CRH acts through CRH_1 receptors to produce a number of anxiety- and depression-like symptoms, which have led to the consideration of CRH_1 receptors as potential drug targets. Several small non-peptide molecules that are able to pass the blood–brain barrier have entered clinical development. One agent, NBI-30775/R121919, was reported to have a clinical profile comparable to paroxetine *(87)*. This compound was administered to 24 patients with a major depressive episode primarily for a safety and tolerability study. The drug was found to be tolerated by patients and did not interfere with cortisol secretion at baseline or following an exogenous CRH challenge *(88)*. Significant reductions in both patient- and clinician-rated depression and anxiety scores were found. Of interest is that mood symptoms worsened following drug discontinuation. CRH_1 receptor antagonism for the treatment of depression has demonstrated potential therapeutic value and merits further examination.

GR antagonists: One drug in this group has been studied, although with only small samples and case reports. The medication, mifepristone, is a powerful progesterone and glucocorticoid receptor antagonist, also known as RU-486. One case of Cushing's disease was successfully treated, and an incidental finding was the patient's suicidal depression resolved *(89)*. A small brief, double-blind, placebo-controlled cross-over study demonstrated substantial improvements in depression symptoms when mifepristone was administered *(90)*. Because of controversies associated with the abortifacient effects of this drug, however, its clinical utility for the treatment of depression is limited.

Steroid-synthesis inhibitors: In the 1970s, depressed Cushing's patients were treated with metyrapone, which blocks the synthesis of cortisol and causes a compensatory increase in ACTH secretion. A subsequent case report using metyrapone and two small double-blind studies on ketoconazole (which also blocks cortisol synthesis) in non-Cushing's depressed patients suggested that steroid-synthesis inhibition might be an effective treatment strategy. Recently, a double-blind trial investigated the use of metyrapone for augmentation treatment in depression *(91)*. Metyrapone induced increases of plasma ACTH and the cortisol precursor 11-deoxycortisol and the neurosteroid DHEA (which itself has anxiolytic and antidepressant properties). Added to selective serotonin inhibitor antidepressants, more patients in the metyrapone-treated group responded and showed an earlier onset of action, in some cases beginning in the first week. Metyrapone-enhanced antidepressant efficacy occurred independently of basal morning plasma cortisol concentrations. The mechanism of action of this effect remains unknown, but metyrapone decreases cortisol levels in both the plasma as well as the brain. Inhibition of cortisol synthesis in the hippocampus leads to up-regulation of mineralocorticoid receptors (MR), a finding demonstrated for many antidepressant medications *(92)*. Increased MR in the hippocampus leads to decreased CRH mRNA in the hypothalamus and resetting of the HPA axis. Additionally, metyrapone increases cell numbers in the dentate gyrus of the hippocampus of mice, possibly mediated through the production of DHEA, facilitating hippocampal feedback restoration to the HPA axis.

Pharmacogenomics: In the not too distant future, we may be able to select antidepressants based on pharmacogenomic profiles. For example, the most studied polymorphism in the pharmacogenomics of antidepressant response is 5-HTTLPR, located in a repeat region of the promoter of the serotonin transporter gene. In Caucasian and Chinese subjects, most studies on the effect of 5-HTTLPR on response to selective serotonin-reuptake inhibitors (SSRIs) in unipolar depressed patients have shown significant associations of the "long" variant (L allele) of the polymorphism with better treatment outcome. Associations with response to antidepressants other than SSRIs have been mostly negative. Knowing that an individual has the L allele may favor the initiation of an SSRI. Ongoing pharmacogenomic projects are evaluating the idea that genetic variations in pharmacokinetic targets may be used to develop drug recommendations that aim at decreasing adverse drug reactions (ADRs) and at increasing remission of depressive symptoms by antidepressant treatment. It is possible that genetic screening for metabolizing enzymes could help improve treatment outcome and lower health care costs if treatment assignment avoids drugs that would be out of the therapeutic window.

Psychotherapies

Aversive experiences both in utero and the neonatal period in rodents resulted in elevated HPA responses to subsequent stress *(93)*. This is similar to the long-lasting effects on the stress response in humans who experienced early traumatic events. Interestingly, nurturing experiences can up-regulate glucocorticoid receptors in the hippocampus, thus terminating the stress response *(94)*. This suggests a possible biological mechanism of action for the psychotherapeutic experience.

Current clinical research has also indicated benefits from psychological therapies. The introduction or inclusion of various types of behavioral interventions into the management of diabetes has been demonstrated to improve metabolic control as well as quality of life. To date, however, there has been little empirical support for the successful use of non-pharmacological therapies (psychotherapies, relaxation) for the management of depression specifically in persons with diabetes. Non-pharmacologic interventions are particularly useful in the initial management of patients who may have mild depressive symptoms and are concerned about taking medications or in older adults who may take multiple medications for co-occurring illnesses.

Other forms of psychotherapy, specifically cognitive-behavioral psychotherapy have been shown useful in the treatment of depression in persons with diabetes. Cognitive-behavioral therapy (CBT) is characterized by implementing behavioral strategies to engage patients in social and physical activities as well as employing problem-solving and cognitive methods to identify and replace maladaptive thought patterns with more adaptive and useful thoughts. Several studies have demonstrated that individuals who received CBT have reduced cortisol response which is a measure of HPA-axis activity *(95)*. Further, Lustman and colleagues (1998) *(96)* performed a randomized, controlled investigation of the use of cognitive-behavioral therapy for depression in patients with type II diabetes. CBT was found to be an effective treatment for depression and also led to a significant decrease in HgbA1c levels compared to the control group.

Collaborative Care Models

Collaborative care models have used case management, in conjunction with problem-solving therapy, for the treatment of depression in diabetic populations *(9)*. Systematic, between-visit patient monitoring appears to be essential for improving outcomes in patients with depression and diabetes, as these patients are more likely to require regular monitoring and follow up, and collaborative care models adhere to systematic monitoring. Several of these models, which integrate mental health and primary care, have specifically targeted persons with diabetes and depression (IMPACT, pathways) *(97–100)*. Both of these models report significantly improved depressive outcomes in patients with diabetes and minimal improvement in hemoglobin A1C levels *(98, 99)*. Another collaborative care model, PROSPECT, which was initiated as a suicide prevention program in primary care, recently reported that persons with diabetes and depression who participated in the collaborative care intervention were significantly less likely to die than depressed diabetic patients who did not participate in the intervention *(100)*.

REFERENCES

1. Rubin RR., Ma Y, Marrero DG, et al. Elevated depression symptoms, antidepressant medicine use, and the risk of developing diabetes during the Diabetes Prevention Program. Diabetes Care 2008; 31:420–426.
2. Kessler RC, Berglund P, Demler O, et al. The epidemiology of major depressive disorder: results from the National Comorbidity Survey Replication. JAMA 2003; 289:3095–3105.
3. Boyle JP, Honeycutt AA, Narayan V, et al. Projection of diabetes burden through 2050: impact of changing demography and disease prevalence in the United States. Diabetes Care 2001; 24:1936–1940.
4. Jacobson AM, Samson JA, Weinger K, Ryan CM. Diabetes, the brain and behavior: is there a biological mechanism underlying the association between diabetes and depression? International Review of Neurobiology 2002; 51:455–479.
5. Anderson RJ, Freedland KE, Clouse RE, et al. The prevalence of comorbid depression in adults with diabetes. Diabetes Care 2004; 24:1069–1078.
6. Gavard JA, Lustman PJ, Clouse RE. Prevalence of depression in adults with diabetes: an epidemiological evaluation. Diabetes Care 1993; 16:1167–1178.
7. Harris MD. Psychosocial aspects of diabetes with an emphasis on depression. Curr Diabetes Rep 2003; 3:49–55.
8. Lustman PJ & Gavard JA. Psychosocial aspects of diabetes in adult populations. In National Diabetes Data Group. Diabetes in America, 2nd Edition. NIH Publication #95-1468, 1995.
9. Katon WJ, Rutter C, Simon G, et al. The association of comorbid depression with mortality in patients with type 2 diabetes. Diabetes Care 2005; 28:2668–2672.
10. Bogner HR, Morales KH, Post EP, Bruce ML. Diabetes, depression and death: a randomized controlled trial of a depression treatment program for older adults based in primary care (PROSPECT). Diabetes Care 2007; 30:3005–3010.
11. Lustman PJ, Clouse RE, Carney RM. Depression and the reporting of diabetes symptoms. Int J Psychiatry Med 1988; 18:295–303.
12. Simon GE, Von Korff M, Barlow W. Health care costs of primary care patients with recognized depression. Arch GenPsychiatry 1995; 52:850–856.
13. Unutzer J, Patrick DL, Simon G, et al. Depressive symptoms and the cost of health services in HMO patients aged 65 years and older : a four-year prospective study. JAMA 1997; 277:1618–1623.
14. Piette JD, Richardson C, Valenstein M. Addressing the needs of patients with multiple chronic illnesses: the case of diabetes and depression. Am J Managed Care 2004; 10(part 2):152–162.
15. de Groot M, Anderson R, Freedland KE. Association of depression and diabetes complications: a meta-analysis. Psychosom Med 2001; 63:619–630.
16. Cohen ST, Welch G, Jacobson AM, deGroot M, Samson J. The association of lifetime psychiatric illness and increased retinopathy in patients with type I diabetes mellitus. Psychosomatics 1997; 38:98–108.
17. Geringer ES, Perlmuter LC, Stern TA, Nathan DM. Depression and diabetic neuropathy: a complex relationship. J Geriatr Psychiatry Neurol 1988; 1:11–15.
18. Egede LE, Zheng D, Simpson K. Comorbid depression is associated with increased health care use and expenditures in individuals with diabetes. Diabetes Care 2002; 25:464–470.
19. Ciechanowski PS, Katon WJ, Russo JE, et al. The relationship of depressive symptoms to symptom reporting, self-care and glucose control in diabetes. Gen Hosp Psychiatry 2003; 25:246–252.
20. Fultz NH, Ofstedal MB, Herzog AR, et al. Additive and interactive effects of comorbid physical and mental conditions on functional health. J Aging Health 2003; 15:465–481.
21. Ciechanowski PS, Katon WJ, Russo JE. Depression and diabetes: impact of depressive symptoms on adherence, function and costs. Arch Int Med 2000; 160:3278–3285.

22. Lustman PJ & Clouse RE. Depression in diabetic patients: the relationship between mood and glycemic control. J Diabetes Complications 2005; 19:113–122.

23. Lustman PJ, Anderson RJ, Freedland KE, et al. Depression and poor glycemic control: a meta-analytic review of the literature. Diabetes Care 2000; 23:434–442.

24. Saydah SH, Brancati FL, Golden SH, et al. Depressive symptoms and the risk of Type II diabetes mellitus in a US sample. Diabetes Metab Res Rev 2003; 19:202–208.

25. Strawbridge WJ, Deleger S, Roberts RE, et al. Physical activity reduces the risk of subsequent depression for older adults. Am J Epidemiology 2002; 156:328–334.

26. Hu FB. Walking: the best medicine for diabetes? Arch Int Med 2003; 163:1397–1398.

27. Lustman PJ, Williams MM, Sayuk GS, Nix BD, Clouse RE. Factors influencing glycemic control in Type 2 diabetes during acute- and maintenance-phase treatment of major depressive disorder with bupropion. Diabetes Care 2007; 30:459–466.

28. Brown LC, Majumdar SR, Johnson JA. Type of antidepressant therapy and risk of Type 2 diabetes in people with depression. Diabetes Res Clin Pract 2008; 79:61–67.

29. Spitzer RL, Kroenke K, Williams JBW. Validation and utility of a self-report version of the PRIME-MD. JAMA 1999; 282:1737–1744.

30. Golden SH, Lazo M, Carnethon M, et al. Examining a bidirectional association between depressive symptoms and diabetes. JAMA 2008; 299:2751–2759.

31. Rasgon N, Jarvik L. Insulin resistance, affective disorders, and Alzheimer's disease: review and hypothesis. J Gerontol: Medical Sciences 2004; 59A:178–183.

32. Carnethon MR, Kinder LS, Fair JM, et al. Symptoms of depression as a risk factor for incident diabetes: findings from the National Health and Nutrition Examination Epidemiologic follow-up study, 1971–1992. Am J Epidemiol 2003; 158:416–423.

33. Kaholokula JK, Haynes SN, Grandinetti A, et al. Biological, psychosocial and sociodemographic variables associated with depressive symptoms in persons with Type II diabetes. J Behavioral Med 2003; 26:435–458.

34. Maraldi C, Volpato S, Pennix BW, et al. Diabetes Mellitus, glycemic control, and incident depressive symptoms among 70- to 79-year-old persons. Arch Intern Med 2007; 167: 1137–1144.

35. Fisher L, Chesla CA, Mullan JT, et al. Contributors to depression in Latino and European-American patients with Type II diabetes. Diabetes Care 2001; 24:1751–1757.

36. Arroyo C, Hu FB, Ryan LM, et al. Depressive symptoms and risk of Type 2 diabetes in women. Diabetes Care 2004; 27:129–133.

37. Carthenon MR, Biggs ML, Barzilay JI, et al. Longitudinal association between depressive symptoms and incident Type 2 diabetes mellitus in older adults: the cardiovascular health study. Arch Int Med 2007; 167:802–807.

38. Engum A. The role of depression and anxiety in onset of diabetes in a large population-based study. J Psychosom Res 2007; 62:31–38.

39. Kiecolt-Glaser JK, Glaser R. Depression and immune function: central pathways to morbidity and mortality. J Psychosom Res 2002; 53:873–876.

40. Duncan BB, Schmidt MI, Pankow JS, et al. Low-grade systemic inflammation and the development of type 2 diabetes: the atherosclerosis risk in communities study. Diabetes 2003; 52:1799–1805.

41. Musselman DL, Betan E, Larsen H, Phillips LS. Relationship of depression to diabetes type 1 and type 2: epidemiology, biology and treatment. Biol Psychiatry 2003; 54:317–329.

42. Van Tilburg M, McCaskill CC, Lane JD. Depressed mood is a factor in glycemic control in type 1 diabetes. Psychosom Med 2001; 63:551–555.

43. Gross R, Olfson M, Gameroff MJ, et al. Depression and glycemic control in Hispanic primary care patients with diabetes. J Gen Intern Med 2005; 20:460–466.

44. Talbot F., Nouwen A. A review of the relationship between depression and diabetes in adults: is there a link? Diabetes Care 2000; 23:1556–1562.

45. Campbell S, Marriott M, Nahmias C, MacQueen GM. Lower hippocampal volume in patients suffering from depression: A meta-analysis. Am J Psychiatry 2004; 161: 598–607.

46. Videbech P, Ravnkilde B. Hippocampal volume and depression: A meta-analysis of MRI studies. Am J Psychiatry 2004; 161:1957–1966.

47. Sheline YI, Sanghavi M, Mintun MA, Gado MH: Depression duration but not age predicts hippocampal volume loss in medically healthy women with recurrent major depression. J Neurosci 1999; 19:5034–5043.

48. MacQueen GM, Campbell S, McEwen BS, et al. Course of illness, hippocampal function and hippocampal volume in major depression. Proc Natl Acad Sci USA 2003; 100: 1387–1392.

49. Hsieh MH, McQuoid DR, Levy RM, Payne ME, MacFall JR, et al. Hippocampal volume and antidepressant response in geriatric depression. In J Geriatr Psychiatry 2002; 17: 519–525.

50. Botteron KN, Raichle ME, Drevets WC, Heath AC, et al. Volumeteric reduction in left subgenual prefrontal cortex in early onset depression. Biol Psychiatry 2002; 51:342–344.

51. Bremner JD, Vythilingham M, Vermetten E, et al. Reduced volume of orbitofrontal cortex in major depression. Biol Psychiatry 2002; 51:273–279.

52. Rajkowska GR, Migel-Hidalgo JJ, Wei J, Dilley G, Pittman SD, et al. Morphometric evidence for neuronal and glial prefrontal cell pathology in major depression. Biol Psychiatry 1999; 45:1085–1098.

53. Cotter D, Mackay D, Landau S, et al. Reduced glial cell density and neuronal size in the anterior cingulate cortex in major depressive disorder. Arch Gen Psychiatry 2001; 58: 545–553.

54. denHeijer T, Vermeer SE, vanDijk, EJ, Prins ND, et al. Type 2 diabetes and atrophy of medial temporal lobe structures on brain MRI. Diabetologia 2003; 46:1604–1610.

55. Convit A, DeLeon, MJ, Tarshish C, DeSanti S, et al. Specific hippocampal volume reductions in individuals at risk for Alzheimer's disease. Neurobiol Aging 1997; 18:131–138.

56. Musen G, Lyoo IK, Sparks CR, Weinger K, et al. Effects of type 1 diabetes on gray matter density as measured by voxel-based morpohometry. Diabetes 2006; 55:326–333.

57. Carroll BJ, Cassidy F, Naftolowitz D, et al. Pathophysiology of hypercortisolism in depression. Acta Psychiatr Scand 2007; 115(Suppl. 433):90–103.

58. Alonso G. Prolonged corticosterone treatment of adult rats inhibits the proliferation of oligodendrocyte progenitors present throughout white and gray matter regions of the brain. Glia 2000; 31:219–231.

59. Pariante CM, Miller AH. Glucocorticoid receptors in major depression: relevance to pathophysiology and treatment. Biol Psychiatry 2001; 49:391–404.

60. MacEwen BS, Magarionos AM. Stress and hippocampal plasticity: implications for the pathophysiology of affective disorders Hum Psychopharmacol 2001; 16(Suppl. 1): S7-S19.

61. van den Biggelaar AH, Gussekloo J, de Craen AJ. Inflammation and interleukin-1 signaling network contribute to depressive symptoms but not cognitive decline in old age. Exp Gerontol 2007; 42:693–701.

62. Irwin MR, Miller AH. Depressive disorders and immunity: 20 years of progress and discovery. Brain Behav Immun 2007; 21:374–383.

63. Bremmer MA, Beekman AT, Deeg DJ, et al. Inflammatory markers in late-life depression: results from a population-based study. J Affect Disord 2008; 106:249–255.

64. Tuglu C, Kara SH, Caliyurt O, Vardar E, Abay E. Increased serum tumor necrosis factor-alpha levels and treatment response in major depressive disorder. Psychopharmacology (Berl) 2003; 170:429–433.

65. Myint AM, Leonard BE, Steinbusch HW, Kim YK. Th1, Th2, and Th3 cytokine alterations in major depression. J Affect Disord 2005; 88:167–173.

66. Berton O, McClung CA, DiLeone RJ, Vaishnav K, et al. eddential role of BDNF in the mesolimbic dopamine pathway in social defeat stress. Science 2006; 311:864–868.

67. Sheline YI, Mintun MA, Barch DM, Wilkins C, et al. Decreased hippocampal 5-HT2A receptor binding in older depressed patients using the (18F)Altanserin positron emission tomography. Neuropsychopharmacology 2004; 29:235–241.

68. Mann JJ, Malone KM, Diehl DJ, Perel J, Cooper TB, Mintun MA. Demonstration in vivo of reduced serotonin responsivity in the brain of untreated depressed patients. Am J Psychiatry 1996; 153:174–182.

69. Frasure-Smith N, Leseperance F, Talajic M. Depression and 18 month prognosis after myocardial infarction. Circulation 1995; 91:999–1005.

70. Lesperance F, Frasure-Smith N, theroux P, Irwin M: the association between major depression and levels of soluble intercellular adhesion molecule 1, interleukin-6 and C-reactive protein in patients with recent acute coronary syndromes. Am J Psychiatry 2004; 161: 271–277.

71. Skilton MR, Nakhala S, Sieveking DP, Caterson ID, et al. Pathophysiological levels of the obesity related peptides resistin and ghrelin increase adhesion molecule expression on human vascular endothelial cells. Clin Exp Pharmacol Physiol 2005; 32:839–844.

72. vonKanel R, bellingrath S, Kudielda BM. Association between burnout and circulating levels of pro-and anti-inflammatory cytokines in schoolteachers. J Psychosom Res 2008; 65(1): 51–59.

73. Steffens DC, Potter GG. Geriatric depression and cognitive impairment. Psychological Med 2008; 38:163175.

74. Shah PJ, Ebmeier KP, Glabus MF, Goodwin GM. Cortical grey matter reductions associated with treatment-resistant chronic unipolar depression: controlled magnetic resonance imaging study. Br J Psychiatry 1998; 172:527–532.

75. Kessing LV. Cognitive impairment in the euthymic phase of affective disorder. Psychol Med 1998; 28:1027–1038.

76. Steffens DC, Payne ME, Greenberg DL, Byrum CE, et al. Hippocampal volume and incident dementia in geriatric depression. Am J Geriatr Psychiatry 2002; 10:62–71.

77. Lustman PJ, Clouse RE. Treatment of depression in diabetes: impact on mood and medical outcome. J Psychosomatic Res 2002; 53:917–924.

78. Katon WJ, Von Korff M, Lin EH, et al. The Pathways Study: a randomized trial of collaborative care in patients with diabetes and depression. Arch Gen Psychiatry 2004; 61: 1042–1049.

79. Williams J Jr, Katon W, Lin E, et al. Effectiveness of depression care management for older adults with coexisting depression and diabetes mellitus. Ann Intern Med 2004; 140: 1015–1024.

80. Llorente MD, Malphurs J (Eds) Psychiatric Disorders and Diabetes Mellitus. London, UK: Informa Healthcare; 2007.

81. Goodnick PJ. Use of antidepressants in treatment of comorbid diabetes mellitus and depression as well as in diabetic neuropathy. Ann Clin Psychiatry 2001; 123:31–41.

82. Goodnick PJ, Kumar A, Henry JH, et al. Sertraline in coexisting major depression and diabetes mellitus. Psychopharmacol Bull 1997; 33:261–264.

83. Goodnick PJ. Use of antidepressants in treatment of comorbid diabetes mellitus and depression as well as in diabetic neuropathy. Ann Clin Psychiatry 2001; 13:31–41.

84. O'Kane M, Wiles PG, Wales JK. Fluoxetine in the treatment of obese type 2 diabetic patients. Diabet Med 1994; 11:105–110.

85. Lustman PJ, Griffith LS, Clouse RE, et al. Effects of nortriptyline on depression and glycemic control in diabetes: results of a double-blind, placebo-controlled trial. Psychosom Med 1997; 59:241–250.

86. Santarelli L, Saxe M, Gross C, Surget A, et al. Requirement of hippocampal neurogenesis for the behavioral effects of antidepressants. Science 2003; 301:805–809.

87. Ising M, Holsboer F. CRH1 receptor antagonists for the treatment of depression and anxiety. Exp Clin Psychopharmacol 2007; 15(6):519–528.

88. Zobel AM, Nickel T, Kunzel HE, Ackl N, et al. Effects of the high-affinity corticotrophin-releasing hormone receptor 1 antagonist R121919 in major depression: the first 20 patients treated. J Psychiatric Res 2000; 34:171–181.

89. Nieman LK, Chrousos GP, Kellner C, Spitz IM, et al. Successful treatment of Cushing's syndrome with the glucorticoid antagonist RU 486. J Clin Endocrinol Metabl 1985; 61: 536–540.

90. Flores BH, Kenna H, Keller J, Solvason HB, Schatzberg AF. Clinical and biological effects of mifepristone treatment for psychotic depression. Neuropsychopharmacology 2006; 31:628–636.
91. Jahn H, Schick M, Kiefer F, Kellner M, et al. Metyrapone as additive treatment in major depression: a double-blind and placebo-contralled trial. Arch Gen Psychiatry 2004; 61:1235–1244.
92. Seckl JR, Fink G. Antidepressants increase glucocorticoid and mineralocorticoid receptor mRNA expression in rat hippocampus in vivo. Neuroendocrinology 1992; 55:621–626.
93. Fride E, Dan Y, Feldon J, Halevy G, et al. Effects of prenatal stress on vulnerability to stress in prepubertal and adult rats. Physiol Behav 1986; 37:681–687.
94. Maccari S, Piazza PV, Kabbaj M, et al. Adoption reverses the long-term impairment in glucocorticoid feedback induced by prenatal stress. J Neurosci 1995; 15:110–116.
95. Golden SH. A review of the evidence for a neuroendocrine link between stress, depression and diabetes mellitus. Curr Diabetes Rep 2007; 3:252–259.
96. Lustman PJ, Griffith LS, Freedland KE, et al. Cognitive behavior therapy for depression in type 2 diabetes mellitus: a randomized, controlled trial. Ann Intern Med 1998; 129:613–621.
97. Unutzer J, Katon W, Callahan CM, et al. for IMPACT investigators. Collaborative care management of late-life depression in the primary care setting: a randomized controlled trial. JAMA 2002; 288:2836–2845.
98. Katon WJ, Von Korff M, Lin EH, et al. The Pathways Study: a randomized trial of collaborative care in patients with diabetes and depression. Arch Gen Psychiatry 2004; 61:1042–1049.
99. Williams JW, Katon W, Lin EH, et al. The effectiveness of depression care management on diabetes-related outcomes in older patients. Ann Intern Med 2004; 140:1015–1024.
100. Katon W, Von Korff M, Lin E, et al. Improving primary care treatment of depression among patients with diabetes mellitus: the design of the Pathways Study. Gen Hosp Psychiatry 2003; 25:158–168.

15 Central Nervous System Involvement in Diabetic Neuropathy

Dinesh Selvarajah, Iain D. Wilkinson, Rajiv A. Gandhi, and Solomon Tesfaye

ABSTRACT

Diabetic neuropathy is a severe, disabling chronic condition that affects a significant number of individuals with diabetes. Long considered a disease of the peripheral nervous system, there is mounting evidence of central nervous system involvement. Recent advances in neuroimaging methods have led to a better understanding and refinement of how diabetic neuropathy affects the central nervous system. Recognition that diabetic neuropathy is, in part, a disease

From: *Contemporary Diabetes: Diabetes and the Brain*
Edited by: G. J. Biessels, J. A. Luchsinger (eds.), DOI 10.1007/978-1-60327-850-8_15
© Humana Press, a part of Springer Science+Business Media, LLC 2009

which affects the whole nervous system should trigger a critical rethinking of this disorder, opening a new direction for further research.

Key words: Diabetes mellitus; Diabetic neuropathy; Central nervous system; Thalamus; Magnetic resonance imaging; Cerebral perfusion.

INTRODUCTION

As has been reviewed in the previous chapters, diabetes causes significant central nervous system (CNS) complications, resulting in important functional impairments *(1)*. Involvement of the CNS in diabetic peripheral neuropathy (DPN) is also increasingly being recognised. Recent developments in non-invasive magnetic resonance (MR) imaging have enabled the in vivo study of various components of the CNS at different stages of DPN. In this chapter we focus on human DPN studies utilising MR investigations of the CNS.

SPINAL CORD INVOLVEMENT IN DIABETIC NEUROPATHY

Previously considered a disease of the peripheral nervous system (PNS), there is mounting evidence to support concomitant involvement of the CNS in diabetic neuropathy. Involvement of the spinal cord has been reported in post-mortem studies, which demonstrated axonal loss, gliosis, and demyelination within the spinal cord *(2–6)*. However, many of these studies did not examine patients with diabetic neuropathy specifically; therefore, it is not possible to conclude whether these changes were due to neuropathy or diabetes.

The reason why some patients develop painful neuropathic symptoms is far from clear. These can occur with little objective evidence of peripheral nerve dysfunction and can be extremely distressing and difficult to treat. Electrical spinal cord stimulation has been used to alleviate pain, which is unresponsive to conventional treatment *(7)*. However, it has been observed that this technique is ineffective in subjects with severe loss of vibration and joint position sense, which has led to the suggestion that the spinal cord may have a role in pain modulation. In a preliminary study, using a non-invasive MR imaging technique, Eaton et al. explored possible involvement of the spinal cord in DPN *(8)*. Onmeasuring cross-sectional area of the spinal cord at three different levels (lower cervical, upper, and lower thoracic regions), they reported significantly lower cord area in the cervical and upper thoracic regions in subjects with established-DPN compared to healthy non-diabetic controls indicating extensive disease in these areas. Diabetic subjects with no-DPN appeared to have intermediate cord area measurements between non-diabetic controls and established-DPN. These results would suggest that the abnormalities previously reported in post-mortem studies do reflect a neuropathic process affecting the spinal cord. One theory postulates that damage to the peripheral nerve causes secondary spinal cord 'shrinkage' due to degeneration or atrophy. Another theory is that the primary insult may be to the CNS, with the well-documented peripheral changes occurring as secondary phenomena. It is also conceivable that both peripheral and CNS involvement occur concomitantly resulting in the findings documented.

In order to examine these theories further, and as the relevance of these findings to the pathogenesis of DPN is dependent on whether spinal cord shrinkage occurs early, a larger, adequately powered study was conducted. In this study 98 subjects with type 1 diabetes were subdivided into three sub-groups (no-DPN, subclinical-DPN, and established-DPN), and spinal cord area measurements were performed at the level C2/C3 (9). Diabetic sub-group measurements were compared with 24 non-diabetic healthy controls and 8 subjects with hereditary sensory motor neuropathy (HSMN). The latter group was chosen to serve as disease controls because it is well recognised to affect only the PNS and vascular factors have not been implicated in its pathogenesis. In this larger study, the results of the pilot study were confirmed and, more importantly, also clearly demonstrated that spinal cord atrophy is an early process being present not only in established-DPN but also even in subjects with relatively modest impairments of nerve function (subclinical-DPN) (Fig. 1). It was also demonstrated that a significant trend of lower cord cross-sectional area with more severe neuropathy occurred across diabetic groups indicating a continuing loss of cord area as the disease progresses. Significant correlations were found between cord area and neurophysiological parameters of neuropathy severity. Cord area was not significantly different between age-matched and sex-matched non-diabetic controls and diabetic subjects without DPN. Approximately 26% and 9% of patients with clinical-DPN and subclinical-DPN, respectively, were found to have spinal cord atrophy (Fig. 2) (9). In contrast, unlike DPN, subjects with HSMN (neuropathy control group) had normal cord areas suggesting that the pathological process here is confined to the peripheral nerve.

The findings of this clinical study show that the neuropathic process in diabetes is not confined to the peripheral nerve and does involve the spinal cord. Worryingly, this occurs early in the neuropathic process. Even at the early DPN stage, extensive and perhaps even irreversible damage may have occurred. Indeed, with these results in mind, it is not surprising that the variety of therapeutic options so far attempted in DPN have not been successful (10). The absence of spinal cord involvement in HSMN argues against a 'dying back' mechanism, i.e. peripheral nerve damage causing secondary spinal cord 'shrinkage' in a progressive 'dying back' fashion, in DPN.

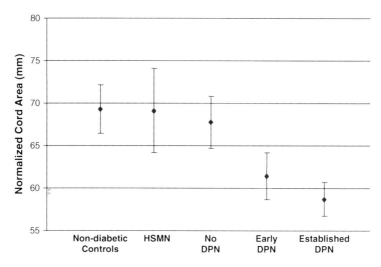

Fig. 1. Normalised spinal cord area (mm, mean ± 95% confidence interval) per group, adjusted for age, height, and weight. From Selvarajah et al. *(54)*. Copyright © 2006 American Diabetes Association. Reprinted from *Diabetes Care* with permission from The American Diabetes Association.)

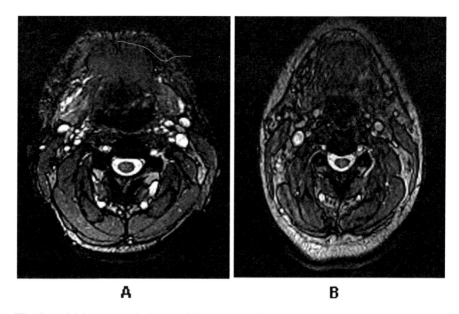

A   **B**

Fig. 2. Axial images at the level of disk space C2/C3 showing a section of the cervical cord in a non-diabetic age-matched control (**A**) and (**B**) a subject with established-DPN illustrating differences in cord size and shape.

Hence, it is likely that the insult of diabetes is generalised, concomitantly affecting the PNS and CNS. The significant correlation between neurophysiological parameters and cord area in DPN supports this. Given these findings we believe a more thorough appreciation of the nature and extent of DPN is essential to the understanding and treatment of this condition.

BRAIN MR SPECTROSCOPY IN DPN

Findings from the spinal cord studies described above suggest that the metabolic insult of diabetes has a generalised effect on the whole nervous system and has made us question whether the brain too may be involved.

Anatomical studies have demonstrated that the ascending sensory pathways of the spinal cord terminate within the thalamus before high-order sensory projections are sent to the cortex (11). Recent studies have shown that the thalamus does not merely act as a sensory relay station but also modulates/processes the information that is presented to the cortex (12). Hence, in the presence of sensory nerve dysfunction that accompanies painless-DPN, the specific aim of this study was to investigate whether thalamic function is also impaired.

The investigative modality used to test this hypothesis was proton magnetic resonance spectroscopy (H-MRS). In vivo H-MRS is a non-invasive technique that can provide metabolic information from different body tissues, including the brain. In the latter context, it has been used to study the classification and pathophysiology of various neurological conditions including neoplasms, viral and retroviral infections, ischaemia, demyelination, some forms of epilepsy, and dementias. Spectroscopy and imaging can be performed during the same subject examination, the information yielded by H-MRS often being considered an adjunct to that provided by imaging (13). Indeed, in some pathologies, neurochemical abnormalities may be present on H-MRS prior to abnormalities being detected on imaging (14). Conventional MRI and H-MRS rely on the same physical principles to collect the MR signal, but differ in the way the data are encoded, displayed, and interpreted. Proton magnetic resonance spectroscopy produces spectra that contain several resonances or peaks. In brain parenchyma, the three major peaks detected are due to N-acetyl groups, total creatine (Cr), and choline (Cho)-containing compounds (Fig. 3).

Immunohistochemical studies have suggested that N-acetyl aspartate (NAA), the major constituent of the N-acetyl group resonance at long echo time (TE), is localised exclusively in neurons and their processes throughout the CNS (15–17). In vivo cerebral NAA determined using H-MRS has been shown to correlate with histological neuronal density in a variety of animal

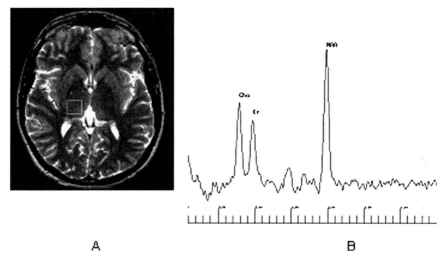

Fig. 3. (A) Axial section of the brain with voxel from which the proton magnetic resonance spectrum is obtained and positioned to encompass the ventroposterior thalamic subnucleus. **(B)** Example of proton magnetic resonance spectrum acquired at long echo time (200 ms). NAA, *N*-acetyl aspartate, Cho, choline, and Cr, creatine. (From Selvarajah et al. *(55)*. Reprinted from *Diabetologia* with kind permission from Springer Verlag.)

models *(18)*. It is also used as a surrogate neuronal marker for the assessment ofneuroprotective therapeutic compounds/strategies in humans *(19)*. It is generally accepted that the NAA resonance on H-MRS can provide a useful marker for brain neuronal and axonal integrity in vivo *(20–23)*.

Recent H-MRS studies have mostly focused on the metabolic impact of diabetes on the developing brain *(24)* and the cerebral consequences of hypoglycaemia *(25)* or diabetic ketoacidosis *(26)*. Observations of cerebral NAA (a marker of neuronal integrity and function) that have been reported are contradictory. Kreis and Ross found several metabolic abnormalities in the brain of subjects with diabetes. In particular, they found a significantly lower *N*-acetyl (NA): creatine in the parietal region of subjects with diabetes compared with that in age-matched control subjects *(27)*. This contrasts with a study by Geissler et al. which found no differences in NA signal between subjects with diabetes and healthy volunteers in either the parietal or the occipital lobes *(28)*. Neither of these studies performed assessments to quantify DPN so it remains unclear if the changes observed are the result of diabetes or the consequence of neuropathy. It should also be noted that different H-MRS acquisition techniques were utilised between these two studies, which may contribute to these disparate findings.

An H-MRS study was conducted which utilised NAA resonance as a surrogate marker for neuronal function to test the hypothesis that damage to
the peripheral sensory nerves caused by diabetes mellitus may be accompanied by thalamic neuronal dysfunction (29). This study also aimed to
characterise the relationship between thalamic neuronal biochemistry and
traditional neurophysiological assessments of the peripheral nerves reflecting severity of painless-DPN.

In this preliminary study, 18 male subjects with type 1 diabetes (8 no-
DPN, 10 established-DPN) and 6 age- and sex-matched non-diabetic healthy
controls underwent H-MRS of the thalamus (see Fig. 3). The main finding was a significantly lower long TE (135 ms) thalamic NAA/Cho ratio
in the group of patients with DPN compared to patients with no-DPN and
healthy controls (Fig. 4). The data also demonstrated significant correlations
between short TE (20 ms) signal from NAA and neurophysiological markers
(overall neuropathy composite score and individual nerve function tests) of
DPN severity.

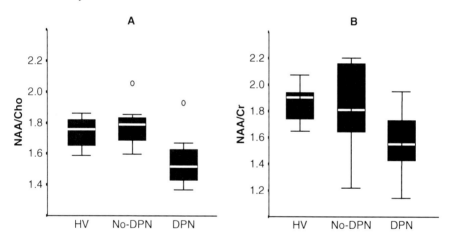

Fig. 4. Mean *N*-acetyl aspartate/choline [NAA/Cho (**A**)] and *N*-acetyl aspartate/creatine
[NAA/Cr (**B**)] ratios at long echo time in healthy volunteers (HV), diabetic patients with
neuropathy (DPN) and no neuropathy (no-DPN). (From Selvarajah et al. *(55)*. Reprinted
from *Diabetologia* with kind permission from Springer Verlag.)

These findings may reflect thalamic neuronal dysfunction in DPN. The
mechanism of thalamic involvement is unclear. One possible explanation for
thalamic neuronal dysfunction in DPN may be that loss of afferent input, as a
result of peripheral nerve damage, subsequently causing changes to occur at
progressively higher levels in the CNS. Correlations observed between NAA
acquired at short TE, duration of diabetes and severity of neuropathy would
seem to support this. Another possible explanation is that the observed
changes in the thalamus may be occurring concomitantly to the changes seen

in the PNS. Nonetheless, thalamic neuronal involvement whether early, late, or concomitant, is likely to result in disturbed sensory gating in DPN. This may have consequences on sensory perception and pain modulation. Further studies utilising these techniques on a subgroup of patients with painful-DPN are necessary to elucidate this.

Taken together with the previously described early spinal cord involvement in DPN, the possibility of thalamic sensory neuronal dysfunction suggests that abnormalities in the sensory system are not merely confined to the peripheral nerves but involves the spinal cord and brain. Prospective studies are required to determine at what stage during the course of the disease these abnormalities occur. It is noteworthy that a variety of therapeutic interventions specifically targeted at peripheral nerve damage in DPN have thus far been ineffective, and it is possible that this may in part be due to inadequate appreciation of the full extent of CNS involvement in DPN.

In a larger follow-up study, 110 subjects with type 1 diabetes and 20 healthy non-diabetic controls underwent detailed clinical and neurophysiological assessments and were subdivided into 4 neuropathy subgroups (20 no-DPN, 30 subclinical-DPN, 30 painful-DPN, and 30 painless-DPN) *(30)*. Each subject then underwent H-MRS of the thalamic nucleus and somatosensory cortex to measure established markers (NAA) of neuronal function using long TE (135 ms) and neuronal integrity using short TE (20 ms) acquisition technique. In the thalamus, at long TE, subjects with painless-DPN had significantly lower NAA ratios compared to other groups. There were no significant intergroup differences in thalamic short TE. In the somatosensory cortex, no intergroup differences were seen at long TE. At short TE, painless-DPN had significantly lower NAA compared to non-diabetic controls and no-DPN. Subjects with painful-DPN had intermediate levels of short TE NAA.

These results appear to confirm the findings of the initial study and imply change in thalamic neuronal physiology or function, rather than neuronal loss in painless but not painful-DPN. It is possible that relative preservation of thalamic neuronal function is necessary for the transmission of abnormal peripheral signals to higher centres and the perception of chronic pain in diabetes. The results within the somatosensory cortex, in contrast, are suggestive of neuronal loss in subjects with DPN and may be reflecting local cerebral parenchymal atrophy.

In a comparable study, Sorensen et al. performed H-MRS on three brain regions (thalamus, anterior cingulate cortex, and dorsolateral prefrontal cortex) in 26 subjects with diabetes and 14 healthy controls *(31)*. Subjects with diabetes were subdivided into painful-DPN ($n = 12$) and painless-DPN ($n=14$). The investigators reported significant reductions in thalamic NAA in subjects with painful symptoms compared with those without. There were no metabolite differences in the dorsolateral prefrontal cortex and anterior cingulate cortex between study groups. These findings are contrary to those reported by Gandhi et al. *(30)*, whose study consisted of greater numbers of subjects who underwent more detailed assessments to quantify the presence and assess the severity of neuropathy.

Diffusion tensor imaging (DTI) is a modality of MR imaging that measures the anisotropy of parenchymal water diffusion, providing a unique insight into neurocellular architecture, in vivo. Information from DTI can yield models, which reflect the make-up of axonal pathways (tractography) within the CNS. Using this technique, Wilkinson et al. reported a lower number of axonal fibre tracts within the spinal-corticosomatosensory pathways in subjects with DPN compared with healthy volunteers (Fig. 5) *(32)*. Abnormalities were present in both first- (spino-thalamic) and second-order (thalamo-cortical) neurons within the CNS. Additional data are currently being acquired to ascertain whether (i) tractographic abnormalities are present in diabetic subjects with no-DPN and (ii) differences can be observed between those with painful and painless-DPN. This information further underlines the need to map out CNS involvement in DPN.

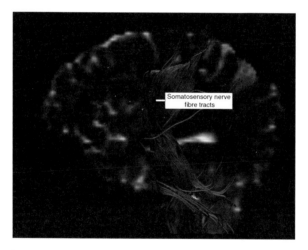

Fig. 5. Magnetic resonance tractography image showing a three-dimensional representation of modelled sensory nerve fibre tracts passing from the brainstem to the right somatosensory cortex.

MR PERFUSION IMAGING IN DPN

The presence of thalamic sensory neuronal dysfunction in DPN suggests that sensory system involvement is not limited to the spinal cord, but that other important somatosensory pathways may also be involved.

Although the pathogenesis of thalamic involvement in DPN is unknown, it is likely that both vascular and metabolic aetiological factors that have been postulated in the pathogenesis of DPN and other microvascular complications of diabetes (retinopathy and nephropathy) may be involved. A better understanding of the pathogenesis of thalamic dysfunction in DPN may provide new therapeutic targets to treat or prevent this condition.

Advances in modern in vivo MR technology have enabled the acquisition of high-quality multislice echo planar imaging of the brain with subsecond temporal resolution. Chelates of gadolinium, a rare earth metal, are commonly used as exogenous contrast agents in MR imaging, having a modulatory effect on both T1 and T2* of tissue within their sphere of influence. Coupled with fast T2*-weighted imaging technique, the ability to detect the passage of a bolus of exogenous contrast as it passes through the capillary bed, provides a method of spatially mapping the perfusion characteristics of brain parenchyma (33). Utilising dynamic contrast-enhanced MR perfusion imaging; we proceeded to test our hypothesis that DPN is associated with thalamic perfusion abnormalities.

In a recent study, thalamic perfusion was compared between 18 subjects with type 1 diabetes (6 no-DPN, 5 painful-DPN, and 7 painless-DPN) and 5 healthy volunteers (34). Relative cerebral blood volume (rCBV) within

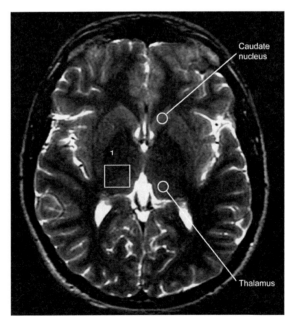

Fig. 6. Cross-sectional image of the cerebral cortex at the level of the thalamus. Circles denote perfusion regions of interests over the thalamus and caudate nucleus.

the thalamus was significantly greater in the painful-DPN group with longer bolus transit time (Fig. 6). Subjects with painless-DPN had a non-significant trend towards the lowest relative cerebral blood flow (rCBF) amongst all the subgroups studied. Inaddition, the perfusion characteristic of the caudate nucleus was assessed, to serve as an internal control deep brain nucleus as it is not directly involved in somatosensory processing. Analysis of these data did not reveal any differences in rCBV, rCBF, or bolus transit time between study groups. Hence unique thalamic pathophysiological microvascular changes have been observed that may provide important clues to the pathogenesis of pain in DPN. The thalamus plays a central role in modulating/processing somatosensory information that is relayed to the cerebral cortices and is therefore possibly more metabolically active in DPN. This greater metabolic activity increases thalamic sensitivity to diabetic metabolic disturbances. Diabetes has been shown to alter endothelial function and permeability of the blood–brain barrier, thus affecting microcirculation and regional metabolism. This increased susceptibility to diabetic metabolic disturbance may then lead to neuronal dysfunction and eventually neuronal loss. Our finding of MR spectroscopic reduction in thalamic NA:Cho ratios in DPN would seem to support this hypothesis.

Several other positron emission tomography (PET) studies have investigated changes in basal regional CBF related to spontaneous continuous non-diabetic neuropathic pain. These studies mainly report a significant decrease in regional CBF in the hemithalamus contralateral to the pain (35). In many instances, this decrease in thalamic activity was reversed by therapeutic interventions providing significant symptomatic relief (36). These results appear contrary to electrophysiological findings in animal and human studies of chronic pain, which have demonstrated abnormal hyperactivity of thalamic neurons (37). There is no satisfactory explanation for the observed relative decrease in thalamic relative CBF in subjects with neuropathy pain (38). Some investigators have postulated that this decrease may be a compensatory mechanism for inhibiting excessive nociceptive inputs or to the uncoupling between blood flow and neuronal activity in subjects experiencing neuropathic pain (39). The observed decrease in thalamic activity appears to be reversible following various types of analgesic procedures, suggestive of functional impairment rather than a degenerative process.

Increases in relative CBF have been reported in the anterior insula, posterior parietal cortex, inferior and lateral prefrontal cortex, and the anterior cingulated cortex in several other non-diabetic neuropathic pain studies (40). These data suggest that changes in basal brain activity in subjects with chronic neuropathic pain involve only a small portion of the 'pain matrix' (described below) associated with acute pain (38). Further studies with better characterised neuropathic assessments are required to confirm the pattern of brain activity associated with spontaneous neuropathic pain. Given the complex, multidimensional clinical entity, that is, painful-DPN, it is likely to be mediated by a number of diverse pathophysiological brain mechanisms and possess a unique 'pain matrix' of its own. A greater understanding of the specific features of painful-DPN will help advance our understanding of the mechanisms of this troublesome complication of diabetes and may result in the development of more rationale (mechanism-based) treatment approaches.

fMRI AND PAINFUL-DPN

The exact pathophysiological mechanisms of neuropathic pain remain unknown although based on experiments in animal models both peripheral and central mechanisms have been postulated (41). However, there are no consistent differences in peripheral nerve morphological parameters between painful-DPN and painless-DPN. It is likely that the pathophysiological changes resulting in pain may in part lie elsewhere within the nervous system. Recent advances in neuroimaging methods have led to better understanding and refinement of how pain is presented to the cerebral cortex. One scientific development that fuelled recent advances in our understanding of the function of the human brain has been the functional magnetic resonance imaging (fMRI). The technique relies on mapping localised changes in magnetic susceptibility that occur following the haemodynamic response to neuronal/synaptic activity. Small susceptibility changes (which depend on alteration of the localised ratio of oxy- to deoxy-haemoglobin, hence the acronymn BOLD or blood oxygen-level dependant fMRI) lead to small signal changes on susceptibility-weighted imaging at high temporal resolution (usually echo-planar imaging or EPI). These are detected, due to small differences in contrast-to-noise, following multiple data averaging strategies and statistical analysis. Brain regions whose signal signatures significantly correlate with the stimulus are those that are defined as being 'active' during a task or presentation of a stimulus. This has led to the characterisation of a network of brain areas that consistently activate in response to acute pain, forming the 'pain matrix' (Fig. 7) (42). These areas include primary and secondary somatosensory cortex, insular, anterior cingulated and prefrontal cortices, and the thalamus (42). Other regions such as basal ganglia, cerebellum, amygdala, hippocampus, and areas within the parietal and temporal cortices can also be active depending on the particular set of circumstances for that individual (43). These studies, however, have been performed mainly in healthy volunteers following acute pain stimulation, and changes in the brain associated with chronic pain have been less thoroughly investigated.

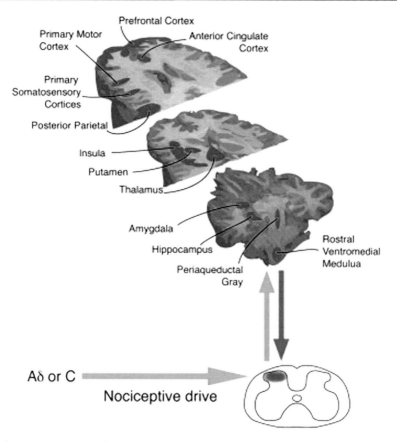

Prefrontal Cortex

Primary Motor
Cortex

Anterior Cingulate
Cortex

Primary
Somatosensory
Cortices

Posterior Parietal

Insula

Putamen

Thalamus

Amygdala

Hippocampus

Periaqueductal
Gray

Rostral
Ventromedial
Medulua

Aδ or C
Nociceptive drive

Fig. 7. Neuroanatomy of pain processing. Main brain regions that activate during a painful experience, highlighted as bilaterally active but with increased activation on the contralateral hemisphere. (Reprinted from Tracey and Mantyh *(56)*, with kind permission from Elsevier.)

Utilising fMRI, a study comprising 18 type 1 diabetic subjects (6 with no-DPN, 6 with painful-DPN, and 6 with painless-DPN) was conducted to test the feasibility of monitoring the brain's response to the presentation of heat-pain in the context of DPN *(43)*. All participants had MR imaging at 3T and a thermode device to the dorsum of the right foot delivered heat-pain stimulation. Our preliminary analysis shows subjects with no-DPN had greater BOLD response than those with painless-DPN. Subjects with painful DPN showed significantly greater response than those with painless-DPN. The primary somatosensory cortex, lateral frontal, and cerebellar regions demonstrated greatest involvement. This may be explained by reduced ascending nociceptive input as a result of neuropathy; however, subjects with painful- and painless-DPN had comparable neuropathy impairment scores based on

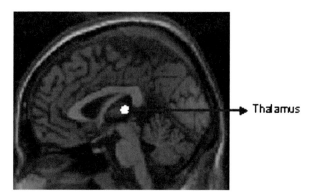

Fig. 8. Area within the thalamus having significant negative correlation between neuropathy composite score and BOLD-fMRI response to hot compared to baseline temperature.

detailed neurophysiological assessments. We also found significant negative correlation between BOLD fMRI response and overall neuropathy score in both the thalamus and left parietal lobe (Fig. 8) *(44)*. Group differences occur within the frontal lobe (high/level perception/cognitive function), the cerebellum (processing speed action), and the thalamus (sensory gateway to the brain) as well as in the sensory cortex. Although similar brain regions are activated in our study with those that comprise the 'pain matrix', there are some clear differences in brain activation patterns. This suggests that a unique network associated with painful-DPN exists, probably involving different mechanisms. In addition, given the subjective nature of the pain experience, an individualised neural 'pain signature' likely exists for each patient. Some authors advocate a move towards this rather than forcing a complex subjective experience into the constraints of a rigid neuroanatomical pain matrix *(45)*.

One component of neuropathic pain is allodynia, which is pain elicited by normally non-painful stimuli, and is frequently associated with spontaneous pain in subjects with diabetes. Numerous studies have been conducted using brush stroke evoked-allodynia in both healthy volunteers (utilising the capsaicin model of neuropathic pain) *(46)* and a variety of clinical non-diabetic neuropathic pain syndromes (central and peripheral) *(47, 48)* to determine whether this aberrant pain results from an abnormal activation of the 'pain matrix'. Instead, these studies revealed different but overlapping patterns of brain activation of the 'pain matrix' with predominant activation of the lateral pain system (thalamus, SI, and SII) and bilateral cortical activation during mechanical allodynia. Prefrontal cortex activation, which is associated with the cognitive/evaluative aspects of pain, was also observed in several studies *(49–51)*. With its regional links with the frontal cortex, the prefrontal cortex may have a role in the descending pain modulatory system (described below).

Many studies have placed greater emphasis on the spatial and temporal representation of nociceptive processing within functionally defined brain regions, without consideration for how their activation in concert causes a perception of pain *(52)*. It is likely that this complex experience emerges from the flow and integration of information among specific brain areas; a better understanding of the temporal integration among these spatially defined brain regions is needed for the development of targeted pharmacological agents *(52)*.

There is a large amount of variability in the patterns of brain activation reported in studies published thus far *(36)*. In the context of DPN, too few neuroimaging studies with small sample sizes have been conducted in non-diabetic neuropathic pain syndromes. In addition, the high level of heterogeneity of neuropathic subtypes and lack of standardised inclusion criteria with detailed neurophysiological assessments may have also contributed to the variation observed *(36)*. In most studies the contralateral side was used as a 'control', and hence painful-DPN largely excluded from these investigations. It is possible that different patterns of abnormal brain activation may be responsible for chronic pain in diabetes. Future studies with larger sample sizes, with standardised, and well-characterised subjects with DPN should be conducted.

DESCENDING PAIN MODULATION

Nociceptive inputs are subjected to modulation by the descending pain modulatory systems prior to arrival at higher cortical centres. This well-characterised functional anatomical network regulates nociceptive processing, largely within the dorsal horn, to produce either facilitation (pronociceptive) or inhibition (antinociceptive) (Fig. 9) *(53)*. The brain regions involved in this descending modulation include the frontal lobe, anterior cingulate cortex, insula, amygdala, hypothalamus, periaqueductal grey, nucleus cuneiformis, and rostral ventromedial medulla. Some components of this network overlap with the pain matrix as ascending pain stimuli are integrated with descending influences from the diencephalon and limbic forebrain. Activation of this network occurs in various circumstances, for example, when concomitant changes in pain ratings are observed when subjects either attend to or are distracted from their pain. Sustained activation of pronociceptive components of this system is thought to play an important role in some states of chronic pain. Recognising the descending modulatory

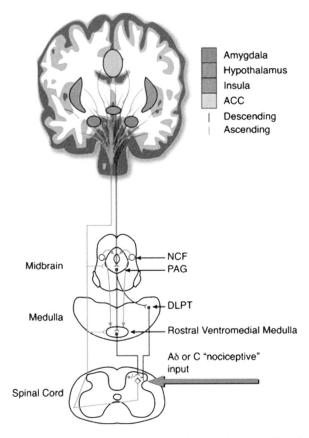

Amygdala
Hypothalamus
Insula
ACC
| Descending
| Ascending

Midbrain
NCF
PAG

Medulla
DLPT
Rostral Ventromedial Medulla

Aδ or C "nociceptive" input

Spinal Cord

Fig. 9. The descending pain modulatory system. NCF (nucleus cuneiformis); PAG (peri-aqueductal grey); DLPT (dorsolateral pontine tegmentum); ACC (anterior cingulate cortex). (Reprinted from Tracey and Mantyh (56), with kind permission from Elsevier.)

system in chronic pain states is likely to be important in future work and treatment developments.

CONCLUSIONS

This chapter focused on the involvement of the CNS in abnormal sensory perception and pain in relation to diabetic neuropathy. From the spinal cord to the brain it has become increasingly apparent that DPN concomitantly affects the CNS and PNS. Recognition that diabetes results in important complications of the CNS should prompt further research into understanding the pathophysiological mechanisms that underpin these effects.

REFERENCES

1. Mijnhout GS, Scheltens P, Diamant M, et al. Diabetic encephalopathy: A concept in need of a definition. Diabetologia 2006; 49:1447–1448.
2. Leichtentritt H. Erkrankung Peripherer nerven und des rucken-marks bei diabetes mellitus. Berlin: G. Schade, 1893:32.
3. Pryce TD. On diabetic neuritis with a clinical and pathological description of three cases of diabetic pseudo-tabes. Brain 1893; 1.
4. Williamson RT. (1904). "Changes in the spinal cord in diabetes mellitus." Br Med J 1904; 1.
5. Reske-Nielsen E, Lundbaek K. Pathological changes in the central and peripheral nervous system of young long-term diabetics. II. The spinal cord and peripheral nerves. Diabetologia 1968; 4:34–43.
6. Reske-Nielsen E, Lundbaek, K, et al. Pathological changes in the central and peripheral nervous system of young long-term diabetics. The terminal neuro-muscular apparatus. Diabetologia 1970; 6:98–103.
7. Tesfaye S, Watt J, et al. Electrical spinal-cord stimulation for painful diabetic peripheral neuropathy. Lancet 1996; 348:1698–1701.
8. Eaton SE, Harris ND, et al.Spinal-cord involvement in diabetic peripheral neuropathy. Lancet 2001; 358:35–36.
9. Selvarajah D, Wilkinson ID, Emery CJ, et al. Early involvement of the spinal cord in diabetic peripheral neuropathy. Diabetes Care 2006; 29:2664–2669.
10. Pfeifer MA, Schumer MP. Clinical trials of diabetic neuropathy: past, present, and future. Diabetes 1995; 44:1355–1361.
11. Wilson P, Kitchener PD, et al. Cutaneous receptive field organization in the ventral posterior nucleus of the thalamus in the common marmoset. J Neurophysiol 1999; 82: 1865–1875.
12. McCormick DA, Bal T. Sensory gating mechanisms of the thalamus. Curr Opin Neurobiol 1994; 4:550–556.
13. Wilkinson ID, Griffiths PD, et al. Proton magnetic resonance spectroscopy of brain lesions in children with neurofibromatosis type 1. Magn Reson Imaging 2001; 19: 1081–1089.
14. Wilkinson ID, Hadjivassiliou M, et al. Cerebellar abnormalities on proton MR spectroscopy in gluten ataxia. J Neurol Neurosurg Psychiatry 2005; 76:1011–1013.
15. Moffett JR, Namboodiri MA, et al.Immunohistochemical localization of N-acetylaspartate in rat brain. Neuroreport 1991; 2:131–134.
16. Simmons ML, Frondoza CG, et al. Immunocytochemical localization of N-acetyl-aspartate with monoclonal antibodies. Neuroscience 1991; 45:37–45.
17. Urenjak J, Williams SR, et al. Proton nuclear magnetic resonance spectroscopy unambiguously identifies different neural cell types. J Neurosci 1993; 13:981–989.
18. Wilkinson ID, Lunn S, et al. Proton MRS and quantitative MRI assessment of the short term neurological response to antiretroviral therapy in AIDS. J Neurol Neurosurg Psychiatry 1997; 63:477–482.
19. Matthews PM, Andermann F, et al. A proton magnetic resonance spectroscopy study of focal epilepsy in humans. Neurology 1990; 40:985–989.
20. De Stefano N, Matthews PM, et al. Reversible decreases in N-acetylaspartate after acute brain injury. Magn Reson Med 1995; 34:721–727.
21. Tsai G, Coyle JT. N-acetylaspartate in neuropsychiatric disorders. Prog Neurobiol 1995; 46:531–540.
22. Hugg JW, Kuzniecky RI, et al. Normalization of contralateral metabolic function following temporal lobectomy demonstrated by 1H magnetic resonance spectroscopic imaging. Ann Neurol 1996; 40:236–239.
23. Nakano M, Ueda H, et al. Measurement of regional N-acetylaspartate after transient global ischemia in gerbils with and without ischemic tolerance: an index of neuronal survival. Ann Neurol 1998; 44:334–340.

24. Sarac K, Akinci A, et al. Brain metabolite changes on proton magnetic resonance spectroscopy in children with poorly controlled type 1 diabetes mellitus. Neuroradiology 2005; 47:562–565.

25. Rankins D, Wellard RM, et al. The impact of acute hypoglycemia on neuropsychological and neurometabolite profiles in children with type 1 diabetes. Diabetes Care 2005; 28:2771–2773.

26. Wootton-Gorges SL, Buonocore MH, et al. Detection of cerebral {beta}-hydroxy butyrate, acetoacetate, and lactate on proton MR spectroscopy in children with diabetic ketoacidosis. Am J Neuroradiol 2005; 26:1286–1291.

27. Kreis R, Ross BD. Cerebral metabolic disturbances in patients with subacute and chronic diabetes mellitus: detection with proton MR spectroscopy. Radiology 1992; 184:123–130.

28. Geissler A, Frund R, et al. Alterations of cerebral metabolism in patients with diabetes mellitus studied by proton magnetic resonance spectroscopy. Exp Clin Endocrinol Diabetes 2003; 111:421–427.

29. Selvarajah D, Wilkinson ID, Emery CJ, Shaw PJ, Griffiths PD, Gandhi R, Tesfaye S. Thalamic neuronal dysfunction and chronic sensorimotor distal symmetrical polyneuropathy in patients with type 1 diabetes mellitus. Diabetologia 2008; 51:2088–2092.

30. Gandhi R, Selvarajah D, Emery CJ, Wilkinson ID, Tesfaye S. Neurochemical abnormalities within sensory pathways in the brain in diabetic neuropathy. Diabetologia 2008; 51(Suppl 1):1–588.

31. Wilkinson ID, Gandhi R, Hutton M, et al. Magnetic resonance diffusion tractography in diabetic neuropathy; imaging the spino-corticosomatosensory pathways. Diabetic Med 2006; 26(1).

32. Sorensen L, Siddall PJ, Trenell MI, Yue DK. Differences in metabolites in pain-processing brain regions in patients with diabetes and painful neuropathy. Diabetes Care 2008; 31: 980–981.

33. Østergaard L. Cerebral perfusion imaging by bolus tracking. Top Magn Reson Imaging 2004; 15:3–9.

34. Selvarajah D, Wilkinson ID, Griffiths PD, Emery CJ, Tesfaye S. Raised thalamic blood volume in painful diabetic neuropathy: clues to the pathogenesis of neuropathic pain in diabetes. Diabetologia 2008; 51(Suppl 1):1–588.

35. Laterre EC, De Volder AG, Goffinet AM. Brain glucose metabolism in thalamic syndrome. J Neurol Neurosurg Psychiatry 1988; 51:427–428.

36. Di Piero V, Jones AK, Iannotti F, Powell M, Perani D, Lenzi GL, Frackowiak RS. Chronic pain: a PET study of the central effects of percutaneous high cervical cordotomy. Pain 1991; 46:9–12.

37. Hua SE, Garonzik IM, Lee JI, Lenz FA. Microelectrode studies of normal organization and plasticity of human somatosensory thalamus. J Clin Neurophysiol 2000; 17: 559–574.

38. Moisset X, Bouhassira D. Brain imaging of neuropathic pain. Neuroimage 2007; Suppl 1: 80–88.

39. Iadarola MJ, Max MB, Berman KF, Byas-Smith MG, Coghill RC, Gracely RH, Bennett GJ. Unilateral decrease in thalamic activity observed with positron emission tomography in patients with chronic neuropathic pain. Pain 1995; 63:55–64.

40. Hsieh JC, Belfrage M, Stone-Elander S, Hansson P, Ingvar M. Central representation of chronic ongoing neuropathic pain studied by positron emission tomography. Pain 1995; 63:225–236.

41. Cervero F, Laird JM. From acute to chronic pain: mechanisms and hypotheses. Prog Brain Res 1996; 110:3–15.

42. Melzack R. From the gate to the neuromatrix. Pain 1999; 6:121–126.

43. Apkarian AV, Bushnell MC, Treede RD, Zubieta JK. Human brain mechanisms of pain perception and regulation in health and disease. Eur J Pain 2005; 9:463–484.

44. Wilkinson ID, Gandhi R, Hunter MD, Selvarajah D, Emery CJ, Griffiths PD, Tesfaye S.A functional magnetic resonance imaging study demonstrating alterations in brain responses to acute pain stimulation in diabetic neuropathy. Diabetologia 2007; 50(Suppl 1):1–538.

45. Brooks J, Tracey I. From nociception to pain perception: imaging the spinal and supraspinal pathways. J Anat 2005; 207:19–33.
46. Valeriani M, Arendt-Nielsen L, Le Pera D, et al. Short-term plastic changes of the human nociceptive system following acute pain induced by capsaicin. Clin Neurophysiol 2003; 114:1879–1890.
47. Petrovic P, Ingvar M, Stone-Elander S, Petersson KM, Hansson P. A PET activation study of dynamic mechanical allodynia in patients with mononeuropathy. Pain 1999; 83:459–4570.
48. Peyron R, García-Larrea L, Grégoire MC, et al. Allodynia after lateral-medullary (Wallenberg) infarct. A PET study. Brain 1998; 121:345–356.
49. Witting N, Kupers RC, Svensson P, Arendt-Nielsen L, Gjedde A, Jensen TS. Experimental brush-evoked allodynia activates posterior parietal cortex. Neurology 2001; 57:1817–1824.
50. Becerra L, Morris S, Bazes S, et al. Trigeminal neuropathic pain alters responses in CNS circuits to mechanical (brush) and thermal (cold and heat) stimuli. J Neurosci 2006; 26: 10646–10657.
51. Schweinhardt P, Glynn C, Brooks J, et al. An fMRI study of cerebral processing of brush-evoked allodynia in neuropathic pain patients. Neuroimage 2006; 32:256–265.
52. Tracey I, Mantyh PW. The cerebral signature for pain perception and its modulation. Neuron 2007; 55:377–391.
53. Fields HL, Basbaum AI. Central nervous system mechanisms of pain modulation. In: Melzack R, Wall P, eds. Textbook of Pain. London: Churchill Livingstone; 2003:125–142.
54. Selvarajah D, Wilkinson ID, Emery CJ, Harris ND, Shaw PJ, Witte DR, Griffiths PD, Tesfaye S. Early involvement of the spinal cord in diabetic peripheral neuropathy. Diabetes Care 2006; 29:2664–2669.
55. Selvarajah D, Wilkinson ID, Emery CJ, Shaw PJ, Griffiths PD, Gandhi R, Tesfaye S. Thalamic neuronal dysfunction and chronic sensorimotor distal symmetrical polyneuropathy in patients with type 1 diabetes mellitus. Diabetologia 2008; 51:2088–2092.
56. Tracey I, Mantyh PW. The cerebral signature for pain perception and its modulation. Neuron 2007; 55:377–391.

V   EXPERIMENTAL MODELS AND PATHOPHYSIOLOGY

16 Animal Models

Geert Jan Biessels

Contents

Abstract

Clinical research has delineated the nature and severity of acute and chronic cerebral disturbances in relation to abnormal glucose metabolism, as reviewed in the previous chapters of this book. By comparison, insight into the pathophysiology is still limited and evidence for effective treatment is largely lacking. Studies in animal models may help to fill in these gaps in our knowledge. This chapter gives an overview of rodent models that are in use for studies into the impact of acute and chronic disturbances of glucose metabolism on the brain. Strengths and limitations of available models will be addressed and methods to assess cerebral function in these models will be reviewed.

Key words: Rodent models; Rat; Mouse; Transgenic animals; Streptozotocin; Learning and memory; Experimental diabetes.

From: *Contemporary Diabetes: Diabetes and the Brain*
Edited by: G. J. Biessels, J. A. Luchsinger (eds.), DOI 10.1007/978-1-60327-850-8_16
© Humana Press, a part of Springer Science+Business Media, LLC 2009

INTRODUCTION

Over the past decades, clinical research has clearly delineated the nature and severity of acute and chronic cerebral complications in patients with diabetes. The relation between hyperglycemia and clinical outcome after stroke is also well documented. In contrast, insight into the role of aberrant glucose metabolism in the pathophysiology of these conditions is still limited and evidence for effective treatment is largely lacking. This is inherent to the fact that the vast majority of the currently available clinical studies are observational. Given the complexity of the topic, with a multifactorial pathophysiology where it is often difficult to identify cause and effect, it is unlikely that the gaps in our knowledge will be filled in by clinical studies alone. Further fundamental research is therefore needed. Although studies in cell model systems or other in vitro techniques may be of value, at present the impact of systemic abnormalities in glucose metabolism on the central nervous system can only be fully appreciated in vivo. Therefore, to further unravel the pathophysiology and develop treatments, studies in animal models are warranted. Skeptics might argue that the use of such models in related fields, such as research on stroke or on diabetic neuropathy, has not yet had a major impact on daily clinical care for patients. Nevertheless, in my view, studies in animal models may make a valuable contribution to this field, as long as one keeps ethical, theoretical, and practical limitations in mind.

This chapter gives an overview of rodent models that are currently in use for studies into the impact of acute and chronic disturbances of glucose metabolism on the brain, with emphasis on models for the long-term effects of type 1 and type 2 diabetes. Strengths and limitations of available models will be addressed and methods to assess cerebral function in these models will be reviewed.

RODENT MODELS OF HYPOGLYCEMIA AND DIABETIC KETOACIDOSIS

The timing, duration, frequency, and level of hypoglycemia can be readily manipulated in animals that are either normoglycemic or hyperglycemic prior to the induction of hypoglycemia. Consequently, rodent models have been used extensively to study the acute and long-term consequences of hypoglycemia on the brain (1, 2). Hypoglycemia can be induced by subcutaneous or intravenous insulin injection (3). Insulin dosage depends on the strain, weight, and age of the animal and on whether the animal has (had) access to food. The dose of insulin can be titrated to obtain the required severity of hypoglycemia.

In rats, deep (blood glucose < 1.0 mmol/l) and prolonged hypoglycemia, up to a level were the electroencephalogram (EEG) becomes isoelectric, is associated with neuronal cell death in several brain regions, including the hippocampus and the cortex (4). However, the long-term consequences of repeated episodes of hypoglycemia that are less extreme are less straightforward. For example, repeated hypoglycemia to a level of 2.5–3.0 mmol/l appears to improve cognitive performance of rats when they are subsequently tested under normoglycemic conditions (3, 5). The mechanisms underlying this improvement are not completely understood, but may involve adaptation of cerebral glucose uptake, altered neurotransmitter metabolism, or long-term effects of a hypoglycemia-induced stress response. Most importantly, similar improvements of cognition after repeated moderate hypoglycemia have not been reported in humans. This may hamper the translation of behavioral observations in these models of repeated hypoglycemia to the human situation.

The effect of ketoacidosis on the brain has not been studied extensively in rodents. Rodents with chemically induced insulin deficiency, despite having elevated ketone levels, generally do not develop severe ketoacidosis spontaneously and do not require insulin treatment to survive. Nevertheless, ketoacidosis can be induced in such animals by additional experimental manipulations, such as deprivation of drinking water (6–9). In models with immune-mediated destruction of β-cells withdrawal of insulin treatment does lead to ketoacidosis (10).

MODELS FOR HYPERGLYCEMIA AND STROKE

Clinical studies clearly show that admission hyperglycemia is related to the outcome after stroke (Chapter 9). It is less clear, however, if this relation is causal, i.e., high admission glucose causes poor outcome. Issues that need to be resolved are as follows: (i) whether stroke-related hyperglycemia reflects pre-existent metabolic abnormalities, such as impaired glucose tolerance, (ii) whether such pre-existent metabolic abnormalities already compromise the brain, which might explain the relatively poorer functional outcome in relation to hyperglycemia, (iii) if hyperglycemia in the days after the initial event is still harmful to the brain or may even represent a compensatory event for reductions in energy supply to the ischemic area, and (iv) if correction of hyperglycemia improves outcome. Studies in animal models can help to clarify these issues.

The timing and severity of hyperglycemia in relation to stroke can be readily manipulated in rodent models. A range of rodent models of stroke is available (11). A detailed discussion of the pros and cons of these models can be found elsewhere (12, 13). This paragraph only deals with induction of hyperglycemia in these models. Hyperglycemia can be induced within minutes in rodents by an intraperitoneal injection of a concentrated glucose solution *(14–16)*, prior to stroke or at any time after the stroke. Hyperglycemia can also be maintained for a prolonged period prior to the induction of a stroke. A stable elevation of blood glucose levels can, for example, be achieved within days after injection of β-cytotoxic compounds *(14)*. If so desired, glucose levels can also be rapidly normalized again by intravenous insulin infusion *(17)* and chronic hyperglycemia may also be combined with other conditions that co-occur with disturbances in glucose metabolism in patients, such as hypertension.

RODENT MODELS OF DIABETES

Animal models of diabetes can be divided into those in which animals are rendered diabetic by specific experimental procedures, such as specific diets, pancreatectomy, exposure to viruses, or administration of β-cytotoxic agents, and those in which animals develop diabetes spontaneously, due to a genetic predisposition *(18)*. Originally, this latter category of models was achieved through selective breeding (e.g., BB/Wor or Zucker rats). Over the past decades, the development of powerful genetic manipulation techniques has given rise to a huge range of new models with specific genetic deficits in insulin signaling and glucose metabolism pathways (Table 1) *(19)*.

This chapter does not offer an exhaustive list of all currently available rodent models, but rather aims to highlight models that have already been used in the study of cerebral complications of diabetes or have specific features that make them attractive for future studies in this field.

β-Cytotoxic Agents

Alloxan and streptozotocin (STZ) are β-cytotoxic agents that are widely used to induce diabetes in rodents *(20, 21)*. While early studies on cerebral complications of diabetes used either of these two agents, recent studies mostly use STZ.

Alloxan can be injected intravenously, intraperitoneally, or subcutaneously. The dose required to induce diabetes depends on the animal species, route of administration, and nutritional status *(21)*. After injection alloxan is taken up by the β-cells. Intracellularly, it gives rise to several processes, including oxidation of essential –SH groups, inhibition of glucokinase, generation of free radicals, and disturbances in intracellular calcium homeostasis *(21)*. The selectivity of alloxan action for the β-cells is, however, not quite satisfactory. Alloxan is also taken up by other tissues, such as the liver. Although these other tissues appear to be more resistant to alloxan toxicity in

Table 1
Rodent models of cerebral complications of diabetes

Model	Mechanism DM	Glucose levels	Insulin levels	Available studies* (n)	Cognition	Plasticity
Alloxan	β-Cell toxicity	↑↑	↓↓	~30	Active avoidance task ↓	?
Streptozotocin	β-Cell toxicity	↑↑	↓↓	>100	Water maze or a spatial-object learning task ↓	Hippocampal LTP ↓
BB/Wor rat	β-cell autoimmunity	↑↑	↓↓↓	~15	Water maze ↓	?
NOD mouse	β-cell autoimmunity	↑↑	↓↓↓	~5	?	Hippocampal LTP ↓
Zucker fa/fa rat	Defective leptin receptor	=/↑	↑↑	~10	Water maze ↓, delayed alternation task ↓	Hippocampal LTP ↓
Diabetic Zucker rat	fa/fa rat, inbred for hyperglycemia	↑↑	↑↑	~5	Water maze =	Hippocampal LTP =

(continued)

Table 1
(continued)

Model	Mechanism DM	Glucose levels	Insulin levels	Available studies* (n)	Cognition	Plasticity
db/db mouse	Defective leptin receptor	=; ↑↑ with age	↑↑; ↓ with age	~10	Water maze ↓	?
GK rat	Inbred for glucose intolerance	↑	↑	~10	Water maze or radial maze ↓	Hippocampal LTP ↓
OLETF rat	Defective CCK-A receptor	=; ↑ with age	↑; ↓ with age	~5	Taste aversion task ↑, lever-press task ↓	?

*This column provides an estimate of the number of studies in each of the models that addressed different aspects of cerebral function or structure (excluding studies published before 1990 and studies that primarily assessed the role of the brain in peripheral metabolism). For further explanation see text.

The table summarizes characteristics of rodent models that have been used to study cerebral complications of diabetes. =: Normal; ↑: moderately increased/enhanced; ↑↑: markedly increased; ↓: moderately decreased/impaired; ↓↓: markedly decreased. Findings on cognition and plasticity in these models are listed in the last two columns.

comparison to pancreatic β-cells, extrapancreatic effects of alloxan cannot be excluded *(21)*. Another disadvantage is that the range of the diabetogenic dose of alloxan is narrow and even light overdosing may be generally toxic and is associated with mortality probably due to renal tubular cell necrosis *(21)*. While a substantial number of studies have addressed neurochemical changes in the brain of alloxan-diabetic rodents, few studies have examined the effects on cognition. Water maze learning was reported to be intact 1 week after diabetes induction *(22)*, whereas active avoidance learning was impaired 6 weeks after diabetes induction *(23)*.

The STZ-model has been used extensively in studies into the pathophysiology of diabetes and its complications. This glucosamine-nitrosourea compound can be injected intravenously, subcutaneously, or intraperitoneally. The nitrosourea moiety of STZ is responsible for its cellular toxicity, which is mediated through a decrease in NAD levels and the formation of intracellular free radicals *(20, 21, 24)*. The deoxyglucose moiety of STZ facilitates its transport across the cell membrane, in which the GLUT-2 glucose transporter appears to play an essential role *(24)*. The insulin-producing β-cells of the islets of Langerhans combine a high expression of GLUT-2 transporters with a relatively low NAD content, making them particularly vulnerable to STZ toxicity *(20, 24)*. The absence of GLUT-2 glucose transporters in the blood–brain barrier *(25)* limits STZ access to the brain after systemic injection. Direct effects of STZ on the brain after systemic administration, if any, will therefore be limited. This is supported by the observations that the alterations in cognition and synaptic plasticity that occur weeks after the actual STZ injection can be prevented by insulin treatment *(26)*. The dosage window for STZ to obtain stable hyperglycemia is rather narrow, albeit relatively wider than alloxan *(21)*. At relatively low dosages a substantial number of injected animals will not become hyperglycemic, whereas at the upper margin of the dosage window animals die, often of nephrotoxicity. Factors that affect STZ toxicity are age, species, and strain of the rodents. Dose finding studies are recommended before one embarks on large-scale experiments with this agent.

STZ-diabetic rodents are hypoinsulinemic, but do not require insulin treatment to survive. Blood glucose levels are 20–25 mmol/l (normal 5 mmol/l). These high blood glucose levels lead to marked polydipsia and polyuria. The animals generally lose weight. Despite the weight loss, STZ-diabetic animals can be kept for months, although severe cachexia can develop in a proportion of the animals in chronic experiments. This makes the animals vulnerable and is associated with increased mortality. It is possible to treat/prevent cachexia with a low daily dose of insulin. This can be achieved with injections, but the use of subcutaneous implants that release a constant dose of insulin for several weeks may also be considered. In our hands a daily dose of 0.5–1 U of insulin to a mature Wistar rat prevents cachexia without an evident lowering of the level of hyperglycemia (unpublished observations).

Like diabetic patients, STZ-diabetic rats develop end-organ damage affecting the eyes, kidneys, heart, blood vessels, and nervous system. The main advantages of the STZ-model are that it is well characterized and that diabetes can be induced at any given age, thus allowing, for example, studies of the interaction of diabetes and aging. Another advantage of the STZ model is that it can be readily combined with other (genetic) models. Experimenters who use animals that are not yet fully grown at the time of diabetic induction should be aware of the fact that maturation effects can be a confounding factor.

Functional changes in the brain in STZ-diabetic rats have now been assessed by a substantial number of studies (27, 28). Decrements in cognitive performance have been noted that develop in the course of months. These decrements mainly involve performance on relatively complex behavioral tasks, such as a water maze or a spatial-object learning task (29–32). Performance on relative simple tasks, such as passive avoidance paradigms, is preserved (or even improved) (27) (see Box 1). The severity of hyperglycemia is an important factor in the development of the deficits, which can be prevented, but not completely reversed, with intensive insulin treatment (27).

BOX 1 TESTING COGNITION IN DIABETIC RODENTS

Outside the field of diabetes an almost infinite number of behavioral paradigms have been developed to examine cognitive functioning in rodents. There are, however, certain caveats when one wishes to apply these paradigms to diabetes. The majority of rodent models of diabetes are characterized by often rather extreme disturbances of glucose metabolism and related abnormalities in energy balance, leading to the rapid development of end-organ complications. This affects the overall vitality of the animals, levels of stress and response to stressful stimuli, locomotion (e.g., reduced muscle mass, neuropathy), sensory systems (e.g., reduced eyesight, skin sensation), and many other aspects of physical and mental functioning. It will be evident that many of these disturbances can affect performance in behavioral tasks and as such may be regarded as confounders if one aims to assess cognition. [For a more detailed discussion of confounders in behavioral learning tasks see (33, 34)].

The nature of the stimulus used in the behavioral paradigm is an important factor. There are clear indications that stressful stimuli, which are often part of learning paradigms, elicit larger physiological responses in STZ-diabetic rodents than in non-diabetic rodents (35). Thus, the enhanced retention of simple passive avoidance in diabetic rodents (36) has been ascribed to an increased sensitivity to foot shock (37). These altered responses to foot shock, or other painful stimuli, may be due to the complex interplay of abnormalities in peripheral [e.g., neuropathy (38)] or central [altered mood and behavior (55)] pain perception. It will be evident that such effects confound experiments that aim to assess the impact of diabetes on cognition. An alternative strategy is to use positive reinforcement for a learning task, such as rewards with food or drink. It should be noted, however, that in such tasks food and water are often withheld from the animals for several hours prior to the test, to increase motivation for the reward. Again this can lead to a different level of motivation in diabetic rodents due to the excessive food and water requirements of these animals. Nevertheless, the level of thirst or hunger can be titrated through modification of the withdrawal period in the diabetic animals (30).

The key message is that there are many potential confounders in behavioral experiments with diabetic rodents. It is therefore essential to use a task that allows dissecting out the cognitive component of the performance of the animals. Ideally, such a task has a control condition that entails all the sensory, motor, and behavioral elements of the condition in which cognition is assessed. The Morris water maze, for example (39), is such a task. In the "learning version" of this task the rodent has to learn the spatial location of an escape platform that is hidden on a fixed position in a circular water pool. Spatial learning in this task involves multiple cognitive components such as problem-solving, enhanced selective attention, formation of internal representations of the external world, and storage and retrieval of relevant information (40). In the "control version" of the task the platform is visible just above the surface of the water. If animals have a normal performance on this task their motivation and swimming capacity are apparently intact. Moreover, if one monitors the search pattern of the animals in the "learning version" of the task one can assess both swimming speed and the search strategy (Fig. 1). Another example of a test that may be of use in diabetic animals is the so-called can test, a spatial/object learning and memory task, without the use of aversive stimuli (30). In this task the rat has to learn to identify a rewarded can (containing water) based on its surface and/or position in an open field. The cognitive demand of the task can easily be modified by increasing the complexity, while motor and motivational aspects of task performance are essentially similar across different task conditions.

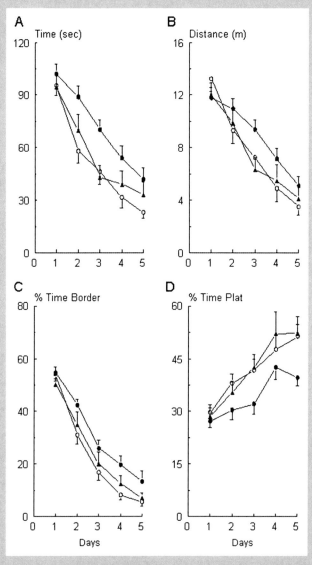

Fig. 1. Example of a behavioral test in STZ-DM rats: the Morris water maze. The water maze *(39)* consisted of a large circular black pool (210 cm diameter,

50 cm height, filled to a depth of 30 cm with water (28±1°C)), placed in a darkened room, and illuminated by sparse red light. A submerged escape plat-form was hidden on a fixed location. Without pretraining, animals were given three acquisition trials per day on 5 consecutive days. Diabetes duration was 10 weeks. One group of rats was treated with subcutaneous insulin implants after confirmation of diabetes. (A) Latencies to reach the platform; (B) dis-tances swum to reach the platform; (C) percentage of time spent in the bor-der zone of the pool; (D) percentage of time in central zone spent in cor-rect quadrant of the pool. o: Control rats ($n=18$), •: diabetic rats ($n=18$), ▲: insulin-treated diabetic rats ($n=12$). The performance of diabetic rats was impaired compared to controls. Insulin treatment prevented deficits in water maze learning in diabetic rats. Untreated diabetic vs. control: latencies: $p <$ 0.001; distance (days 3–5): $p < 0.05$; border: $p < 0.01$; quadrant: $p < 0.001$. Untreated vs. insulin-treated diabetic: latencies: $p < 0.01$; distance (days 3–5): $p < 0.05$; border: $p = 0.06$; quadrant: $p < 0.005$. Insulin-treated diabetic vs. controls: not significant. Data are mean ± SEM. Note that the measurement of swimming distance and search pattern provide important additional information. While increased latencies might reflect reduced swimming speed due to motor deficits or altered motivation, the aberrant search pattern is more likely to reflect abnormal comprehension and acquisition of the task. (Adapted from Biessels et al. (26), with kind permission from Elsevier.)

In view of the crucial role of the hippocampus in memory formation (41), several groups have studied dynamic changes in synaptic strength in the hippocampus in STZ-diabetic rats, in search of a neural correlate of the impaired cognition. Indeed, a complex pattern of changes in synaptic plas-ticity has been observed in hippocampal slices. A deficit in the expression of N-methyl-d-aspartate (NMDA)-dependent long-term potentiation (LTP) in the CA1 field gradually develops and reaches a maximum at 12 weeks after diabetes induction (29, 42, 43). The relevance of this observation lays in the fact that hippocampal LTP is generally accepted as a model system to study information storage in the brain at the cellular level (44). The severity of the LTP deficit is related to the severity of hyperglycemia (29). Insulin treatment is able to prevent the development of the changes in LTP but is less effective against existing deficits. In contrast to LTP, expression of long-term depression (LTD) is enhanced in the CA1 field following low-frequency stimulation of slices from diabetic rats (27, 43). It is interesting to note that both the learning deficits and the facilitation of LTD and impair-ment of LTP in STZ-diabetic rats are accentuated by aging (45). Functional abnormalities in the brain and spinal cord of STZ-diabetic rats have also been noted with neurophysiological techniques (see Box 2). Over the course of months STZ-diabetic rats develop increased latencies of visual- and auditory-evoked potentials and reduced conduction velocities in the spinal cord (46–48).

BOX 2 NEUROPHYSIOLOGICAL ASSESSMENT: EVOKED POTENTIALS

Assessment of evoked potential latencies is a common tool in neurophysiological studies of central nervous system involvement in patients with diabetes. Evoked potentials are the electrical manifestations of the brain's response to an external stimulus, such as a flash of light or a sound click. In patients with diabetes, the latencies of evoked potentials of different modalities, including visual-evoked potentials (VEPs), brainstem auditory-evoked potentials (BAEPs), and somatosensory-evoked potentials (SSEPs), are increased *(49)*. Evoked-potential measurements can also be used to monitor CNS involvement in experimentally diabetic rodents. Such measurements allow monitoring of the course of development of CNS abnormalities *(48)* or the effects of therapeutic intervention *(50)*. In rodents BAEPs and VEPs can be measured longitudinally through implantation of recording electrodes into the skull *(48)* or through repeated placement of subcutaneous electrodes (Fig. 2) *(51)*.

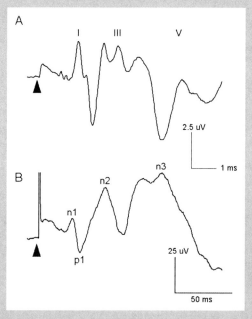

Fig. 2. Typical recordings of a BAEP (**A**) and a VEP (**B**) from a rat. The black triangles indicate presentation stimulus; relevant peaks are indicated: I, III and

V in the brainstem auditory-evoked potential (BAEP); n1, p1, n2, and n3 in the visual-evoked potential (VEP). Although some uncertainty remains as to the precise location of the generators of these waves, BAEP wave I is assumed to be generated in the auditory nerve, wave III in the superior olivary complex, and wave V in the lateral lemniscus or the inferior colliculus *(87–89)*. Hence, the latency of wave I and the interpeak latencies I–III and III–V were used as a measure of the function of the auditory nerve, the pontomedullary region, and the rostral pontine and midbrain region, respectively. For the VEP, peaks n1 and p1 have been suggested to be generated in the primary and secondary visual cortex, whereas n2 and n3 may be generated in associative cortical areas beyond the classically defined visual cortex *(90)*. Adapted from Biessels et al. *(48)*.

If one wishes to measure evoked-potential latencies to monitor the effects of diabetes on the central nervous system in rodents, it is important to consider the potential confounding effects of maturation and growth. The latencies of evoked potentials reflect the sum of the time for perception in sensory organs, axonal conduction in the peripheral and central components of the sensory pathways, and the time for synaptic transmission. The length of the peripheral and central components of the sensory pathways increases with growth of the animal, leading to an increase in latencies, while maturation of axons and myelin sheets will increase conduction velocity along the pathways, thus reducing latencies. The majority of experimental studies in diabetes use immature rodents. Diabetes can disturb both growth of the animal and the maturation of the nervous system. Differences in latencies relative to age-matched non-diabetic rodents may thus reflect the combined effects of impaired growth and maturation and those of diabetes per se *(48)*. In this respect, studies in animals that are mature at the time of diabetes onset may give more straightforward results.

Histological studies of the brain and spinal cord in STZ-diabetic rats are still relatively scarce. While early studies reported structural abnormalities, such as loss of cortical neurons, after many months of diabetes *(52, 53)*, more recent studies show that ultrastructural changes, at the synaptic level, may develop within a week *(54, 55)*.

In the context of this book it is also appropriate to mention studies that administer STZ through intracerebroventricular injection *(56, 57)*. After such injections, local concentrations of STZ in the brain will be much higher than after systemic injection, not only because of the dose (5% of the systemic dose in a confined tissue compartment that contains less than 1% of the body mass of an adult rat), but also because of the barrier function of the blood–brain barrier after systemic administration. Intracerebroventricular

STZ injections alter glucose metabolism within the brain, while leaving systemic glucose levels unaffected, and are associated with behavioral abnormalities *(56, 57)*. Because of these features, intracerebroventricular STZ injection has been put forward as a model of Alzheimer's disease *(58)*. It should be noted, however, that given the pharmacological properties of STZ, as an alkylating agent, damage to cell types in the brain that take up STZ is likely to be widespread and to involve much more than just "abnormal glucose metabolism." Thus far this model has been used by a limited number of research groups and it may need further characterization.

Spontaneously Diabetic Rodent Models

BB/WOR RATS AND NOD MICE

The BB/Wor rat and NOD mouse models mimic several aspects of type 1 diabetes in humans [For reviews and discussion see *(20, 59–62)*].

The BB/Wor rat is an inbred Wistar strain that spontaneously develops diabetes, due to immune-mediated destruction of β-cells *(20, 59)*. Intense mononuclear infiltration within and around the islets of Langerhans can be observed 2–3 weeks prior to the onset of overt diabetes *(59)*. Insulin treatment is required for survival. Extrapancreatic inflammatory changes have also been reported. These include lymphocytic infiltration of the thymus, albeit without the development of frank hypothyroidism *(59)*.

The NonObese Diabetic (NOD) mouse model is also characterized by immune-mediated destruction of β-cells. These animals also require insulin for survival, but they are less prone to ketoacidosis than BB/Wor rats *(20)*. The NOD mouse is a favored model for investigations into the etiology of autoimmune, T-cell-mediated type 1 diabetes in humans, because relative to the BB/Wor model the genome of NOD mice is better-defined, more monoclonal reagents for the analysis of immune system components are available and maintenance costs are considerably lower.

The number of studies that have assessed the functional and structural integrity of the brain in these models is still relatively small. In BB/Wor rats impairments in water maze performance are observed after 8 months, but not after 2 months of diabetes *(63)*. Observations on hippocampal LTP are not yet available from the BB/Wor rat model, but a study in NOD mice reported that LTP was disturbed relative to control mice, possibly due to changes in glutamatergic neurotransmission *(64)*. Hippocampal neurogenesis is also reduced in NOD mice *(65)*, a finding that has also been reported in STZ-diabetic rats *(66)*.

ZUCKER RATS AND DB/DB MICE

Zucker rats come in different strains. Zucker fa/fa rats have an autosomal recessive mutation of the *fa*-gene, encoding for the leptin receptor. The animals are hyperphagic, hyperlipidemic, and obese *(20, 67)*. They also express peripheral insulin resistance, hyperinsulinemia, and an impaired glucose tolerance. Hyperglycemia is usually mild. A substrain of fa/fa rats has been inbred for hyperglycemia, leading to the so-called diabetic Zucker rat (ZDF/DRT-fa) model *(20)*.

The features of the db/db mouse closely mimic those of the fa/fa rat, with an autosomal recessive mutation in the diabetes (*db*) gene, encoding for the leptin receptor. Young db/db mice are hyperinsulinemic, hyperphagic, and obese *(20, 67)*. Animals become progressively hyperglycemic. At an age of 3–6 months insulin levels start to decline and the animals develop pancreatic β-cell atrophy.

Behavioral and electrophysiological findings in these models of insulin resistance vary. An initial study in ZDF rats reported no impairments in Morris water maze performance up to 8 weeks after the onset of hyperglycemia, apart from a modest reduction in swimming speed *(68)*. Expression of LTP in hippocampal slices from these animals was also preserved *(68)*. In contrast, a study in Zucker fa/fa aged 6 months with relatively mild hyperglycemia (~10 mmol/l) did report impaired cognitive performance on a delayed alternation task *(69)*. In our lab we have tested obese hyperinsulinemic Zucker fa/fa rats with modest hyperglycemia (9 mmol/l vs. 5 mmol/l in fa/– controls) and observed impairments in both water maze performance and hippocampal LTP (unpublished observations). After 8 months of hyperglycemia ZDF rats do develop neuronal loss in the CA1 field of the hippocampus, albeit to a lesser extent than BB/Wor rats *(70)*.

In db/db mice acquisition of a conditioned taste aversion learning task appears to be preserved, but its extinction is accelerated *(71)*. Moreover, performance of these mice in the Morris water maze is impaired *(32)*.

Other Models

The Otsuka Long–Evans Tokushima fatty (OLETF) rat is characterized by mild obesity and an impaired glucose tolerance as early as at 2 months of age. Next, hypertriglyceridemia and slight hypercholesterolemia develop, followed by hyperinsulinemia, hyperglycemia, and ultimately (at 10 months of age) hypoinsulinemia, requiring insulin therapy for survival *(20, 67)*. Genetically, this model is characterized by a reduced expression of the cholecystokinin (CCK)-A receptor gene *(72)*.

Behavioral studies in OLETF rats have been performed with relatively young (age 2–5 months) animals that had not yet developed increased fasting plasma glucose values. At this age, performance on an inhibitory avoidance test is preserved *(73)*, or even improved *(72)*, whereas performance on more complex tasks, such as a Morris water maze or a radial maze, is impaired *(72, 74)*. The improved performance in the avoidance task was attributed to increased sensitivity to aversive stimuli *(72)*, analogous to observations in STZ-diabetic rats with these kind of behavioral paradigms (see Box 1). In OLETF rats aged 3 months, LTP expression in the dentate gyrus of the hippocampus is impaired *(74)*.

The Goto–Kakizaki (GK) rat is a substrain of Wistar rats which has been established by selective breeding with glucose intolerant animals *(20, 67)*. The animals are non-obese, insulin resistant with modest hyperinsulinemia and hyperglycemia (±10 mmol/l). The severity of diabetes does not increase with age. In GK rats, acquisition of a conditioned taste aversion learning task is enhanced *(75)*, whereas performance on a lever-press task, a behavioral paradigm which allows the study of response–reinforcement learning, was impaired *(76)*.

The Akita mouse model expresses an autosomal dominant inherited form of diabetes characterized by hyperglycemia and severe insulin deficiency due to degradation of β-cells as a result of intracellular accumulation of misfolded proinsulin 2 *(77)*. In Akita mice, Morris water maze performance (with a longitudinal testing protocol that differs from the aforementioned studies) is preserved, even after prolonged hyperglycemia *(78)*.

Clinical Relevance

Table 1 summarizes an overview of several rodent models that have been used to assess the effects of diabetes on the brain. Observations regarding cognition and plasticity in models characterized by hyperglycemia and insulin deficiency (i.e., alloxan or STZ-diabetes, BB/Wor rats, NOD-mice), often referred to as models of type 1 diabetes, are quite consistent. With respect to clinical relevance, it should be noted that the level of glycemia in these models markedly exceeds that observed in patients. Moreover, changes in cognition as observed in these models are much more rapid and severe than in adult patients with type 1 diabetes *(79–81)*, even if the relatively shorter lifespan of rodents is taken into account. Finally, the majority of experiments are being performed in relatively young animals. Thus, potential effects of experimental diabetes on brain maturation may affect the results. In my view these models of "type 1 diabetes" may help to understand the pathophysiology of the effects of severe chronic hyperglycemia–hypoinsulinemia on the brain, but mimic the impact of type 1 diabetes on the brain in humans only to a limited extent.

Abnormalities in cognition and plasticity have also been noted in the majority of models characterized by insulin resistance, hyperinsulinemia, and (modest) hyperglycemia (e.g., Zucker fa/fa rat, Diabetic Zucker rat, db/db mouse, GK rat, OLETF rat), often referred to as models of type 2 diabetes. With regard to clinical relevance, it is important to note that although the endocrinological features of these models do mimic certain aspects of type 2 diabetes, the genetic defect that underlies each of them is not the primary defect encountered in humans with type 2 diabetes. Some of the genetic abnormalities that lead to a "diabetic phenotype" may also have a direct impact on the brain. For example, leptin and CCK, the receptors of which are defective in, respectively, the Zucker and OLETF rat, are both known to have modulatory effects on learning and memory. This may explain why some studies using these models report abnormalities in cognition and plasticity, even in the absence of hyperglycemia *(72, 74)*. In addition, in the majority of available models insulin resistance and associated metabolic abnormalities develop at a relatively early age. Although this is practical for research purposes it needs to be acknowledged that type 2 diabetes is typically a disease of older age in humans. Moreover, clinically relevant cognitive deficits mainly occur in older patients with type 2 diabetes *(82, 83)*. It is therefore still too early to determine the clinical significance of the available models in understanding the impact of type 2 diabetes on the brain. Further efforts into the development of a valid model are warranted. These efforts should not only focus on models that reflect the endocrinological features of type 2 diabetes, but also take into account the age of the population involved, and the associated co-morbidity. Type 2 diabetes typically develops in the context of a cluster of vascular and metabolic risk factors (including hypertension, dyslipidemia, and obesity) referred to as the "metabolic syndrome." The metabolic syndrome itself, with or without hyperglycemia, is associated with atherosclerotic cardiovascular disease, ischemic stroke, and cognitive decline and dementia *(84)*. A key question is therefore whether diabetes per se or other factors from the metabolic syndrome are the prime determinants of impaired cognition in type 2 diabetes. Hopefully, rodent models can help to answer this question.

Future Perspectives

As indicated in the previous section, none of the available models mimic either type1 or type 2 diabetes and associated cerebral complications in every aspect. The question is, however, what one might expect from a rodent model of cerebral complications of a complex endocrinological disease in humans. Rather than focusing on the shortcomings of rodent models it might be more worthwhile to zoom in on the elements of these models that can help to further our insight into the impact of diabetes on the brain. As I indicated in the introduction of this chapter, a key problem in clinical studies is the complexity and multifactorial nature of cerebral complications in relation to diabetes. Metabolic factors in patients (e.g., glucose levels, insulin levels, insulin sensitivity) are strongly interrelated and related to other factors that may affect the brain (e.g., blood pressure, lipids, inflammation, oxidative stress). Derangements in these factors in the periphery and the brain may be dissociated, for example, through the role of the blood–brain barrier, or adaptations of transport across this barrier, or through differences in receptor functions and post-receptor signaling cascades in the periphery and the brain. The different forms of treatments that patients receive add to the complexity. A key contribution of animal studies may be to single out individual components and study them in isolation or in combination with a limited number of other factors in a controlled fashion. One may, for example, wish to study the effects of abnormalities in insulin signaling on the brain in the absence of systemic abnormalities in insulin sensitivity and associated metabolic abnormalities *(85)*. One may also wish to assess the effects of hyperglycemia alone or in combination with factors that may accentuate glucose-mediated damage such as the level of expression of the receptor for advanced glycation end-products (RAGE) *(86)*. In fact, the possibilities are infinite.

The experimental studies that have been performed over the past decades, as reviewed in this chapter, show that it is possible to examine some of the aspects of cerebral complications of diabetes in rodents. However, much refinement will be needed to obtain clinically meaningful insights. The challenges for future studies are to ask the right research questions, to develop the right models according to these questions, and to strive for further improvement of the standards for range and quality of the animal data *(12)*.

REFERENCES

1. Auer RN. Progress review: hypoglycemic brain damage. Stroke 1986; 17:699–708.
2. Auer RN. Hypoglycemic brain damage. Metab Brain Dis 2004; 19:169–175.
3. McNay EC, Sherwin RS. Effect of recurrent hypoglycemia on spatial cognition and cognitive metabolism in normal and diabetic rats. Diabetes 2004; 53:418–425.
4. Auer RN, Olsson Y, Siesjo BK. Hypoglycemic brain injury in the rat: correlation of density of brain damage with the EEG isoelectric time: A quantitative study. Diabetes 1984; 33:1090–1098.
5. McNay EC, Williamson A, McCrimmon RJ, Sherwin RS. Cognitive and neural hippocampal effects of long-term moderate recurrent hypoglycemia. Diabetes 2006; 55:1088–1095.
6. Beech JS, Williams SC, Iles RA, et al. Haemodynamic and metabolic effects in diabetic ketoacidosis in rats of treatment with sodium bicarbonate or a mixture of sodium bicarbonate and sodium carbonate. Diabetologia 1995; 38:889–898.

7. Federiuk IF, Casey HM, Quinn MJ, Wood MD, Ward WK. Induction of type-1 diabetes mellitus in laboratory rats by use of alloxan: route of administration, pitfalls, and insulin treatment. Comp Med 2004; 54:252–257.

8. Haas MJ, Pun K, Reinacher D, Wong NC, Mooradian A.D. Effects of ketoacidosis on rat apolipoprotein A1 gene expression: a link with acidosis but not with ketones. J Mol Endocrinol 2000; 25:129–139.

9. Lam TI, Anderson SE, Glaser N, O'Donnell ME. Bumetanide reduces cerebral edema formation in rats with diabetic ketoacidosis. Diabetes 2005; 54:510–516.

10. Guberski DL, Butler L, Manzi SM, Stubbs M, Like AA. The BBZ/Wor rat: clinical characteristics of the diabetic syndrome. Diabetologia 1993; 36:912–919.

11. Small DL, Buchan AM. Animal models. Br Med Bull 2000; 56:307–317.

12. Sena E, van der Worp HB, Howells D, Macleod M. How can we improve the pre-clinical development of drugs for stroke? Trends Neurosci 2007; 30:433–439.

13. Dirnagl U. Bench to bedside: the quest for quality in experimental stroke research. J Cereb Blood Flow Metab 2006; 26:1465–1478.

14. Duckrow RB, Beard DC, Brennan RW. Regional cerebral blood flow decreases during chronic and acute hyperglycemia. Stroke 1987; 18:52–58.

15. Liu L, Wang Z, Wang X, et al. Comparison of two rat models of cerebral ischemia under hyperglycemic conditions. Microsurgery 2007; 27:258–262.

16. Kikano GE, LaManna JC, Harik SI. Brain perfusion in acute and chronic hyperglycemia in rats. Stroke 1989; 20:1027–1031.

17. Biessels GJ, Stevens EJ, Mahmood SJ, Gispen WH, Tomlinson DR. Insulin partially reverses deficits in peripheral nerve blood flow and conduction in experimental diabetes. J Neurol Sci 1996; 140:12–20.

18. Mordes JP, Rossini AA. Animal models of diabetes. Am J Med 1981; 70:353–360.

19. LeRoith D, Gavrilova O. Mouse models created to study the pathophysiology of Type 2 diabetes. Int J Biochem Cell Biol 2006; 38:904–912.

20. Shafrir E. Diabetes in animals: contribution to the understanding of diabetes by study of its etiopathology in animal models. In: Porte JR D, Sherwin RS, eds. Ellenberg and Rifkin's Diabetes Mellitus; Theory and Practice. Stamford: Appleton & Lange; 1997:301–348.

21. Szkudelski T. The mechanism of alloxan and streptozotocin action in B cells of the rat pancreas. Physiol Res 2001; 50:537–546.

22. Xie W, Du L. High-cholesterol diets impair short-term retention of memory in alloxan-induced diabetic mice, but not acquisition of memory nor retention of memory in prediabetic mice. Life Sci 2005; 77:481–495.

23. Kucukatay V, Agar A, Gumuslu S, Yargicoglu P. Effect of sulfur dioxide on active and passive avoidance in experimental diabetes mellitus: relation to oxidant stress and antioxidant enzymes. Int J Neurosci 2007; 117:1091–1107.

24. Schnedl WJ, Ferber S, Johnson JH, Newgard CB. STZ transport and cytotoxicity. Specific enhancement in GLUT2- expressing cells. Diabetes 1994; 43:1326–1333.

25. Kumagai AK. Glucose transport in brain and retina: implications in the management and complications of diabetes. Diabetes Metab Res Rev 1999; 15:261–273.

26. Biessels GJ, Kamal A, Urban IJ, Spruijt BM, Erkelens DW, Gispen WH. Water maze learning and hippocampal synaptic plasticity in streptozotocin-diabetic rats: effects of insulin treatment. Brain Res 1998; 800:125–135.

27. Gispen WH, Biessels GJ. Cognition and synaptic plasticity in diabetes mellitus. Trends Neurosci 2000; 23:542–549.

28. Trudeau F, Gagnon S, Massicotte G. Hippocampal synaptic plasticity and glutamate receptor regulation: influences of diabetes mellitus. Eur J Pharmacol 2004; 490:177–186.

29. Biessels GJ, Kamal A, Ramakers GM, et al. Place learning and hippocampal synaptic plasticity in streptozotocin-induced diabetic rats. Diabetes 1996; 45:1259–1266.

30. Popovic M, Biessels GJ, Isaacson RL, Gispen WH. Learning and memory in streptozotocin-induced diabetic rats in a novel spatial/object discrimination task. Behav Brain Res 2001; 122:201–207.

31. Lupien SB, Bluhm EJ, Ishii DN. Systemic insulin-like growth factor-I administration prevents cognitive impairment in diabetic rats, and brain IGF regulates learning/memory in normal adult rats. J Neurosci Res 2003; 74:512–523.
32. Stranahan AM, Arumugam TV, Cutler RG, Lee K, Egan JM, Mattson MP. Diabetes impairs hippocampal function through glucocorticoid-mediated effects on new and mature neurons. Nat Neurosci 2008; 11(3):309–317.
33. Squire LR, Knowlton B, Musen G. The structure and organization of memory. Annu Rev Psychol 1993; 44:453–495.
34. Chabot C, Massicotte G, Milot M, Trudeau F, Gagne J. Impaired modulation of AMPA receptors by calcium-dependent processes in streptozotocin-induced diabetic rats. Brain Res 1997; 768:249–256.
35. Kamal A, Biessels GJ, Urban IJA, Gispen WH. Hippocampal synaptic plasticity in streptozotocin-diabetic rats: impairment of long-term potentiation and facilitation of long-term depression. Neuroscience 1999; 90:737–745.
36. Bliss TV, Collingridge GL. A synaptic model of memory: long-term potentiation in the hippocampus. Nature 1993; 361:31–39.
37. Kamal A, Biessels GJ, Duis SEJ, Gispen WH. Learning and hippocampal synaptic plasticity in streptozotocin-diabetic rats: interaction of diabetes and ageing. Diabetologia 2000; 43:500–506.
38. Carsten RE, Whalen LR, Ishii DN. Impairment of spinal cord conduction velocity in diabetic rats. Diabetes 1989; 38:730–736.
39. Rubini R, Biasiolo F, Fogarolo F, Magnavita V, Martini A, Fiori MG. Brainstem auditory evoked potentials in rats with streptozotocin-induced diabetes. Diabetes Res Clin Pract 1992; 16:19–25.
40. Biessels GJ, Cristino NA, Rutten G, Hamers FPT, Erkelens DW, Gispen WH. Neurophysiological changes in the central and peripheral nervous system of streptozotocin-diabetic rats: course of development and effects of insulin treatment. Brain 1999; 122: 757–768.
41. Mukai N, Hori S, Pomeroy M. Cerebral lesions in rats with streptozotocin-induced diabetes. Acta Neuropathol (Berl) 1980; 51:79–84.
42. Jakobsen J, Sidenius P, Gundersen HJ, Osterby R. Quantitative changes of cerebral neocortical structure in insulin-treated long-term streptozotocin-induced diabetes in rats. Diabetes 1987; 36:597–601.
43. Reagan LP, Magarinos AM, Mcewen BS. Neurological changes induced by stress in streptozotocin diabetic rats. Ann N Y Acad Sci 1999; 893:126–137.
44. Reagan LP, Grillo CA, Piroli GG. The As and Ds of stress: Metabolic, morphological and behavioral consequences. Eur J Pharmacol 208; 585:64–75.
45. Mayer G, Nitsch R, Hoyer S. Effects of changes in peripheral and cerebral glucose metabolism on locomotor activity, learning and memory in adult male rats. Brain Res 1990; 532:95–100.
46. Nitsch R, Hoyer S. Local action of the diabetogenic drug, streptozotocin, on glucose and energy metabolism in rat brain cortex. Neurosci Lett 1991; 128:199–202.
47. Hoyer S, Lee SK, Loffler T, Schliebs R. Inhibition of the neuronal insulin receptor. An in vivo model for sporadic Alzheimer disease? Ann N Y Acad Sci 2000; 920:256–258.
48. Crisa L, Mordes JP, Rossini AA. Autoimmune diabetes mellitus in the BB rat. Diabetes Metab Rev 1992; 8:9–37.
49. Atkinson MA, Leiter EH. The NOD mouse model of type 1 diabetes: as good as it gets? Nat Med 1999; 5:601–604.
50. Roep BO, Atkinson M. Animal models have little to teach us about type 1 diabetes: 1. In support of this proposal. Diabetologia 2004; 47:1650–1656.
51. Leiter EH, von Herrath M. nimal models have little to teach us about type 1 diabetes: 2. In opposition to this proposal. Diabetologia 2004; 47:1657–1660.
52. Li ZG, Zhang W, Grunberger G, Sima AA. Hippocampal neuronal apoptosis in type 1 diabetes. Brain Res 2002; 946:221–231.

53. Valastro B, Cossette J, Lavoie N, Gagnon S, Trudeau F, Massicotte G. Up-regulation of glutamate receptors is associated with LTP defects in the early stages of diabetes mellitus. Diabetologia 2002; 45:642–650.
54. Beauquis J, Saravia F, Coulaud J, et al. Prominently decreased hippocampal neurogenesis in a spontaneous model of type 1 diabetes, the nonobese diabetic mouse. Exp Neurol 2008; 210:359–367.
55. Jackson-Guilford J, Leander JD, Nisenbaum LK. The effect of streptozotocin-induced diabetes on cell proliferation in the rat dentate gyrus. Neurosci Lett 2000; 293:91–94.
56. Janssen U, Phillips AO, Floege J. Rodent models of nephropathy associated with type II diabetes. J Nephrol 1999; 12:159–172.
57. Belanger A, Lavoie N, Trudeau F, Massicotte G, Gagnon S. Preserved LTP and water maze learning in hyperglycaemic-hyperinsulinemic ZDF rats. Physiol Behav 2004; 83: 483–494.
58. Winocur G, Greenwood CE, Piroli GG, et al. Memory impairment in obese Zucker rats: An investigation of cognitive function in an animal model of insulin resistance and obesity. Behav Neurosci 2005; 119:1389–1395.
59. Li ZG, Zhang W, Sima AA. The role of impaired insulin/IGF action in primary diabetic encephalopathy. Brain Res 2005; 1037:12–24.
60. Ohta R, Shigemura N, Sasamoto K, Koyano K, Ninomiya Y. Conditioned taste aversion learning in leptin-receptor-deficient db/db mice. Neurobiol Learn Mem 2003; 80:105–112.
61. Li XL, Aou S, Hori T, Oomura Y. Spatial memory deficit and emotional abnormality in OLETF rats. Physiol Behav 2002; 75:15–23.
62. Matsushita H, Akiyoshi J, Kai K, et al. Spatial memory impairment in OLETF rats without cholecystokinin-a receptor. Neuropeptides 2003; 37:271–276.
63. Nomoto S, Miyake M, Ohta M, Funakoshi A, Miyasaka K. Impaired learning and memory in OLETF rats without cholecystokinin (CCK)-A receptor. Physiol Behav 1999; 66: 869–872.
64. Marfaing-Jallat P, Portha B, Pénicaud L. Altered conditioned taste aversion and glucose utilization in related brain nuclei of diabetic GK rats. Brain Res Bull 1995; 37:639–643.
65. Moreira T, Malec E, Ostenson CG, Efendic S, Liljequist S. Diabetic type II Goto-Kakizaki rats show progressively decreasing exploratory activity and learning impairments in fixed and progressive ratios of a lever-press task. Behav Brain Res 2007; 180:28–41.
66. Izumi T, Yokota-Hashimoto H, Zhao S, Wang J, Halban PA, Takeuchi T. Dominant negative pathogenesis by mutant proinsulin in the Akita diabetic mouse. Diabetes 2003; 52:409–416.
67. Choeiri C, Hewitt K, Durkin J, Simard CJ, Renaud JM, Messier C. Longitudinal evaluation of memory performance and peripheral neuropathy in the Ins2(C96Y) Akita mice. Behav Brain Res 2004; 157:31–38.
68. The Diabetes Control and Complications Trial/Epidemiology of DiabetesInterventions and Complications (DCCT/EDIC) Study Research Group. Long-term effect of diabetes and its treatment on cognitive function. N Engl J Med 2007; 356:1842–1852.
69. Brands AMA, Biessels GJ, De Haan EHF, Kappelle LJ, Kessels RPC. The effects of Type 1 diabetes on cognitive performance: a meta-analysis. Diabetes Care 2005; 28:726–735.
70. Brands AM, Kessels RP, Hoogma RP, et al. Cognitive performance, psychological well-being, and brain magnetic resonance imaging in older patients with type 1 diabetes. Diabetes 2006; 55:1800–1806.
71. Biessels GJ, Deary IJ, Ryan CM. Cognition and diabetes: a lifespan perspective. Lancet Neurol 2008; 7:184–190.
72. Ryan CM, Geckle M. Why is learning and memory dysfunction in Type 2 diabetes limited to older adults? Diabetes Metab Res Rev 2000; 16:308–315.
73. Kalmijn S, Foley D, White L, et al. Metabolic cardiovascular syndrome and risk of dementia in Japanese-American elderly men. The Honolulu-Asia aging study. Arterioscler Thromb Vasc Biol 2000; 20:2255–2260.
74. Grillo CA, Tamashiro KL, Piroli GG, et al. Lentivirus-mediated downregulation of hypothalamic insulin receptor expression. Physiol Behav 2007; 92:691–701.

75. Toth C, Rong LL, Yang C, et al. Receptor for advanced glycation end products (RAGEs) and experimental diabetic neuropathy. Diabetes 2008; 57:1002–1017.
76. Gerlai R. Behavioral tests of hippocampal function: simple paradigms complex problems. Behav Brain Res 2001; 125:269–277.
77. van der Staay FJ. Assessment of age-associated cognitive deficits in rats: a tricky business. Neurosci Biobehav Rev 2002; 26:753–759.
78. Rowland NE, Bellush LL. Diabetes mellitus: stress, neurochemistry and behavior. Neurosci Biobehav Rev 1989; 13:199–206.
79. Bellush LL, Rowland NE. Stress and behavior in streptozotocin diabetic rats: biochemical correlates of passive avoidance learning. Behav Neurosci 1989; 103:144–150.
80. Flood JF, Mooradian AD, Morley JE. Characteristics of learning and memory in streptozotocin-induced diabetic mice. Diabetes 1990; 39:1391–1398.
81. Calcutt NA. Experimental models of painful diabetic neuropathy. J Neurol Sci 2004; 220:137–139.
82. Morris RGM, Garrud P, Rawlins JNP, O'Keefe J. Place navigation is impaired in rats with hippocampal lesions. Nature 1982; 297:681–683.
83. Bannerman DM., Good MA, Butcher SP, Ramsay M, Morris RG. Distinct components of spatial learning revealed by prior training and NMDA receptor blockade. Nature 1995; 378:182–186.
84. Di Mario U, Morano S, Valle E, Pozzessere G. Electrophysiological alterations of the central nervous system in diabetes mellitus. Diabetes Metab Rev 1995; 11:259–278.
85. Biessels GJ, Smale S, Duis SEJ, Kamal A, Gispen WH. The effect of gamma-linolenic acid -- alpha-lipoic acid on functional deficits in the peripheral and central nervous system of streptozotocin-diabetic rats. J Neurol Sci 2001; 182:99–106.
86. Manschot SM, Gispen WH, Kappelle LJ, Biessels GJ. Nerve conduction velocity and evoked potential latencies in streptozotocin-diabetic rats: effects of treatment with an angiotensin converting enzyme inhibitor. Diabetes Metab Res Rev 2003; 19:469–477.
87. Shaw NA. The auditory evoked potential in the rat – a review. Prog Neurobiol 1988; 31:19–45.
88. Strachan MW. Insulin and cognitive function. Lancet 2003; 362:1253.
89. Wada SI, Starr A. Generation of auditory brain stem responses (ABRs). III. Effects of lesions of the superior olive, lateral lemniscus and inferior colliculus on the ABR in guinea pig. Electroencephalogr Clin Neurophysiol 1983; 56:352–366.
90. Barth DS, Goldberg N, Brett B, Di S. The spatiotemporal organization of auditory, visual, and auditory-visual evoked potentials in rat cortex. Brain Res 1995; 678:177–190.

17

Pathobiology of Diabetic Encephalopathy in Animal Models

Anders A.F. Sima

CONTENTS

ABSTRACT

This review will compare longitudinally the cognitive deficits and associated metabolic and structural abnormalities in two models with spontaneous onset of type 1 and type 2 diabetes, respectively. From these studies it is becoming increasingly evident that the cerebral dysmetabolism differs in many respects as to underlying mechanisms leading up to progressive cognitive dysfunction, although mechanistic overlaps exist between the two models. In the type 1 model, insulin deficiency appears to play a prominent role in degenerative and apoptotic phenomena of neuronal populations and white matter constituents. In these processes, undoubtedly, hyperglycemia and its downstream metabolic aberrations are also active participants.

In the type 2 model, which reflects closely the situation in human type 2 diabetes, the underlying mechanisms appear more complex and are likely to include components of the metabolic syndrome such as hypercholesterolemia and hypertension. This model displays increased activity of the amyloidogenic processing of APP with subsequent accumulation of A(amyloid)β products. This together with central insulin resistance is likely to be responsible for increased presence of hyperphosphorylated tau. Hence, in this model similarities

From: *Contemporary Diabetes: Diabetes and the Brain*
Edited by: G. J. Biessels, J. A. Luchsinger (eds.), DOI 10.1007/978-1-60327-850-8_17
© Humana Press, a part of Springer Science+Business Media, LLC 2009

with factors responsible for the progressive degenerative changes characterizing Alzheimer's disease are obvious. Although information to date is rather limited in genetically unmanipulated models of diabetes, available information stresses differences in the pathogeneses responsible for diabetic encephalopathy in the two types of diabetes will be reviewed.

Key words: Diabetic encephalopathy; Type 1 diabetes; Type 2 diabetes; Morris water maze; Neuronal apoptosis; Amyloidogenesis; BB/Wor-rat; BBZDR/Wor-rat.

INTRODUCTION

Diabetic encephalopathy is now recognized as a complication of diabetes resulting in progressive cognitive deficits. It affects both type 1 and type 2 diabetes, although underlying mechanisms are likely to differ and the outcomes are different in the two types of diabetes. The term *primary diabetic encephalopathy* has been proposed to include encephalopathic abnormalities related to impaired insulin action and hyperglycemia, whereas *secondary diabetic encephalopathy* is the result of diabetic vascular disease (1). It is obvious that substantial overlaps may exist between this conceptual division.

Only during the last decade have various pathogenetic mechanisms started to be addressed experimentally (2–4). Like the peripheral neuropathic complications (5, 6) and the encephalopathic complications in humans (7–10), responsible mechanisms and resulting pathologies in diabetic encephalopathy differ in experimental models of type 1 and type 2 diabetes (11–14).

Type 1 diabetes is characterized by insulin and C-peptide deficiencies and hyperglycemia. Several recent studies of type 1 diabetic patients (15–17) and a meta-analysis of 33 studies (10) suggest that hyperglycemia is a major culprit underlying cognitive deficits. Age of onset of type 1 diabetes has been shown to have an impact on cognitive dysfunction, this being greater with onset at a younger age, potentially interfering with the metabolically demanding so-called brain growth spurts during development and compromising "cognitive reserve" (18–21).

Another potential mechanism not always considered is impaired insulin action (see Chapter 18). Apart from insulin's immediate glucose regulatory effects, it possesses a myriad of regulatory molecular effects. In and by itself insulin is a potent neurotrophic factor and has gene regulatory effects on other neurotrophic factors and their receptors (1, 22–26). Together with intrinsically synthesized insulin in the brain, it regulates neuronal glucose metabolism via insulin-dependent GLUTs and has direct regulatory effects on neurotransmitter synthesis. It also shows, as does insulinomimetic C-peptide, strong anti-apoptotic effects *(13, 26–29)*.

Differences in the profiles of cognitive dysfunction developing in type 2 diabetes, as compared to those of type 1 diabetes, suggest that different and/or additional pathogenetic components are involved. Type 2 diabetes is characterized by insulin resistance with ensuing impairment of insulin signaling, hyperinsulinemia, and hyperglycemia. Additional contributing factors commonly accompanying type 2 diabetes are hypercholesterolemia, hyperlipidemia, and hypertension, which together constitute the metabolic syndrome. To this, age alone may be contributing to cognitive impairment in type 2 diabetes.

In type 1 diabetes, perturbed cognitive function involves intelligence, attention, processing speed, spatial learning, and long-term memory, whereas learning abilities per se appear to be spared (see Chapter 11) *(10, 30, 31)*. On the other hand, neuropsychological deficits in type 2 diabetes tend to involve verbal and recent memory and information processing *(2, 32)* and are hence different from those in type 1 diabetes (see Chapter 12). What accounts for these differences is not known. It is probably not incorrect to suggest that the pathogenetic factors underlying cognitive dysfunction in type 2 diabetes are more complex and varied and it cannot be accounted for by hyperglycemia and insulin resistance alone. The exploration of additional pathogenetic factors is just starting to evolve. It is even possible that other components of the metabolic syndrome such as elevated cholesterol levels and hypertension with ensuing vascular defects may be major contributing components. Several studies have recently demonstrated evidence supporting a linkage between type 2 diabetes and Alzheimer's disease and vascular dementia (see Chapter 13) *(7, 8, 33–35)*

As mentioned above, the cognitive deficits accompanying human type 1 and type 2 diabetes are different, and this appears to be true also for experimental models of type 1 and type 2 diabetes. Following is a review of the relatively sparse information on possible mechanisms underlying the progressive development of cognitive dysfunction in non-genetically manipulated models of the two types of diabetes.

TYPE 1 DIABETES

The two rodent models most commonly used for this kind of study include streptozotocin-induced diabetes in rodents and the spontaneously diabetic BB/Wor-rat. The first model develops incomplete insulin deficiency and severe hyperglycemia and is sustained without insulin supplementation. The second model develops acutely an immune-mediated β-cell destruction with complete insulin (and C-peptide) deficiency and requires daily insulin supplementation for its survival (see Chapter 16) *(36)*. Hence, the overriding metabolic abnormalities in these type 1 diabetic models are hyperglycemia and insulin deficiency.

Cerebral-Evoked Potentials

Electrophysiological changes arising from various brain regions, reflected by somatosensory-, visual- and auditory-evoked potentials occur in spontaneously diabetic BB/Wor-rats and the streptozotocin (STZ)-induced diabetic rats *(3, 37)*. Like peripheral neuropathies occurring in these models, they are followed by progressive axonal degenerative changes and eventually axonal loss in the spinal cord dorsal columns and in the optic nerve *(38, 39)*. Interestingly, such changes can be modified by insulin treatment and by aldose reductase inhibition *(3, 40)*, paralleling the effects on peripheral neuropathy.

Cognitive Deficits

Several studies examining behavioral learning have shown progressive deficits in diabetic rodents, whereas simple avoidance tasks are preserved. Impaired spatial learning and memory as assessed by the Morris water maze paradigm occur progressively in both the spontaneously diabetic BB/Wor-rat and STZ-induced diabetic rodents *(1, 11, 12, 22, 41, 42)*. The cognitive components reflected by impaired Morris water maze performances involve problem-solving, enhanced attention and storage, and retrieval of information *(43)*. In the BB/Wor-rat significant deficits in latencies start to evolve after 4 months diabetes duration and progress to significant deficits in 8-month diabetic rats (Fig. 1) *(1, 3, 12, 13)*.

Assessments using the radial-arm maze paradigm have shown that the cognitive sphere affected early, already at 3 months of diabetes in the BB/Wor-rat, involves memory retention *(44)*. Insulin treatment of STZ-rats demonstrates significant prevention of Morris water maze deficits and intervention with insulin prevents further progression of cognitive function *(11)*. These beneficial effects are in part likely to be due to replacement of insulin

Fig. 1. Latencies in seconds to reach the submersed platform from the four quadrants of the Morris water maze *(13)* in control and type 1 diabetic BB/Wor-rats, after 2, 4, 6, and 8 months (**A–D**) of diabetes. The animals were placed in a circular pool of water with a constant temperature of 28°C. A platform was submerged 3 cm below the water 10 cm from the edge of the pool. The pool was divided into four quadrants and the time to reach the platform (latencies from each quadrant) was measured. Animals were trained

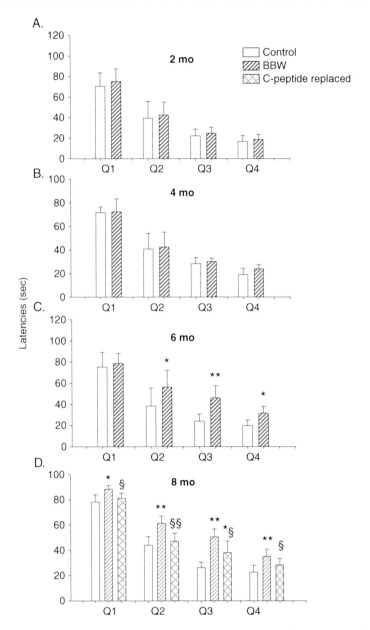

Fig. 1. (continued) to reach the platform from the four quadrants for 2 consecutive days each week for 2 weeks prior to testing. They were then given three acquisition trials per day. Note: significant delays in latencies are noticed only after 6 months of diabetes (**C**). In (**D**) control and diabetes latencies are compared with those of diabetic (hyperglycemic) C-peptide replaced rats, showing complete prevention of cognitive deficits as assessed by the Morris water maze paradigm. $^*p < 0.01$; $^{**}P < 0.001$ vs. control rats; $^§p < 0.05$; $^{§§}p < 0.01$ vs. untreated BB/Wor-rats.

itself rather than due to its glucose regulatory effects. This reasoning is based on data following C-peptide replacement in the BB/Wor-rat. C-peptide does not effect hyperglycemia *(13, 45)*. Replacement of insulinomimetic C-peptide from onset of diabetes prevents the cognitive decline noticed after 8 months of diabetes (see Fig. 1). These effects are most likely due to the dehexamerization effect of C-peptide on insulin resulting in monomeric insulin, thereby enhancing and prolonging its availability for non-glycemia-mediated regulatory functions *(11, 45–47)* *(see below)*.

Changes in synaptic strength and plasticity are believed to underlie information storage and retrieval *(41, 48)*. Several studies of synaptic plasticity have demonstrated progressive deficits in *N*-methyl-D-aspartate (NMDA)-dependent long-term potentiation in hippocampal CA_1 followed by impairment of NMDA-independent long-term potentiation in hippocampal CA_3 *(49)*. A recent study reported beneficial effects of an NMDA receptor agonist on learning and memory in STZ-diabetic rats *(50)*. These progressive deficits are believed to be postsynaptic in nature, possibly involving postsynaptic membrane excitability or cellular signaling mechanisms *(49, 51)*. As potential mechanisms, modulations of GABA-mediated inhibition or changes in adenosine sensitivity have been suggested *(49–52)*. However, the underlying molecular abnormalities in these dynamic and progressive processes have not been fully elucidated and are likely to be multifactorial involving Ca^{2+}-dependent processes, modulation of α-amino-3-hydroxy-5-methyl-4-isoxazole propionic acid (AMPA), and glutamate receptor subunits *(51, 53, 54)* [see *(41)* for review].

Pathogenetic Mechanisms in Type 1 Diabetic Encephalopathy

The pathobiological mechanisms underlying peripheral neuropathic changes in type 1 diabetes, such as hyperglycemia and insulin deficiency, are likely to be operable also in the development of type 1 diabetic encephalopathy *(1, 22, 24, 55)*.

Hyperglycemia

In recent positron emission tomography (PET) and autoradiography studies using the 2 deoxy-2[*(18)*-F]-fluoro-d-glucose (18F-FDG) tracer, we have demonstrated more than a doubling in glucose uptake in both hippocampus and frontal cortex of diabetic rats despite a decreased uptake rate constant (Sima et al., unpublished data), thereby overriding the regulatory effects by endothelial glucose transporters (GLUTs) *(56)*. These initial studies therefore indicate excess glucose exposure to the brain under diabetic condition in the BB/Wor-rat. Excess glucose is converted through the polyol pathway to sorbitol and fructose *(57)* with consequently increased production of

Type 1 Diabetes

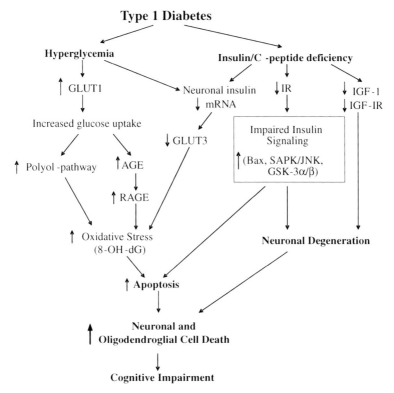

Fig. 2. Suggested pathogenetic mechanisms underlying diabetic encephalopathy in type 1 diabetes. Hyperglycemia leads to dysregulation of endothelial GLUTs with increased glucose uptake into the brain. This in turn results in activation of the polyol pathway and increased production of AGE and increased expression of RAGE, resulting in oxidative stress and contributing to neuronal and oligodendroglial apoptosis (see text). Impaired availability of insulin and insulinomimetic C-peptide results in impaired expression of neuronal insulin and suppression of the insulin and IGF-1 receptors. Resulting decreases in their signaling activities generate proapoptotic factors (see Fig. 4) with ultimate upregulation of caspase 3 and apoptotic neuronal and oligodendroglial cell death. These combined influences in type 1 diabetes result in cortical and white matter degenerative changes and progressive cognitive decline.

advanced glycation end products (AGEs) *(58)*, upregulation of the multi-ligand receptor RAGE *(59)*, oxidative and nitrosative stresses *(60, 61)*, and apoptosis (Fig. 2) *(12, 14, 24)*. However, it should be kept in mind that some of these components are also influenced by impaired insulin and insulin-like growth factor-1 (IGF-I) signaling (see below and Fig. 2).

Like other microvascular beds in neural tissues, the cerebral microvasculature is responsible for the integrity of the blood–brain barrier (BBB) and undergoes changes in streptozotocin-induced diabetes *(62, 63)*. With duration of diabetes its permeability increases even to small molecules like sucrose *(64)*. This has been associated with decreased expression of cell adhesive molecules such as occludin, which constitutes a component of tight junctions *(63, 65)*. Interestingly, insulin treatment attenuates the BBB disruption *(64)*, which appears to be analogous to the protective effects of insulinomimetic C-peptide on peripheral nerve barriers *(11)*. In addition to these changes affecting the cerebral microvasculature, impaired cerebral blood flow occurs in STZ-diabetic rats *(67–69)*.

The expression of the multiligand RAGE is upregulated in brains from the BB/Wor-rat. Like in humans, it is localized to capillary endothelial cells, astrocytes, and neurons *(69–72)*. Besides hyperglycemia, the upregulation of RAGE is likely to be initiated by hyperketonemia and resulting oxidative stress, as well as stress kinases from impaired insulin signaling *(71, 73)*. In agreement with a contributory component through impaired insulin signaling is the finding that insulinomimetic C-peptide prevents upregulation of RAGE in the white matter of the BB/Wor-rat *(44)*. Further factors likely to be involved in stimulation of RAGE include 3-deoxyglucosone (3-DG) methylglyoxal resulting from degradation of glycated proteins, tumor necrosis factor (TNF)-α, and C-reactive protein *(12, 13, 74–76)*. The increased expression of RAGE in astrocytes may impact on glutamate-mediated modulation of synaptic activity in hippocampal neurons*(77)* and result in amplification and sustenance of a perpetuating loop for oxidative stress *(78)* and initiation of apoptosis *(79)*. Oxidative stress is a central component in the genesis of diabetic complications, diabetic encephalopathy being no exception. Oxidative stress is generated by hyperglycemia and activation of the polyol pathway, by impaired insulin signaling and via upregulation of RAGE. Various modes of antioxidant treatments have demonstrated beneficial effects on RAGE *(59)*, hippocampal glial fibrillary acid protein *(80)*, and hippocampal synaptic plasticity *(81)*. It is therefore obvious that hyperglycemia and its metabolic consequences play important roles in a number of metabolic abnormalities underlying cognitive dysfunction.

Impaired Insulin Action

In previous studies, we *(45, 66, 82–85)* and others *(86)* have shown that impaired insulin action contributes significantly to diabetic neuropathies. Apart from the immediate glucose regulatory effects, insulin possesses a myriad of regulatory effects. Insulin is in and by itself a potent neurotrophic factor and has gene regulatory effects on other tyrosine kinase-mediated neurotrophic factors and their receptors such as IGFs, nerve growth factor (NGF), and neurotrophin-3 (NT-3) *(23, 55, 86, 87)*. Together with intrinsically synthesized insulin in the CNS, it regulates functions of neuronal glucose metabolism via insulin-dependent GLUTs (see Fig. 2), it has regulatory effects on neurotransmitter synthesis such as acetylcholine *(28)* and provides anti-apoptotic functions *(23, 55, 88)*. To maintain the non-glucose lowering effects of insulin over time, proinsulin C-peptide has been shown to enhance insulin signaling in a sustainable fashion without effecting hyperglycemia *(46, 55, 89)*. The sustained insulin effects necessary for gene and molecular regulatory functions are related to C-peptide's longer half-life compared to insulin *(84, 87)* and are mediated by its dehexamerization effects on insulin providing monomeric insulin, hence resulting in amplification of sustained insulin action *(47, 55)*.

Recent voxel-based morphometric studies in type 1 diabetic subjects have shown modest volume reduction of cortical gray matter *(90)* and ventricular dilation suggesting white matter atrophy *(9)*. Studies in the STZ-rat over 20 years ago reported loss of neocortical neurons *(91, 92)*. Neuronal pathology has been studied longitudinally in the type 1 diabetic BB/Wor-rat. Both Northern and Western blots have demonstrated significant decreases in the expression of insulin-receptor, IGF-I and IGF-II receptors in hippocampus after 2 months diabetes duration, a time point at which no cognitive deficits or neuronal loss is obtainable *(12)*. These changes are followed by upregulation of proapoptotic Bax, increased expression of caspase 3 activity, TUNEL-positive neurons, as well as increased nucleosomal DNA fragmentation in hippocampus and frontal cortex of 8-month diabetic rats *(13)*, in association with prolonged latencies in the Morris water maze and significant neuronal loss in hippocampal CA_1 and CA_2 (Figs. 3 and 4) *(12, 13)*. These data suggest increasing apoptotic activity and neuronal death with duration of diabetes. This is further substantiated by increased expression of caspase 12, the FAS/TNF receptor family, and NGFRp75 *(13)*, suggesting that both oxidative stress and endoplasmic reticulum dysfunction are involved in apoptotic neuronal death. Substitution with C-peptide from onset of diabetes has profound preventive effects on cognitive dysfunction, apoptosis-related molecular changes as well as neuronal loss (see Figs. 1, 3, and 4) *(13)*. These findings are consistent with the anti-apoptotic effects of insulin and C-peptide, being mediated via PI-3 kinase stimulation and a series of intermediate metabolites such as p38 activation as well as disinhibition of IκB and translocation of NF-κ(kappa)B, upregulation of Bax, and inhibition of jun NH_2-terminal kinase (JNK) phosphorylation *(12, 23)*. It is therefore obvious that insulin deficiency and the downstream consequences on its signaling pathway contribute significantly to apoptotic stresses and eventually to apoptotic neuronal cell death of vulnerable populations.

As mentioned earlier, white matter changes occur in type 1 diabetic encephalopathy in humans. Recent studies in the BB/Wor-rat demonstrate apoptotic stresses of white matter oligodendroglia with loss of myelinating

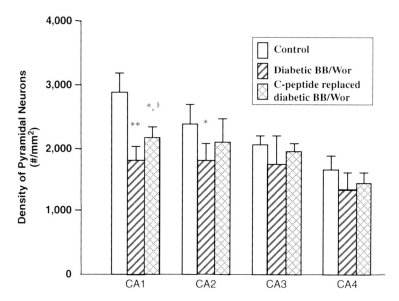

Fig. 3. Densities of pyramidal cell neurons in hippocampal CA_1–CA_4 in 8 months type 1 diabetic BB/Wor-rats. The data are compared to those of age-matched non-diabetic control rats and diabetic rats receiving complete replacement of insulinomimetic C-peptide from onset of diabetes. Note significant losses of CA_1 and CA_2 neurons in non-treated diabetic animals, which were significantly ($p<0.05$) prevented by C-peptide replacement. (From Sima and Li *(13)*. Copyright © 2005 American Diabetes Association. From *Diabetes*®, Vol. 54, 2005, 1497–1505 *(13)*. Reproduced with permission from the American Diabetes Association.) ${}^{**}p<0.001$; ${}^{*}P < 0.01$ vs. controls; ${}^{§}p < 0.05$ vs. BB/Wor-rats.

glia and profound white matter astrogliosis. Interestingly, these changes seem to precede those affecting neuronal populations as indicated by significant oligodendroglial cell loss at 3 months of diabetes that then progresses with duration of diabetes in the BB/Wor-rat *(44)*.

Hypothalamic–Pituitary–Adrenal Axis

Recent studies in diabetic rodents have demonstrated hyperactivity of the hypothalamic–pituitary axis with increased secretion of corticosterone and activation of cerebral corticorticoid and glucocorticoid receptors *(93, 94)* with potentially adverse effects on hippocampal activity *(95)*. It has been demonstrated that hypothalamic neuropeptide upregulation is associated with impaired hippocampal neurogenesis *(96, 97)*, plasticity, and learning and that such changes are reversible following normalization of corticosterone levels *(97)*.

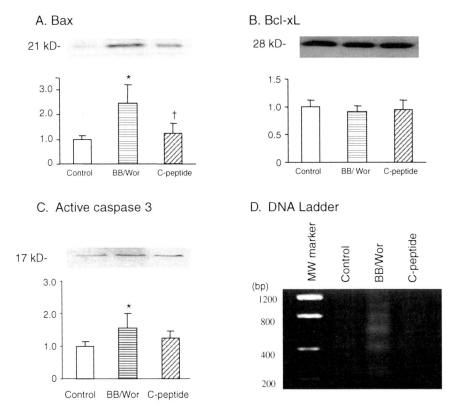

Fig. 4. Protein expression of Bax (**A**) and Bcl-xL (**B**) in hippocampi of type 1 diabetic BB/Wor-rats, age-matched non-diabetic control rats, and rats replenished with C-peptide. At 8 months there was significant upregulation of Bax in untreated diabetic rats. C-peptide replacement resulted in a significant prevention of Bax upregulation. Diabetes or C-peptide replacement showed no effects on Bcl-xL. Upregulation of Bax was associated with significant upregulation of active caspase 3 (**C**) and DNA laddering (**D**) in hippocampi of diabetic BB/Wor-rats, both of which were prevented by C-peptide substitution from onset of diabetes. Adapted from Sima and Li *(13)*. Copyright © 2005 American Diabetes Association. From *Diabetes*®, Vol. 54, 2005, 1497–1505 *(13)*. Reproduced with permission from the American Diabetes Association. *$p < 0.01$ vs. controls; †$p < 0.05$ vs. BB/Wor-rats.

TYPE 2 DIABETES

There is a growing wealth of data indicating that brain insulin deficiency and brain insulin resistance are related to sporadic late-onset Alzheimer's disease (see Chapter 18) *(98–100)*. Neuronal glucose metabolism is regulated by neuronal insulin and the neuron-specific GLUT-3 (see Fig. 2) *(101, 102)*. Impaired insulin signaling will result in perturbations of protein kinase B (PKB) (Akt) and glycogen synthase kinase-3

(GSK-3α/β) with potential consequences for the regulation of A(amyloid)β peptides *(103)* and tau phosphorylation *(14, 104, 105)*. Apart from brain insulin resistance, additional metabolic changes may contribute to the increased incidence of Alzheimer's disease in type 2 diabetes and metabolic syndrome. Elevated cholesterol levels are associated with the formation of caveolae, invaginations of cellular membranes enriched in cholesterol and sphingolipids *(106)*. The associated upregulation of caveolin-1 signaling has been postulated to influence the activity of several growth factor receptors localized to caveolae, like those of insulin and IGF-I *(107, 108)*. Increased expression of caveolin-1 signaling is linked to upregulation of APP and β-secretase *(109, 110)*. On the other hand, α-secretase responsible for the non-amyloidogenic soluble amyloid precursor protein (sAPPα) is located outside the caveolae (Fig. 5).

Several experimental models of Alzheimer's disease are available, but none exists that is truly mimicking the occurrence of Alzheimer's disease in type 2 diabetes, unrelated to genetic manipulations. However, rats treated with intracerebroventricular STZ injections have been proposed as a model *(99, 111)*. Although this model results in decreased brain glucose utilization and increased lactate release and cognitive deficits, it does not reflect the whole spectrum of the metabolic perturbations in the brain associated with type 2 diabetes.

Amyloidogenesis in Type 2 BBZDR/Wor-Rat

To examine underlying linkages between long-standing type 2 diabetes and Alzheimer's disease under experimental conditions, we have examined the spontaneously type 2 diabetic BBZDR/Wor-rat. It spontaneously develops type 2 diabetes around the age of 75 days, which is preceded by obesity and maintains hyperglycemic levels (20–25 mmol/l), without diabetogenic agents or high-caloric feeding. It is the product of inbreeding of the Zucker-derived *fa/fa* allele on the BB background *(112)*. It develops peripheral and central insulin resistance, hyperinsulinemia, hypercholesterolemia, and late in the course of diabetes hypertension *(14, 112, 113)*. It has been used extensively to delineate differences in the pathogeneses and expressions of peripheral neuropathies as compared to those occurring in type 1 BB/Wor-rat [reviews see *(6)* and *(114)*].

At 8 months of untreated diabetes, BBZDR/Wor-rats show a 24% increase in body weight, an almost fourfold increase in glyHb, 25% increase in plasma insulin, 2.3-fold increase in plasma cholesterol levels but a 25% decrease in plasma IGF-I levels *(14)*. Examination of the frontal cortex shows a significant neuronal loss, being most pronounced in the layers II–IV (Fig. 6), which is associated with a significant loss in synaptic densities and

Type 2 diabetes and AD

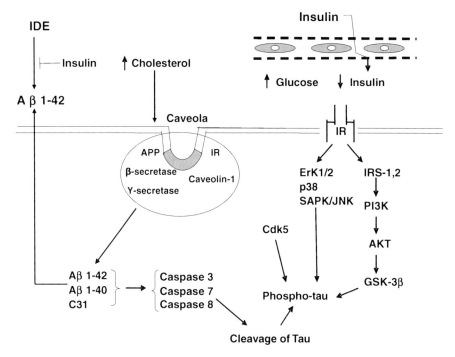

Fig. 5. Suggested mechanisms by which insulin resistant type 2 diabetes induces mechanisms resulting in increased amyloidogenic processing of APP and increased phospho-tau. Under hyperinsulinemic conditions CNS levels of insulin are decreased (see text). As demonstrated in the BBZDR/Wor-rats, there is in addition resistance of insulin signaling *(14)*. These perturbations in insulin signaling activity results in activation of several stress kinases such as GSK-3β, cdk5, MAP kinases, and SAPK/JNK. These proline-directed serine/threonine kinases phosphorylate tau at pathologically relevant sites (see text). Hypercholesterolemia and endogenously increased cholesterol synthesis result in upregulation of not only APP but also the enzymes β-secretase and γ-secretase responsible for the cleavage of APP into A(amyloid)β fragments. The production of A(amyloid)β_{1-42}, A(amyloid)β_{1-40}, and CTF A(amyloid)β fragments induces several apoptotic pathways which through their proteolytic effects cleave tau making it susceptible to phosphorylation and polymerization. Another mechanism that may be responsible for extracellular A(amyloid)β deposition is the competition between insulin and A(amyloid)β for IDE (see text).

an eightfold increase in degenerating cortical neurites. These pathological changes are accompanied by significant upregulation of APP, β-secretase, A(amyloid)β, and A(amyloid)β COOH-terminal fragment (CTF) expressions (Fig. 7). Interestingly the non-amyloidogenic sAPPα is also significantly increased *(14)*. Immunocytochemically, A(amyloid)β is confined to

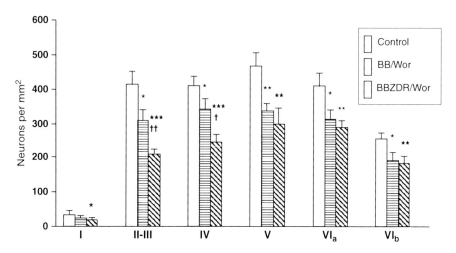

Fig. 6. Neuronal densities in frontal cortex of 8 months type 2 BBZDR/Wor-rats and type 1 BB/Wor-rats compared to age-matched control rats. Note significant neuronal loss in all layers of frontal cortex in type 2 rats, being most pronounced in layers II–IV. The neuronal loss in hyperglycemia and duration-matched type 1 rats was significantly milder. (Copyright © 2007 American Diabetes Association. From *Diabetes*®, Vol. 56, 2007, 1817–1824 *(14)*. Reproduced with permission from the American Diabetes Association.) *$p < 0.05$; **$p < 0.01$; ***$p < 0.001$ vs. control rats; †$p < 0.01$; ††$p < 0.005$ vs. BB/Wor-rats.

neuronal cell bodies and does not appear to accumulate in the neuropil. Amyloidogenic APP handling in this type 2 model is significantly more expressed than in the type 1 counterpart. Although not examined in this setting, one may speculate that hyperinsulinemia in the type 2 model may compete for insulin-degrading enzyme (IDE), resulting in decreased degradation of A(amyloid)β *(115)*. Furthermore, increased circulating insulin levels will saturate endothelial transfer, potentially resulting in decreased insulin exposure to cell constituent behind the BBB. Decreased insulin signaling activity and associated activation of stress kinases such as p38 and JNK promote abnormal processing of APP *(116, 117)*. Impaired insulin action activates the FAS/TNF (CD95) receptor family as well as NGFRp75. FAS activation leads via FADD to activation of caspase 8 or caspase-independent apoptosis. Caspase 8 has been implied in the C-terminal splicing of APP to CTF and further processing of intracellular APP to soluble A(amyloid)β_{1-42} *(118, 119)* by increased activity of β-secretase *(120)*.

Tau Expression in Type 2 BBZDR/Wor-Rats

In the type 2 diabetic BBZDR/Wor-rats, the expression of frontal cortex insulin receptor is unaltered compared to non-diabetic age-matched

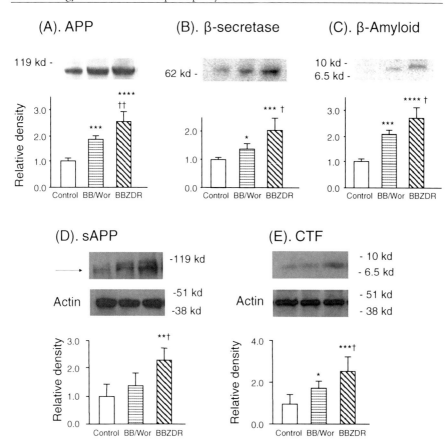

Fig. 7. APP amyloidogenic metabolism in type 1 BB/Wor-rats and type 2 BBZDR/Wor-rats. In the type 2 model there is a significantly higher upregulation of APP in frontal cortex, followed by significantly greater expression of β-secretase, β-amyloid, and A(amyloid)β C-terminal fragments (CTS). Interestingly, the amyloidogenic processing of APP is not normal in the type 1 model. This may be related to the compromised insulin signaling activity occurring in type 1 diabetes but for different reasons (see text). The non-amyloidogenic extracaveolar processing of APP to sAPPα was increased in type 2 but not in type 1 diabetic rats. (Copyright © 2007 American Diabetes Association. From *Diabetes*®, Vol. 56, 2007, 1817–1824 *(14)*. Reproduced with permission from the American Diabetes Association.) *$p<0.05$; **$p<0.01$; ***$p<0.005$; ****$p<0.001$ vs. control rats; †$p<0.05$; ††$p<0.01$ vs. BB/Wor-rats.

rats whereas the IGF-I receptor is significantly downregulated *(14)*. These changes may reflect associated caveolin signaling in caveolae, which enhances the expression of the insulin receptor, whereas it suppresses other growth factor receptors including that of IGF-1 *(121, 122)*. However, impaired insulin signaling in the presence of normally expressed insulin receptor is reflected in significantly decreased phosphokinase B (PKB)

(Akt) and glycogen synthase kinase (GSK)-3α/β *(14)*. This impairment of insulin signaling and activation of so-called tau kinases in particular GSK-3α/β, but also cyclin-dependent kinase (cdk)5, extracellular signal regulated kinase/mitogen-activated protein kinases(ERK/MAPKs) cascade and p38, is associated with increased expression and immunostaining of phospho-tau *(14)*. The significant decrease seen in synaptic density mentioned above is in keeping with the toxic effects of the increased A(amyloid)β load and increased phospho-tau.

Compared to duration- and hyperglycemia-matched type 1 diabetic BB/Wor-rats, the latter shows milder but still increased expression of amyloidogenic APP, β-secretase, and A(amyloid)β, but no significant increase in phospho-tau *(14)*.

Recent in vitro studies in SH-SY5Y cells examining the effects of high glucose (30 mM) and high cholesterol (7 μ(mu)g/ml) demonstrate increased expression of APP and increased amyloidogenesis in both situations, although no synergistic or additive effects on β-amyloid expression was obtained under the combined conditions *(107)*.

A(amyloid)$β_{1-42}$ induces several apoptotic pathways. Particularly caspases 3, 7, and 8 have been invoked in the proteolytic cleavage of the tau protein *(123)*. The apoptotic stressors exert these functions before the cell undergoes apoptotic cell death, a phenomenon that appears to be regulated by upregulation of contraregulatory proteins, such as heat shock proteins 27 and 70, which have recently been demonstrated in diabetic peripheral nerve *(124, 125)*. So for instance, caspase 3 cleaves tau at Asp 421 *(126)*. It has been suggested that phosphorylation of tau at Ser 422 by SAPK/JNK or ERK regulates the cleavage at Asp 421 by caspase 3. Once cleaved, the inhibitory domain of the tau C-terminal is lost, allowing the N-terminal fragment to phosphorylate and polymerize more rapidly *(127, 128)*. The accumulation of both soluble A(amyloid)$β_{1-42}$ and hyperphosphorylated tau leads to neurite and neuronal degeneration as demonstrated in the BBZDR/Wor-rat *(14, 129–131)*. The apoptogenicity of the pathologic metabolites of abnormal APP processing will eventually lead to programmed cell death *(14, 132–134)*.

It therefore appears that this animal model which closely replicates human type 2 diabetes develops the characteristic Alzheimer changes such as increased A(amyloid)β products, like A(amyloid)$β_{1-42}$ and CTF, and phospho-tau associated with substantial neurite degeneration and cortical neuronal loss, which have not been previously reported in spontaneously type 2 diabetic rodents. This model may therefore serve as an eloquent model for further study of the relationships between type 2 diabetes and Alzheimer's disease.

CONCLUSIONS

The research into the associations between diabetes, cognitive dysfunction, and Alzheimer's disease is rapidly evolving and exciting areas of biomedical research with tremendous implication as to how we will be able to treat and prevent these common disorders. This short review mainly focused on two models of spontaneous diabetes, which closely mimic the underlying pathophysiological mechanisms characterizing two main diabetic disorders in humans.

It is clear that although overlaps exist between the diabetic encephalopathies developing in type 1 and type 2 diabetes, there are also distinct differences. In type 1 diabetes, glycotoxicity and impaired insulin action appear to be the main players resulting in oxidative stress, abnormal blood flow, accumulation of RAGE and impaired trophic support with combined effects on apoptotic stressors, and consequent neuronal and white matter loss. Of potential significant value is that at least under experimental conditions, the supplementation of insulinomimetic C-peptide prevents the components that can be ascribed to insulin deficiencies. These findings may be analogous to the significant interventional effects of C-peptide replacement in patients with type 1 diabetic neuropathy *(135, 136)*.

The situation in type 2 diabetic encephalopathy appears to be more complex, since several factors may be involved such as hyperinsulinemia, hyperglycemia, and most likely also hypercholesterolemia, which in concert appear to affect APP metabolism in favor of amyloidogenesis. Oxidative stresses, RAGE formation, and phospho-tau expression result in part from cerebral insulin resistance. To this, other factors such as age alone, hypertension, and genetic factors are likely to add to the susceptibility for the development of Alzheimer's disease in diabetic humans.

REFERENCES

1. Sima AAF, Kamiya H, Li ZG. Insulin, C-peptide hyperglycemia and central nervous system complications in diabetes. Europ J Pharmacol 2004; 490:187–197.
2. Biessels GJ. Diabetic encephalopathy. In: Veves A, Malik RA eds. Diabetic Neuropathy, Clinical Management. Totowa, NJ: Humana Press; 2007:187–205.
3. Biessels GJ, Cristino NA, Rutten G, Hamers FPT, Erkelens DW, Gispen WH. Neurophysiological changes in the central and peripheral nervous system of streptozotocin-diabetic rats: course of development and effect of insulin treatment. Brain 1999; 122:757–768.
4. Sima AAF, Zhang W, Li ZG, Kamiya H. The effects of C-peptide on type 1 diabetic polyneuropathies and encephalopathy in the BB/Wor-rat. Exp Diab Res 2008:ID 230458, 13pp. (online publ.).
5. Sima AAF, Zhang W, Kamiya H. Metabolic-functional-structural correlations in somatic neuropathies in the spontaneously type 1 and type 2 diabetic BB-rats. In: Veves A, Malik RA, eds. Diabetic Neuropathy, Clinical Management. Totowa, NJ: Humana Press; 2007:133–152.

6. Sima AAF. Heterogeneity of diabetic neuropathy. Frontiers of Bioscience 2008; 13: 4809–4816.
7. Ott A, Stolk RP, van Harskamp F, Pols HA, Hofman A, Breteler MM. Diabetes mellitus and risk of dementia: the Rotterdam study. Neurology 1999; 58:1937–1941.
8. Arvanitakis Z, Wilson RS, Bievias JL, Evans DA, Bennett DA. Alzheimer's disease and decline in cognitive function. Arch Neurol 2004; 61:661–666.
9. Ryan CM. Why is cognitive dysfunction associated with the development of diabetes early in life? The diathesis hypothesis. Pediatr Diab 2006; 7:289–297.
10. Brands AMA, Biessels GJ, de Haan EHF, Kappelle LJ, Kessels RPC. The effects of type 1 diabetes on cognitive performance. A meta-analysis. Diabetes Care 2005; 28:726–735.
11. Biessels GJ, Kamal A, Urban IJ, Spruijt BM, Erkelens DW, Gispen WH. Water maze learning and hippocampal synaptic plasticity in streptozotocin-diabetic rats: effects of insulin treatment. Brain Res 1998; 800:125–135.
12. Li Z, Zhang W, Grunberger G, Sima AAF. Hippocampal neuronal apoptosis in type 1 diabetes. Brain Res 2002; 946:212–231.
13. Sima AAF, Li ZG. The effect of C-peptide on cognitive dysfunction and hippocampal apoptosis in type 1 diabetes. Diabetes 2005; 54:1497–1505.
14. Li ZG, Zhang W, Sima AAF. Alzheimer-like changes in rat models of spontaneous diabetes. Diabetes 2007; 56:1817–1824.
15. Kramer L, Fasching P, Madl C, et al. Previous episodes of hypoglycemic coma are not associated with permanent cognitive brain dysfunction in IDDM patients on intensive insulin treatment. Diabetes 1998; 47:1909–1914.
16. Diabetes Control and Complications Trial Research Group. Effects of intensive diabetes therapy on neuropsychological function in adults in the Diabetes Control and Complications Trial. Ann Intern Med 1996; 124:379–388.
17. Reichard P, Pihl M. Mortality and treatment side-effects during long-term intensified conventional insulin treatment in the Stockholm Diabetes Intervention Study. Diabetes 1994; 43:313–317.
18. Rovet JF, Ehrlich RM, Hoppe MG. Intellectual deficits associated with the early onset of insulin-dependent diabetes mellitus in children. Diabetes Care 1987; 10:510–515.
19. Dobbing J, Sands J. Vulnerability of developing brain. IX. The effect of nutritional growth retardation on the timing of brain growth spurt. Biol Neonate 1971; 19:363–378.
20. Schoenle EJ, Schoenle D, Molinari L, Largo RH. Impaired intellectual development in children with type 1 diabetes: association with HbA1c, age at diagnosis and sex. Diabetologia 2002; 45:108–114.
21. Ryan CM, Geckle MO, Orchard TJ. Cognitive efficiency declines over time in adults with type 1 diabetes: effects of micro- and macrovascular complications. Diabetologia 2003; 46:940–948.
22. Li ZG, Zhang W, Sima AAF. The role of impaired insulin/IGF action in primary diabetic encephalopathy. Brain Res 2005; 1037:12–24.
23. Li ZG, Zhang W, Sima AAF. C-peptide enhances insulin-mediated cell growth and protection against high glucose induced apoptosis in SH-SY5Y cells. Diab Metab Res Rev 2003; 19:375–385.
24. Li ZG, Sima AAF. C-peptide and CNS complications in diabetes. Exp Diab Res 2004; 5: 79–90.
25. Brands AMA, Kessels RPC, de Haan EHF, Kappelle LJ, Biessels GJ. Cerebral dysfunction in type 1 diabetes: effects of insulin, vascular risk factors and blood glucose levels. Eur J Pharmacol 2004; 490:159–168.
26. Zhao WQ, Chen H, Quon MJ, Alkou DL. Insulin and the insulin receptor in experimental models of learning and memory. Eur J Pharmacol 2004; 490:71–81.
27. Wozniak M, Rydzewski B, Baker SP, Raijada MK. The cellular and physiological action of insulin in the central nervous system. Neurochem Int 1993; 22:1–10.
28. Park CR. Cognitive effects of insulin in the central nervous system. Neurosci Biobehav Rev 2001; 25:311–323.

29. Kern W, Peters A, Fruehwald-Schultes B, Deininger E, Born J, Fehm HL. Improving influence of insulin on cognitive functions in humans. Neuroendocrinology 2001; 74: 270–280.

30. Northam EA, Anderson PJ, Jacobs R, Hughes M, Warne GL, Werther GA. Neuropsychological profiles of children with type 1 diabetes 6 years after disease onset. Diabetes Care 2001; 24:1541–1546.

31. Bjorgaas M, Gimse R, Vik T, Sand T. Cognitive function in type 1 diabetic children with and without episodes of severe hypoglycemia. Acta Paediatr 1997; 86:148–153.

32. Awad N, Gagnon M, Messier C. The relationship between impaired glucose tolerance, type 2 diabetes and cognitive function. J Clin Exp Neuropsychol 2004; 26:1044–1080.

33. Peila R, Rodriquez BL, Lanner LJ. Type 2 diabetes, APOE gene and risk for dementia and related pathologies: The Honolulu-Asia Aging Study. Diabetes 2002; 51:1256–1262.

34. Yoshitake T, Kiyohara Y, Kato I, et al. Incidence and risk factors of vascular dementia and Alzheimer's disease in a defined elderly Japanese population. The Hisayama Study. Neurology 1995; 445:1161–1168.

35. Leibson CL, Rocca WA, Hanson VA, Cha R, Kokmen E, O'Brien PC, Palumbo PJ. The risk of dementia among persons with diabetes mellitus: a population-based cohort study. Ann NY Acad Sci 1997; 26:422–427.

36. Mordes JP, Bortell R, Groen H, Guberski D, Rossini AA, Greiner DL. Autoimmune diabetes mellitus in the BB rat. In: Sima AAF, Shafrir E eds. Animal Models of Diabetes. A Primer. Amsterdam: Harwood Acad. Publ.; 2001:1–42.

37. Sima AAF, Zhang WX, Cherian PV, Chakrabarti S. Impaired visual evoked potentials and primary axonopathy of the optic nerve in the diabetic BB/W-rat. Diabetologia 1992; 35: 602–607.

38. Chakrabarti S, Zhang WX, Sima AAF. Optic neuropathy in the diabetic BB-rat. Nervous system and fuel hemostatis. Adv Exp Biol Med 1991; 291:257–264.

39. Sima AAF, Yagihashi S. Central-peripheral distal axonopathy in the spontaneously diabetic BB-rat: Ultrastructural and morphometric findings. Diab Res Clin Prac 1986; 1:289–298.

40. Kamijo M, Cherian PV, Sima AAF. The preventive effect of aldose reductase inhibition on diabetic optic neuropathy in the BB/W-rat. Diabetologia 1993; 36:893–898.

41. Gispen WH, Biessels GJ. Cognition and synaptic plasticity in diabetes. Trends Neurosci 2000; 23:542–549.

42. Flood JF, Mooriadian AD, Morley JE. Characteristics of learning and memory in streptozotocin-induced diabetic mice. Diabetes 1990; 39:1391–1398.

43. Bannerman DM, Good MA, Butcher SP, Ramsay M, Morris RG. Distinct components of spatial learning revealed by prior training and NMDA receptor blockade. Nature 1995; 378:182–186.

44. Sima AAF, Zhang W, Hoffman W. Apoptosis of oligodendroglia cells contribute to white matter changes in type 1 diabetic encephalopathy. Neurodiab Orvieto, Italy; 2008.

45. Sima AAF, Zhang WX, Sugimoto K, et al. C-peptide prevents and improves chronic type 1 diabetic neuropathy in the BB/Wor-rat. Diabetologia 2001; 44:889–897.

46. Grunberger G, Qiang X, Li ZG, et al. Molecular basis for the insulinomimetic effects of C-peptide. Diabetologia 2001; 44:1247–1257.

47. Shafqat J, Melles E, Sigmundsson K, et al. Proinsulin C-peptide elicits disaggregation of insulin resulting in enhanced physiological insulin effects. Cell Mol Life Sci 2006; 63: 1805–1811.

48. Bliss TV, Collingridge GL. A synaptic model of memory: long term potentiation in the hippocampus. Nature 1993; 361:31–39.

49. Kamal A, Biessels GJ, Urban IJ, Gispen WH. Hippocampal synaptic plasticity in streptozotocin-diabetic rats: impairment of long-term potentiation and facilitation of long-term depression. Neuroscience 1999; 90:737–745.

50. Grzeda E, Wiśniewska RJ, Wiśniewski K. Effect of an NMDA receptor agonist on T-maze and passive avoidance test in 12-week streptozotocin-induced diabetic rats. Pharmacol Rep 2007; 59(6):656–663.

51. Chabot C, Massicotte G, Milot M, Trudeau F, Gagné J. Impaired modulation of AMPA receptors by calcium-dependent processes in streptozotocin-induced diabetic rats. Brain Res 1997; 768:249–256.

52. de Mendonca A, Ribeiro JA. Endogenous adenosine modulates long-term potentiation in the hippocampus. Neuroscience 1994; 62:385–390.

53. Gagné J, Milot M, Gélinas S, et al. Binding properties of glutamate receptors in streptozotocin-induced diabetes in rats. Diabetes 1997; 46:841–846.

54. Biessels GJ, ter Laak MP, Kamal A, Gispen WH. Effects of the Ca(2+) antagonist nimodipine on functional deficits in the peripheral and central nervous system of streptozotocin-diabetic rats. Brain Res 2005; 1035 (1):86–93.

55. Sima AAF, Kamiya H. Is C-peptide replacement the missing link for successful treatment of neurological complications in type 1 diabetes? Current Drug Targets 2008; 49:37–46.

56. Choeiri C, Stoines W, Miki T, Seino S, Messier C. Glucose transporter plasticity during memory processing. Neuroscience 2005; 130:591–600.

57. Sredy J, Sawicki DR, Notvest RR. Polyol pathway activity in nervous tissues of diabetic and galactose-fed rats: effect of dietary galactose withdrawal or tolrestat intervention therapy. J Diab Comp 1991; 5:2–7.

58. Ryle C, Leow CK, Donaghy M. Non-enzymatic glycation of peripheral and central nervous system proteins in experimental diabetes mellitus. Muscle Nerve 1997; 20:577–584.

59. Aragano M, Mastrocola R, Medana C, et al. Upregulation of advanced glycated products receptor in the brain of diabetic rats is prevented by antioxidant treatment. Endocrinology 2005; 146:5561–5567.

60. Kumar JS, Menon VP. Effect of diabetes on levels of lipid peroxides and glycolipids in rat brain. Metabolism 1993; 42:1435–1439.

61. Pop-Busui R, Sima AAF, Stevens M. Oxidative stress and diabetic neuropathy. Diab Metab Res Rev 2006; 22:257–273.

62. Mooradian AD, Haas MJ, Batejko O, Hovsepyan M, Feman SS. Statins ameliorate endothelial barrier permeability changes in the cerebral tissue of streptozotocin-induced diabetic rats. Diabetes 2005; 54(10):2977–2982.

63. Hawkins BT, Lundeen TF, Norwood KM, Brooks HL, Egleton RD. Increased blood-brain barrier permeability and altered tight junctions in experimental diabetes in the rat: contribution of hyperglycaemia and matrix metalloproteinases. Diabetologia 2007; 45(1):202–211.

64. Huber JD, VanGilder RL, Houser KA. Streptozotocin-induced diabetes progressively increases blood-brain barrier permeability in specific brain regions in rats. Am J Physiol Heart Circ Physiol 2006; 291:H2660–H2668.

65. Chehade JM, Haas MJ, Mooradian AD. Diabetes-related changes in rat cerebral occludin and ZO-1 expression. Neurochem Res 2002; 27:249–252.

66. Sima AAF, Zhang W, Li ZG, Murakawa Y, Pierson CR. Molecular alterations underlie nodal and paranodal degeneration in type 1 diabetic neuropathy and are prevented by C-peptide. Diabetes 2004; 53:1556–1563.

67. Jakobsen J, Nedergaard M, Aarlew-Jensen M, Diemer NH. Regional brain glucose metabolism and blood flow in streptozotocin-induced diabetic rats. Diabetes 1990; 39:437–440.

68. Li ZG, Britton M, Sima AAF, Dunbar J. Diabetes enhances apoptosis induced by cerebral ischemia. Life Sci 2004; 76:249–262.

69. Manschot SM, Biessels GJ, Cameron NE, et al. Angiotensin converting enzyme inhibition partially prevents deficits in water maze performance, hippocampal synaptic plasticity and cerebral blood flow in streptozotocin-diabetic rats. Brain Res 2003; 966(2):274–282.

70. Hoffman WH, Casanova MF, Cudrici CD, et al. Neuroinflammatory response of the choroid plexus epithelium in fatal diabetic ketoacidosis. Exp Mol Pathol 2007; 83:65–72.

71. Hoffman WH, Artlett CM, Zhang W, et al.. Receptor for advanced glycation end products and neuronal deficit in the fatal brain edema of diabetic ketoacidosis. Brain Research 2008:E. Pub., Aug. 26.

72. Toth C, Martinez J, Zochodne DW. RAGE, diabetes, and the nervous system. Curr Mol Med 2007; 7(8):766–776.

73. Jani SK, McVie R, Bocchini Jr JA. Hyperketonemia (ketosis), oxidative stress and type 1 diabetes. Pathophysiology 2006; 13:163–170.

74. Baynes JW, Requena JR. Studies in animal models on the role of glycation and advanced glycation end-products (AGE's) in the pathogenesis of diabetic complications: pitfalls and limitations. In: Sima AAF ed. Chronic Complications in Diabetes. Amsterdam: Harwood Acad. Publ.; 2000:43–70.

75. Makherjee TK, Mukhopadhyay S, Hoidal JR. The role of reactive oxygen species in TNF α-dependent expression of the receptor for advanced glycation end products in human umbilical vein endothelial cells. Biochem Biophys Acta 2005; 1744:213–223.

76. Zhang Y, Li SH, Liu SM, et al. C-reactive protein upregulates receptor for advanced glycation end products expression in human endothelial cells. Hypertension 2006; 48:504–511.

77. Araque A, Parpura V, Sanzgiri RP, Haydon PG. Glutamate-dependent astrocyte modulation of synaptic transmission between cultured hippocampal neurons. Eur J Neurosci 1998; 10:2129–2142.

78. Yau SD, Schmidt AM, Anderson GM, et al. Enhanced cellular oxidant stress by the interaction of advanced glycation end products with their receptor/binding proteins. J Biol Chem 1994; 269:9889–9897.

79. Vance JE. Phosphatidylserine and phosphatidyl-ethanolamine in mammalian cells: two metabolically related aminophospholipids. J Lipid Res Jan. 19, 2008 [E pub].

80. Baydas G, Nedzvetskii VS, Tuzcu M, Yasar A, Kirichenko SV. Increase in glial fibrillary acidic protein and S-100B in hippocampus and cortex of diabetic rats: effects of vitamin E. Eur J Pharmacol 2003; 461:67–71.

81. Biessels GJ, Smale S, Duis SE, Kamal A, Gispen WH. The effect of gamma-linoleic acid-alpha-lipoic acid on functional deficits in the peripheral and central nervous systems of streptozotocin-diabetic rats. J Neurol Sci 2001; 182:99–106.

82. Stevens MJ, Zhang W, Li F, Sima AAF. C-peptide corrects endoneurial blood flow but not oxidative stress in type 1 BB/Wor-rats. Am J Physiol 2004; 287:E497–E505.

83. Kamiya H, Zhang W, Sima AAF. C-peptide prevents nociceptive sensory neuropathy in type 1 diabetes. Ann Neurol 2004; 56:827–835.

84. Zhang W, Kamiya H, Ekberg K, Wahren J, Sima AAF. C-peptide improves chronic diabetic neuropathy in type 1 diabetic BB-Wor-rats: the effects of varying dose regiments. Diab Metab Res Rev 2007; 23:63–70.

85. Kamiya H, Zhang W, Ekberg K, Wahren J, Sima AAF. C-peptide reverses nociceptive neuropathy in type 1 diabetic BB/Wor-rat. Diabetes 2006; 55:3581–3587.

86. Brussee V, Cunningham FA, Zochodne DW. Direct insulin signaling of neurons reverses diabetic neuropathy. Diabetes 2004; 53:1824–1830.

87. Sima AAF, Kamiya H. Insulin, C-peptide and diabetic neuropathy. Science Med 2004; 10:308–319.

88. Wozniak M, Rydzewski B, Baker SP, Raijada MK. The cellular and physiological action of insulin in the central nervous system. Neurochem Int 1993; 22:1–10.

89. Grunberger G, Sima AAF. The C-peptide signaling. Exp Diab Res 2004; 5:25–36.

90. Musen G, Lyool K, Sparks CR, et al. Effect of type 1 diabetes on gray matter density as measured by voxel-based morphometry. Diabetes 2006; 55:326–333.

91. Jakobsen J, Sidenius P, Gundersen HJ, Østerby R. Quantitative changes of cerebral neocortical structure in insulin treated long-term streptozotocin-induced diabetes in rats. Diabetes 1987; 36:597–601.

92. Mukai N, Hori S, Pomeroy M. Cerebral lesions in rats with streptozotocin-induced diabetes. Acta Neuropath (Berl) 1980; 51:79–84.

93. Reul JM, Gesing A, Droste S, et al. The brain mineralocorticoid: greedy for ligand, mysterious in function. Eur J Pharmacol 2000; 405:235–249.

94. de Kloet ER, de Rijk R. Signaling pathways in brain involved in predisposition and pathogenesis of stress-related disease: genetic and kinetic factors affecting the MR/GR balance. Ann NY Acad Sci 2004; 1032:14–34.

95. de Kloet ER, Vreugdenhil E, Oitzl MS, Joels M. Brain corticosteroid receptor balance in health and disease. Endo Rev 1998; 19:269–301.

96. Revsin Y, Saravia F, Roig P, et al. Neuronal and astroglial alterations in the hippocampus of a mouse model for type 1 diabetes. Brain Res 2005; 1038:22–31.

97. Stranahan AM, Arumugam TV, Cutler RG, Lee K, Egan JM, Mattson MP. Diabetes impairs hippocampal function through glucocorticoid-mediated effects on new and mature neurons. Nature Neurosci 2008; 11:309–317.

98. Fulop T, Larbi A, Donziech N. Insulin receptor and aging. Pathol Biol 2003; 51:574–580.

99. Hoyer S. Glucose metabolism and insulin receptor signal transduction in Alzheimer's disease. Eur J Pharmacol 2004; 490:115–125.

100. de la Monte SM, Wands JR. Review of insulin and insulin-like growth factor expression, signaling, and malfunction in the central nervous system: relevance to Alzheimer's disease. J Alzheimer Dis 2005; 7:45–61.

101. Salkovic-Petrisic M, Tribl R, Schmidt M, Hoyer S, Riederer P. Alzheimer-like changes in protein kinase B and glycogen synthase kinase-3 in rat frontal cortex and hippocampus after damage to the insulin signaling pathway. J Neurochem 2006; 96:1005–1015.

102. Reagan LP, Magariños AM, Lucas LR, Van Beuren A, McCall AL, McEwen BS. Regulation of GLUT-3 glucose transporter in the hippocampus of diabetic rats subjected to stress. A J Physiol (Endocr Metab 39) 1999; 276:E879–E886.

103. Phiel CJ, Wilson CA, Lee VMY, Klein PS. GSK-3α regulates production of Alzheimer's disease amyloid-β peptides. Nature 2003; 423:435–439.

104. Ishiguro K, Shiratsuchi, A, Sato S, et al. Glycogen synthase kinase 3 beta is identical to tau protein kinase I generating several epitopes of paired helical filaments. FEBS Lett 1993; 325:167–172.

105. Clodfelder-Miller BJ, Zmijewska AA, Johnson GV, Jope RS. Tau is hyperphosphorylated at multiple sites in mouse brain in vivo after streptozotocin-induced insulin deficiency. Diabetes 2006; 55(12):3320–3325.

106. Haley RW. Is there a connection between concentration of cholesterol circulating in plasma and the rate of neurite plaques formation in Alzheimer's disease? Arch Neurol 2000; 57:1410–1412.

107. Sima AAF, Zhang W. High glucose and cholesterol enhances caveolin-1 expression and amyloidogenic APP metabolism in SH-SY5Y cells (abstract). Proc. 18th Neurodiab Meeting, Orvieto, Italy, 2008.

108. Kimura A, Mora S, Shigematsu S, Pessin JE, Saltiel AR. The insulin receptor catalyzes the tyrosine phosphorylation of caveolin-1. J Biol Chem 2002; 277:30153–30158.

109. Ridell DR, Christie G, Hussain I, Dingwall C. Compartmentalization of beta secretase (Asp2) into low-buoyant density, noncaveolar lipid rafts. Curr Biol 2001; 11:1288–1293.

110. Ghribi O, Larsen B, Schrag M, Herman MM. High cholesterol content in neurons increases BACE, beta-amyloid and phosphorylated tau levels in rabbit hippocampus. Exp Neurol 2006; 200:460–467.

111. Sharma M, Gupta YK. Intracerebroventricular injection of streptozotocin in rats produces both oxidative stress in the brain and cognitive impairment. Life Sci 2001; b8: 1021–1029.

112. Sima AAF, Merry AC, Hall DE, Grant M, Murray FT, Guberski D. The BB/Z^{DR}-rat; A model for type II diabetic neuropathy. Exp Clin Endocrin Diab 1997; 105:63–64.

113. Sima AAF, Zhang W, Xu G, Sugimoto K, Guberski DL, Yorek MA. A comparison of diabetic polyneuropathy in type-2 diabetic BBZDR/Wor-rat and in type 1 diabetic BB/Wor-rat. Diabetologia 2000; 43:786–793.

114. Sima AAF. Diabetic neuropathy differs in type 1 and type 2 diabetes. Ann NY Acad Sci 2006; 1084:235–249.

115. Farris W, Mansourian S, Chang Y, et al. Insulin-degrading enzyme regulates the levels of insulin, amyloid beta-protein, and the beta-amyloid precursor protein intracellular domain in vivo. Proc Natl Acad Sci USA 2003; 100:4162–4167.

116. Petanceska SS, Gandy S. The phosphotidylinositol 3-kinase inhibitor Wortmannin alters the metabolism of the Alzheimer's amyloid precursor protein. J Neurochem 1999; 73: 2316–2320.

117. Johnson GVW, Bailey CDC. The p38 MAP kinase signaling pathway in Alzheimer's disease. Exp Neurol 2003; 183:262–268.
118. Lu DC, Rabizadeh S, Chandra S, et al. A second cytotoxic proteolytic peptide derived from amyloid β-protein precursor. Nature Med 2000; 6:397–404.
119. Galvan V, Chen S, Lu D, et al. Caspase cleavage of members of the amyloid precursor family of proteins. J Neurochem 2003; 82:283–294.
120. Tamagno E, Bardini P, Obbili A, et al. Oxidative stress increases expression of BACE in NT2 neurons. Neurobiol Dis 2002; 10:279–288.
121. Cohen AW, Combs TP, Scherer PE, Lisanti MP. Role of caveolin and caveolae in insulin signaling and diabetes. Am J Phys Endocrinol Metab 2003; 28:E1151–E1160.
122. Nyström FH, Chen H, Long LN, Li Y, Quon MJ. Caveolin-1 interacts with the insulin receptor and can differentially modulate insulin signaling in transfected Coc-7 cells and rat adipose cells. Mol Endocrinol 1999; 13:2013–2024.
123. Gamblin TC, Chen F, Zambrano A, et al. Caspase cleavage of tau: linking amyloid and neurofibrillary tangles in Alzheimer's disease. PNAS 2003; 100:10032–10037.
124. Kamiya H, Zhang W, Sima AAF. Degeneration of Golgi and neuronal loss in DRG's in diabetic BB/Wor-rats. Diabetologia 2006; 49:2763–2774.
125. Cheng C, Zochodne DW. Sensory neurons with activated caspase-3 survive long-term experimental diabetes. Diabetes 2003; 52:2363–2371.
126. Oddo S, Caccamo A, Shepheard JD, et al. Triple-transgenic model of Alzheimer's disease with plaques and tangles: Intracellular Aβ and synaptic dysfunction. Neuron 2003; 39: 409–421.
127. Ivins KJ, Thornton PL, Rohn TT, Colman CW. Neuronal apoptosis induced by beta-amyloid is mediated by caspase-8. Neurobiol Dis 1999; 6:440–449.
128. Matsui T, Ramasamy K, Ingelsson M, et al. Coordinated expression of caspase 8, 3 and 7 mRNA in temporal cortex of Alzheimer disease: relationship to formic acid extractable Aβ$_{42}$ levels. J Neuropath Exp Neurol 2006; 65:508–515.
129. Hoyer S. The brain insulin signal transduction system and sporadic (type II) Alzheimer disease: an update. J Neurol Transm 2000; 109:341–360.
130. Selkoe DJ. Alzheimer's disease: genes, proteins and therapy. Physiol Rev 2001; 81:741–766.
131. Lee VM, Goedert M, Trojanowski JQ. Neurodegenerative tauopathies. Annu Rev Neurosci 2001; 24:1121–1159.
132. Bayer TA, Wirths O, Majtenyi K, et al. Key factors in Alzheimer's disease: beta amyloid precursor protein processing, metabolism and intraneuronal transport. Brain Pathol 2001; 11:1–11 (Review).
133. Uetzuki T, Takemoto K, Nishimura I, et al. Activation of neuronal caspase-3 by intracellular accumulation of wild-type Alzheimer amyloid precursor protein. J Neurosci 1999; 19: 6955–6964.
134. Geschvind M, Huber G. Apoptotic cell death induced by β-amyloid 1–42 peptide is cell dependent. J Neurochem 1995; 65:292–300.
135. Ekberg K, Brismar T, Johansson BL, Jonsson B, Lindström P, Wahren J. Amelioration of sensory nerve dysfunction by C-peptide in patients with type 1 diabetes. Diabetes 2003; 52:536–541.
136. Ekberg K, Johansson BL. Effect of C-peptide on diabetic neuropathy in patients with type 1 diabetes. Exp Diab Res 2008:2008.457912 (online publ.)

18 The Role of Insulin Resistance in Age-Related Cognitive Decline and Dementia

G. Stennis Watson and Suzanne Craft

CONTENTS

ABSTRACT

The role of insulin in peripheral energy metabolism has been well described, and converging evidence has identified a role for insulin in central nervous system functions. Epidemiological studies support an important relationship between diabetes and other insulin-resistant conditions, and cognitive

From: *Contemporary Diabetes: Diabetes and the Brain*
Edited by: G. J. Biessels, J. A. Luchsinger (eds.), DOI 10.1007/978-1-60327-850-8_18
© Humana Press, a part of Springer Science+Business Media, LLC 2009

functioning. For example, diabetes increases the risk for memory loss, and treating diabetes can reverse memory loss. These studies have also identified a reciprocal relationship between insulin resistance and dementia, such that one condition increases the risk for the other. A substantial body of work has explored the role of insulin in regulating brain glucose metabolism, memory function, inflammatory responses, and amyloid concentrations. Knowledge of these relationships has suggested that increasing brain insulin activity may have a beneficial impact on memory and may serve as the basis for novel therapeutic strategies for Alzheimer's disease. Three such strategies include intranasal administration of insulin, drugs that improve insulin sensitivity, and diet and exercise

Key words: Alzheimer's disease; Apolipoprotein E; Beta amyloid; Diabetes; Diet and exercise; Glucose; Inflammation; Insulin; Insulin resistance; IGF-1; Intranasal; Memory; PPAR-γ.

INTRODUCTION

Peripheral glucose metabolism and insulin sensitivity are key determinants of cognitive functioning in aging. This fact is hardly surprising, given that the brain consumes the largest proportion of the body's glucose supply and is dependent on glucose received from the periphery. Despite this close association, neuroscientists and diabetologists virtually ignored insulin as a neuromodulator. Thirty years ago, Havrankova and colleagues demonstrated the presence of insulin and insulin receptors in rodent brain *(1, 2)*. More recently, we and other investigators have documented a role for insulin both in the normal regulation of memory and in the pathophysiology associated with memory loss and Alzheimer's disease and mild cognitive impairment (MCI), which is widely believed to be a prodromal phase of Alzheimer's disease *(3)*. A growing body of evidence suggests that one way in which insulin influences memory is by modulating glucose metabolism in the brain. In addition, insulin may influence memory via effects on neuronal plasticity, neurotransmitters, inflammatory responses, and dementia-related proteins such as beta amyloid (Aβ). Furthermore, both peripheral and central nervous system (CNS) concentrations of insulin and glucose appear to contribute to normal memory and other cognitive functions, as well as to memory loss and dementia. For example, patients with type 2 diabetes mellitus (T2DM) have an enhanced risk of memory decline, and normalizing blood glucose levels can facilitate memory. Moreover, the risk for dementia, a disease of profound memory loss, is increased by T2DM. Therefore, strategies that improve glucose metabolism or insulin action may provide symptomatic relief or exert disease-altering effects in the crucial war against dementia.

GLUCOSE AND MEMORY

The beneficial effects of glucose administration on memory have been well documented, as reviewed by Messier *(4)*. Nearly three decades ago, Lapp demonstrated in teenagers that acute glucose administration could facilitate memory *(5)*. Since then, researchers have shown in animals and humans that the beneficial effects of elevating plasma glucose levels on learning and memory are dependent on an optimal dose, the type of sugar, task demands, gender, age, cognitive status, and the relative timing of glucose administration and task *(3, 4)*. These glucose effects are consistent with observations that the brain supply of glucose is derived from peripheral circulation and that glucose is the brain's principal energy substrate *(6)*. Glucose-induced memory facilitation has been observed in both healthy older adult humans and persons with Alzheimer's disease *(3, 7)*. For example, Craft et al. gave patients with Alzheimer's disease an oral glucose load of 75 g and showed improved memory for patients with a specific glucoregulatory profile.

In contrast to acute hyperglycemia, chronic hyperglycemia exerts detrimental effects on cognition. T2DM and its precursor, impaired glucose tolerance, are common among aging adults. Adults above age 60 run a one in five chance of having T2DM *(8)* and a one in three chance of having either impaired glucose tolerance or T2DM *(9)*. Most, though not all, studies have detected cognitive changes associated with T2DM *(10–13)*. In older adults with T2DM, the most common cognitive deficit is a decline in list learning *(12)*; other areas affected by diabetes may include attention, manual dexterity, reasoning, and psychomotor speed *(10–13)*. Furthermore, there is evidence from rodents and humans that abnormal glucoregulation in the absence of diabetes can impair memory and global cognitive functioning *(14–16)*. It is important to note that cognitive deficits associated with diabetes may, in part, be reversible with treatment for diabetes *(11, 17–19)*.

DIABETES AND DEMENTIA

Several well-designed epidemiological studies support the notion that T2DM likely increases the risk for dementia. Investigators in Honolulu Asia Aging Study reported that T2DM increased the incidence of Alzheimer's disease and vascular dementia among Japanese-Americans *(20)*. Consistent with these findings, investigators for the Mayo and Rotterdam groups reported that the presence of T2DM increased the risk for Alzheimer's disease, independent of vascular dementia *(21, 22)* and Luchsinger et al. reported that hyperinsulinemia, a condition associated with early T2DM and impaired glucose tolerance, increased the risk for both memory impairment and Alzheimer's disease *(15)*. Autopsy studies have not confirmed this relationship between Alzheimer's disease and T2DM *(23)*. Therefore, diabetes may increase the risk for serious memory loss, presenting very much like Alzheimer's disease with a different pathophysiology than typical Alzheimer's disease. Convergent evidence supports the notion that insulin plays a role in both the beneficial effects of acute hyperglycemia and the detrimental effects of chronic hyperglycemia on cognition. As we previously noted, an acute rise in plasma glucose is rapidly followed by a rise in plasma insulin. Therefore, the beneficial effects attributed to increased plasma glucose levels may, in part, reflect effects of increased plasma insulin levels. (We will present evidence supporting this possibility in the following section.) However, detrimental effects may follow chronic glucose and insulin elevations. In T2DM, hyperglycemia is produced by two deficits: insulin resistance and insufficient compensatory insulin secretion by pancreatic β cells. Insulin resistance, or reduced insulin sensitivity, is characterized by a reduction in the ability of insulin to promote glucose disposal. Consequently, more insulin is needed to promote glucose utilization. This heightened compensatory response results in elevated plasma levels of glucose and insulin in patients with impaired glucose tolerance and early T2DM.

INSULIN IN THE PERIPHERY AND THE CNS

It has long been established that insulin plays a crucial role in peripheral energy regulation. In a tightly controlled system, plasma glucose levels are kept remarkably constant in healthy human beings. Carbohydrate consumption initiates a rise in plasma glucose levels, which in turn, stimulates insulin secretion by the pancreas. As blood glucose levels begin to fall, counterregulatory hormones are secreted, and plasma glucose concentrations are returned to normal pre-prandial levels. Therefore, there are normal fluctuations in plasma insulin levels throughout the day. As we will see, these peripheral fluctuations may have important implications for central nervous system functioning.

In the past three decades, a rapidly expanding body of literature has evolved that supports the notion that insulin contributes to normal brain functioning. In 1978, Havrankova and colleagues reported that insulin and insulin's receptors are selectively distributed in the brains of rats *(1, 2)* and humans *(24, 25)*. The greatest insulin binding is found in the olfactory bulb, cortex, hippocampus, hypothalamus, amygdale, and septum *(1, 2, 26, 27)*, with insulin receptors located on neuronal and astroglial synapses *(28)*. Although there are some suggestions that the adult brain may produce insulin *(29)*, the vast majority of brain insulin is derived from circulating insulin secreted by pancreatic β cells. In brief, insulin in peripheral circulation is transported rapidly across the blood–brain barrier by a saturable receptor-mediated transport system. When plasma insulin levels are raised by intravenous infusion, spinal fluid levels of insulin increase within 90 min *(30)*. Consequently, postprandial increases in insulin levels likely increase central nervous system insulin levels.

Once in the brain, insulin regulates a variety of functions, including cognition. For example, our work has shown that an optimal insulin dose facilitates memory and attention in patients with Alzheimer's disease and in healthy older adults *(30–34)*. In a typical experiment, we administered a fixed dose of insulin and a variable dose of dextrose, which allowed us to raise plasma insulin to postprandial levels and to maintain euglycemia. Under these conditions, patients and controls experienced an improvement in memory and selective attention. It may be argued that the infusion of dextrose actually accounted for cognitive facilitation; however, results of two studies suggest that it is the insulin per se that is responsible for cognitive facilitation. In one study by Park and colleagues, insulin administered into the cerebral ventricles without glucose supplementation facilitated performance of a passive avoidance task *(35)*. In a separate study, Craft and colleagues compared the cognitive effects of insulin administration (with dextrose supplementation to maintain euglycemia) with glucose administration when the endogenous insulin response was suppressed; participants were patients with Alzheimer's disease, relative to saline control, insulin but not glucose facilitated memory *(32)*.

MECHANISMS CONTRIBUTING TO BRAIN INSULIN EFFECTS

The cognitive effects of insulin reflect several mechanisms, including molecular plasticity, neurotransmitter changes, and glucose metabolism.

Glucose, transported across the blood–brain barrier, is the principal energy substrate for the brain *(6)*. Therefore, it would make intuitive sense that global changes in glucose transport and metabolism would result in cognitive improvement or impairment. Although there is evidence that low doses of exogenous insulin can mediate brain glucose metabolism, it is not likely that insulin has a principal effect on glucose transport into the brain *(36)*. On the other hand, it is likely that insulin has an effect on local glucose metabolism in areas that are important to cognitive function. As previously noted, insulin and insulin receptors are localized to the hippocampus and cerebral cortex. Additionally, insulin-sensitive glucose transporters are co-localized to these same areas *(37)*. These glucose transporters are normally found inside the cells; in the presence of insulin, they are relocated to the cell membrane in order to increase glucose uptake. In rats, hyperinsulinemia can modulate local cerebral glucose metabolism *(38, 39)*.

In addition to changes in glucose metabolism, insulin also modulates levels of neurotransmitters, including acetylcholine, norepinephrine, and dopamine, which affect memory and attention. Acetylcholine is known to have profound effects on memory. For example, blocking acetylcholine receptors impairs memory *(3)*. The observation that cholinergic neurotransmission is essential for memory forms the basis for the most commonly accepted treatments for Alzheimer's disease, namely cholinesterase inhibitors. At least one study has shown that low dose of insulin can ameliorate the amnestic effects of a cholinergic receptor antagonist *(40)*. Insulin also modulates norepinephrine concentrations in rodent brains *(41, 42)*. Collectively, these studies suggest that the insulin increases synaptic concentrations of norepinephrine by reducing reuptake by norepinephrine transporters. Recently, we reported that an intravenous infusion of a high physiologic dose of insulin yielded an increase in both insulin and norepinephrine concentrations in spinal fluid in healthy older adults *(43)*.

Finally, insulin may modulate molecular mechanisms associated with memory. Zhao et al. showed that training rats on a spatial learning task produced a rapid increase in insulin receptor expression in the hippocampus and dentate gyrus and induced *tyr* phosphorylation *(44)*. Other investigators have shown that insulin influences long-term potentiation (LTP) and long-term depression (LTD), which are thought to be models of learning at the molecular level *(45)*. Insulin may increase the probability of LTP by inducing cell membrane expression on NMDA receptors *(46)*. In contrast, streptozotocin administration, which induces irreversible hypoinsulinemia, makes LTP less likely *(47)*. Taken together, these observations are consistent with the hypothesis that insulin plays a role in normal memory functioning through effects at the molecular level.

INSULIN AND DEMENTIA

Thus far, we have examined the relationship between insulin and normal memory, and now we turn to the relationship between insulin and dementia. As we have seen, diabetes increases the risk for both cognitive decline and dementia. It is important to keep in mind that T2DM represents both abnormal glycemic regulation and abnormal insulin activity. This section will examine the relationship between Alzheimer's disease, the most common form of dementia among older adults, and insulin abnormalities. First, we turn to a brief discussion on Alzheimer's disease. Then, we will turn to the discussion on insulin resistance and Alzheimer's disease.

Alzheimer's Disease

Dementia is a pathological condition characterized by deficits in memory, another area of cognitive functioning, and social or occupational functioning. The most common form of dementia among older adults is Alzheimer's disease. The most prominent symptom of Alzheimer's disease is a loss of declarative memory, which begins insidiously and invariably progresses, usually until the person with Alzheimer's disease has no memory for self or others. Structural brain imaging frequently shows progressive atrophy of the hippocampus, a structure known to play an essential role in the formation of declarative memory *(3)*. Furthermore, functional imaging has revealed a decrease in glucose metabolism in the hippocampus, superior and middle temporal gyri, and the cingulate gyrus *(48)*. Other hallmark pathologies of Alzheimer's disease are the formation of amyloid plaques, neurofibrillary tangles, generalized cerebral atrophy, and neurotransmitter changes.

Insulin and Apolipoprotein E (APOE) Genotype

The most important genetic risk factor for Alzheimer's disease is apolipoprotein E *(APOE)*, which likely functions to shift the age of onset of Alzheimer's disease by several years. There are three isoforms of the *APOE* gene; *APOE* ε3, which is the most common isoform and is considered to have a relative risk of 1.0, *APOE* ε2, which is the least common and is thought to convey a reduced risk for Alzheimer's disease, and *APOE* ε4, which dose-dependently increases the risk for Alzheimer's disease *(49)*. Interestingly, this genotype may modulate the relationship between metabolic abnormalities and Alzheimer's disease. For example, we have previously reported that *APOE* genotype distinguished groups of Alzheimer's patients on several metabolic measures, including insulin sensitivity (assessed by the rate of glucose disposal during a hyperinsulinemic–euglycemic clamp procedure), plasma insulin concentrations, and the ratio of insulin in spinal fluid to insulin in plasma *(31–34, 50)*. Furthermore, we have observed that *APOE* differentiated groups of patients with Alzheimer's disease regarding the optimal insulin dose producing facilitation of memory and attention *(31, 51)*. Finally, possession of the ε4 allele influenced the insulin-related processing of the amyloid precursor protein from which the Aβ peptide is derived. Interestingly, patients possessing the ε4 allele were more insulin sensitive on metabolic measures and were more sensitive to insulin dose effects than were their counterparts who did not possess the ε4 allele. These observations raise the intriguing possibility that treatment for Alzheimer's disease may need to consider this genetic factor.

Insulin Resistance and Neurodegenerative Disease

In recent years, a number of investigators have reported insulin defects in Alzheimer's disease. Notably, patients with Alzheimer's disease may have reduced insulin-mediated glucose disposal, indicative of insulin resistance, or may be at risk for abnormal glucose metabolism (11, 52). Converging evidence is consistent with the hypothesis that brain insulin signaling is abnormal in patients with Alzheimer's disease (29). De la Monte and other investigators have reported reductions in the following components of the insulin signaling pathway: tyrosine kinase activity, insulin concentration, IRS mRNA, IRS-associated phosphatidylinositol 3-kinase, and activated phosphor-Akt (24, 53, 54). These abnormalities are sufficient to influence energy production, oxidative stress, cell survival, GSK-3β activation, and advanced glycation of proteins (29). De la Monte and colleagues have proposed that these insulin signaling abnormalities are so profound that they constitute "type 3 diabetes" or brain insulin resistance associated with Alzheimer's disease (25). When they modeled type 3 diabetes in rodents, using streptozotocin administration, they found changes in the brain similar to those found in patients with Alzheimer's disease: atrophy; increased levels of activated GSK-3β, phospho-tau, and β-amyloid (Aβ); and decreased expression of a number of genes (55).

Insulin and β-Amyloid

The principal constituent of neuritic plaques is β-amyloid, primarily the more toxic species, Aβ42. Aβ is produced in the brain, where it may remain as amyloid deposits or from where it may be cleared by degradation or transported across the blood–brain barrier into the peripheral sink (56). Insulin plays several roles in regulating levels of β-amyloid including promoting the release of Aβ from the intracellular compartment and accelerating Aβ trafficking to the plasma membrane (57). These observations suggest that insulin potentially may increase Aβ levels. Conversely, Aβ degradation may depend in part on insulin . Both Aβ and insulin are degraded by insulin-degrading enzyme, which is highly expressed in brain and liver (58–60). Notably, insulin-degrading enzyme has a preferential affinity for insulin over Aβ. Consequently, it is likely that excess insulin in the brain could result in decreased Aβ degradation. Consistent with these observations, increasing insulin levels should result in increased Aβ levels. Indeed, when we administered insulin to healthy older adults and maintained euglycemia, we found that both Aβ and insulin levels were increased in spinal fluid and that reduced memory facilitation was associated with increased Aβ levels (61). Furthermore, body mass index, a measure that is highly related to insulin resistance, was associated with plasma Aβ42 levels, such that body mass index rose as plasma Aβ levels rose *(62)*.

Insulin Resistance and Inflammation

Inflammation appears to play a crucial role in Alzheimer's disease. It has been reported that patients with Alzheimer's disease have elevated levels of interleukin 6 (IL-6) and F-2 isoprostane, a marker of lipid peroxidation, in spinal fluid and tumor necrosis factor-α (TNF-α) in spinal fluid and plasma *(63–65)*. Several observations implicate insulin as a regulator of inflammation in patients with Alzheimer's disease. First, insulin has dual competing effects on inflammation in the periphery: whereas low insulin doses are associated with an anti-inflammatory response *(66)*, chronic hyperinsulinemia is associated with a proinflammatory response *(67)*, and exogenous insulin can increase the proinflammatory reaction to an endotoxin such as lipopolysaccharide *(68)*. Second, moderate doses of systemically administered insulin can induce a rapid proinflammatory response. For 16 healthy older adults, we raised plasma insulin levels to about 80 μ(mu)U/ml while maintaining normal blood sugar levels. After 90 min of insulin infusion, lumbar spinal fluid was acquired. Relative to saline, insulin induced marked increases in spinal fluid concentrations of IL-1α, IL-1β, IL-6, TNF-α, and F-2 isoprostane. Third, a reciprocal relationship exists between Aβ and inflammation. On the one hand, soluble Aβ oligomers induce a rapid inflammatory response in vitro, which leads to increased levels of the proinflammatory cytokines IL-1β and IL-6 *(69)*. Aβ also induces glial activation, cytokine gene expression, and expression of COX-2 *(70)*. On the other hand, the production of Aβ from the amyloid precursor protein (APP) is governed, in part, by IL-1β and IL-6, which act to increase concentrations of Aβ42, the most toxic Aβ isoform *(71, 72)*. The net result is a "cytokine cycle," leading to increased Aβ and IL-1β/IL-6.

Insulin, Obesity, and Free Fatty Acids (FFA)

Obesity is a major risk factor for metabolic (or insulin resistance) syndrome. As body mass index (BMI, a weight-to-height ratio) increases, the risk for hyperinsulinemia, hyperglycemia, hypertension, and dyslipidemia also increases. It has recently been reported that BMI can modulate plasma concentrations of Aβ42, the longer and more toxic species of the Aβ family. In a group of healthy adults, Aβ42 was strongly correlated with both BMI ($r = 0.55$) and fat mass ($r = 0.60$) *(62)*. Consistent with these data, longitudinal data support the notion that a higher BMI is predictive of incident Alzheimer's disease in Swedish adults ranging in age from 70 to

88 *(73)*. Finally, we have reported that BMI modulated the relationship between insulin-induced memory facilitation and plasma levels of Aβ42 ($r = 0.49$) *(61)*.

FFAs likely provide a connection between obesity and insulin resistance. Elevated FFAs are common in people with obesity or insulin resistance, and normalization of FFA levels typically leads to a dramatic improvement in insulin sensitivity *(74)*. Furthermore, high fasting FFA levels are associated with progression to diabetes *(75, 76)*. FFAs are also associated with inflammation. For example, TNF-α, a proinflammatory cytokine expressed in adipocytes, has a role in regulating glucose uptake that may be mediated in part by FFAs. Insulin resistance is associated with overexpression of TNF-α in adipocytes, and reducing TNF-α levels has a beneficial effect on insulin resistance *(77)*. FFAs are also expressed in the brain where they may play several important roles. Following head injury, brain levels of FFAs rise, suggesting that FFAs may be part of the body's normal response to brain trauma *(78)*. Additionally, FFAs inhibit mitochondrial respiration, suggesting that FFAs play a role in energy metabolism at the subcellular level *(79)*. This has direct relevance to Alzheimer's disease, a condition in which cerebral glucose metabolism is reduced. Also of direct relevance to Alzheimer's disease, insulin-degrading enzyme is inhibited by FFAs. As previously noted, insulin-degrading enzyme degrades both insulin and Aβ. Therefore, it is possible that high levels of FFAs would lead to reduced degradation of Aβ.

Summary

Thus far, we have reviewed evidence suggesting that there is a relationship among glucose, insulin, and memory, that impaired glucose metabolism and insulin action are associated with changes in cognitive functioning, and that insulin abnormalities may contribute to the pathophysiology and cognitive symptoms of Alzheimer's disease, the most common form of dementia in older adults. We have also considered mechanisms that may account for the relationship between insulin and Alzheimer's disease. In the next section, we will discuss several potential treatments for Alzheimer's disease based on improving insulin action in the periphery and the brain.

NOVEL TREATMENT STRATEGIES FOR ALZHEIMER'S DISEASE

In this final section, we will discuss three novel treatment strategies for Alzheimer's disease and for its prodromal stage, mild cognitive impairment (Table 1). The three strategies have a common thesis that improving insulin sensitivity will have a beneficial effect on patients with memory loss.

Table 1
Novel therapeutic strategies for Alzheimer's disease and mild cognitive impairment

Strategy	Target	Therapeutic action
Intranasal insulin administration	Raises brain insulin levels without affecting plasma glucose or insulin levels	Increases brain insulin activity Modulates Aβ levels (Modulates local cerebral glucose metabolism?)
PPAR-γ agonist administration (rosiglitazone, pioglitazone)	Improves peripheral insulin sensitivity	Lowers plasma insulin and glucose levels (Increases rate of insulin transport into brain?) Modulates Aβ levels Modulates inflammatory response Modulates cerebral glucose metabolism Modulates peripheral (and central?) lipid storage
Lifestyle modification (healthy diet and exercise)	Improves peripheral insulin sensitivity	Lowers plasma insulin and glucose levels (Increases rate of insulin transport into brain?) Modulates plasma and brain Aβ levels, α- and γ-secretase activities, neuritic plaque deposition Modulates growth factor secretion and hippocampal Neurogenesis

The first of these strategies, intranasal insulin administration, builds on our work with intravenous insulin infusion in the hyperinsulinemic–euglycemic clamp model. The second of these strategies employs an insulin-sensitizing agent, rosiglitazone, to increase insulin efficiency. The third strategy, diet and exercise, is a powerful intervention against diabetes to reduce insulin resistance.

Intranasal Insulin Administration and Treatment of Alzheimer's Disease

We have previously reported that intravenous infusion of insulin facilitates memory and attention in patients with Alzheimer's disease and in healthy older adults *(30)*. Therefore, this is a useful strategy to explore the effects of insulin on cognition, inflammatory responses, and Aβ responses to increased plasma and brain insulin levels *(43, 61, 80)*. There are, however, several practical issues that limit the usefulness of intravenous insulin infusion as a therapeutic strategy. One important limitation is that chronically raising plasma insulin levels could potentially induce insulin resistance and thus produce exactly the opposite of desired effects. Furthermore, these infusions must be done in a clinic or other controlled environment. Consequently, we sought other means of elevating brain insulin levels without using a peripheral infusion.

Intranasal Administration of Drugs

Intranasal insulin administration offers a practical and efficacious alternative to intravenous infusion. In separate studies, Kern and Born demonstrated that small molecule neuropeptides are rapidly transported from the nasal cavity into the central nervous system *(81, 82)*. Specifically, Born and colleagues demonstrated that intranasal delivery of small molecule neuropeptides (insulin, vasopressin, and MSH/ACTH) results in increased lumbar spinal fluid levels in about 10 min. For each of the peptides, the area under the curve showed large increases in spinal fluid but not in serum *(81)*. These data imply that transport of small molecule neuropeptides from the nasal cavity into brain and spine is rapid and efficient; however, these data do not allow us to ascertain the specific transport pathway. Work by other investigators suggests that neuropeptide transport originating in the nasal cavity follows two different extra-axonal pathways: the trigeminal pathway that leads to the brainstem and spinal column and the olfactory pathway that leads to the olfactory bulbs in the rostral brain regions *(83)*.

We and other investigators have demonstrated rapid functional effects following intranasal insulin administration in younger and older adult humans. Intranasal insulin administration is associated with changes in auditory-evoked brain potentials (AEPs) *(82)* and memory facilitation in younger and older adults *(51, 84–88)*. We have found that intranasal insulin administration facilitates memory in the patients and not in the healthy older adults *(51, 87, 88)*. Response to intranasal insulin administration may also vary by gender *(86)*. These observations (that intranasal insulin administration delivers insulin into the brain, but not peripheral circulation, alters brain electrical responses, and facilitates memory) suggest that intranasal insulin administration has therapeutic potential in the treatment of Alzheimer's disease. To date, three studies have considered the effects of intranasal insulin in patients with Alzheimer's disease. These three studies are reviewed in the following section.

Intranasal Insulin Administration and Alzheimer's Disease

This first study was designed to characterize intranasal insulin dose effects in older adults with and without impaired memory. Our hypotheses were that insulin would facilitate memory for patients and controls. Participants were 26 (14 ε4−, 12 ε4+) memory-impaired older adults and 35 (27 ε4−, 8 ε4+) normal controls. Of 26 memory-impaired participants, 13 had probable Alzheimer's disease and 13 had amnestic mild cognitive impairment, a condition widely believed to be a prodrome of Alzheimer's disease. On 3 separate days, participants received saline or one of two insulin doses (20 or 40 IU) in randomized order. Cognitive testing was initiated 15 min after insulin administration. The primary endpoint was performance on two measures of verbal memory (story recall, word list recall). As predicted, both insulin doses facilitated memory for patients not possessing the *APOE* ε4 allele (ε4−). In contrast, patients possessing the *APOE* ε4 allele (ε4+) showed a dose-dependent decline on word list recall and no insulin effect on story recall. Neither insulin dose affected memory for healthy older adults. Although inconsistent with our predictions, these findings were anticipated by findings from a previously reported intravenous insulin administration study in which ε4+ patients and healthy older adults experienced effects on memory, attention, and plasma APP concentrations at a lower dose than did ε4− patients. As predicted, plasma glucose and insulin levels were affected by insulin administration.

A subsequent study examined the effects of four insulin doses on verbal memory. Participants were 33 older adults with memory-impairment (11 ε4−, 22 ε4+; 13 with Alzheimer's disease and 20 with amnestic mild cognitive impairment) and 59 cognitively intact older adults (48 ε4−, 11 ε4+). On 4 separate days, participants received saline or one of four insulin doses (10, 20, 40, or 60 IU) in randomized order. In other respects, the design followed the previous study. Cognitive results were remarkably similar to findings in the previous study. *APOE* ε4− patients demonstrated facilitation of immediate and delayed word recall when they received 20 IU of insulin, but not higher or lower doses. On immediate story recall, *APOE* ε4− patients also demonstrated facilitation of immediate story recall with the three lowest insulin doses. Insulin did not affect memory for controls or ε4+ patients. Insulin's effects on plasma levels of A β42 differed by diagnostic group and by *APOE* genotype. Among memory-impaired individuals, the lowest insulin dose increased plasma Aβ42 levels regardless of the genotype; the highest insulin dose also increased Aβ42 levels in memory-impaired individuals without the ε4 allele. Among cognitively intact adults, lower Aβ42 levels were seen in individuals without the ε4 allele. Also, in the ε4– group, escalating insulin doses produced an inverted U-shaped curve, such that the two lowest insulin doses significantly lowered Aβ42 levels. Thus, results from this study corroborate findings from the previous study: intranasal insulin administration facilitates verbal declarative memory for memory-impaired individuals who do not possess the *APOE* ε4.

This third study examined the effects of chronic daily dosing with intranasal insulin administration. Participants were 25 memory-impaired older adults who were randomized to receive either saline ($n = 12$) or 20 IU of insulin ($n = 13$) twice daily for 21 days. The primary endpoint was verbal memory, specifically, the proportion of information retained after a delay. Secondary endpoints included performance on measures of attention and functional status and the changes in plasma levels of Aβ40 and Aβ42. Participants having received insulin retained significantly more information after a delay, in comparison with participants having received only saline. Insulin administration also produced an interesting effect on plasma Aβ levels: Aβ40 levels increased, but Aβ42 levels did not increase, thus yielding an increased ratio of Aβ40-to-Aβ42. Furthermore, insulin treatment was associated with improved attention and functional status.

Summary

Collectively, these studies support the notion that intranasal insulin administration may offer a novel therapeutic strategy for treating patients with Alzheimer's disease. Insulin administration consistently facilitated verbal memory in the three studies. These, of course, are small pilot studies, and they serve to raise as many questions as they answer. These questions include, "What is the optimal drug dose... delivery system ... dosing schedule?" and "Who will benefit most from intranasal insulin administration?" One of the most intriguing suggestions to come out of these studies is that *APOE* genotype exerts a powerful influence on insulin treatment outcomes. In two of the three studies, memory facilitation was observed only in memory-impaired participants who did not possess the *APOE* ε4 allele. In contrast, insulin administration did not facilitate memory in participants who were cognitively intact and may have had a detrimental impact on memory-impaired subjects who were *APOE* ε4+. Thus, these studies suggest that the effectiveness of insulin and perhaps other medications may depend on a patient's genetic background. Clearly, more work is needed to determine the answers to this question. Finally, plasma Aβ is a target of growing interest. At this point, investigators are not certain about the natural course of circulating Aβ. As more is known about the course of Aβ in healthy older adults and older adults with Alzheimer's disease, it may become possible to plan interventions that target this peptide.

PEROXISOME PROLIFERATOR-ACTIVATED RECEPTOR (PPAR-γ) AGONISTS AND TREATMENT OF ALZHEIMER'S DISEASE

Drugs of the PPAR-γ class have been approved by the FDA to treat T2DM for approximately a decade. Members of this class currently in clinical use include rosiglitazone and pioglitazone. They are ligand-activated nuclear transcription factors that improve insulin sensitivity. PPAR-γ, expressed in adipocytes, regulates adipogenesis and increases the uptake of fatty acids into adipocytes. Thus, PPAR-γ agonists reduce the burden of fatty acid uptake for striated muscles, which likely explains their insulin-sensitizing characteristics. PPAR-γ agonists also reduce visceral fat stores, which are relocated to subcutaneous stores, and they reduce the expression of TNF-α *(89)*. Furthermore, these compounds produce anti-inflammatory responses in rats and humans *(90, 91)*. An interesting characteristic of PPAR-γ agonists is that they have little immediate effect on plasma glucose or insulin levels, since they do not stimulate insulin secretion by the pancreas or glucose production by the liver. Ultimately, these drugs lower both plasma glucose and plasma insulin levels, which are marks of a successful treatment response. To date, they have proven to be effective treatments for T2DM.

PPAR-γ in the CNS

In the brain, PPAR-γ is localized to neurons and astrocytes *(92)*, where it is responsible for regulating cell survival and inflammatory responses. In brief, PPAR-γ is associated with lower levels of iNOS expression and microglial activation *(93–95)*. Furthermore, Aβ induces a variety of proinflammatory responses (monocyte differentiation glial activation, and cytokine gene expression), which are modulated by PPAR-γ agonists *(70)*. Although equivocal, PPAR-γ may affect processing and deposition of Aβ, likely through effects on β-secretase.

PPAR-γ is also involved in the regulation of energy metabolism via increased glucose metabolism and direct effects on mitochondria *(96)* that possibly increase astrocytic lactate production and glucose consumption *(97)*. Additionally, PPAR-γ agonists may promote cell health through anti-inflammatory actions directed toward mitochondria. These agonists initiate a protective cascade that increases Iκ(kappa)B expression and blocks NFκ(kappa)B expression thereby reducing inflammatory gene expression and inflammatory responses. Therefore, PPAR-γ is a novel therapeutic target for Alzheimer's disease that may reflect diverse affects, including improving energy metabolism, improving glucose uptake, and mounting an anti-inflammatory response.

PPAR-γ and the Treatment of Alzheimer's Disease

To date, there have been two reported therapeutic trials of a PPAR-γ agonist to treat Alzheimer's disease. The first trial, conducted by our group, was a small pilot trial involving 30 persons with mild cognitive impairment or early Alzheimer's disease (98). The second was a much larger trial conducted in Europe with patients with Alzheimer's disease (99). Both trials showed therapeutic potential; however, the trial by Risner et al. suggested that treatment effects are dependent on APOE genotype.

Our pilot study was a 6-month randomized, placebo-controlled trial in which 20 participants received a daily dose of 4 mg of rosiglitazone, and 10 participants took matched placebo. They completed cognitive testing at baseline months 2, 4, and 6. Primary endpoints were performance on a measure of declarative memory (word list learning) and plasma Aβ levels. Groups were well matched at baseline. As predicted, participants in the placebo group showed declining memory over the 6-month trial. In contrast, participants taking rosiglitazone showed stable memory over the same time period. Thus, the rosiglitazone group improved relative to the placebo group. When we compared performance on declarative memory measures with treatment response to rosiglitazone (indexed by fasting insulin levels), we found that participants with the most improvement in memory also showed the best treatment response to rosiglitazone. On a secondary endpoint, performance on a measure of selected attention, participants showed a similar pattern: the rosiglitazone group was stable over time, whereas the placebo group declined over time. Additionally, better response to treatment was associated with better selective attention. When we examined treatment affects on Aβ40 and Aβ42, plasma levels of these peptides dropped over 6 months in the placebo group; however, rosiglitazone prevented the decline. It has been reported that plasma Aβ levels rise in the earliest stages of Alzheimer's disease and begin to fall some time later (100). In keeping with this notion, preventing a fall in plasma Aβ levels may be therapeutic.

In the industry-sponsored, intent-to-treat study *(99)*, 511 participants with mild-to-moderate probable Alzheimer's received one of three doses of rosiglitazone (2, 4, 8 mg per day) or matched placebo; 322 participants had *APOE* genotyping. Performance on the AD Assessment Scale-Cognitive (ADAS-Cog) was the primary endpoint. Primary analyses conducted with the entire sample failed to detect effects of rosiglitazone. In contrast, secondary analyses which separated participants into $\varepsilon 4+$ and $\varepsilon 4-$ groups detected improvement in the $\varepsilon 4-$ group taking the highest dose of rosiglitazone.

Taken together, these two studies offer promise for rosiglitazone as a novel therapeutic agent for Alzheimer's disease. Our pilot study detected affects on memory, attention, and $A\beta$ levels. The study by Risner et al. raises the provoking suggestion that *APOE* genotype mediates therapeutic response to certain medications (pharmacogenetics), making *APOE* an important variable both to understand the mechanisms of drug actions and to plan successful treatment strategies. Currently, there are several ongoing studies with rosiglitazone that will help clarify the extent to which rosiglitazone has therapeutic potential in the treatment of Alzheimer's disease.

Summary

Rosiglitazone may offer a promising novel therapeutic strategy for the treatment of Alzheimer's disease. Several different mechanisms may account for its actions, the most prominent of which is its ability to improve insulin sensitivity. Other mechanisms include regulation of energy metabolism and inflammatory responses. There are, however, drawbacks to pharmacotherapy that should be considered. Medications typically elicit a broad spectrum of effects, both desired and unwanted. For example, rosiglitazone is known to increase the risk for edema and anemia, and adversely affect cardiovascular function. In contrast, therapeutic strategies that do not rely on medications may offer a lower side-effect profile. Therefore, equivalent non-pharmacologic strategies, when available, may be preferable to pharmacologic strategies.

DIET, EXERCISE, AND ALZHEIMER'S DISEASE

Diet and exercise constitute a powerful intervention to reduce the risk of conversion from impaired glucose tolerance (a prodromal phase of T2DM) to T2DM, as shown by results of two large-scale studies *(101, 102)*. In one, a North American trial known as the Diabetes Prevention Program *(101)*, 522 overweight middle-aged adults with impaired glucose tolerance were randomized to either an active intervention (metformin or diet/exercise) or the control group. Metformin, a standard anti-diabetic medication, and diet/exercise reduced the risk of incident diabetes; however, the risk reduction was much greater for participants in the diet/exercise group than for participants in the metformin group. Similarly, investigators of the Finnish Diabetes Prevention Study reported that healthy lifestyle modification (i.e., diet and exercise) could reduce the risk for incident diabetes. Furthermore, participants with the highest compliance to the diet and exercise regimen had the lowest risk of incident diabetes (102). Taken together, these two studies provide conclusive evidence that lifestyle modification (diet/exercise) is an effective therapeutic strategy. Earlier, we discussed findings supporting the notion that T2DM and insulin-resistant conditions in the absence of diabetes impair memory and other cognitive functions (13–16) and that effectively treating diabetes can improve cognition (11, 18, 10). Collectively, these observations suggest that diet and exercise should have a positive impact on cognition.

We have reported that a 6-month lifestyle intervention resulted in physical and cognitive improvement in a sample of Japanese-Americans with impaired glucose tolerance (98). In brief, participants were randomized to receive either a low-fat diet paired with aerobic exercise (1 h three times per week; active treatment group) or a typical American diet paired with stretching (control group). Relative to the control intervention, the active intervention reduced body mass index and increased the proportion of story information recalled after a delay. When we compared treatment-related changes in memory with treatment-related changes in glucose-stimulated plasma insulin levels (acquired at the end of a standard oral glucose tolerance test), improved story recall was associated with lower glucose-stimulated insulin levels, suggesting that memory improvement increased in conjunction with lower insulin levels (a marker of insulin effectiveness). Thus, diet and exercise can regulate both metabolic and cognitive aspects of diabetes and other insulin-resistant conditions. Next, we will consider the case for using lifestyle modification to treat Alzheimer's disease.

Epidemiological work supports the notion that exercise may be a prophylactic treatment for Alzheimer's disease (103). In the Adult Changes in Thought (ACT) Study, 1,740 cognitively intact, older adults were followed biennially to detect incident dementia; 158 participants developed dementia. The risk for incident dementia was significantly lower among participants who exercised three times per week or more (13.0 per 1,000 person years) than for participants who exercised fewer than three times per week (19.7 per thousand person years). The relationship between exercise frequency and the risk for incident Alzheimer's disease was similar to that for incipient dementia. Consequently, these authors hypothesized that frequent exercise would reduce the risk for incident dementia and incident Alzheimer's disease.

Animal studies point to possible mechanisms that may account for the beneficial actions of lifestyle modification on the risk for dementia and Alzheimer's disease. Medial temporal atrophy, an important feature of Alzheimer's disease, partially explains the characteristic memory loss. Reducing this atrophy potentially may limit memory loss. Exercise increases the rate of cell proliferation in the dentate gyrus, a brain area that participates in the making of new memories *(104)*. Interestingly, exercise increased cell proliferation in older rats (62 weeks), as well as in younger animals (4 or 8 weeks). Other investigators have reported that exercise increases secretion of neurotrophic factors including insulin-like growth factor-1 (IGF-1) *(105)*. They observed that subcutaneous administration of IGF-1 during exercise training increased expression of new hippocampal neurons in adult rats; however, blocking the brain uptake of circulating IGF-1 inhibited expression of new neurons. They concluded that neurotrophic factors such as IGF-1 are associated with hippocampal neurogenesis. These observations suggest that it may be possible to reduce hippocampal atrophy through exercise.

Lifestyle modification may also produce beneficial effects related to Aβ. For example, it has been shown that high fat feeding, which can induce insulin resistance *(106)*, can promote amyloidosis in transgenic mice *(14)* and that caloric restriction can reduce amyloid pathology in the same mouse model *(107)*. In Tg2576 mice, a common model of Alzheimer's disease, diet-induced insulin resistance increased brain levels of Aβ40 and Aβ42, as well as increased amyloid plaque burden *(14)*. Furthermore, these peptide changes were accompanied by an increase in γ-secretase activity and decrease in insulin-degrading enzyme activity. Finally, a number of changes in the insulin receptor-mediated signal transduction pathway were observed. Investigators from the same group subsequently reported that caloric restriction promoted α-secretase activity, which reduced Aβ generation and neuritic plaque deposition *(107)*.

Thus, diet and exercise may decrease the risk of incident dementia and Alzheimer's disease as effectively as pharmacotherapies. Furthermore, the financial burden for diet and exercise can be much lower than the cost of medication, the risk for serious adverse events can be much lower than with medication, and diet and exercise are readily available to most people. The greatest drawback is long-term compliance with lifestyle modification.

SUMMARY

In previous sections, we have discussed the relationship among insulin, insulin resistance, memory, and Alzheimer's disease. In this last section, we discussed three potential treatments for Alzheimer's disease based on our knowledge of the role of insulin in central nervous system functions: intranasal insulin administration, PPARγ agonists, and lifestyle modification (diet/exercise). These three potential therapies have a common theme that improving insulin action should improve memory and may have an effect on neurobiological processes associated with age-related cognitive decline and Alzheimer's disease. Thus, these studies serve two important functions. First, they provide converging evidence that insulin resistance can be a pathogenic factor for memory loss and Alzheimer's disease and suggest several mechanisms to account for this relationship. Second, and perhaps most importantly, they use this knowledge to explore promising avenues for novel therapies for Alzheimer's disease.

REFERENCES

1. Havrankova J, Roth J, Brownstein M. Insulin receptors are widely distributed in the central nervous system of the rat. Nature 1978; 272(5656):827–829.
2. Havrankova J, Schmechel D, Roth J, Brownstein M. Identification of insulin in rat brain. Proc Natl Acad Sci USA 1978; 75(11):5737–5741.
3. Watson GS, Craft S. Modulation of memory by insulin and glucose: neuropsychological observations in Alzheimer's disease. Eur J Pharmacol 2004; 490(1–3):97–113.
4. Messier C. Glucose improvement of memory: a review. Eur J Pharmacol 2004; 490(1–3):33–57.
5. Lapp JE. Effects glycemic alterations and noun imagery on the learning of paired associates. J Learn Disabil 1981; 14:35–38.
6. Magistretti PJ. Brain energy metabolism. In: Squire LR, Bloom FE, McConnell SK, Roberts JL, Spitzer NC, Zigmond MJ, eds. Fundamental Neuroscience 2nd ed. San Diego, CA: Academic Press; 2003:339–360.
7. Manning CA, Ragozzino ME, Gold PE. Glucose enhancement of memory in patients with probable senile dementia of the Alzheimer's type. Neurobiol Aging 1993; 14(6):523–528.
8. Harris MI, Flegal KM, Cowie CC, et al. Prevalence of diabetes, impaired fasting glucose, and impaired glucose tolerance in U.S. adults. The Third National Health and Nutrition Examination Survey, 1988–1994. Diabetes Care 1998; 21(4):518–524.
9. Prevalence of diabetes and impaired fasting glucose in adults–United States, 1999–2000. MMWR. Morb Mortal Wkly Rep 2003; 52 (35): 833–837.
10. Gregg EW, Yaffe K, Cauley JA, et al. Is diabetes associated with cognitive impairment and cognitive decline among older women? Study of Osteoporotic Fractures Research Group. Arch Intern Med 2000; 160(2):174–180.
11. Meneilly GS, Cheung E, Tessier D, Yakura C, Tuokko H. The effect of improved glycemic control on cognitive functions in the elderly patient with diabetes. J Gerontol 1993; 48(4):M117–M121.
12. Ryan CM, Geckle M. Why is learning and memory dysfunction in Type 2 diabetes limited to older adults? Diabetes Metab Res Rev 2000; 16(5):308–315.
13. Strachan MW, Deary IJ, Ewing FM, Frier BM. Is type II diabetes associated with an increased risk of cognitive dysfunction? A critical review of published studies. Diabetes Care 1997; 20(3):438–445.

14. Ho L, Qin W, Pompl PN, et al. Diet-induced insulin resistance promotes amyloidosis in a transgenic mouse model of Alzheimer's disease. FASEB J 2004; 18(7):902–904.
15. Luchsinger JA, Tang MX, Shea S, Mayeux R. Hyperinsulinemia and risk of Alzheimer disease. Neurology 2004; 63(7):1187–1192.
16. Vanhanen M, Koivisto K, Kuusisto J, et al. Cognitive function in an elderly population with persistent impaired glucose tolerance. Diabetes Care 1998; 21(3):398–402.
17. Gradman TJ, Laws A, Thompson LW, Reaven GM. Verbal learning and/or memory improves with glycemic control in older subjects with non-insulin-dependent diabetes mellitus. J Am Geriatr Soc 1993; 41(12):1305–1312.
18. Naor M, Steingruber HJ, Westhoff K, Schottenfeld-Naor Y, Gries AF. Cognitive function in elderly non-insulin-dependent diabetic patients before and after inpatient treatment for metabolic control. J Diabetes Complications 1997; 11(1):40–46.
19. Ryan CM, Freed MI, Rood JA, Cobitz AR, Waterhouse BR, Strachan MW. Improving metabolic control leads to better working memory in adults with type 2 diabetes. Diabetes Care 2006; 29(2):345–351.
20. Peila R, Rodriguez BL, Launer LJ. Type 2 diabetes, APOE gene, and the risk for dementia and related pathologies: The Honolulu-Asia Aging Study. Diabetes 2002; 51(4):1256–1262.
21. Leibson CL, Rocca WA, Hanson VA, et al. The risk of dementia among persons with diabetes mellitus: a population-based cohort study. Ann NY Acad Sci 1997; 826:422–427.
22. Ott A, Stolk RP, van Harskamp F, Pols HA, Hofman A, Breteler MM. Diabetes mellitus and the risk of dementia: The Rotterdam Study. Neurology 1999; 53(9):1937–1942.
23. Arvanitakis Z, Schneider JA, Wilson RS, et al. Diabetes is related to cerebral infarction but not to AD pathology in older persons. Neurology 2006; 67(11):1960–1965.
24. Frolich L, Blum-Degen D, Bernstein HG, et al. Brain insulin and insulin receptors in aging and sporadic Alzheimer's disease. J Neural Transm 1998; 105(4–5):423–438.
25. Rivera EJ, Goldin A, Fulmer N, Tavares R, Wands JR, de la Monte SM. Insulin and insulin-like growth factor expression and function deteriorate with progression of Alzheimer's disease: link to brain reductions in acetylcholine. J Alzheimers Dis 2005; 8(3):247–268.
26. Baskin DG, Figlewicz DP, Woods SC, Porte D, Jr, Dorsa DM. Insulin in the brain. Annu Rev Physiol 1987; 49:335–347.
27. Unger JW, Livingston JN, Moss AM. Insulin receptors in the central nervous system: localization, signalling mechanisms and functional aspects. Prog Neurobiol 1991; 36(5):343–362.
28. Abbott MA, Wells DG, Fallon JR. The insulin receptor tyrosine kinase substrate p58/53 and the insulin receptor are components of CNS synapses. J Neurosci 1999; 19(17):7300–7308.
29. de la Monte SM, Wands JR. Review of insulin and insulin-like growth factor expression, signaling, and malfunction in the central nervous system: relevance to Alzheimer's disease. J Alzheimers Dis 2005; 7(1):45–61.
30. Watson GS, Craft S. The role of insulin resistance in the pathogenesis of Alzheimer's disease: implications for treatment. CNS Drugs 2003; 17(1):27–45.
31. Craft S, Asthana S, Cook DG, et al. Insulin dose-response effects on memory and plasma amyloid precursor protein in Alzheimer's disease: interactions with apolipoprotein E genotype. Psychoneuroendocrinology 2003; 28(6):809–822.
32. Craft S, Asthana S, Newcomer JW, et al. Enhancement of memory in Alzheimer disease with insulin and somatostatin, but not glucose. Arch Gen Psychiatry 1999; 56(12):1135–1140.
33. Craft S, Asthana S, Schellenberg G, et al. Insulin metabolism in Alzheimer's disease differs according to apolipoprotein E genotype and gender. Neuroendocrinology 1999; 70(2):146–152.
34. Craft S, Newcomer J, Kanne S, et al. Memory improvement following induced hyperinsulinemia in Alzheimer's disease. Neurobiol Aging 1996; 17(1):123–130.
35. Park CR, Seeley RJ, Craft S, Woods SC. Intracerebroventricular insulin enhances memory in a passive-avoidance task. Physiol Behav 2000; 68(4):509–514.
36. Bingham EM, Hopkins D, Smith D, et al. The role of insulin in human brain glucose metabolism: an 18fluoro-deoxyglucose positron emission tomography study. Diabetes 2002; 51(12):3384–3390.

37. Apelt J, Mehlhorn G, Schliebs R. Insulin-sensitive GLUT4 glucose transporters are colocalized with GLUT3-expressing cells and demonstrate a chemically distinct neuron-specific localization in rat brain. J Neurosci Res 1999; 57(5):693–705.

38. Doyle P, Cusin I, Rohner-Jeanrenaud F, Jeanrenaud B. Four-day hyperinsulinemia in euglycemic conditions alters local cerebral glucose utilization in specific brain nuclei of freely moving rats. Brain Res 1995; 684(1):47–55.

39. Marfaing P, Penicaud L, Broer Y, Mraovitch S, Calando Y, Picon L. Effects of hyperinsulinemia on local cerebral insulin binding and glucose utilization in normoglycemic awake rats. Neurosci Lett 1990; 115(2–3):279–285.

40. Blanchard JG, Duncan PM. Effect of combinations of insulin, glucose and scopolamine on radial arm maze performance. Pharmacol Biochem Behav 1997; 58(1):209–214.

41. Figlewicz DP, Bentson K, Ocrant I. The effect of insulin on norepinephrine uptake by PC12 cells. Brain Res Bull 1993; 32(4):425–431.

42. Figlewicz DP, Szot P, Israel PA, Payne C, Dorsa DM. Insulin reduces norepinephrine transporter mRNA in vivo in rat locus coeruleus. Brain Res 1993; 602(1):161–164.

43. Watson GS, Bernhardt T, Reger MA, et al. Insulin effects on CSF norepinephrine and cognition in Alzheimer's disease. Neurobiol Aging 2006; 27(1):38–41.

44. Zhao W, Chen H, Xu H, et al. Brain insulin receptors and spatial memory. Correlated changes in gene expression, tyrosine phosphorylation, and signaling molecules in the hippocampus of water maze trained rats. J Biol Chem 1999; 274(49):34893–34902.

45. van der Heide LP, Kamal A, Artola A, Gispen WH, Ramakers GM. Insulin modulates hippocampal activity-dependent synaptic plasticity in a N-methyl-d-aspartate receptor and phosphatidyl-inositol-3-kinase-dependent manner. J Neurochem 2005; 94(4):1158–1166.

46. Skeberdis VA, Lan J, Zheng X, Zukin RS, Bennett MV. Insulin promotes rapid delivery of N-methyl-D- aspartate receptors to the cell surface by exocytosis. Proc Natl Acad Sci USA 2001; 98(6):3561–3566.

47. Di Luca M, Ruts L, Gardoni F, Cattabeni F, Biessels GJ, Gispen WH. NMDA receptor subunits are modified transcriptionally and post-translationally in the brain of streptozotocin-diabetic rats. Diabetologia 1999; 42(6):693–701.

48. Garrido GE, Furuie SS, Buchpiguel CA, et al. Relation between medial temporal atrophy and functional brain activity during memory processing in Alzheimer's disease: a combined MRI and SPECT study. J Neurol Neurosurg Psychiatry 2002; 73(5):508–516.

49. Corder EH, Saunders AM, Strittmatter WJ, et al. Gene dose of apolipoprotein E type 4 allele and the risk of Alzheimer's disease in late onset families. Science 1993; 261(5123): 921–923.

50. Craft S, Peskind E, Schwartz MW, Schellenberg GD, Raskind M, Porte D, Jr. Cerebrospinal fluid and plasma insulin levels in Alzheimer's disease: relationship to severity of dementia and apolipoprotein E genotype. Neurology 1998; 50(1):164–168.

51. Reger MA, Watson GS, Frey WH, 2nd, et al. Effects of intranasal insulin on cognition in memory-impaired older adults: modulation by APOE genotype. Neurobiol Aging 2006; 27(3):451–458.

52. Razay G, Wilcock GK. Hyperinsulinaemia and Alzheimer's disease. Age Ageing 1994; 23(5):396–399.

53. Frolich L, Blum-Degen D, Riederer P, Hoyer S. A disturbance in the neuronal insulin receptor signal transduction in sporadic Alzheimer's disease. Ann NY Acad Sci 1999; 893: 290–293.

54. Steen E, Terry BM, Rivera EJ, et al. Impaired insulin and insulin-like growth factor expression and signaling mechanisms in Alzheimer's disease–is this type 3 diabetes? J Alzheimers Dis 2005; 7(1):63–80.

55. Lester-Coll N, Rivera EJ, Soscia SJ, Doiron K, Wands JR, de la Monte SM. Intracerebral streptozotocin model of type 3 diabetes: relevance to sporadic Alzheimer's disease. J Alzheimers Dis 2006; 9(1):13–33.

56. Marques M, Kulstad JJ, Savard CE, et al. Peripheral A-beta levels regulate A-beta clearance from the central nervous system. J Alzheimers Dis: in press.

57. Gasparini L, Gouras GK, Wang R, et al. Stimulation of beta-amyloid precursor protein trafficking by insulin reduces intraneuronal beta-amyloid and requires mitogen-activated protein kinase signaling. J Neurosci 2001; 21(8):2561–2570.

58. Authier F, Posner BI, Bergeron JJ. Insulin-degrading enzyme. Clin Invest Med 1996; 19(3):149–160.

59. Sudoh S, Frosch MP, Wolf BA. Differential effects of proteases involved in intracellular degradation of amyloid beta-protein between detergent-soluble and -insoluble pools in CHO-695 cells. Biochemistry (Mosc) 2002; 41(4):1091–1099.

60. Zhao L, Teter B, Morihara T, et al. Insulin-degrading enzyme as a downstream target of insulin receptor signaling cascade: implications for Alzheimer's disease intervention. J Neurosci 2004; 24(49):11120–11126.

61. Watson GS, Peskind ER, Asthana S, et al. Insulin increases CSF Abeta42 levels in normal older adults. Neurology 2003; 60(12):1899–1903.

62. Balakrishnan K, Verdile G, Mehta PD, et al. Plasma Abeta42 correlates positively with increased body fat in healthy individuals. J Alzheimers Dis 2005; 8(3):269–282.

63. Cacquevel M, Lebeurrier N, Cheenne S, Vivien D. Cytokines in neuroinflammation and Alzheimer's disease. Curr Drug Targets 2004; 5(6):529–534.

64. Montine TJ, Kaye JA, Montine KS, McFarland L, Morrow JD, Quinn JF. Cerebrospinal fluid abeta42, tau, and f2-isoprostane concentrations in patients with Alzheimer disease, other dementias, and in age-matched controls. Arch Pathol Lab Med 2001; 125(4):510–512.

65. Tarkowski E, Blennow K, Wallin A, Tarkowski A. Intracerebral production of tumor necrosis factor-alpha, a local neuroprotective agent, in Alzheimer disease and vascular dementia. J Clin Immunol 1999; 19(4):223–230.

66. Dandona P. Endothelium, inflammation, and diabetes. Curr Diab Rep 2002; 2(4):311–315.

67. Krogh-Madsen R, Plomgaard P, Keller P, Keller C, Pedersen BK. Insulin stimulates interleukin-6 and tumor necrosis factor-alpha gene expression in human subcutaneous adipose tissue. Am J Physiol Endocrinol Metab 2004; 286(2):E234–E238.

68. Soop M, Duxbury H, Agwunobi AO, et al. Euglycemic hyperinsulinemia augments the cytokine and endocrine responses to endotoxin in humans. Am J Physiol Endocrinol Metab 2002; 282(6):E1276–E1285.

69. White JA, Manelli AM, Holmberg KH, Van Eldik LJ, Ladu MJ. Differential effects of oligomeric and fibrillar amyloid-beta 1–42 on astrocyte-mediated inflammation. Neurobiol Dis 2005; 18(3):459–465.

70. Combs CK, Johnson DE, Karlo JC, Cannady SB, Landreth GE. Inflammatory mechanisms in Alzheimer's disease: inhibition of beta-amyloid-stimulated proinflammatory responses and neurotoxicity by PPARgamma agonists. J Neurosci 2000; 20(2):558–567.

71. Buxbaum JD, Oishi M, Chen HI, et al. Cholinergic agonists and interleukin 1 regulate processing and secretion of the Alzheimer beta/A4 amyloid protein precursor. Proc Natl Acad Sci USA 1992; 89(21):10075–10078.

72. Papassotiropoulos A, Hock C, Nitsch RM. Genetics of interleukin 6: implications for Alzheimer's disease. Neurobiol Aging 2001; 22(6):863–871.

73. Gustafson D, Rothenberg E, Blennow K, Steen B, Skoog I. An 18-year follow-up of overweight and risk of Alzheimer disease. Arch Intern Med 2003; 163(13): 1524–1528.

74. Santomauro AT, Boden G, Silva ME, et al. Overnight lowering of free fatty acids with Acipimox improves insulin resistance and glucose tolerance in obese diabetic and nondiabetic subjects. Diabetes 1999; 48(9):1836–1841.

75. Knowler WC, Pettitt DJ, Saad MF, Bennett PH. Diabetes mellitus in the Pima Indians: incidence, risk factors and pathogenesis. Diabetes Metab Rev. 1990; 6(1):1–27.

76. Paolisso G, Tataranni PA, Foley JE, Bogardus C, Howard BV, Ravussin E. A high concentration of fasting plasma non-esterified fatty acids is a risk factor for the development of NIDDM. Diabetologia 1995; 38(10):1213–1217.

77. Craft S. Insulin resistance and Alzheimer's disease pathogenesis: potential mechanisms and implications for treatment. Curr Alzheimer Res 2007; 4(2):147–152.

78. Dhillon HS, Carman HM, Zhang D, Scheff SW, Prasad MR. Severity of experimental brain injury on lactate and free fatty acid accumulation and Evans blue extravasation in the rat cortex and hippocampus. J Neurotrauma 1999; 16(6):455–469.

79. Hillered L, Chan PH. Role of arachidonic acid and other free fatty acids in mitochondrial dysfunction in brain ischemia. J Neurosci Res 1988; 20(4):451–456.

80. Fishel MA, Watson GS, Montine TJ, et al. Hyperinsulinemia provokes synchronous increases in central inflammation and beta-amyloid in normal adults. Arch Neurol 2005; 62(10):1539–1544.

81. Born J, Lange T, Kern W, McGregor GP, Bickel U, Fehm HL. Sniffing neuropeptides: a transnasal approach to the human brain. Nat Neurosci 2002; 5(6):514–516.

82. Kern W, Born J, Schreiber H, Fehm HL. Central nervous system effects of intranasally administered insulin during euglycemia in men. Diabetes 1999; 48(3):557–563.

83. Thorne RG, Pronk GJ, Padmanabhan V, Frey WH, 2nd. Delivery of insulin-like growth factor-I to the rat brain and spinal cord along olfactory and trigeminal pathways following intranasal administration. Neuroscience 2004; 127(2):481–496.

84. Benedict C, Hallschmid M, Hatke A, et al. Intranasal insulin improves memory in humans. Psychoneuroendocrinology 2004; 29(10):1326–1334.

85. Benedict C, Hallschmid M, Schmitz K, et al. Intranasal insulin improves memory in humans: superiority of insulin aspart. Neuropsychopharmacology 2007; 32(1):239–243.

86. Benedict C, Kern W, Schultes B, Born J, Hallschmid M. Differential sensitivity of men and women to anorexigenic and memory-improving effects of intranasal insulin. J Clin Endocrinol Metab 2008; 93(4):1339–1344.

87. Reger MA, Watson GS, Green PS, et al. Intranasal insulin administration dose-dependently modulates verbal memory and plasma amyloid-beta in memory-impaired older adults. J Alzheimers Dis 2008; 13(3):323–331.

88. Reger MA, Watson GS, Green PS, et al. Intranasal insulin improves cognition and modulates beta-amyloid in early AD. Neurology 2008; 70(6):440–448.

89. Ferre P. The biology of peroxisome proliferator-activated receptors: relationship with lipid metabolism and insulin sensitivity. Diabetes 2004; 53(Suppl 1):S43–S50.

90. Gurnell M. PPARgamma and metabolism: insights from the study of human genetic variants. Clin Endocrinol (Oxf) 2003; 59(3):267–277.

91. Sidhu JS, Cowan D, Kaski JC. The effects of rosiglitazone, a peroxisome proliferator-activated receptor-gamma agonist, on markers of endothelial cell activation, C-reactive protein, and fibrinogen levels in non-diabetic coronary artery disease patients. J Am Coll Cardiol 2003; 42(10):1757–1763.

92. Moreno S, Farioli-Vecchioli S, Ceru MP. Immunolocalization of peroxisome proliferator-activated receptors and retinoid X receptors in the adult rat CNS. Neuroscience 2004; 123(1):131–145.

93. Heneka MT, Klockgether T, Feinstein DL. Peroxisome proliferator-activated receptor-gamma ligands reduce neuronal inducible nitric oxide synthase expression and cell death in vivo. J Neurosci 2000; 20(18):6862–6867.

94. Kitamura Y, Kakimura J, Matsuoka Y, Nomura Y, Gebicke-Haerter PJ, Taniguchi T. Activators of peroxisome proliferator-activated receptor-gamma (PPARgamma) inhibit inducible nitric oxide synthase expression but increase heme oxygenase-1 expression in rat glial cells. Neurosci Lett 1999; 262(2):129–132.

95. Uryu S, Harada J, Hisamoto M, Oda T. Troglitazone inhibits both post-glutamate neurotoxicity and low-potassium-induced apoptosis in cerebellar granule neurons. Brain Res 2002; 924(2):229–236.

96. Dello Russo C, Gavrilyuk V, Weinberg G, et al. Peroxisome proliferator-activated receptor gamma thiazolidinedione agonists increase glucose metabolism in astrocytes. J Biol Chem 2003; 278(8):5828–5836.

97. Feinstein DL, Spagnolo A, Akar C, et al. Receptor-independent actions of PPAR thiazolidinedione agonists: is mitochondrial function the key? Biochem Pharmacol 2005; 70(2):177–188.

98. Watson GS, Cholerton BA, Reger MA, et al. Preserved cognition in patients with early Alzheimer disease and amnestic mild cognitive impairment during treatment with rosiglitazone: a preliminary study. Am J Geriatr Psychiatry 2005; 13(11):950–958.

99. Risner ME, Saunders AM, Altman JF, et al. Efficacy of rosiglitazone in a genetically defined population with mild-to-moderate Alzheimer's disease. Pharmacogenomics J 2006; 6(4):246–254.

100. Mayeux R, Honig LS, Tang MX, et al. Plasma A[beta]40 and A[beta]42 and Alzheimer's disease: relation to age, mortality, and risk. Neurology 2003; 61(9):1185–1190.

101. Knowler WC, Barrett-Connor E, Fowler SE, et al. Reduction in the incidence of type 2 diabetes with lifestyle intervention or metformin. N Engl J Med 2002; 346(6):393–403.

102. Tuomilehto J, Lindstrom J, Eriksson JG, et al. Prevention of type 2 diabetes mellitus by changes in lifestyle among subjects with impaired glucose tolerance. N Engl J Med 2001; 344(18):1343–1350.

103. Larson EB, Wang L, Bowen JD, et al. Exercise is associated with reduced risk for incident dementia among persons 65 years of age and older. Ann Intern Med 2006; 144(2):73–81.

104. Kim YP, Kim H, Shin MS, et al. Age-dependence of the effect of treadmill exercise on cell proliferation in the dentate gyrus of rats. Neurosci Lett 2004; 355(1–2):152–154.

105. Trejo JL, Carro E, Torres-Aleman I. Circulating insulin-like growth factor I mediates exercise-induced increases in the number of new neurons in the adult hippocampus. J Neurosci 2001; 21(5):1628–1634.

106. Kaiyala KJ, Prigeon RL, Kahn SE, Woods SC, Schwartz MW. Obesity induced by a high-fat diet is associated with reduced brain insulin transport in dogs. Diabetes 2000; 49(9): 1525–1533.

107. Wang J, Ho L, Qin W, et al. Caloric restriction attenuates beta-amyloid neuropathology in a mouse model of Alzheimer's disease. FASEB J. 2005; 19(6):659–661.

Subject Index

From: *Contemporary Diabetes: Diabetes and the Brain*
Edited by: G. J. Biessels, J. A. Luchsinger (eds.), DOI 10.1007/978-1-60327-850-8
© Humana Press, a part of Springer Science+Business Media, LLC 2009

Insulin-dependent diabetes mellitus
(IDDM), 4
Insulin detemir, 24–25
Insulin-induced hypoglycemia, symptoms,
137
Insulin injection systems, for diabetic
patients, 26
Insulin-like growth factor-1 (IGF-I), 415
Insulin resistance, 191, 224, 225, 238, 298,
325–331, 334, 335, 347, 436,
440, 441
role in age related cognitive decline and
dementia, 434
brain insulin effects, 437–438
diabetes and dementia, 435–436
glucose and memory, 435
insulin and dementia, 438–442
in periphery and CNS, 436–437
Insulin therapy, 23–25
Insulin-treated diabetes
and driving, 153
hypoglycemia, 142
risk factors, 143
Intelligence, types, 80–81
See also Cognitive function, assessment
Intensive care unit (ICU), 221, 233, 238
International Diabetes Federation (IDF),
35, 36
International Stroke Trial, 63
International Stroke Trial and the Chinese
Acute Stroke Trial, 63
Intra-arterial thrombolysis, in ischemic
stroke treatment, 62–63
Ischemic brain injury, causes, 58–59
Ischemic stroke, acute
causes, 59
contraindications to intravenous
thrombolysis, 62
diagnosis, 59–61
epidemiology, 58
medical complications, 66–71
pathophysiology, 58–59
secondary prevention, 71
treatment, 61–66
See also Type 1 diabetes (T1D); Type 2
diabetes (T2D)
Ischemic stroke, hyperglycemia
etiology
inflammation, 224

stress response, 222–224
unrecognized insulin resistance
measurement, 224–225
risk factors, 220
See also Hyperglycemia, in acute stroke

J
Jun NH$_2$-terminal kinase (JNK), 417

K
Kaufman Adult Intelligence Test (KAIT), 81
Ketoacidosis, see Diabetic ketoacidosis

L
LADA, see Latent-onset autoimmune
diabetes
in adults
Laser photocoagulation, efficacy, 12
Latent-onset autoimmune diabetes in
adults, 5
LDL cholesterol goals modification, risk
categories, 47
Long-acting insulin glargine, 25
Long-term depression (LTD), 397, 438
Long-term potentiation (LTP), 397, 438
Low blood glucose, see Hypoglycemia

M
Macrovascular complications, of diabetes,
16–17
Magnetic resonance imaging (MRI),
60, 282
Major depressive disorder (MDD), 348, 349
Management, see Diabetes management
MCI, see Mild cognitive impairment
Mechanical clot disruption, in ischemic
stroke treatment, 63
Medial temporal lobe atrophy (MTA), 115
Mesial temporal sclerosis, 260
Meta-analytic technique, advantage, 279
See also Type 1 diabetes (T1D), cognitive
impairments in adults
Metabolic disorders, 3, 33, 34, 375
Metabolic syndrome (MS), 190–192
and AD, 334–335
and cognition, 300–302
criteria, 299
Metformin, for T1D patients, 25
MICRO-HOPE Study, 46